Blackwell's Five-Minute
Veterinary Consult

**Clinical Companion**

# Small Animal Toxicology

Blackwell's Five-Minute
Veterinary Consult

# Clinical Companion

# Small Animal Toxicology

## Third Edition

## Edited by

**Lynn R. Hovda, RPh, DVM, MS, DACVIM**
Director of Veterinary Medicine
SafetyCall International, LLC and Pet Poison Helpline, Minneapolis, Minnesota, USA

and

Adjunct Assistant Professor
Department of Veterinary and Biomedical Sciences, College of Veterinary Medicine
University of Minnesota, St. Paul, Minnesota, USA

**Ahna G. Brutlag, DVM, MS, DABT, DABVT**
Senior Director of Veterinary Services and Senior Veterinary Toxicologist
SafetyCall International, LLC and Pet Poison Helpline, Minneapolis, Minnesota, USA

and

Adjunct Assistant Professor
Department of Veterinary and Biomedical Sciences, College of Veterinary Medicine
University of Minnesota, St. Paul, Minnesota, USA

**Robert H. Poppenga, DVM, PhD, DABVT**
Head, Toxicology Section
California Animal Health and Food Safety Laboratory System
School of Veterinary Medicine, University of California, Davis
Davis, California, USA

**Steven E. Epstein, DVM, DACVECC**
Professor of Clinical Small Animal Emergency and Critical Care
Department of Veterinary Surgical and Radiological Sciences
School of Veterinary Medicine, University of California, Davis
Davis, California, USA

WILEY Blackwell

*Library of Congress Cataloging-in-Publication Data*

Names: Hovda, Lynn R., 1951– editor. | Brutlag, Ahna G., 1979– editor. |
   Poppenga, Robert H., editor. | Epstein, Steven E., editor.
Title: Blackwell's five-minute veterinary consult clinical companion. Small
   animal toxicology / edited by Lynn R. Hovda, Ahna G. Brutlag, Robert H.
   Poppenga, Steven E. Epstein.
Other titles: Small animal toxicology | Five minute veterinary consult.
Description: Third edition. | Hoboken, New Jersey : Wiley-Blackwell, [2024] |
   Series: Blackwell's five-minute veterinary consult | Includes
   bibliographical references and index.
Identifiers: LCCN 2023046417 (print) | LCCN 2023046418 (ebook) |
   ISBN 9781394158720 (paperback) | ISBN 9781394158737 (adobe pdf) |
   ISBN 9781394159864 (epub)
Subjects: MESH: Poisoning–veterinary | Drug-Related Side Effects and
   Adverse Reactions–veterinary | Animals, Domestic
Classification: LCC SF757.5 (print) | LCC SF757.5 (ebook) | NLM SF 757.5 |
   DDC 636.089/59–dc23/eng/20231129
LC record available at https://lccn.loc.gov/2023046417
LC ebook record available at https://lccn.loc.gov/2023046418

Cover Design: Wiley
Cover Images: Courtesy of Lynn Hovda and Elise Roschen

Set in 10/12pts Berkeley by Straive, Pondicherry, India

SKY10077220_061124

# Dedications

The third edition of this textbook, dedicated solely to small animal toxicology, is an extension of *Blackwell's Five-Minute Consult: Canine and Feline* by Drs Larry Tilley and Frank Smith. We remain grateful for their vision that fostered this textbook as well as others in the series. The editors of the third edition would like to acknowledge the work of the prior editors, in particular Dr Gary Osweiler whose leadership in establishing the first edition was invaluable. We are also indebted to the prior authors for their assistance and to the current authors for providing additional knowledge to make the third edition much more comprehensive. We would be remiss if we didn't recognize the veterinary students and veterinarians in practice who each day challenge us to become better teachers, clinicians, and toxicologists.

To Gary Osweiler, a friend and mentor, who sadly passed away far too soon, and to all my veterinary colleagues at Pet Poison Helpline, whose keen minds continue to stimulate growth in all of us. Finally, to Bob, my husband, and Tyne, my daughter, the cornerstones of my world.

*Lynn R. Hovda*

To my parents, Gwen and Paul Brutlag, for guiding and encouraging my unconventional explorations, and to my husband Nathan Clough, for your constant love, support, and extraordinary wit. Additionally, to my talented and passionate colleagues at Pet Poison Helpline and SafetyCall – I'm so grateful for you.

*Ahna G. Brutlag*

I'd like to dedicate this edition to all of my colleagues with a passion for the discipline of veterinary toxicology. We are a mutually supportive group of individuals who are always eager to share our knowledge with small animal clinicians and pet owners. I'd also like to acknowledge the wonderful support and joy that my wife, Amy, and two daughters, Mia and Zoe, have given me over the years.

*Robert H. Poppenga*

I want to dedicate my portion of this book to my family. In particular, to my mother, Roberta Epstein, without whose support I would not be where I am today. Additionally, to my mentors over the years whose teaching and encouragement guided my career – Drs Janet Aldrich, Kate Hopper, and Steven Haskins.

*Steven E. Epstein*

# Contents

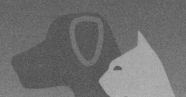

# List of Contributors

**Colleen M. Almgren, DVM, PhD, DABT, DABVT**
Veterinary Toxicologist
SafetyCall International, LLC and Pet Poison Helpline
Minneapolis, Minnesota, USA

**Sarah Alpert, DVM, DABT**
Senior Consulting Veterinarian, Clinical Toxicology
SafetyCall International, LLC and Pet Poison Helpline
Minneapolis, Minnesota, USA

**Rebecca Anderson, DVM**
Associate Veterinarian, Industry
SafetyCall International, LLC and Pet Poison Helpline
Minneapolis, Minnesota, USA

**Catherine Angle, DVM, MPH**
Owner of Padfoot Veterinary Care, LLC
Anoka, Minnesota, USA

**Itamar Aroch, DVM, DECVIM-CA**
The Veterinary Teaching Hospital
Koret School of Veterinary Medicine
The Hebrew University of Jerusalem, Israel

**Sarah L. Babcock, DVM, JD**
President
Animal & Veterinary Legal Services, PLLC
Harrison Township, Michigan, USA

**Jessie Barber, DVM**
Associate Veterinarian
SafetyCall International, LLC and Pet Poison Helpline
Minneapolis, Minnesota, USA

**Nicola Bates, BSc (Brunel), BSc (Open), MSc, MA, SRCS**
Research Lead
Veterinary Poisons Information Service (VPIS)
London, UK

**Adrienne Bautista, DVM, PhD, DABVT**
Scientific Communications Veterinarian
Royal Canin USA Inc
Saint Charles, Missouri, USA

**Jami Becker, DVM, DACVECC**
Emergency and Critical Care Resident
Austin Veterinary Emergency and Specialty Center
Austin, Texas, USA

**Karen Bischoff, DVM, MS, DABVT**
Diagnostic Toxicologist/Senior Extension Associate
New York Animal Health Diagnostic Center /Cornell University
Ithaca, New York, USA

**David R. Brown, MS, PhD**
Professor of Pharmacology
University of Minnesota, College of Veterinary Medicine
St. Paul, Minnesota, USA

**Ahna G. Brutlag, DVM, MS, DABT, DABVT**
Senior Director of Veterinary Services and Senior Veterinary Toxicologist
SafetyCall International, LLC and Pet Poison Helpline
Minneapolis, Minnesota, USA

and

Adjunct Assistant Professor
Department of Veterinary and Biomedical Sciences
College of Veterinary Medicine, University of Minnesota
St. Paul, Minnesota, USA

**Alessia Cenani, DVM, MS, DACVAA, CVA**
Assistant Professor of Clinical Anesthesiology
School of Veterinary Medicine
University of California, Davis
Davis, California, USA

**Dana L. Clarke, VMD, DACVECC**
Assistant Professor of Interventional Radiology and Critical Care
University of Pennsylvania School of Veterinary Medicine
Philadelphia, Pennsylvania, USA

**Seth L. Cohen, DVM**
Medical Director
VCA North Shore Animal Hospital
Vancouver, British Columbia, Canada

**Crystal Davis, BVM&S**
Associate Veterinarian
SafetyCall International, LLC and Pet Poison Helpline
Minneapolis, Minnesota, USA

**David C. Dorman, DVM, PhD, DABVT, DABT, ERT**
Professor of Toxicology
College of Veterinary Medicine
North Carolina State University
Raleigh, North Carolina, USA

**Eric K. Dunayer, MS, VMD, DABT, DABVT**
Retired
Urbana, Illinois, USA

**Steven E. Epstein, DVM, DACVECC**
Professor of Clinical Small Animal Emergency and Critical Care
School of Veterinary Medicine
University of California, Davis
Davis, California, USA

**James N. Eucher, DVM, DHSc, MS, MPH, DABT**
Senior Toxicologist
WuXi AppTec
St. Paul, Minnesota, USA

**Kate Farrell, DVM, DACVECC**
Assistant Professor of Clinical Small Animal Emergency and Critical Care
School of Veterinary Medicine
University of California, Davis
Davis, California, USA

**Charlotte Flint, DVM, DABT, DABVT**
Veterinarian
Mission Animal Hospital
Eden Prairie, Minnesota, USA

**Anna Folska, PharmD**
Senior Clinical Toxicologist
SafetyCall International, LLC and Pet Poison Helpline
Minneapolis, Minnesota, USA

**Scott Fritz, DVM, DABVT**
Clinical Assistant Professor
Kansas State University College of Veterinary Medicine
Manhattan, Kansas, USA

**Sarah Gray, DVM, DACVECC**
Emergency and Critical Care Specialist
Horizon Veterinary Specialists
Ventura, California, USA

**Amanda Gross, DVM**
Associate Veterinarian, Industry
Veterinary Pharmacovigilance Officer
SafetyCall International, LLC and Pet Poison Helpline
Minneapolis, Minnesota, USA

**Alonso Guedes, DVM, MS, PhD, DACVAA**
Associate Professor, Comparative Anesthesia and Pain Medicine
Veterinary Clinical Sciences Department
College of Veterinary Medicine
University of Minnesota
Minneapolis, Minnesota, USA

**Sharon Gwaltney-Brant, DVM, PhD, DABVT, DABT**
Consultant
Veterinary Information Network
Mahomet, Illinois, USA

**Heather Handley, DVM**
Senior Consulting Veterinarian, Clinical Toxicology
SafetyCall International, LLC and Pet Poison Helpline
Minneapolis, Minnesota, USA

**Cristine Hayes, DVM, DABT, DABVT**
Medical Director
ASPCA Animal Poison Control Center
Champaign, Illinois, USA

**Sabrina N. Hoehne, Dr. med. vet., DACVECC, DECVECC**
Assistant Professor of Small Animal Emergency and Critical Care
Washington State University College of Veterinary Medicine
Pullman, Washington, USA

**Susan Holland, DVM, DABT**
Consulting Veterinarian, Clinical Toxicology
SafetyCall International, LLC and Pet Poison Helpline
Minneapolis, Minnesota, USA

**Holly Hommerding, DVM, DABT, DABVT**
Senior Consulting Veterinarian, Clinical Toxicology
SafetyCall International, LLC and Pet Poison Helpline
Minneapolis, Minnesota, USA

**Erica J. Howard, DVM**
Associate Veterinarian, Clinical Toxicology
SafetyCall International, LLC and Pet Poison Helpline
Minneapolis, Minnesota, USA

**Lynn R. Hovda, RPh, DVM, MS, DACVIM**
Director of Veterinary Medicine
SafetyCall International, LLC and Pet Poison Helpline
Minneapolis, Minnesota, USA

and

Adjunct Assistant Professor
Department of Veterinary and Biomedical Sciences
College of Veterinary Medicine, University of Minnesota
St. Paul, Minnesota, USA

**Tyne K. Hovda, DVM**
Resident in Anesthesiology
North Carolina State University
Raleigh, North Carolina, USA

**Tiffany Hughes, DVM**
Associate Veterinarian, Clinical Toxicology
SafetyCall International, LLC and Pet Poison Helpline
Minneapolis, Minnesota, USA

**Sandra James-Yi, DVM, PhD, DABT, DABVT**
Director, Product Safety Compliance and Outreach
Nu Skin Enterprises, Inc.
Provo, Utah, USA

**Karl E. Jandrey, DVM, MAS, DACVECC**
Professor, Clinical Small Animal Emergency and Critical Care
School of Veterinary Medicine
University of California, Davis
Davis, California, USA

**Shannon Jarchow, DVM**
Associate Veterinarian, Clinical Toxicology
SafetyCall International, LLC and Pet Poison Helpline
Minneapolis, Minnesota, USA

**Sarah K. Jarosinki, DVM, DACVAA**
Veterinary Specialty Hospital North County
San Marcos, California, USA

**Tracy Julius, DVM, DACVECC**
Director of Emergency and Critical Care
Animal Emergency and Referral Center of Minnesota
Oakdale, Minnesota, USA

**Megan Kaplan, DVM, DACVECC**
Emergency and Critical Care Specialist
Premier Veterinary Group
Chicago, Illinois, USA

**Dijana Katan, DVM, MPH, DABT**
VCA Ocean Beach Animal Hospital
Longview, Washington, USA

**Daniel E. Keyler, RPh, PharmD, FAACT**
Senior Consulting Clinical Toxicologist
SafetyCall International, LLC and Pet Poison Helpline
Minneapolis, Minnesota, USA

and

Adjunct Clinical Professor
Department of Experimental and Clinical Pharmacology
University of Minnesota
Minneapolis, Minnesota, USA

**Sigal Klainbart, DVM, MVPH, DACVECC, DECVECC**
The Veterinary Teaching Hospital
Koret School of Veterinary Medicine
The Hebrew University of Jerusalem, Israel

**Pamela Kloepfer, DVM**
Associate Veterinarian
SafetyCall International, LLC and Pet Poison Helpline
Minneapolis, Minnesota, USA

**Philip Krawec, DVM, DACVECC**
Clinical Assistant Professor, Small Animal Emergency and Critical Care
University of Tennessee Veterinary Medical Center
Knoxville, Tennessee, USA

**Deepa A. Kuttappan, DVM, PhD, DABT**
Study Director (Toxicology)
Labcorp Early Drug Development
Greenfield, Indiana, USA

**Deanna Lombardo, DVM, DACVECC**
Emergency and Critical Care Specialist
VCA R.I.V.E.R.
Chattanooga, Tennessee, USA

**Alicia Mastrocco, DVM, DACVECC**
Staff Criticalist, Emergency and Critical Care
The Animal Medical Center
New York, USA

**Katrina L. Mealey, DVM, PhD, DACVIM, DACVCP**
Director, Program in Individualized Medicine
College of Veterinary Medicine
Washington State University
Pullman, Washington, USA

**Charlotte Means, DVM, DABVT, DABT**
Director of Toxicology
ASPCA Animal Poison Control Center
Champaign, Illinois, USA

**Sarah Musulin, DVM, DACVECC**
Clinical Associate Professor, Emergency and Critical Care
Director of Emergency Services
North Carolina State University
Raleigh, North Carolina, USA

**Katherine L. Peterson, DVM, DACVECC**
Emergency and Critical Care Specialist
BluePearl Veterinary Partners
Duluth, Minnesota, USA

**Michael E. Peterson, DVM, MS**
Staff Veterinarian
Reid Veterinary Hospital
Albany, Oregon, USA

**Helen Philp, BVMS, DACVECC**
Staff Veterinarian – Small Animal Emergency and Critical Care
School of Veterinary Medicine
University of California, Davis
Davis, California, USA

**Amanda Poldoski, DVM**
Associate Manager of Veterinary and Regulatory Affairs
Senior Consulting Veterinarian, Clinical Toxicology
SafetyCall International, LLC and Pet Poison Helpline
Minneapolis, Minnesota, USA

**Robert H. Poppenga, DVM, PhD, DABVT**
Head, Toxicology Section
California Animal Health and Food Safety Laboratory
School of Veterinary Medicine
University of California, Davis
Davis, California, USA

**Birgit Puschner, DVM, PhD, DABVT**
Dean and Professor
College of Veterinary Medicine
Michigan State University
East Lansing, Michigan, USA

**Tiffany Romelhardt, DVM**
Associate Veterinarian, Industry
Veterinary Pharmacovigilance Officer
SafetyCall International, LLC and Pet Poison Helpline
Minneapolis, Minnesota, USA

**Tommaso Rosati, DVM, DACVECC, DECVECC**
Senior Clinician
Small Animal Emergency and Intensive Care
University of Zurich
Zurich, Switzerland

**Wilson K. Rumbeiha, DVM, PhD, DABT, DABVT**
Professor of One Environmental Health Toxicology
Department of Molecular Biosciences
School of Veterinary Medicine
University of California, Davis
Davis, California, USA

**Laurence M. Saint-Pierre, DVM, DACVECC**
Staff Veterinarian – Small Animal Emergency and Critical Care
School of Veterinary Medicine
University of California, Davis
Davis, California, USA

**Julie Schildt, DVM, DACVECC**
Clinical Associate Professor
University of Tennessee College of Veterinary Medicine
Knoxville, Tennessee, USA

**Renee D. Schmid, DVM, DABT, DABVT**
Manager, Veterinary Medicine and Professional Services
Senior Veterinary Toxicologist
SafetyCall International, LLC and Pet Poison Helpline
Minneapolis, Minnesota, USA

**Ashley Smit, DVM, DABT**
Consulting Veterinarian, Clinical Toxicology
SafetyCall International, LLC and Pet Poison Helpline
Minneapolis, Minnesota, USA

**Laura Stern, DVM, DABVT**
Director, APCC Training
ASPCA Animal Poison Control Center
Champaign, Illinois, USA

**Chelsea Sykes, DVM**
California Animal Health and Food Safety Laboratory
School of Veterinary Medicine
University of California, Davis
Davis, California, USA

**Patricia Ann Talcott, MS, DVM, PhD, DABVT**
Clinical Professor and Veterinary Diagnostic Toxicologist, Washington Animal Disease
Diagnostic Laboratory
Department of Integrative Physiology and Neuroscience
College of Veterinary Medicine, Washington State University
Pullman, Washington, USA

**Wan Khoon Avalene Tan, BVSc, PGCertSci, DACVECC**
Senior Lecturer in Emergency and Critical Care Veterinary Teaching Hospital
School of Veterinary Science
Massey University
Palmerston North, New Zealand

**Dominic Tauer, DVM, DABT, DABVT**
Veterinary Toxicologist
SafetyCall International, LLC and Pet Poison Helpline
Minneapolis, Minnesota, USA

**John H. Tegzes, MA, VMD, DABVT, FNAP**
Interim Dean, College of Veterinary Medicine
Western University of Health Sciences
Pomona, California, USA

**Renee Tourdot, DVM, DABT, DABVT**
Senior Toxicologist
ASPCA Animal Poison Control Center
Champaign, Illinois, USA

**Rebecca A.L. Walton, DVM, DACVECC**
Staff Criticalist
VCA West Los Angeles
Los Angeles, California, USA

**Kirsten Waratuke, DVM, DABT, DABVT**
Associate Director of Quality Assurance
ASPCA Animal Poison Control Center
Champaign, Illinois, USA

**Ginger Watts Brown, DVM, DABT, DABVT**
Director, APCC Team
ASPCA Animal Poison Control Center
Champaign, Illinois, USA

**Tina Wismer, DVM, MS, DABVT, DABT**
Senior Director of Toxicology
ASPCA Animal Poison Control Center
Champaign, Illinois, USA

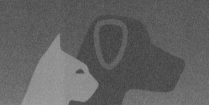

The third edition of *Blackwell's Five-Minute Veterinary Consult Clinical Companion: Small Animal Toxicology* improves on the second edition yet still follows the lead of the successful *Five-Minute Veterinary Consult: Canine and Feline*, 7th edition. The Five-Minute concept of providing essential and relevant information in an organized and easy-to-access format continues in this textbook. In addition, the format of the focused and relevant information can provide excellent support for teaching veterinary toxicology in a professional curriculum. *Blackwell's Five-Minute Veterinary Consult Clinical Companion: Small Animal Toxicology* provides selected details and expanded coverage of toxicology that meet the needs of contemporary small animal toxicology care. The coverage is organized by traditional categories of overview, etiology/pathophysiology (including mechanism of action, pharmacokinetics or toxicokinetics, toxicology, and systems affected), signalment/history, clinical features, key differential diagnoses, diagnostics, and therapeutics. Incorporated is information essential to toxicology evaluation such as dosage, absorption, distribution, metabolism, excretion, toxic doses, prevention, and possible outcomes.

*Blackwell's Five-Minute Veterinary Consult Clinical Companion: Small Animal Toxicology* is designed to aid in the identification of harmful exposures from many natural, synthetic, and consumer products, while subsequently providing the reader with the necessary information to identify and confirm clinical poisoning. In addition, further information discussing prompt detoxification and supportive therapy, as well as specific antidotes, if known, or drug therapies, are reviewed. This book provides a logical, consistent, and sufficiently detailed resource to reach an appropriate clinical decision making accessing specific information quickly and efficiently.

## ORGANIZATION AND FORMAT

The first section of the book, Clinical Toxicology, provides organized and detailed information on the determination of effective detoxification and effective life support measures which are often responsible for saving animals' lives even before a diagnosis can be confirmed. A separate chapter on antidotes provides rapid and useful information for known toxicants and another chapter aids the clinician in dealing with unknown poisons. The chapter on laboratory diagnostics provides the clinician with both clinical and postmortem tests as well as a chart of selected clinical laboratory tests supporting a toxicological diagnosis. Two newer chapters incorporate much needed information on pet foods and medico-legal considerations.

The second section of this book, Specific Toxins and Toxicants, is organized around broad categories of toxicants generally familiar to clients and veterinarians alike. This section details 120 individual topics representing current toxins or toxicants in small animal toxicology. Many of the chapters contain groups of easily identifiable toxins. The selection of these topics is based on evidence from published literature, animal poison control center databases, and advice from colleagues and professionals at veterinary colleges throughout North America. The multiple author format and use of four distinct editors provides a broad range of experiences by those whose professional careers are in the clinical specialties of emergency and critical care, internal medicine, and toxicology.

Section 3, Reference Information, provides useful information, including abbreviations, important resources for toxicology, sample calculations, and tables summarizing anthelmintics, common metals, plants, and topical toxins.

## KEY FEATURES

Within each major category of toxins or toxicants, individual chapters are arranged alphabetically to provide consistent access to the topics. Specific headings within each chapter are similar to common clinical organization of information and augmented by essential toxicological categories. These sections include Definition/Overview, Etiology/Pathophysiology, Signalment/History, Clinical Features, Differential Diagnosis, Diagnostics, Therapeutics, and Comments (including prevention and avoidance, possible complications, and expected course and prognosis). Each chapter provides up to five pertinent and clinically relevant references for additional direction to the clinician or student.

*Lynn R. Hovda, Ahna G. Brutlag,*
*Robert H. Poppenga, and Steven E. Epstein*

# Clinical Toxicology

# Chapter 1

# Decontamination and Detoxification of the Poisoned Patient

## DEFINITION/OVERVIEW

- Decontamination and detoxification are essential processes in the management of an animal which has been poisoned. Poisoning can result from exposure to a variety of harmful substances, including chemicals, medications, and environmental toxicants.
- Decontamination and detoxification aim to remove or neutralize the toxic substance from the animal's body to prevent further harm and promote recovery.
- Decontamination involves the physical removal of the toxicant from the patient's body, while detoxification refers to the use of medications or other substances to neutralize the toxic effects of the poison. Decontamination may need to occur for the eyes, skin, or the gastrointestinal tract.
- Detoxification may involve the administration of antidotes or supportive therapies to manage the patient's symptoms and prevent further harm.
- The effectiveness of decontamination and detoxification depends on several factors, including the type of toxicant, the route of exposure, and the time elapsed since the poisoning occurred. Rapid and appropriate intervention is essential to minimize the potential for serious or life-threatening complications.

## OCULAR DECONTAMINATION

- The goal of ocular decontamination is to reduce tissue damage by removing the offending product from the eye.
- This is accomplished by flushing the eye at home or in the veterinary clinic with sterile saline (e.g., contact lens solution) or warm water for 15–20 minutes. There may need to be a rest period for compliance of the animal to accomplish the total lavage time.
- High-pressure sprays should be avoided (e.g., detachable kitchen sink heads).
- Prevention of further iatrogenic trauma to the eye can be accomplished by placing an Elizabethan collar.
- If decontamination is carried out by the pet owner, the animal should be brought to a veterinarian and evaluated for corneal ulceration.

## DERMAL DECONTAMINATION

- The goal of dermal decontamination is to prevent oral ingestion and transdermal absorption of a poison.
- Proper personal protective equipment should be used by pet owners and veterinary staff to prevent their exposure. This may include gloves, face shield or eye protection, facemask, apron, etc.

*Blackwell's Five-Minute Veterinary Consult Clinical Companion: Small Animal Toxicology*, Third Edition.
Edited by Lynn R. Hovda, Ahna G. Brutlag, Robert H. Poppenga, and Steven E. Epstein.
© 2024 John Wiley & Sons, Inc. Published 2024 by John Wiley & Sons, Inc.

- When an oil-based toxicant is on the animal, they should be bathed with warm water and a liquid dish degreasing soap. The patient should be bathed and rinsed multiple times as soon after exposure as possible. Avoid pet or human shampoos, as they are typically insufficient to remove the majority of an oil-based product.
- When a dry substance is present, the animal may be vacuumed or brushed to remove prior to bathing.
- If an irritating or corrosive substance is on the skin, careful, gentle decontamination must occur. The skin should be thoroughly flushed with copious amounts of warm water for 15–20 minutes, making sure not to traumatize the area with abrasive scrubbing or high-pressure water sprays.

## EMESIS

- Emesis is generally most effective if performed within 1–2 hours of ingestion.
- Exceptions to this are:
  - Acetaminophen and ethylene glycol, which are very rapidly and completely absorbed.
  - Many liquid medications are rapidly absorbed.
  - Situations where emesis may be effective after 1-2 hours.
    - Large blocks of toxicants (e.g., rodenticides), or ingestion of substances that can form concretions (e.g., xylitol-containing gum, fish oil capsules, etc.).
    - Chocolate as it increases pyloric sphincter tone.
    - Fruits (e.g., grapes or raisins) or eaten right after a meal.
    - Toxicants that delay gastric emptying (e.g., opioids, some antidepressants, some blood pressure medications, etc.).
- In a barium sulfate ingestion model in dogs, it has been reported that recovery rates of gastric contents following induction of emesis with apomorphine were 54-87%, while a mean estimated recovery was only 52% in a clinical study.
- Induction of emesis typically yields higher recovery rates than gastric lavage.
- Prior to induction of emesis, a history of what was ingested and screening for contraindications for emesis should be performed.
- Contraindications for emesis include:
  - Inability to protect their airway.
    - Altered mentation or unconsciousness patients.
    - Animals with laryngeal paralysis.
    - Megaesophagus/pharyngeal weakness.
  - Ingestion of caustic or corrosive substances (e.g., acids, alkalis, etc.).
  - Ingestion of petroleum products (e.g., gasoline, motor oil, etc.) can result in aspiration of the material into the lungs, which can lead to respiratory distress.
  - Ingestion of toxicants associated with sharp or pointed objects.
  - Actively seizuring, or a history of seizures (relative contraindication).

### At-home Emesis

- Currently there are no over-the-counter emetic agents recommended for at-home use. Medications that have been used include 3% hydrogen peroxide, table salt, dish soap, 7% syrup of ipecac. Of these, the most acceptable is 3% hydrogen peroxide.
  - Induction of emesis with 3% hydrogen peroxide in dogs has been noted to induce gross esophageal and gastric lesions at appropriate doses, and a severe necroulcerative gastritis in a cat, necessitating euthanasia.
  - It should be noted that many animals have induction of emesis with 3% hydrogen peroxide with no clinical signs.

- Table salt should be avoided due to the risks of hypernatremia, persistent emesis, and hematemesis.
- Dish soap (e.g., Dawn®, Joy®) may be more benign and less efficacious than other methods of at-home emesis. It is dosed at 10 mL/kg of a mixture of three tablespoons of dish soap to 8 ounces of water. *Dish washer soap must be avoided* due to its caustic nature.
- 7% syrup of ipecac *is not recommended* in veterinary or human medicine. Potential complications from syrup of ipecac administration include:
    - Lack of effectiveness in approximately 50% of small animals.
    - Protracted emesis, severe hematemesis, lethargy, diarrhea, depression.
    - Potential cardiotoxic arrhythmogenic action.
- The decision on whether to induce emesis at home or wait until a patient can reach a veterinary office is multifactorial. Considerations include the time it takes to reach veterinary care, onset of action of potential toxicant, ability to administer 3% hydrogen peroxide (e.g., owner comfort in administering, availability in home, etc.) and if contraindications are present.
- For animals that have needed induction of emesis multiple times, ropinirole (Clevor®) can be prescribed for at-home use.

## Emetic Agents

- 3% hydrogen peroxide.
    - Hydrogen peroxide is thought to act as an emetic by direct gastric irritation. Higher concentrations *should not* be used.
    - In cats, the use of hydrogen peroxide as an emetic *is not* recommended. It is not as effective in cats compared to dogs.
    - Dose: 1–2 mL/kg PO, maximum of two doses (1 tablespoon = 15 mL).
    - Emesis usually occurs within 10 minutes.
    - Care is needed to avoid aspiration during administration. Typically, it is administered with a turkey baster, syringe, or spoon.
- Apomorphine.
    - Apomorphine acts directly on the CTZ and works in dogs but not cats.
    - Dose: dogs 0.02–0.04 mg/kg IV or IM, or direct application of the tablet form onto the subconjunctival sac or gingival mucosa. If subconjunctival or gingival apomorphine is used, thorough flushing must be performed after the patient vomits.
    - Emesis typically occurs within 4–6 minutes.
    - If emesis does not occur, a second dose can be tried if given IV or IM. If emesis does not occur after a second dose, alternative medications should be used, or consider gastric lavage.
    - If a patient exhibits excessive CNS sedation or respiratory depression after apomorphine administration, naloxone can be used as a reversal (dose 0.01–0.04 mg/kg, IV, IM, SQ). However, naloxone will not reverse the emetic effect of apomorphine due to different receptor effects.
- Ropinirole.
    - Ropinirole is a dopamine agonist selectively affecting the D2 receptor and available as a topical eye drop (Clevor®) and can be used to induce emesis in dogs but not cats.
    - Dose administration in dogs is split between both eyes, 1–8 drops depending on body size.
    - Emesis usually occurs within 10–15 minutes and is effective on the first dose in 85–87% of dogs.
    - If emesis is not induced, a second dose can be used, or apomorphine tried if available.

- No statistically significant difference has been found between it and IV/IM apomorphine, but studies have been underpowered to detect this.
- Alpha-2-adrenergic agonists.
  - Xylazine and dexmedetomidine have been used to induce emesis in cats.
  - Xylazine dose in cats is 0.22–0.44 mg/kg IM.
  - Dexmedetomidine dose in cats is 5.0–7.0 mcg/kg IM.
  - Xylazine has been reported to induce emesis in 43–60% of cats while dexmedetomidine is effective in 58–81% of cats and typically takes approximately 10 minutes.
  - Given availability and the suggestion for better efficacy, dexmedetomidine is more commonly administered.
  - Typically, emesis (if it occurs) is followed by sedation if the reversal agent is not administered. Cardiovascular and respiratory depression may also occur.
  - Xylazine should be reversed with yohimbine 0.05–0.1 mg/kg IM for doses of xylazine listed above.
  - Dexmedetomidine (0.5 mg/mL) should be reversed with equal volumes of atipamezole (5 mg/mL), or 0.05–0.07 mg/kg atipamezole for doses listed above.
- Tranexamic acid.
  - Tranexamic acid is an antifibrinolytic drug that when administered rapidly can induce emesis in dogs by stimulating a pathway involving tachykinin neurokinin 1.
  - Dose: dogs 50 mg/kg IV administered over 2–3 minutes induced emesis in approximately 85% of dogs within six minutes.
  - If emesis does not occur within 10 minutes, a second dose of 20–30 mg/kg IV can be administered.
  - Potential adverse effects reported include seizures.
  - Tranexamic acid has been used for its antifibrinolytic effects in cats at 10 mg/kg, but no reports on its use as an emetic have been published.

# ADSORBENTS AND CATHARTICS

## Activated Charcoal

- The goal of activated charcoal (AC) is to act as an adsorbent and to prevent systemic absorption of a toxicant. It is the primary treatment of choice for decontamination of the veterinary poisoned patient.
- AC contains carbon moieties that adsorb compounds with varying affinity, binding nonpolar compounds well.
- Heavy metals (e.g., zinc, iron, etc.) and alcohols (e.g., ethylene glycol, xylitol, methanol, isopropyl alcohol, ethanol) typically are not absorbed by AC.
- The interaction between the bound toxicant and AC could potentially undergo desorption (where the toxicant unbinds from the AC over time); hence, a cathartic is often added to help promote fecal expulsion and decrease GI tract transit time.
- Administration of AC with a cathartic as long as six hours past ingestion may still be beneficial with toxicosis, particularly if the product has delayed release (e.g., extended or sustained release) or undergoes enterohepatic recirculation.
- The use of AC with a magnesium-containing cathartic should be undertaken judiciously in cats.
- Dose: 1–2 g of AC per kg of body weight orally with the first dose containing a cathartic.
- Drugs undergoing enterohepatic recirculation (e.g., theobromine, bromethalin, etc.), with a long half-life (naproxen), or delayed-release products will require multidose administration of AC, with subsequent doses not containing a cathartic.

- Additional doses of AC should ideally not contain a cathartic, due to increased risks for dehydration via fluid losses from the GI tract.
- Adverse effects of AC administration include diarrhea (when contains a cathartic), electrolyte derangements, hyperlactatemia and hyperosmolality, and a report of small intestinal obstruction in dog with repeated doses.
- Few animals will ingest AC voluntarily without the addition of food. The addition of food causes a clinically insignificant reduction of the absorptive capacity. Alternatives for animals who will not voluntarily ingest AC include syringe feeding or large-bore nasogastric tube administration.
- To prevent dehydration and hypernatremia, the patient should be given free access to water.
- Administration of an antiemetic may help prevent emesis of the AC and allow for rapid return to oral water.
    - Maropitant 1 mg/kg, IV q 24 hours has been successfully used in this scenario.
- Activated charcoal should be used with care in patients with dehydration or electrolyte derangements and the need for fluid therapy should be evaluated in these patients.
- Contraindications for AC include a compromised airway (risk for aspiration pneumonia), known perforation of the GI tract, caustic substance ingestion, and hydrocarbon toxicosis (due to increased risk for aspiration pneumonia).

## Cholestyramine
- Cholestyramine is a medication used to bind bile acids, lower cholesterol, and treat certain types of diarrhea.
- Cholestyramine can be dosed at 0.3–1 g/kg every 6–8 hours with toxicants that undergo enterohepatic recirculation or biliary elimination.
    - It is most likely to be helpful in vitamin $D_3$, microcystin, and bromethalin toxicosis.
- Little is known about the success of cholestyramine in veterinary medicine, and it should not routinely be used as a substitute for AC.

## Cathartics
- Cathartics are designed to decrease the transit time of substances in the GI tract and promote fecal excretion of the toxicant.
- The two most common types of cathartics used in veterinary medicine are nonabsorbable saccharides (e.g., sorbitol), and nonabsorbable salts (e.g., magnesium sulfate).
- Dose: sorbitol 70% solution, 1–2 mL/kg, PO or 250 mg/kg magnesium sulfate diluted to a 20% solution PO.
- Adverse effects of sorbitol administration: vomiting, dehydration, secondary hypernatremia, abdominal cramping or pain, and possible hypotension.
- The use of cathartics alone is no longer recommended or beneficial.

## GASTRIC LAVAGE

- Gastric lavage can be utilized if there is a contraindication to induction of emesis, or induction of emesis was unsuccessful.
- Recovery rates of toxicants are consistently lower than with emesis in people and dogs.
- Gastric lavage should be considered when:
    - Symptomatic patients need decontamination (e.g., metaldehyde toxicosis presenting with seizures).

- Recent (<1–2 hours) ingestion of a life-threatening dose of toxicants that has no antidote.
- Material is not easily absorbed (e.g., lily flower, oleander leaves, etc.).
- Patient has a high risk of aspiration pneumonia with induction of emesis.
- Contraindications for gastric lavage include:
  - Corrosive agents.
  - Hydrocarbon ingestion.
- To perform gastric lavage, the patient must first be anesthetized and maintained on intravenous or inhalational anesthesia. An endotracheal tube should be placed and the cuff inflated and verified to not be leaking at 20 cmH$_2$O pressure in the anesthesia circuit. Frequently, an antiemetic is administered prior to induction of anesthesia to prevent vomiting at the time of induction, or in recovery.
- The orogastric tube of the largest diameter appropriate for the patient should be selected and premeasured to the 13th rib. A piece of tape can be used to mark this distance.
- The orogastric tube should be lubricated and inserted to the stomach. Its presence can be verified by direct external visualization, or auscultation of gas bubbles over the stomach as air is blown into the tube.
- Once the orogastric tube is properly placed and verified, the stomach is emptied (Figure 1.1a). Then a pump (Figure 1.1b) can be used, or gravity with a funnel to administer approximately

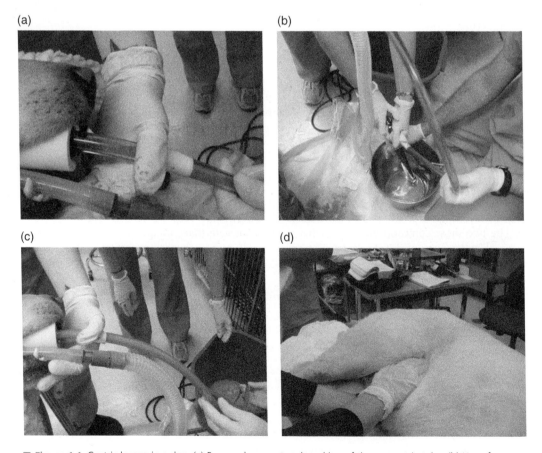

(a)  (b)  (c)  (d)

■ **Figure 1.1** Gastric lavage in a dog. (a) Proper placement and marking of the orogastric tube. (b) Use of a pump to administer warm water into the stomach. (c) Siphon action of water to facilitate withdrawal of gastric contents. (d) Frequent palpation of stomach to ensure it is not overdistended.

20 mL/kg warm water into the stomach. The pump can be removed and the tube lowered below the patient to drain the water and contents from the stomach (Figure 1.1c). This process can be repeated multiple times until only clear water remains. During the process, the patient's stomach should be palpated frequently to ensure overdistention does not occur (Figure 1.1d).

- The gastric lavage fluid should be examined for the presence of toxicants (e.g., plant material, mushrooms, rodenticides, medications, etc.), and can be saved for toxicological testing if needed.
- Prior to removal of the orogastric tube, AC or cholestyramine can be administered.
- The orogastric tube should be kinked prior to removal to prevent contents from the tube from leaking into the esophagus during the removal process.
- The patient can then be recovered from anesthesia, ideally in sternal recumbency with their head elevated.

## DIURESIS

- The main use of fluid diuresis in toxicities is to increase elimination of substances that are renally cleared from the body.
- Highly protein-bound substances (e.g., NSAIDs) do not benefit from fluid diuresis.
- Results of early studies have failed to show a benefit.
- Toxicants in which fluid diuresis is most likely to be beneficial include:
  - Amphetamines.
  - Lithium.
  - Bromide.
  - Phenobarbital.
  - Salicylates.
- If fluid diuresis is attempted, balanced electrolyte solutions (e.g., Lactated Ringer's solution, Plasma-Lyte-148®) are commonly used unless a high chloride concentration is indicated (bromide toxicosis) and then 0.9% saline may be utilized at 4–8 mL/kg/h IV.
- Furosemide at 1–2 mg/kg IV q 6–8 hours may be added to help prevent overhydration or treat it if it occurs.
- Adverse effects of fluid diuresis include:
  - Fluid overload.
  - Electrolyte and acid–base disturbances (hypokalemia, metabolic acidosis, etc.).

## INTRAVENOUS LIPID EMULSION

- Intravenous lipid emulsion (ILE) therapy was first used to treat cardiac arrest from bupivacaine toxicosis in a human and has become the standard of care to treat local anesthetic systemic toxicity.
- ILE has been used to treat a multitude of veterinary toxicities with little evidence of efficacy or improving case outcomes.
  - Current veterinary evidence includes multiple case reports which garner the critique of selection bias (e.g., only cases in which therapy was perceived as successful are reported).
    - Some case reports do include pharmacokinetic evidence; however, often multiple therapies are utilized concurrently.
  - High-level evidence exists only as a randomized controlled trial in permethrin toxicosis in cats.

- ILE therapy in veterinary medicine, outside permethrin toxicosis, should be reserved for severe poisonings that are not responsive to standard medical therapy or where euthanasia is being considered because of poor prognosis or financial constraints.
- ILE is available in 10–30% solutions (20% is most widely used), and is composed of neutral, medium- to long-chain triglycerides derived from combinations of plant oils (e.g., soybean, safflower), egg phospholipids, and glycerin.
- The mechanism of action is not fully elucidated at this time, but two theories predominate.
  - The "lipid sink/shuttle" theory involves creating a lipid phase in the bloodstream sequestering lipophilic drugs, preventing them from reaching their target sites or shuttles them from target sites such as the brain or heart and transports toxicants to muscle or adipose tissue until they can be metabolized or excreted.
  - The other theory is that lipids can increase cardiac performance which likely plays a role in toxicants like the local anesthetics causing cardiovascular collapse.
- Initially ILE was thought to work better for toxicities with high lipid solubility as measured by the octanol/water partition coefficient (LogP), but an apparent benefit in nonlipophilic toxicities (e.g., baclofen, which has a negative LogP) indicates that other properties of the toxicant are important.
- A list of toxicants in which ILE have an apparent benefit is beyond the scope of this chapter and when thought to be of benefit is covered in individual chapters.
- The ideal dose of ILE has not been determined; however, a 20% solution is recommended for treatment of toxicities. Possible doses are:
  - 1.5 mL/kg IV fast bolus (if cardiac arrest or life-threatening situation) followed by 0.25 mL/kg/min IV for 30–60 minutes.
    - The clinician should recognize that this CRI rate delivers the initial bolus of 1.5 mL/kg over six minutes and the intent of the bolus is to rapidly achieve plasma levels.
  - If not in cardiac arrest, 0.25 mL/kg/min for 30–60 minutes IV.
    - If the patient is still experiencing severe clinical signs and the plasma is not lipemic, this dose can be repeated in 4–6 hours.
  - In humans, a 1.5 mL/kg intravenous bolus with an additional 0.25 mL/kg/min over three minutes, then 0.025 mL/kg/min up to 6.5 hours has been utilized as well.
- The use of an in-line filter might avoid lipid emboli creating adverse effects.
- Maximum dosing of 10–15 mL/kg/day of 20% lipid has been recommended as a nutritional supplement in parenteral nutrition; however, higher doses have been well tolerated on a single day for treatment of toxicosis.
- Generally, ILE therapy is well tolerated. Adverse effects include:
  - Pancreatitis.
  - Corneal lipidosis.
  - Facial pruritus and type I hypersensitivity.
  - Hemolysis.
  - Possible acute respiratory distress syndrome (ARDS).
  - Interference with laboratory tests.
  - Fat overload syndrome and death (accidental overdose of ILE).

## EXTRACORPOREAL THERAPY

- Extracorporeal therapy (ECT) for toxicities consists of hemodialysis (HD), hemoperfusion (HP), and therapeutic plasma exchange (TPE).
- TPE can be performed manually or automated on a specialized machine, while other extracorporeal modalities can only be performed with a machine.

- There is little definitive evidence for the use of ECT in veterinary medicine; however, for many toxicants based on human literature, it is considered the standard of care when available (e.g., ethylene glycol).
  - Multiple case reports exist in veterinary medicine where ECT appeared to be beneficial. However, the effect on pharmacokinetic parameters other than simple plasma clearance measurements and the contribution of endogenous clearance in these cases is unknown. There is also likely selection bias similar to ILE therapy.
    - o Propylene glycol.
    - o Barbiturates.
    - o Cannabinoids.
    - o Methotrexate.
    - o NSAIDs.
    - o Vincristine.
- As during the treatment process, a portion of the blood is extracorporeal, a minimum patient size may be needed depending on the modality used (often >5 kg).
  - It is possible to treat smaller patients, but this will depend on the modality (primarily the extracorporeal circuit size), the experience of the operator, availability of blood products for priming, and the cardiovascular stability of the patient.
- Treatment with ECT for a toxicity should be considered for toxicants that are primarily limited to the vascular space and have low volumes of distribution (preferably <1 L/kg, but up to <2 L/kg).
  - If the volume of distribution is >2 L/kg, then prolonged treatment and processing of multiple blood volumes are necessary to achieve a significant decrease in total body drug concentration. This may not exceed endogenous clearance in which case ECT is unlikely to be of benefit.
- If the protein binding is >95% or the molecular weight (MW) of the toxicant is >50 kDa, TPE is the preferred methodology (e.g., vincristine). For effective TPE, a small volume of distribution (ideally <0.5 L/kg) is necessary.
- If the protein binding is >80–95% or the MW is 10–50 kDa, then hemoperfusion will likely be utilized (e.g., phenobarbital). The efficacy of hemoperfusion is dictated by the affinity of the toxicant for the adsorbent.
- If the protein binding is <80% or the MW is <500 Da to 1 kDa, then hemodialysis will likely be utilized. (e.g., ethylene glycol, baclofen).
- If the above criteria are met, consultation with a referral center capable of performing ECT is recommended.
- Conventional decontamination should be performed pending decision making regarding ECT.

## Abbreviations

- AC = activated charcoal
- CTZ = chemoreactive trigger zone
- ECT = extrcorporeal therapy
- HD = hemodialysis
- HP = hemoperfusion
- ILE = intravenous lipid emulsion
- NSAID = nonsteroidal anti-inflammatory drug
- TPE = therapeutic plasma exchange

## Suggested Reading

Epstein SE, Hopper K, Farrell KS. Manual plasma exchange to treat an accidental overdose of intravenous lipid emulsion in a dog with baclofen toxicosis. *J Am Vet Med Assoc* 2022;260(6):650–656.

Gwaltney-Brant S, Meadows I. Intravenous lipid emulsions in veterinary clinical toxicology. *Vet Clin North Am Small Anim Pract* 2018;48(6):933–942.

Mauro KD, McClosky ME. Extracorporeal therapies for blood purification. In: Silverstein DC, Hopper K (eds) *Small Animal Critical Care Medicine*, 3rd edn. St Louis: Elsevier, 2022.

Niedzwecki AH, Book BP, Lewis KM, Estep JS, Hagan J. Effects of oral 3% hydrogen peroxide used as an emetic on the gastroduodenal mucosa of healthy dogs. *J Vet Emerg Crit Care* 2017;27:178–184.

Suokko M, Saloranta L, Lamminen T, Laine T, Elliott J. Ropinirole eye drops induce vomiting effectively in dogs: a randomised, double-blind, placebo-controlled clinical study. *Vet Rec* 2020;186(9):283.

**Author**: Steven E. Epstein, DVM, DACVECC
**Consulting Editor**: Steven E. Epstein, DVM, DACVECC

# Chapter 2

# Emergency Management of the Poisoned Patient

 ## DEFINITION/OVERVIEW

- Management of the acutely poisoned patient includes initial telephone triage, appropriate communication and history gathering from the pet owner, thorough physical examination, and initial stabilization.
- Prompt decontamination and detoxification of the patient should be performed, when appropriate. Please see Chapter 1, Decontamination and Detoxification of the Poisoned Patient, for more information.
- Initial stabilization of the emergent patient should include the ABCDs.
  - Airway.
  - Breathing.
  - Circulation.
  - Dysfunction.
- Appropriate diagnostic testing (e.g., CBC, chemistry, venous blood gas analysis, electrolytes, urinalysis) should be performed, as this may help guide therapy or assist in the diagnosis of an unknown toxicosis.
- Appropriate monitoring of the critically ill, poisoned patient may include the following.
  - Continuous electrocardiogram (ECG).
  - Blood pressure monitoring (BP).
  - Pulse oximetry (SpO$_2$).
  - Blood gas analysis.
- If an antidote (e.g., fomepizole, 2-PAM, atropine, vitamin K$_1$) or reversal agent (e.g., naloxone, flumazenil, yohimbine, atipamezole) is available, it should be initiated promptly for the specific toxicant.
- Note, the majority of toxicants do *not* have a readily available antidote; therefore, the use of decontamination and symptomatic supportive care is warranted.

## ABCDS of the Poisoned Patient

### Airway
- Any patient presenting comatose, unconscious, or neurologically impaired with an absent gag reflex should be intubated with an endotracheal tube, connected to an oxygen source, and treated with positive pressure ventilation (PPV) or manual delivery of breaths (see Breathing).

### Breathing
- The patient should be evaluated for signs of respiratory distress or lack of any chest wall movement to indicate ineffective breathing.
- If the patient is not breathing, immediate intubation and PPV are indicated at 10–20 bpm, with a tidal volume of approximately 10 mL/kg.

*Blackwell's Five-Minute Veterinary Consult Clinical Companion: Small Animal Toxicology*, Third Edition. Edited by Lynn R. Hovda, Ahna G. Brutlag, Robert H. Poppenga, and Steven E. Epstein.
© 2024 John Wiley & Sons, Inc. Published 2024 by John Wiley & Sons, Inc.

- If clinical signs of respiratory distress are present, the patient should be treated immediately with supplemental oxygen.
- Obtaining a sample for blood gas analysis (venous or arterial) to help diagnose hypoventilation ($PaCO_2$ >45 mmHg or $PvCO_2$ >50 mmHg) or hypoxemia ($PaO_2$ <80 mmHg) may be helpful.
- If hypoventilation or hypoxemia is present, identifying the etiology rapidly may assist the clinician in identifying a treatment plan (e.g., hypoventilation from opioids can be reversed with naloxone, pulmonary hemorrhage from anticoagulant rodenticide ingestions may need a plasma transfusion, etc.).
- Mechanical ventilation may be indicated when the $PaCO_2$ >60 mmHg or $PvCO_2$ >65 mmHg and the cause cannot be rapidly reversed, or when the $PaO_2$ <60 mmHg despite oxygen supplementation.
- Readers are referred to the references on mechanical ventilation for more information.

## Circulation

- Altered circulation secondary to inadequate perfusion is often due to hypovolemia, or a direct effect of various toxicants such as beta-blockers, calcium channel blockers, etc.
- The patient should be assessed for effective circulation based on the following physical examination parameters: mentation, mucous membrane color, capillary refill time, heart rate, pulse quality and pressure, and core versus body temperature.
- Patients judged to be in circulatory shock should have appropriate therapy initiated promptly. This may include the following:
  - Fluid therapy to treat hypovolemia.
  - Vasopressor or positive inotrope infusions.
  - See section on Cardiovascular support below for more details.

## Dysfunction

- Neurological dysfunction may be due to various toxicants causing depression, agitation, or seizures.
- On initial presentation, the poisoned patient should be evaluated for gross neurological disability. If abnormalities are present, a full neurological examination should be performed if possible.
- Poisoned patients with neurological disease should have prompt assessment of metabolic parameters (e.g., blood glucose concentration, PCV/TP, calcium concentration) to help determine if the clinical signs are a direct effect of the toxicant or due to a secondary effect (e.g., hypoglycemia, hypocalcemia, etc.).
- Treatment for the neurologically impaired poisoned patient includes decreasing intracranial pressure, increasing perfusion to the brain, and immediate treatment of seizure activity.
- For more information on treatment for neurological disorders, please see Neurological Support later in this chapter.

## SUPPORTIVE CARE AND TREATMENT

- As stated previously, very few toxicities have antidotes, and treatment is often symptomatic and supportive, including the following:
  - Monitoring and supportive care.
  - Cardiovascular support.
    - Fluid therapy.
    - Antiarrhythmia therapy.
    - Vasopressor and positive inotrope therapy.
  - Neurological support.

## Monitoring and Supportive Care

- Monitoring of the poisoned patient may include any of the following:
  - ECG.
  - BP.
  - Pulse oximetry.
  - Blood gas analysis.

### Continuous ECG

- Specific toxicants that may require the use of ECG monitoring include cardiac medications (e.g., beta-blockers, calcium channel blockers, digoxin), albuterol, SSRIs, amphetamines, caffeine, lamotrigine, cardiac glycoside-containing plants, *Bufo* toads, amitraz, etc.
- If abnormalities are identified, a continuous ECG should be used to look for the presence of dysrhythmias, bradycardia, or tachycardia that may warrant treatment.
- In general, the following parameters should warrant treatment if detected on an ECG:
  - Dog: HR <50 bpm or >180 bpm.
  - Cat: HR <120 bpm or >240 bpm.
  - R on T phenomenon (often predisposing to serious ventricular arrhythmias like ventricular fibrillation).
  - Runs of ventricular tachyardia >180 bpm for 60 seconds or longer.
  - When abnormalites are present that are associated with clinical signs of poor perfusion or hypotension.
- For more information on general treatment for arrhythmias, please see Cardiovascular Support later in this chapter. Readers are also directed to a veterinary cardiology or critical care book for more details due to the large scope of information.

### Blood Pressure (BP)

- If abnormalities are present on cardiovascular examination, then blood pressure monitoring is indicated. Poisoned patients may be either hypotensive or hypertensive depending on the toxicant.
- Blood pressure can be monitored by direct arterial blood pressure, Doppler, or oscillometric measurement.
  - Direct arterial blood pressure is advantageous because it is continuous and very accurate, but it is invasive, requires specialized equipment, requires a high level of skill to maintain and place an arterial line, and if disconnected (and unobserved), can lead to catastrophic bleeding.
  - Indirect blood pressure monitoring can be performed with oscillometric or Doppler monitoring and is often more economical.
- In the poisoned patient, hypotension may be seen from the following toxicants.
  - Cardiac medications (e.g., beta-blockers, calcium channel blockers, cardiac glycoside-containing plants, *Bufo* toads, others), resulting in arrhythmias or severe bradycardia, which results in poor cardiac contractility, decreased afterload, and decreased systemic vascular resistance.
  - Beta-agonists (e.g., albuterol, salmeterol, clenbuterol), resulting in severe tachycardia, which prevents adequate ventricular filling and secondary hypotension.
  - Sedatives (e.g., baclofen, opioids, others), resulting in severe sedation and CNS depression.
  - Anticoagulant rodenticides (e.g., bromadiolone, brodifacoum, etc.), which can result in hemorrhagic shock secondary to coagulopathy and secondary bleeding.
- If the patient is hypotensive (MAP <60 mmHg or systolic <90 mmHg), appropriate volume resuscitation should occur with IV fluid therapy, provided cardiogenic shock has been ruled out (see below for more details).

- In the poisoned patient, hypertension may be seen from the following toxicants: SSRIs, amphetamines, caffeine, theobromine, decongestants, phenylpropanolamine, others.
- Nontoxicant-related causes for hypertension in veterinary medicine include pain, fear, renal disease, cardiac disease, endocrine disease (e.g., hyperadrenocorticism, hyperthyroidism), immune-mediated hemolytic anemia, pheochromocytoma, etc.
- Patients with a blood pressure higher than a MAP >140 mmHg or systolic >180–200 mmHg should be promptly treated.
    - The use of judicious sedation/analgesia, anxiolytics, anticonvulsants, vasodilators, or ACE inhibitors may be necessary.
    - If the hypertension is toxicant related and concurrent agitation is simultaneously observed, the use of sedation is recommended for patients with stable cardiovascular systems.
    - In the poisoned patient, persistent hypertension typically responds well to aggressive, frequent sedation of the patient. However, if the patient is persistently hypertensive despite multiple doses of sedation, the additional use of antihypertensives may be necessary to prevent vascular injury, retinal detachment, or ischemic injury. Antihypertensives include:
        - Amlodipine (calcium channel blocker).
            - Dog: 0.1–0.25 mg/kg, PO q 12–24 hours PRN to effect.
            - Cat: 0.625 mg *total* per cat, PO q 12–24 hours PRN to effect.
            - Use cautiously in patients with cardiac or hepatic disease. Do not use in hypotensive patients or those with toxicants that may result in hypotension (e.g., calcium channel blockers, beta-blockers, etc.).
        - Clevidipine (calcium channel blocker).
            - Dog and cats: 0.5 to 5 mcg/kg/min IV CRI titrated to effect.

## Pulse Oximetry

- Pulse oximeters are noninvasive, easy-to-use bedside monitors that measure $SpO_2$ rather than $SaO_2$ (oxygen saturation). A pulsatile tissue bed is required for an accurate reading. Measurements can be taken on the lip, tongue, pinnae, base of tail, toe web, vulva, prepuce, or rectum (with a rectal probe).
- Reliable pulse oximetry readings are affected by ambient light, hypotension, poor perfusion, pigmentation, icterus, and nail polish.
- An accurate HR and strong signal *must* correlate with the pulse oximeter before a reliable reading can be taken.
- Normal pulse oximetry (without oxygen supplementation) is ≥95–100%. A pulse oximetry reading of 90% correlates with a $PaO_2$ of 60 mmHg (normal 80–100 mmHg), consistent with severe hypoxemia.
- Pulse oximetry is useful in the poisoned patient when dyspnea, tachypnea, abnormal lung sounds, or respiratory distress is evident.

## Blood Gas Analysis

- Venous or arterial blood gas analysis is the determination of the pH, $PaO_2$ (arterial), $PCO_2$ (venous or arterial), base excess, and bicarbonate concentration of blood. Plasma lactate and electrolyte concentrations frequently accompany blood gas testing to give a more complete picture of the animal's metabolic status.
- Blood gas analysis can be beneficial in the poisoned patient to evaluate the severity of acid–base imbalances. There are four main causes of a metabolic acidosis that is associated with an elevated anion gap.
    - Lactic acidosis (may be falsely elevated in ethylene glycol toxicosis).
    - Uremic acidosis (e.g., acute kidney injury [AKI]).

- Diabetic ketoacidosis.
- Toxicants (e.g., ethylene glycol, salicylates, methanol, etc.).

■ Blood gas analysis may also help to determine the severity of a patient's respiratory disease as noted above.

## Cardiovascular Support

### Fluid Therapy

■ Fluid therapy, a cornerstone therapy of emergency management of the poisoned patient:
  - corrects hypovolemia and maintains perfusion at a cellular level.
  - corrects dehydration.
  - vasodilates the renal vessels (particularly with nephrotoxic toxins like NSAIDs, lilies, etc.).
  - may treat hypotension (particularly with toxicants such as beta-blockers, calcium channel blockers, others).

■ Poisoned patients with poor signs of perfusion should be assessed for hypovolemia and treated for this on an emergency basis.

■ When volume resuscitating a patient, the following IV fluids can be used:
  - Any balanced, isotonic crystalloid (e.g., Normosol-R®, Plasma-Lyte-148®, Lactated Ringer's solution®): 20–30 mL/kg IV aliquots over 5–15 minutes; repeat 2–3× as needed, monitoring frequently for response to therapy.
  - If no improvement, consider synthetic colloid boluses (e.g., Hetastarch®, VetStarch®): 5 mL/kg IV aliquots over 10–20 minutes.

■ Patients should be evaluated for dehydration based on skin turgor, tacky mucous membrane, and presence of sunken eyes. Depending on the severity of dehydration and illness, patients should be treated with IV fluid replacement.

■ Fluid therapy can also be used to aid in detoxification in certain scenarios by increasing renal excretion of toxicants by forced diuresis.

■ Crystalloids.
  - Any balanced, isotonic buffered solution can be used.
  - Dose: the dose of IV fluids to administer is dependent on the clinical state and physical examination findings of the patient.
  - In a healthy patient, fluid rates of 4–10 mL/kg/h can be used to force renal clearance of the toxicant.
  - Neonates have a higher maintenance fluid rate (80–180 mL/kg/day), and fluid rates should be adjusted accordingly.
  - Patients with cardiac disease or respiratory disease, or those which have ingested toxicants that may increase their risk of pulmonary edema (e.g., TCA antidepressants, phosphide rodenticides) should have judicious fluid administration.
  - Careful assessment of hydration should be made based on PCV/TP, weight gain, and physical examination findings.

### Antiarrhythmia Therapy

■ In patients with cardiac arrhythmias, the use of antiarrhythmic therapy is recommended if it is directly affecting perfusion parameters (e.g., CRT, blood pressure, etc.).
  - Bradyarrhythmias (dog: HR <50 bpm; cat: HR <120 bpm).
    ○ Atropine: 0.02–0.04 mg/kg IV, IM, SQ PRN bradycardia.
    ○ Glycopyrrolate: 0.01–0.02 mg/kg IV, IM, SQ PRN bradycardia.
  - Supraventricular tachyarrhythmias (SVTs) (dog: HR >180 bpm; cat: HR >240 bpm).
    ○ Esmolol: 100–500 mcg/kg IV slow over 2 minutes, then 10–200 mcg/kg/min CRI.
    ○ Diltiazem: 0.05–0.25 mg/kg IV slowly, repeat q 15 minutes to maximum dose of 0.5 mg/kg.

> o Propranolol: 0.02 mg/kg IV slowly over 2–3 minutes, titrate dosage up to effect (to a maximum of 0.1 mg/kg). Can be repeated every 8 hours.
- Ventricular arrhythmias.
  - o Lidocaine:
    - ◇ Dogs: 2–4 mg/kg IV bolus, then 25–100 mcg/kg/min IV CRI.
  - o Procainamide:
    - ◇ Dogs: 2 mg/kg IV bolus, repeated to maximum cumulative dosage of 10 mg/kg, then 25–50 mcg/kg/min IV CRI.

### Vasopressor/Positive Inotrope Therapy

- In patients with cardiovascular collapse (e.g., hypotension, tachycardia, bradycardia, etc.), the appropriate use of IV fluids and/or antiarrhythmic therapy is warranted. In persistently hypotensive patients not responding to boluses of fluids, the use of positive inotropes or vasopressors may be necessary to increase cardiac contractility or blood pressure. Due to the complexity of this topic, readers are directed to the Suggested Reading at the end of this chapter.
  - Dopamine.
    - o 2–10 mcg/kg/min IV CRI to effect (dose for beta effect).
    - o >10 mcg/kg/min IV CRI to effect (dose for alpha effect).
  - Dobutamine.
    - o Dogs: 5–20 mcg/kg/min IV CRI.
    - o Cats: 1–10 mcg/kg/min IV CRI.
  - Norepinephrine: 0.1–1.0 mcg/kg/min IV CRI.
  - Epinephrine: 0.05–0.4 mcg/kg/min IV CRI.
  - Vasopressin: 0.5–4 mU/kg/min IV CRI.

## Neurological Support

- Certain toxicants may result in signs of agitation, CNS depression, or refractory seizures. Examples include 5-FU, amphetamines, SSRIs, baclofen, ivermectin, bromethalin, benzodiazepines, lamotrigine, pyrethrins, organophosphates, metaldehyde, cocaine, mushrooms, salt, blue-green algae, and others.
- In the poisoned patient, it is imperative that appropriate drug therapy be used to stop tremors and seizures immediately. Persistent tremoring and seizuring can result in rhabdomyolysis with secondary AKI, lowering of the seizure threshold, secondary hyperthermia, and secondary DIC. The use of muscle relaxants and anticonvulsant therapy is imperative.
  - Methocarbamol 55–220 mg/kg, IV, PRN to effect.
  - Diazepam 0.25–0.5 mg/kg, IV, PRN to effect.
  - Midazolam 0.1–0.5 mg/kg, IV, PRN to effect, followed by CRI if indicated.
  - Levetiracetam 20–60 mg/kg, IV, PRN to effect.
  - Phenobarbital 4 mg/kg, IV q 4 hours × 4 doses to load; additional doses may be necessary.
- Severely neurologically impaired poisoned patients should be monitored and treated for cerebral ischemia or edema with the following supportive care, if needed.
  - 15–30° head elevation.
  - Oxygen therapy titrated to avoid hypoxemia.
  - Fluid therapy to maintain perfusion, blood pressure.
  - ECG, pulse oximetry, or $CO_2$ monitoring.
  - Frequent neurological examination.
  - Treatment for cerebral edema with mannitol 0.5–1 g/kg, IV slowly over 20–30 minutes PRN.

## CONCLUSIONS

With toxicosis, the majority of toxins do not have a readily available antidote. Symptomatic and supportive care remains the primary goal of emergency management of the poisoned patient.

### Abbreviations

- AKI = acute kidney injury
- BP = blood pressure
- ECG = electrocardiogram
- ICP = intracranial pressure
- MAP = mean arterial presssure
- $PaO_2$ = partial pressure of arterial oxygen
- $P_aCO_2$ = partial pressure of arterial carbon dioxide
- $PCO_2$ = partial pressure of carbon dioxide
- $P_vCO_2$ = partial pressure of venous carbon dioxide
- $SaO_2$ = arterial oxygen saturation
- $SpO_2$ = saturation of arterial blood with oxygen as measured by pulse oximetry
- SVT = supraventricular tachyarrhythmia

### Suggested Reading

deLaforcade A, Silverstein DC. Classification and initial management of shock. In: Silverstein DC, Hopper K (eds) *Small Animal Critical Care Medicine*, 3rd edn. St Louis: Elsevier Saunders, 2023; pp. 37–41.

Hopper K. Mechanical ventilation – core concepts. In: Silverstein DC, Hopper K (eds) *Small Animal Critical Care Medicine*, 3rd edn. St Louis: Elsevier Saunders, 2023; pp. 185–192.

Mellema MS. Initial management of the poisoned patient. In: Peterson ME, Talcott PA (eds) *Small Animal Toxicology*, 3rd edn. St Louis: Elsevier Saunders, 2013; pp. 63–71.

Waddell LS. Hemodynamic monitoring. In: Silverstein DC, Hopper K (eds) *Small Animal Critical Care Medicine*, 3rd edn. St Louis: Elsevier Saunders, 2023; pp. 1030–1036.

### Acknowledgment

The authors and editors acknowledge the prior contributions of Justine A. Lee, DVM, DACVECC, DABT, who authored this topic in the previous edition.

**Author:** Steven E. Epstein, DVM, DACVECC
**Consulting Editor:** Steven E. Epstein, DVM, DACVECC

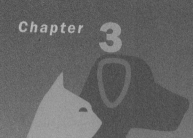

# Chapter 3

# Antidotes and Other Useful Drugs

## DEFNITION/OVERVIEW

- Antidotes are substances used to counteract poisons. Specifically, antidotes are defined as any substance used to relieve or prevent the effects associated with a toxicant.
- Very few antidotes exist in medicine, and those that do are generally not approved for veterinary use. Any use associated with nonveterinary-approved antidotes is considered extra-label. Veterinarians are legally allowed to use medications in an extra-label manner but when doing so assume all the responsibility associated with their use.
- The dosages used are often extrapolated from human literature with very little scientific animal data available.
- Little effort has been made by manufacturers to produce antidotes approved for use in veterinary medicine. There is no financial incentive for them to do this as the use of antidotes is limited, making research and manufacturing cost prohibitive.
- Antidotes can be divided into three broad categories.
  - *Chemical or causal antidotes* are those that work directly on the toxicant. They bind with the toxicant to yield an innocuous compound that is excreted from the body.
  - *Functional antidotes* have no chemical or physical interaction with toxicants but work to lessen the clinical signs associated with intoxication.
  - *Pharmacological or physiological antidotes* work in the body by several different mechanisms. Most commonly, they work directly at the receptor site, generally counteracting toxicosis by producing opposing clinical signs. They may also prevent the formation of toxic metabolites, facilitate a more rapid elimination of a toxicant, or aid in the restoration of normal body function.

## Chemical Antidotes

### Antivenoms

- IV antivenom can be used in dogs and cats to prevent paralysis, coagulopathies, and thrombocytopenia from snake, black widow spider, or scorpion bites. It has no effect on tissue necrosis. Early administration is preferred as it not only lessens the severity of signs but decreases the need for additional doses later.
- Anaphylactoid, anaphylactic, and serum sickness reactions can occur, especially if the animal has received antivenom at a prior time.
- **Elapid antivenom (coral snakes).**
  - North American coral snake antivenin (Wyeth Pharmaceuticals LLC, Antivenin *Micrurus fulvius*) (IgG equine origin) is FDA approved and available for human use in

*Blackwell's Five-Minute Veterinary Consult Clinical Companion: Small Animal Toxicology*, Third Edition. Edited by Lynn R. Hovda, Ahna G. Brutlag, Robert H. Poppenga, and Steven E. Epstein. © 2024 John Wiley & Sons, Inc. Published 2024 by John Wiley & Sons, Inc.

the United States. Product cost is a major consideration. Efficacy with Sonoran coral snake envenomation has not been established.

- Alternative coral snake antivenoms produced in other countries may sometimes be obtained from local zoos. Follow manufacturer's guidelines for preparation and administration.
- Protective cross-reactivity and paraspecific coverage of North American coral snake (excluding the Sonoran coral snake) envenomation has been demonstrated with the following antivenoms:
  - Coralmyn®, polyvalent anti-coral fabotherapic (F(ab')2 equine origin); Instituto Bioclon, Mexico.
  - Anti-coral (elapid) antivenin (IgG equine origin), Costa Rican coral snake antivenin; Instituto Clodomiro Picado, Costa Rica.
  - Australian tiger snake (*Notechis scutatus*) antivenin; CSL Limited, Parkville, Victoria, Australia.

■ **Crotalid antivenom (pit vipers).**
  - Antivenoms listed below provide coverage for all North American pit vipers (Crotalinae: rattlesnakes, copperheads, cottonmouths). All three snake antivenoms specific for veterinary use have been shown to be therapeutically effective. The particular use of any one of the three products may depend on the timely availability of a given product, the patient's medical history (prior exposures/allergic reactions, age, other pathologies), cost differences, and DVM prior experience with use of a given antivenom.
  - Consideration should be given to total fluid volume and animal size when administering any antivenom, particularly in smaller patients.
  - Specific USDA veterinary-approved products available in the USA:
    - Antivenin – (Crotalidae) polyvalent (equine origin) – IgG.
      - Boehringer-Ingelheim, Ridgefield, CT.
      - Canine indication.
      - Dose varies from 1 to 5 vials IV depending on severity of signs.
      - 95% of cases controlled with a single vial.
      - Lyophilized product that requires reconstitution.
    - VenomVet™ Antivenin Polyvalent Crotalidae (F(ab')$_2$, Equine origin) Injectable Solution.
      - MT Venom, LLC, Canoga Park, CA.
      - Species indication not specified.
      - No reconstitution necessary but does require further dilution.
      - Dose 1–2 vials.
    - Rattler Antivenin™ – Antivenin Crotalidae Polyvalent, Equine Origin.
      - Mg Biologics, Ames, IA.
      - Canine and equine indication.
      - Liquid plasma preparation (50 mL IV bag).
      - One or two doses (50–100 mL) are typically adequate.
  - Alternative antivenoms (human) – exact dose not precisely determined for veterinary use:
    - CroFab® Crotalidae polyvalent immune Fab (ovine).
      - BTG International Inc., West Conshohocken, PA.
      - Supplied as a carton of two vials.

- ○ Anavip® – Crotalidae immune (Fab')$_2$: (equine).
    - ◇ Instituto Bioclon, Mexico.
    - ◇ Maintained by multiple hospitals and zoos in United States.
- ■ **Black widow spider antivenom.**
    - • This antivenom is the definitive antidote. It should be reserved for high-risk patients (pediatric, geriatric, metabolically compromised). In one case report, a cat was treated with antivenom 26 hours after becoming clinically compromised and quickly recovered neurological function.
    - • Lycovac antivenin black widow spider (human antivenin, equine origin); Merck, West Point, PA.
        - ○ One vial mixed with 100 mL crystalloid solution given IV slowly with monitoring of the ventral ear pinna for evidence of hyperemia (an indicator of allergic response).
        - ○ One dose is usually sufficient, with a response occurring within 30 minutes.
        - ○ With proper use, reactions are rare. If an adverse reaction occurs, stop antivenin and administer diphenhydramine (2–4 mg/kg IM, lower dose in cats). Wait 5–10 minutes and restart the antivenom at a slower rate.
    - • A second antivenom (Aracmyn®, Instituto Bioclon, Mexico) has completed human trials and is scheduled to be submitted to the FDA for approval in the first quarter of 2023.
        - ○ This is an equine-origin Fab2 antivenin product and may be less likely to trigger an allergic reaction.
- ■ **Scorpion antivenom.**
    - • Anascorp® (*Centruroides* [F(ab')$_2$]; equine origin) antivenin; Instituto Bioclon, Mexico.

## Chelating Agents

- ■ These antidotes are generally used to remove heavy metals from the body. The chelating agent combines with a metal ion to form a complex that is then excreted.
- ■ **Calcium disodium ethylenediaminetetraacetic acid or CaNa$_2$EDTA** (Calcium Disodium Versenate, Bausch Health, others).
    - • Calcium disodium EDTA and *not* disodium EDTA must be used. These two should not be confused.
    - • Labeled for use in pediatric and adult humans with acute and chronic lead poisoning. The use has declined over the years due to side-effects and decreased incidence of lead toxicosis in human beings.
    - • Still widely used in veterinary medicine to chelate lead, zinc, inorganic mercury, and perhaps cadmium, particularly in birds.
    - • Should not be used while lead remains in the GIT as it may enhance the systemic absorption of lead.
    - • Should be used in conjunction with dimercaprol to increase lead excretion and prevent acute neurological signs.
    - • Dose (dogs and cats):
        - ○ Dilute product in 5% dextrose to a final concentration of 2–4 mg/mL prior to use.
        - ○ 25 mg/kg IV or SQ q 6 hours.
        - ○ Maximum recommended daily dose of 2 g/day.
        - ○ Treat for 5 days; rest for 5–7 days; and repeat if needed.
    - • IM injection is painful and not recommended.
    - • Causes GI signs and is very nephrotoxic so care needs to be taken to ensure hydration; should not be used in animals with chronic renal failure.

- **D-penicillamine** (Cuprimine®, Bausch Health; Depen®, Meda Pharmaceuticals).
  - Labeled for use in humans for copper overload.
  - Used in veterinary medicine for acute cadmium, inorganic mercury, lead, and zinc toxicosis, and with chronic copper toxicosis in dogs with inherited copper storage disease.
  - May cause vomiting and depression.
  - Often difficult to obtain and may be expensive, depending on source.
  - Dose (dogs) for at-home therapy after CaNa$_2$EDTA lead treatment: 110 mg/kg/day divided, PO q 6–8 hours for 1–2 weeks.
  - Dose (cats) for at-home therapy after CaNa$_2$EDTA lead treatment and in the presence of elevated blood levels: 125 mg *total* dose, PO q 12 hours for 5 days.
  - Dose (dogs and cats) for copper-associated hepatopathy: 7–15 mg/kg q 12 hours. Give one hour before feeding.
- **Deferoxamine** (Desferal®, Novartis Pharmaceutical Corporation).
  - Labeled in human beings for the treatment of acute iron intoxication and chronic iron overload due to transfusion-dependent anemia.
  - Contraindicated in patients with severe renal disease or anuria and those with high circulating levels of aluminum.
  - Complexes with iron; deferoxamine chelated complex is water soluble and excreted primarily in urine.
  - Dose (dogs and cats): 40 mg/kg IM q 4–8 hours. In critical situations, an IV infusion of 15 mg/kg/h can be used, but the cardiovascular system must be monitored closely during this time. The excreted complex turns the urine pink or salmon colored and is sometimes referred to as the "vin rosé" of iron poisoning. Continue treatment until the urine is clear or serum iron levels are within normal limits.
  - Deferoxamine is most effective if used within the first 24 hours while iron is still in circulation and has not been distributed to tissues.
  - Ascorbic acid: 10–15 mg/kg IM, IV, SQ, PO q 4–6 hours can be used in acute situations *after* all iron has been removed from the GIT to increase the efficacy of deferoxamine but should be used cautiously in chronic iron poisoning as it can cause adverse cardiac effects.
- **Dimercaprol** (BAL in oil, Taylor).
  - Labeled in human beings for use in the treatment of arsenic, gold, and mercury poisoning. Can also be used in acute lead poisoning concomitantly with CaNa$_2$EDTA and for treatment of high copper levels in those animals with copper storage disease.
  - Complex is water soluble and excreted in urine.
  - Dose (dogs and cats):
    - For arsenic toxicosis: 5 mg/kg IM × one dose followed by 2.5 mg/kg IM q 4 hours for 2 days, q 8 hours for 1 day, and q 12 hours until recovered.
    - For lead toxicosis: 2.5–5 mg/kg IM as 10% solution q 4 hours on days 1 and 2, then q 6 hours on day 3.
  - IM injections are painful (peanut oil carrier) and should only be given deep IM.
  - Dimercaprol is nephrotoxic so limit use and monitor BUN and creatinine. Be sure patients are adequately hydrated while product is used.
- **Dimercaptosuccinic acid** (also referred to as DMSA or succimer; Chemet®, Kremer Urban Pharmaceuticals).
  - Labeled for use in pediatric humans for lead poisoning when the blood levels are >45 mcg/mL. Unlabeled use includes mercury and arsenic toxicosis. It has not been shown to be effective for iron poisoning.
  - Used in veterinary medicine for lead or zinc toxicosis.

- Advantages over other chelators:
  - Can be given PO or rectally if GI signs are severe.
  - Incidence of adverse GI signs is much lower.
  - Can be used while lead is still present in the GIT.
  - Has less of an effect on systemic zinc concentrations.
- Disadvantages:
  - Cost – expensive.
  - Availability – often difficult to find.
  - Postchelation lead level rebound can occur.
  - May have a transient increase in AST and ALT.
  - Anecdotal reports of renal failure in cats.
- Dose (dogs and cats): 10 mg/kg PO or rectal q 8 hours × 10 days; retreat only if clinical signs are present.

■ **Trientine** (also known as TETA or 2,2,2 tetramine; Syprine®, Bausch Health).
  - Labeled for use in humans with copper toxicity who cannot tolerate succimer.
  - Used in veterinary medicine as an oral copper chelator in the treatment of copper-associated hepatopathies in dogs.
  - Advantages:
    - Fewer adverse reactions, especially vomiting.
  - Disadvantages:
    - Limited veterinary experience.
    - More expensive than d-penicillamine.
    - Not readily available; need to compound smaller doses.
    - Cannot open capsules to sprinkle on food as topical exposure results in dermatitis.
    - Also chelates zinc, iron, and other minerals so may need to supplement while treating.
    - Possibility of acute kidney injury.
  - Dose (dog):
    - 10–15 mg/kg PO 1–2 hours before meals.
    - 5–7 mg/kg PO BID 1–2 hours before meals (used in dogs with very high copper levels; helps avoid acute kidney injury).

## Others

■ **Digoxin immune Fab fragments** (Digibind®, ovine, Glaxo Smith Kline) and (Digifab®, bovine, BTG Pharmaceuticals).
  - Specific antidote used for digoxin toxicosis. It may also protect from poisoning associated with *Rhinella marina* (*Bufo*) toads and many cardiac glycoside-containing plants, especially foxglove and oleander. See Chapters 68 and 112.
  - Fab fragments should be reserved for the treatment of life-threatening cardiac arrhythmias that do not respond to conventional antiarrhythmic therapy.
  - They are expensive and will likely have to be obtained from a human hospital.
  - Dose depends on the amount ingested and serum digoxin level.
    - If a serum digoxin level is available:
      - ◇ Number of vials = serum digoxin level (ng/mL) × BW (kg)/100.
    - If a serum digoxin level is not available or if treating a *Rhinella marina* (*Bufo*) toad or cardiac glycoside-containing plant toxicosis, start therapy with 1–2 vials and reassess as needed.
■ **Protamine sulfate** (generic, various).
  - Complexes with heparin to form an inactive salt.
  - Useful in heparin overdoses when life-threatening bleeding occurs.

- Rapid onset of action – binding begins 5 minutes after IV administration.
- Dose (dogs and cats):
  - 1 mg protamine sulfate IV per 100 units heparin to be inactivated.
  - Give slowly, no faster than 50 mg per over 10 minutes.
  - Decrease amount of protamine sulfate by 50% for every 30–60 minutes that has passed since heparin overdose given.

## Functional Antidotes

- **Bisphosphonates** (pamidronate – Aredia®; Novartis; zoledronate – Zometa, Novartis; several others).
  - Used as the current antidote for vitamin $D_3$ (cholecalciferol) toxicosis, including cholecalciferol rodenticides and calcipotriene, a human prescription medication for psoriasis.
  - Bisphosphonates are a group of compounds that lower serum calcium levels by binding to hydroxyapatite crystals in the bone.
  - They are expensive and generally must be obtained from a human hospital or drug warehouse.
  - Due to the poor prognosis with hypercalcemia and secondary mineralization, use, despite the cost, is highly recommended early in the treatment of hypercalcemia.
  - Pamidronate dose (dogs and cats):
    - 1.3–2 mg/kg diluted in 250–500 mL 0.9% NaCl, IV slowly over several hours.
    - Monitor serum calcium levels every 12–24 hours and adjust ancillary treatment as needed. If hypercalcemia is still present, a repeated dose of pamidronate may be necessary 3–7 days after the initial dose.
  - Zoledronate (dogs):
    - Dogs: 0.25 mg/kg BW dissolved in 50 mL of 0.9% NaCl as a 15-minute IV constant rate infusion.
    - Dose has not been well established in veterinary medicine and it is possible that other doses may be effective.
- **Cyproheptadine** (various manufacturers).
  - Used for the treatment of serotonin syndrome (e.g., excitation or depression, vocalization, ataxia, hyperthermia, seizures, tremors, vomiting, diarrhea) associated with ingestions of baclofen, SSRIs, and other medications.
  - Antihistamine with serotonin antagonistic properties.
    - Dose (dogs): 1.1 mg/kg PO or rectally q 1–6 hours PRN.
    - Dose (cats): 2–4 mg *total* dose PO or rectally q 4–8 hours PRN.
- **Intravenous lipid emulsion (ILE)** (Intralipid®, Baxter; Liposyn®, Hospira; Medialipide®, Braun).
  - Available in 10% and 20% emulsions.
  - Composed of medium- to long-chain triglycerides derived from plant oils (safflower oil, soybean oil), egg phosphatides, and glycerin.
    - Clinolipid® (Baxter) is somewhat different as it contains olive oil and soybean oil in addition to egg phosphatides.
  - ILE has been used successfully in veterinary medicine to treat toxicosis associated with lipid-soluble drugs such as baclofen, beta-receptor antagonists, calcium channel blockers, lidocaine, loperamide, ivermectin, moxidectin, marijuana, minoxidil, nonsteroidal anti-inflammatory drugs (NSAIDS), permethrin, phenobarbital, synthetic cannabinoids, and tremorgenic mycotoxins as well as ingestion of the toxic plant *Pieris japonica*. Use with other substances such as bromethalin has been more controversial.
  - Other lipid-soluble drugs such as anticonvulsants may be affected by ILE and this needs to be considered when choosing those medications.

- The exact mechanism of how ILE works is unknown, but possible mechanisms include the following:
  - ILE may create a "lipid shuttle" where the body moves toxins to storage tissues like fat and skeletal muscle or to the liver for metabolism or the kidney for elimination.
  - ILE may create a "pharmacological sink" for fat-soluble drugs. In this mechanism, ILE forms a lipid phase into which free drug passes, thereby lowering the tissue drug concentration.
  - ILE may increase intracellular calcium via direct activation of voltage-gated calcium channels. This may restore myocyte function in the drug-depressed myocardium.
  - ILE may provide an additional fatty acid supply to improve cardiac performance or support the myocardial cells by some other method.
- Adverse effects of ILE are infrequent in veterinary medicine. Reported effects in humans include hyperlipidemia, hepatosplenomegaly, jaundice, seizures, hemolytic anemia, prolonged clotting time, thrombocytopenia, and fat embolism.
- Several different treatment suggestions exist.
  - Suggested protocol.
    - ◇ 1.5–4 mL/kg IV bolus of 20% ILE over 1 minute, followed by CRI of 0.25 mL/kg/minute over 30–60 minutes.
    - ◇ Individual boluses of 20% ILE may be repeated as needed up to 7 mL/kg.
  - "Standard" or alternate protocol based on human use.
    - ◇ 1.5 mL/kg IV bolus of 20% ILE over 5–15 minutes, followed immediately with CRI of 0.25 mL/kg/min over 1–2 hours.
    - ◇ May repeat dose in several hours if signs of toxicosis return.

- **Phytonadione** (generic, various manufacturers).
  - Used primarily for the treatment of anticoagulant rodenticide and digoxin toxicity.
  - Analog of systemic vitamin $K_1$, which is required for the synthesis of clotting factors II, VII, IX, and X.
  - Dosing information:
    - 2–5 mg/kg PO every 24 hours or divided twice a day.
    - SQ or IM dosing can be used if need be; IM injection may cause injection site bleeding, especially early in therapy. IV administration is not recommended due to incidence of anaphylactoid reactions.
- **Skeletal muscle relaxants.**
  - **Methocarbamol** (generic, various manufacturers).
    - Used for the treatment of tremors associated with pyrethrins and pyrethroids, tremorgenic mycotoxins, strychnine, and CNS stimulant toxicosis.
    - Central-acting skeletal muscle relaxant.
    - Dose:
      - ◇ Dogs: 55–220 mg/kg slow IV. Labeled not to exceed 330 mg/kg/day but higher doses may be used in severe poisonings if the dog is monitored for CNS and respiratory depression.
      - ◇ Cats: 44 mg/kg slow IV, up to 330 mg/kg/day. Labeled not to exceed 330 mg/kg/day but higher doses may be needed in severe poisonings. Monitor for CNS and respiratory depression when using high doses.
  - **Dantrolene** (Dantrium®, Par Pharmaceuticals; some generics).
    - Used for the treatment of malignant hyperthermia reactions associated with hops (*Humulus lupulus*) or as an adjunct therapy for black widow spider bites.
    - Direct-acting skeletal muscle relaxant.

- o Dose (dogs):
  - ◇ Black widow spider bites: 1 mg/kg IV followed by 1 mg/kg PO q 4 hours as needed.
  - ◇ Hops toxicosis: 2–3 mg/kg IV or 3.5 mg/kg PO.

## Pharmacological or Physiological Antidotes

- ■ Atipamezole, yohimbine, tolazoline.
  - • **Atipamezole** (Antisedan®, Pfizer) is an alpha-2-adrenergic antagonist labeled for reversal of medetomidine and dexmedetomidine. It is used off-label to reverse other alpha-2-adrenergic agonists, including amitraz, clonidine, and xylazine. The half-life is short (2–3 hours) and the drug may need to be repeated if used to reverse longer acting agonists.
    - o Dose (dogs): 50–100 mcg/kg IM.
    - o Dose (cats): 25–50 mcg/kg IM or IV (slow).
    - o Atipamezole has been used anecdotally in dogs by the intranasal route to reverse the effects of xylazine. In one small xylazine study reversal occurred rapidly with few, if any, side-effects.
  - • **Tolazoline** (Tolazine®, Akorn) is an alpha-2-adrenergic antagonist. It is used off-label primarily to reverse xylazine. The effects may be partial and transient and it is rarely used in small animal medicine.
    - o Dose (dogs and cats): 2–4 mg/kg IV (slow).
  - • **Yohimbine** (Yobine®, Lloyd) is an alpha-2-adrenergic antagonist indicated to reverse the effects of xylazine. The half-life is short (1.5–2 hours) and the drug will likely need to be repeated if used to reverse longer acting agonists. Yohimbine has more side-effects at lower doses than atipamezole, including CNS excitation, tremors, and hypersalivation.
    - o Dose (dogs and cats): 0.11 mg/kg IV slowly.
    - o Dose for amitraz toxicity: 0.1 mg/kg IV or 0.25 mg/kg IM.
- ■ Atropine (various manufacturers).
  - • Antimuscarinic agent used for treatment of SLUDGE (salivation, lacrimation, urination, defecation, and gastroenteritis) that accompanies organophosphate (OP) and carbamate insecticide toxicity.
  - • Competes with acetylcholine at the postganglionic parasympathetic sites.
  - • Dose (dogs and cats): 0.2–2 mg/kg. One quarter of the dose should be given IV and the remainder IM or SQ. The dose will likely need to be repeated; heart rate and secretions should be used to guide redosing.
  - • It is important that enough atropine be provided, especially in large overdoses of OP or carbamates. Without adequate therapy for OP toxicosis, patients may drown in their own secretions.
- ■ Ethanol (various manufacturers).
  - • Used as a second-line treatment for ethylene glycol toxicosis. Fomepizole is the preferred treatment.
  - • The mechanism of action is like fomepizole (inhibits alcohol dehydrogenase), but side-effects including CNS depression, metabolic acidosis, and hyperosmolality limit the use.
  - • Many different IV treatment recommendations have been made.
    - o Preferred method: using 7% ethanol (70 mg/mL), load with 8.6 mL/kg (600 mg/kg) slow IV × 1 dose and follow with 1.43 mL/kg/h (100 mg/kg/h) IV CRI for 24–36 hours or until ethylene glycol (EG) test results are negative.
    - o Other methods can be used depending on source and concentration of ethanol source.

&#x25C7; 5.5 mL/kg IV of a 20% ethanol solution every 4 hours × 5 doses; follow with 5.5 mL/kg every 6 hours for 4 more doses *OR*

&#x25C7; CRI at 5.5 mL/kg/h of 5% ethanol solution until EG test is negative *OR*

&#x25C7; 12 mL/kg IV of 5% ethanol solution slow IV followed by 2 mL/kg/h as CRI until EG test is negative.

- **Fomepizole** or 4-MP (Antizol-Vet®, Paladin Labs).
  - Indicated as the specific antidote for animals with ethylene glycol (EG) toxicosis.
  - 4-MP is a competitive inhibitor of alcohol dehydrogenase. The mechanism of action is like ethanol, as it prevents the conversion of EG to toxic metabolites. Unlike ethanol, fomepizole does not result in CNS depression, metabolic acidosis, or hyperosmolality.
  - Labeled for use in dogs, extra-label in cats.
    - Dogs: May be treated as late as 8 hours after ingestion and still survive.
    - Cats: Must be treated *within 3 hours* after ingestion. Cats treated greater than 4 hours after ingestion have a reported mortality rate of 100%.
  - Dose (dogs):
    - 20 mg/kg IV over 15–20 minutes as loading dose; then
    - 15 mg/kg IV at 12 and 24 hours; then
    - 5 mg/kg IV at 36 hours. Repeat EG test.
    - If EG tests remains positive, continue 5 mg/kg IV every 12 hours until negative.
  - Dose (cats):
    - 125 mg/kg slow IV as a loading dose; then
    - 31.25 mg/kg IV at 12, 24, and 36 hours.
- **Flumazenil** (Romazicon®, Anexate®, others).
  - Reversal agent for benzodiazepine (diazepam, midazolam, others) overdoses with marked CNS and respiratory depression that are nonresponsive to conventional therapy.
  - Competitive antagonist at the benzodiazepine receptor site.
  - Use needs to be carefully balanced against the side-effects – lowering of seizure threshold, vomiting, and ataxia.
  - The duration of action is very short (1–2 hours) and often needs to be repeated, especially when longer acting benzodiazepines have been ingested.
  - Dose (dog and cat): 0.01 – 0.2 mg/kg IV, begin with lower amount and increase as needed.
- **Leucovorin** (generic, various manufacturers).
  - Calcium salt of folinic acid used for toxicity associated with folic acid antagonists (methotrexate, pyrimethamine, trimethoprim, ormetoprim).
  - Reduced form of folic acid that does not require conversion by dihydrofolate reductase to become biologically active.
  - Dose (dogs and cats):
    - Pyrimethamine, trimethoprim, ormetoprim: 0.1–0.3 mg/kg PO every 24 hours.
    - Methotrexate: varies depending on methotrexate serum concentrations (25–200 mg/m² IV, IM every 6 hours for up to 8 doses).
- **Methylene blue** (generic, various).
  - Infrequently used to treat methemoglobinemia formed secondary to oxidative agents such as hydroxyurea, nitrates, phenols, naphthalene (moth balls), and phenazopyridine.
  - Use with extreme caution or not at all in cats.
  - Dog dose: 1–1.5 mg/kg as 1% solution IV over several minutes; may be repeated but use with caution as Heinz body anemia may develop.

■ **N-acetylcysteine** (Acetadote®, Cumberland).
- Acetylcysteine (NAC) is used to prevent hepatic necrosis that occurs secondary to acetaminophen toxicosis. It is most effective when used within 8 hours of exposure and should be used within 24 hours to be of value.
- It has also been used successfully as a liver protectant for other hepatotoxins and poisonings, including *Amanita* mushroom, xylitol, and sago palm toxicosis.
- NAC is a sulfhydryl compound that acts to increase glutathione synthesis in the liver, providing an alternate substrate for conjugation of acetaminophen metabolites and restoring glutathione levels.
- Dose (dog and cat): 140 mg/kg IV or PO × 1 dose, then 70 mg/kg IV or PO q 6 hours for 7 doses.
- Specifics of use:
  ○ Dilute to a 5% solution prior to use.
  ○ IV administration is preferred in cats due to low oral bioavailability (20%).
  ○ Other doses have been suggested, most based on extrapolation from human literature. Some recommend higher doses (280 mg/kg) and others additional doses (up to 17 doses) for massive ingestions.
  ○ Emesis frequently occurs with oral dosing, especially after the initial dose, and an antiemetic may be required prior to starting NAC therapy.
■ **Naloxone** (Narcan® and Narcan® Nasal Spray, Emergent BioSolutions; generics).
- Used for the reversal of CNS and respiratory depression associated with opiate and opioid intoxication.
- Pure mu opioid antagonist with no analgesic activity.
- Effectively reverses mu opiate and opioid agonist activity for drugs such as fentanyl and morphine.
- Will not reverse respiratory depression associated with buprenorphine and likely not in butorphanol, pentazocine, and nalbuphine.
- Rapid onset of action (1–5 minutes) and short duration of action (approximately 90 minutes). The dose will generally have to be repeated, especially with longer acting opioids.
- Dose of injectable product (dogs and cats): 0.01–0.04 mg/kg, IV, IM, SQ; may need to use 0.04 mg/kg with larger overdoses; some recommend up to 0.2mg/kg.
  ○ IM and SQ route result in slower onset of action (5 minutes).
- Dose of intranasal spray (dogs): 4 mg total dose from a fixed-dose human product.
  ○ Rapid onset, about 2 minutes.
  ○ No adverse reactions noted in initial study.
■ **Pralidoxime** (2-PAM or protopam chloride, Baxter Healthcare; generics).
- Pralidoxime is used in organophosphate (OP) toxicosis to reactivate cholinesterase enzymes inactivated by the insecticide. It binds to the enzyme, attaches to the OP, and forms a pralidoxime–OP complex that detaches (reactivating the enzyme) and is excreted.
- Helps prevent nicotinic signs and should be used in conjunction with atropine.
- Limited benefits with carbamate toxicosis.
- Generally, pralidoxime should be used within 24 hours of exposure, but may still be effective when given at 36–48 hours.
- There is some evidence that it is also effective when used for treatment of the intermediate syndrome of OP toxicosis.
- Dose (dogs and cats): 20 mg/kg IM or slow IV (over 30 minutes) for first dose. Repeat dose q 6–12 hours, IM or SQ.
- If there is no response after three doses the drug should be discontinued.

- • Rapid IV administration has resulted in tachycardia, neuromuscular blockade, laryngospasm, muscle rigidity, and death.
- ■ **Pyridostigmine** (Mestinon®, Bausch; generics).
  - • Anticholinesterase that directly competes with acetylcholine for attachment to acetylcholinesterase enzyme.
  - • Longer t1/2 (half-life) than other similar drugs.
  - • Rarely used in veterinary medicine for poisonings, but may be effective against a wide variety of overdoses including those from anticholinergic plants (*Cestrum* spp., *Datura* spp.), atropine, ivermectin, some Elapid snake bites, and curare and pancuronium.
  - • Dose 0.01–0.03 mg/kg/h CRI.
- ■ **Pyridoxine** (generic, various manufacturers).
  - • Infrequently used for isoniazid toxicosis in dogs (extra-label use).
  - • Converted in RBCs to pyridoxal phosphate and pyridoxamine.
  - • Enhances excretion.
  - • Dose: 71 mg/kg as 5–10% infusion over 30–60 minutes; if total amount of isoniazid ingested by the animal has been reported, administer on a mg per mg (1:1) basis.
  - • Also used as additional treatment of seizures from hydrazine mushroom (Gyromita spp.) toxicosis (75–150 mg/kg IV).

 **COMMENTS**

- ■ Antidotes, in and of themselves, are not free of side-effects and should never be used indiscriminately. Each case needs to be evaluated on an individual basis and the antidote used with knowledge and forethought.
- ■ Many toxicants lack a true antidote, and symptomatic and supportive care is imperative for survival of the poisoned patient. Refer to Chapter 2, Emergency Management of the Poisoned Patient, for more information on specific supportive care and treatment.
- ■ Many other useful drugs are not mentioned in this chapter, and the reader is directed to the references below for further information.

### Abbreviations

See Appendix 1 for complete list.

### Suggested Reading

Chacko B, Peter JV. Antidotes in poisoning. *Indian J Crit Care Med* 2019;23 (S4):S241–269.

Connally HE, Thrall MA, Hamar DW. Safety and efficacy of high dose fomepizole compared with ethanol as therapy for ethylene glycol intoxication in cats. *J Vet Emerg Crit Care* 2010;20(2):191–206.

Dalefield RR, Oehme F. Antidotes for specific poisons. In: Peterson ME, Talcott PA (eds) *Small Animal Toxicology*, 2nd edn. St Louis: Elsevier, 2006; pp. 459–474.

Fernandez AL, Lee JA, Rahilly L et al. The use of intravenous lipid emulsion as an antidote in veterinary toxicology. *J Vet Emerg Crit Care* 2011;21(4):309–320.

Focken A, Loewen J, Woodsworth J. Evaluating the use of intranasal atipamezole to reverse the sedative effects of xylazine in dogs. *J Vet Emerg Crit Care* 2021;31:S2–S41.

Gerhard C, Jaffey HA. Persistent increase in serum 25-hydroxyvitamin D concentration in a dog following cholecalciferol intoxication. *Front Vet Sci* 2020;6:472.

Gwaltney-Brant S, Meadows I. Intravenous lipid emulsions in veterinary clinical toxicology. *Vet Clin North Am Small Anim Pract* 2018;48(6):265–268.

Heggem-Perry B, McMichael M, O'Brien M et al. Intravenous lipid emulsion therapy for bromethalin toxicity in a dog. *J Am Amim Hosp Assoc* 2016;52(4):265–268.

Khan SA. Common reversal agents/antidotes in small animal poisoning. *Vet Clin North Am Small Anim Pract* 2018;48(6):1081–1085.

Martin-Jimenez T, de Lorimier L, Fan T, Freise J. Pharmacokinetics and pharmacodynamics of a single dose of zoledronate in healthy dogs. *J Vet Pharmacol Ther* 2017;30:492–495.

Pao-Franco A, Hammond N, Weatherton LK et al. Successful use of digoxin-specific immune Fab in the treatment of severe Nerium oleander toxicosis in a dog. *J Vet Emerg Crit Care* 2017;27(5):596–604.

Plumb DC. *Plumb's Veterinary Drug Handbook*, 9th edn. Ames: Blackwell, 2018.

Wahler BM, Lerche P, Pereira CH et al. Pharmacokinetics and pharmacodynamics of intranasal and intravenous naloxone hydrochloride administration in healthy dogs. *Am J Vet Res* 2019;80(7):696–701.

Wismer T. Antidotes. In: Poppenga RH, Gwaltney-Brant S (eds) *Small Animal Toxicology Essentials*. Chichester: Wiley-Blackwell, 2011; pp. 57–70.

**Author**: Lynn R. Hovda, RPh, DVM, MS, DACVIM
**Consulting Editor**: Lynn R. Hovda, RPh, DVM, MS, DACVIM

# Chapter 4

# Identification and Management of the Unknown Toxicant

## DEFINITION/OVERVIEW

- Animals are often presented to the veterinarian with a variety of clinical signs and a complaint by the owner that the animal was "poisoned."
- In reality, the incidence of true poisoning in animals is low. Other processes such as infectious or metabolic diseases, neoplasia, and trauma need to be considered when working through these cases.
- The age-old adage "treat the patient, not the poison" is still the basis of sound veterinary medicine in these cases.
- Obtaining an accurate and complete history is a diagnostic cornerstone and should not be overlooked, even if the animal has life-threatening signs.
- Stabilizing the animal and providing emergency care (see Chapter 2) should be undertaken immediately. If possible, a history should be taken simultaneously by an assistant.
- This, coupled with the physical examination findings, may help determine if a poisoning has occurred as well as suggesting what specific toxicant may have been involved.

## PERTINENT INFORMATION

### History

- Well-planned written protocols should be used to ensure that no details are omitted.
- These should contain, at the very least, client information (i.e., owner, address, contact information); patient information, including species, breed, age, and weight plus any known medical conditions and medications and/or supplements taken, and a brief history of known or potential exposures.
  - Most animal owners are forthcoming with this information; however, this may not always be the case when illicit substances are involved.
- Many owners do not know or do not remember their animal's history and only with careful questioning will this information come to light.
- When questioning owners about known or potential toxicant exposures, it is helpful to be as specific as possible since owners might not be aware of the toxicity of many chemicals, foods, medications, plants, or other natural products.
  - Specific questioning can be facilitated if target organs can be identified and species sensitivities considered. For example, if an animal presents with acute kidney injury, the owners can be asked specifically about possible exposure to ethylene glycol (dogs and cats), grapes/raisins (dogs), or lilies (cats).

*Blackwell's Five-Minute Veterinary Consult Clinical Companion: Small Animal Toxicology*, Third Edition.
Edited by Lynn R. Hovda, Ahna G. Brutlag, Robert H. Poppenga, and Steven E. Epstein.
© 2024 John Wiley & Sons, Inc. Published 2024 by John Wiley & Sons, Inc.

- In addition to baseline information, other animal specific information should be obtained.
  - This may include reproductive status, vaccination history, housing (indoors or outdoors, garage or basement, etc.), environment (city, lake, farm, free roaming, or fenced in yard), any recent travel to an atypical location for the pet, and exposure to other animals.
  - A history of clinical signs should be established, including the estimated time the animal was last observed as "normal," when the clinical signs were first noted, and the progression of signs (worse, better, same).
- Any first aid provided by the owner, such as inducing emesis or bathing the animal, should also be noted as this may have complicated the situation. For example, some pet owners may have administered "home remedies" such as milk, egg whites, table salt, hydrogen peroxide, or charcoal capsules if they think that their pet has been poisoned.

## Physical Examination

- A complete physical examination should be performed, paying particular attention to the cardiovascular, neurological, and respiratory systems.
- Any animal with life-threatening signs should receive immediate emergency care (see Chapter 2) and the physical examination should be completed when the animal is stabilized.
- Superficial physical assessment for toxicant-induced changes should include the color of the skin and mucous membranes; presence of petechiation or ecchymoses; distinctive colors, odors or substances on the breath or body (e.g., garlic or rotten fish smell is suggestive of zinc phosphide); evidence of foreign substances on hair coat (i.e. blue-green algae, solvents, essential oils, ticks, etc.); and evidence of bites or stings (common on the face/neck or front legs/feet).
- The animal should be examined for any signs of trauma, such as hit by a car, or self-inflicted due to a neurological or dermal problem.
- Ocular examination may also be important. Pupil size and response to light should be noted, as well as irritation to the cornea or conjunctiva.

 # DIAGNOSTICS

- Baseline laboratory testing should include blood glucose concentration, a CBC, serum biochemistries, and a urinalysis with a urine specific gravity.
- If possible, stomach contents (from spontaneous or induced emesis or initial gastric lavage fluid), whole blood, serum, and urine should be saved for further testing.
  - In general, obtaining as much sample as possible for testing is desirable since the degree of testing required might be unknown.
  - All samples for toxicological testing can be refrigerated initially and frozen if to be stored for more than one or two days.
- A coagulation panel should be added if hemorrhage occurs easily or if petechiae or ecchymoses were present on physical examination.
- Blood gas analysis and pulse oximetry are required for compromised respiratory systems.
- Urinalysis may include point-of-care tests for common illicit drugs and amanita mushrooms, or presence of crystalluria.
- Other laboratory diagnostics should be ordered as needed based on clinical signs consistent with various intoxications and could include specifics such as carboxyhemoglobin concentration (carbon monoxide poisoning), cholinesterase activity (organophosphate or carbamate poisoning) or individual drug/chemical concentrations (e.g., aspirin, acetaminophen, ethanol, ethylene glycol, iron, etc.).

- Further diagnostics are performed based on the history and physical examination findings.
  - Evaluation of the body temperature is part of a routine physical examination but should be repeated often as some toxicants cause severe hyperthermia (e.g., aspirin, hops, tremorgenic mycotoxins, metaldehyde).
  - Abnormalities noted on cardiac auscultation should be evaluated with an ECG.
  - Radiographic imaging is useful to rule out radiopaque foreign objects or material.

## TOXIDROMES

- Toxidromes are recognizable syndromes resulting from particular toxicants or classes of toxicants.
- They consist of a group of clinical signs or characteristic effects which can aid a practitioner or toxicologist with diagnosis. Toxidromes are analogous to a group of clinical signs associated with certain medical conditions.
  - For example, a dog suffering from bloat or GDV typically exhibits a distended, tympanic abdomen, retching, unproductive vomiting, and hypersalivation.
  - Likewise, a dog presenting with hot, dry, flushed skin, mydriasis, tacky mucous membranes, tachycardia, urinary retention, and lethargy or disorientation might suggest exposure to a toxicant with anticholinergic effects (e.g., Jimson weed or atropine).
- Common toxidromes noted in veterinary toxicology include cholinergic, anticholinergic, sympathomimetic, and serotonin toxidromes.
- The opioid toxidrome is well described in people but, due to significant interspecies variability, the signs are not as reliably similar in veterinary species.

### Cholinergic Toxidrome

- The cholinergic toxidrome is produced by an overstimulation of muscarinic and nicotinic receptors by acetylcholine in the CNS, at neuromuscular junctions, and in the sympathetic and parasympathetic nervous systems. This typically occurs following the inhibition of acetylcholinesterase, the enzyme responsible for breaking down acetylcholine.
  - Acute muscarinic signs include excessive salivation, lacrimation, urination (dribbling), defecation, gastroenteropathy (i.e., SLUDGE), miosis, and coughing or dyspnea (excessive pulmonary excretions).
  - Acute nicotinic signs include muscle tremors (often starting with the head and progressing toward the tail), generalized muscle stiffness/tetany, weakness with potential paresis or paralysis.
- Agents resulting in this toxidrome include organophosphate and carbamate insecticides; muscarinic mushrooms (e.g., *Inocybe* spp., *Clitocybe* spp.); pharmaceuticals used to treat glaucoma, dry mouth, or increase bladder contractility (e.g., carbachol, pilocarpine, bethenachol); and cholinergic plants.
- Atropine is the antidote for muscarinic signs and extremely large doses may be required, especially in cases of severe poisoning (0.1–2.0 mg/kg, give ¼ dose IV, remainder SQ or IM, repeat every 1–2 hours until animal is stable and secretions are controlled).
- Nicotinic signs can be treated with pralidoxime chloride or "2-PAM" (20 mg/kg IV over 15–30 minutes or SQ q 12 hours). Pralidoxime usually needs to be administered within the first 24 hours to effectively treat acute signs. For more information on the treatment of the cholinergic toxidrome, see Chapter 101, Organophosphorus and Carbamate Insecticides.

## Anticholinergic Toxidrome

- The anticholinergic toxidrome is produced by the inhibition of cholinergic neurotransmission at muscarinic receptor sites in the parasympathetic nervous system.
- The common mnemonic used to describe the clinical signs associated with this toxidrome is:
  - **Mad as a hatter** (bizarre behavioral signs)
  - **Blind as a bat** (severe mydriasis which impairs visual focus)
  - **Dry as a bone** (blockade of cholinergic tone to salivary glands results in dry mouth, intense thirst, and difficulty swallowing)
  - **Red as a beet** (erythema, may be missed due to haircoat)
  - **Hot as a pistol** (hyperthermia).
- Additional acute clinical signs may include reduced GI motility, constipation, urinary retention, restlessness, and muscular twitching. These signs may progress to incoordination, paralysis, delirium, and respiratory paralysis.
- Atropine and glycopyrrolate are prototype anticholinergic agents.
  - Other agents resulting in this toxidrome include prescription and OTC anti-motion sickness agents (e.g., scopolamine patches, Dramamine® [dimenhydrinate], meclizine), drugs for overactive bladder syndrome (e.g., Detrol® [tolterodine]), antipsychotics, and many antihistamines (e.g., Benadryl® [diphenhydramine]).
  - There are also many plants with anticholinergic properties including *Datura* spp. (Jimson weed, angel's trumpet), *Atropa belladonna* (deadly nightshade), and *Convolvulus* spp. (bindweed).
- Unlike treatment for the cholinergic toxidrome, treatment for the anticholinergic toxidrome is more focused on supportive care such as IV fluids, diazepam, cooling measures, etc.
  - Physostigmine (canine dose: 1 mg total dose *per dog*, not mg/kg, q 12 hours IV or SQ), a parasympathomimetic drug which stimulates the parasympathetic nervous system, is available but should be reserved for cases where the patient exhibits either extreme agitation and is at risk of injuring itself or others, or where supraventricular tachycardia and sinus tachycardia are nonresponsive to traditional therapy.
  - Pyridostigmine does not readily penetrate into the CNS so is not recommended for use in this scenario.

## Sympathomimetic Toxidrome

- Sympathomimetic agents are stimulant compounds which mimic the effects of the neurotransmitters in the sympathetic nervous system (i.e., epinephrine, norepinephrine, dopamine, etc.).
  - These agents may have a direct effect on alpha- and beta-adrenergic receptors, or may act indirectly by causing the release of norepinephrine from presynaptic nerve endings and/or by preventing the metabolism or reuptake of norepinephrine by inhibiting norepinephrine transporter (NET) activity.
  - Furthermore, these agents may inhibit monoamine oxidase, an enzyme involved in the breakdown of catecholamines.
- Clinical signs associated with the sympathomimetic toxidrome include hypertension, restlessness/hyperactivity/agitation, tachycardia, and mydriasis.
  - Severe cases may display head bobbing, nausea/vomiting, tachydysrhythmias including supraventricular tachycardia and ventricular tachycardia.
  - Severe hypertension may also result in intracranial hemorrhage or renal insufficiency.
  - Reflex bradycardia due to significant hypertension is possible.
  - Prolonged agitation can lead to rhabdomyolysis and hyperthermia.
  - The beta-2 receptor-agonists (e.g., albuterol, clenbuterol) can cause significant electrolyte abnormalities, including severe hypokalemia.

- Unintentional pet exposure to sympathomimetic agents is frequently reported to Pet Poison Helpline, a 24/7 animal poison control center, because these drugs are often found in human OTC nasal decongestants (e.g., Bendaryl-D® and Clartin-D® contain phenylepherine and pseudoephedrine, respectively), weight loss agents, anabolic bodybuilding agents, aphrodisiacs, mood stimulants, and other "energy" supplements designed to promote wakefulness. They are also present in a variety of human and veterinary prescription products such as ADD/ADHD medications (e.g., amphetamines), bronchodilators, and phenylpropanolamine.
- There is no antidote for sympathomimetic agents although helpful baseline treatments include starting with sedation (e.g., acepromazine +/- butorphanol; if unsuccessful proceed to dexmedetomidine). Acepromazine often helps reduce hypertension. Other treatments such as injectable beta-blockers (e.g., esmolol) may be needed to treat tachycardia, and intravenous fluids to maintain perfusion.
  - Benzodiazepines are known to produce paradoxical excitation in these patients and are usually best avoided or used with caution until the clinician is comfortable with the patient's response.
- Vital signs, including blood pressure, must be monitored closely and an ECG should be used if arrhythmias are noted.
  - If hyperthermia develops, cooling measures are recommended but should be stopped once the body reaches 103.5 °F to avoid hypothermia.
- Electrolytes should be monitored closely for hypokalemia if the patient was exposed to a beta-agonist (e.g., dog biting into albuterol inhaler). For more information on specific toxicants and treatment, see chapters on amphetamines, beta-2-receptor agonists, chocolate and caffeine, cocaine, decongestants (pseudoephedrine, phenylephrine), phenylpropanolamine, ephedra (ma huang), and methamphetamine.

## Serotonin Toxidrome

- The serotonin toxidrome, often called serotonin syndrome or hyperactivity syndrome, is caused by overstimulation of postsynaptic serotonin receptors in the CNS.
- The main receptors responsible for serotonin syndrome are thought to be the 5-HT1A type, associated with hyperactivity, hyperreflexia, and anxiety, and the 5-HT2A type, associated with hyperthermia, incoordination, and neuromuscular excitement.
- There are at least four mechanisms by which excessive serotonin concentrations are likely to occur.
  - Decreasing serotonin breakdown (e.g., MAOIs).
  - Decreasing serotonin reuptake at presynaptic sites (e.g., SSRIs, SNRIs, TCAs, tramadol, fentanyl, cocaine, methadone, meperidine, St John's wort, amphetamines, dextromethorphan).
  - Increasing serotonin precursors or agonists (e.g., L-tryptophan, select antimigraine medications, LSD, buspirone).
  - Increasing serotonin release (e.g., amphetamines, cocaine, buspirone, lithium).
- Acute clinical signs associated with the serotonin toxidrome include agitation, vocalization, tremors, muscle rigidity, tachycardia, hypertension, and severe hyperthermia.
  - Other reported signs include abdominal pain, diarrhea, hypersalivation, increased reflexes, ataxia, myoclonus, shivering, increased respiratory rate, transient blindness, seizures, coma, and death.
- Treatment is primarily symptomatic and supportive.
  - Cyproheptadine, a serotonin antagonist, has been used with good results in animals displaying milder signs, especially vocalization (1.1 mg/kg for dog or 2–4 mg total dose per cat given orally or rectally q 4–6 hours until signs resolve).

- Levetiracetam and phenobarbital are preferred for treating seizures over benzodiazepines but either can be used.
- As with the treatment of sympathomimetics, benzodiazepines may cause paradoxical excitation so should be used cautiously until the practitioner can gauge the patient's response.
- Acepromazine can used for sedation; high doses may be needed.
- Other treatments include fluid therapy, blood pressure monitoring, ECG monitoring, and thermoregulation.

■ For more information, see chapters on atypical antipsychotics, club drugs (MDMA, GHB, flunitrazepam, bath salts), lysergic acid diethylamide (LSD), and SSRI and SNRI antidepressants.

## TREATMENT PLAN

### Consultation With Animal Poison Control Center

■ Consultation with an animal poison control center should be undertaken as soon as possible. Their experts, available 24/7, have a vast amount of knowledge and experience in sorting out clinical and historic findings, providing a rule-out list and treatment advice.

■ It is possible that the history and physical exam findings, coupled with laboratory values, may suggest a specific toxicant or toxidrome (see Toxidrome section).
- For instance, metabolic acidosis, an increased serum osmolality, and subsequent elevations in BUN and creatinine are associated with ethylene glycol intoxication, while early and severe hypoglycemia and subsequent elevations in liver enzymes are consistent with xylitol (dogs) or alpha-lipoic acid intoxication (cats or dogs).

### Decontamination

■ The primary goal of decontamination, whether it is ophthalmic, dermatological, respiratory, or gastrointestinal, is to slow or prevent further absorption of a toxicant (see Chapter 1).

■ Care should be taken to protect workers during decontamination as some toxicants such as blue-green algae, cholinesterase-inhibiting insecticides, or zinc phosphide (which creates phosphine gas) are harmful to humans.

■ Ophthalmic decontamination includes immediate lavage of the affected eye(s) for 15–20 minutes followed by a slit lamp examination to evaluate for damage.

■ Moving animals to fresh air or providing oxygen assists with respiratory decontamination.

■ Multiple baths with a mild, degreasing shampoo or liquid hand dishwashing detergent and tepid water followed by thorough rinsing are used to remove and prevent absorption of many dermal toxins.

■ Several factors should be considered prior to undertaking gastrointestinal decontamination.
- Important historical information includes the time since exposure, if emesis was induced at home, and whether there is any underlying medical condition that precludes decontamination (e.g., megaesophagus, seizure disorder, cardiac disease, etc.).
- Induction of emesis is generally not an appropriate form of decontamination to use with an unknown toxicant.
  o It is contraindicated in most symptomatic patients, especially if sedate or seizuring, those with a hydrocarbon odor (e.g., gasoline, kerosene, pesticides), or lesions in mouth or oropharynx (indicative of corrosive injury).
  o Prior spontaneous vomiting is also a relative contraindication.
- Gastric lavage is an effective form of GI decontamination, especially if the practitioner is skilled at doing so, but must be performed quickly following exposure with an inflated ETT in place. It allows for gastric emptying in sedate patients and the administration of activated charcoal (with or without a cathartic) or cholesytramine directly

into the stomach prior to removal of the tube. Activated charcoal is effective for many toxicants, provides rapid adsorption, and quickly moves into the small intestine where most toxicants are systemically absorbed.
- The clinician always needs to balance the use of gastric evacuation procedures (emetics or gastric lavage) with the consequent delay in administering activated charcoal or cholestyramine.

## Case Management

- Case management depends on the history and physical examination but even stable animals should have IV catheter placement for emergency access if needed and a TPR repeated frequently.
- Very few antidotes are available and they are generally useful only for specific toxicants (see Chapter 3).
- Treatments such as intralipid emulsion (ILE) or extracorporeal treatments (ECT) (see Chapter 1) may be helpful for a broader range of toxicants; however, these are not usually recommended as first-line treatments, especially if the toxicant is unknown. In particular, ILE may render other medications, such as anticonvulstants, ineffective.
- If a specific toxicant or toxidrome is identified during the history and physical exam, by diagnostics, or in consultation with an animal poison control center, then an appropriate antidote or treatment such as ILE or ECT may be effective.
  - Even if an antidote is indicated for a particular case, it might be prohibitively expensive, not readily available, or beyond the point of clinical utility. For example, fomepizole, the preferred antidote for ethylene glycol toxicosis, is most effective if administered within 3 hours of ingestion in cats or 3–8 hours of ingestion in dogs.

## Neurological Signs

- If the animal appears heavily sedated or is comatose, a stat blood glucose concentration should be obtained and dextrose administered as needed.
- If there is a potential history of opiate or opioid ingestion, as is indicated by coexisting respiratory and cardiovascular depression, response to a test dose of naloxone can be determined.
- Ingestion of benzodiazepines generally does not cause severe sedation, but if suspected, then flumazenil may be used to reverse the signs and help with the diagnosis.
- Any animal with CNS depression undergoing decontamination via bathing should be monitored closely as hypothermia may spontaneously occur.
- Neurological stimulation in the form of tremors or seizures is typical of toxicants such as concentrated pyrethrins (cats), amphetamines (see Sympathomimetic Toxidrome), caffeine/theobromine, 5-fluorouracil, ivermectin, metaldehyde, and many more.
- If the toxicant is unidentified, it is typically safe to attempt to stabilize the tremoring or seizuring patient with injectable methocarbamol, diazepam, levetiracetam, or barbiturates while simultaneously evaluating a blood glucose concentration and a serum biochemistry panel.

## Gastrointestinal Signs

- These signs are common, nonspecific, and may be due to a variety of toxicants or other etiologies.
- Mild gastroenteritis may require only supportive care but severe signs such as projectile vomiting, melena, HGE, cholinergic signs, etc. require urgent care coupled with IV fluids, appropriate pharmacological treatment, laboratory diagnostics, imaging, etc.
- A test dose of atropine may be useful in animals with typical organophosphate (OP) signs (excessive salivation, lacrimation, urination, diarrhea, gastroenteritis).

## Respiratory Signs

- Relatively few toxicants result in respiratory signs, with the notable offenders being OPs/carbamates (increased pulmonary secretions), direct pulomonary irritants (e.g., smoke, phosphine gas, or choloramine gas which is created by mixing chlorine bleach and ammonia) or toxicants interfering with oxygen transport or hemoglobin binding such as carbon monoxide, cyanide, and hydrogen sulfide.
- Upon presentation, immediate actions should include supplemental oxygen, assessment with pulse oximetry, laboratory diagnostics including gross examination of the blood for methemoglobinemia, blood gas analysis, and thoracic radiographs (once stable).
- Additional treatments such as bronchodilators, atropine, cyanide antidotes, etc. may be warranted based on presentation and diagnostic results.

## Cardiovascular Signs

- Cardiovascular signs are often relatively nonspecific and need to be contextualized with other clinical signs (see Toxidromes).
- Regardless of the cause, the first approach to treatment should be aimed at basic stabilization via IV fluid therapy and potential supplemental oxygen.
- In general, if related to intoxication, acute onset cardiovascular depression or stimulation will be apparent.
- Bradycardia, hypotension, and other signs associated with cardiac depression may be due to toxicants such as alpha-2-adrenergic agonists, amitraz, beta- or calcium channel blockers, cardiac glycosides, opioids, and OPs/carbamates.
  - Based on other clinical signs, agents such as atipamezole, atropine, naloxone, calcium gluconate, and vasopressors should be considered.
  - Reflex bradycardia (i.e., concurrent hypertension) is often due to sympathomimetic agents so treatment should be focused on decreasing the blood pressure instead of raising the heart rate.
- Cardiovascular stimulation including tachycardia and hypertension may be due to toxicants such as albuterol, amphetamines, caffeine/theobromine, metaldehyde, phenylpropanolamine, and many more (see Sympathomimetic Toxidrome).
  - If CV stimulation is coupled with hyperactivity/agitation, focus initial treatment on sedation (i.e., acepromazine for amphetamine intoxication) as this may simultaneously decrease the heart rate and blood pressure.
  - If sedation is not required or CV stimulation is refractory to sedatives, then additional agents such as injectable beta-blockers or vasodilators may be used.
- As with all potential toxicants, treatment should be coupled with pointed historical exposure questions and diagnostics.

## Toxicological Testing

- Although it is helpful to narrow down a list of possible toxicants to select the most appropriate testing, it is possible to rule out exposure to a large number of toxicants through screening approaches for unknown compounds.
- The use of powerful screening tools for both organic and inorganic toxicants is a viable option in many cases of suspected exposure to an unknown chemical.
- Depending on the specifics of a case, testing gastric contents, urine or serum/plasma can be useful.
  - Stomach content is often the sample of choice in cases of acute onset of clinical signs while urine can be a useful sample if clinical signs have been present for several hours up to one or two days.

- It is often recommended to test more than one sample to be as thorough as possible, although costs associated with testing might restrict analysis to one sample. In such a situation, a toxicologist can assist with making the most appropriate sample selection.
- In many cases, toxicological testing takes some time and therefore should not be counted on to help direct early case management.
  - Despite this limitation, test results can sometimes be available within 24 hours.
  - More delayed results are still useful to many pet owners or veterinarians in order to confirm exposure to a toxicant and to prevent further exposure risks to pets and people.
- There are a few useful point-of-care tests that can provide a preliminary diagnosis; such tests are not considered confirmatory and need to be interpreted in conjunction with case history and clinical signs. When possible, POC tests should be verified by confirmatory testing such as mass spectrometry.
  - In addition, many suspected intoxications might result in later litigation, in which case appropriate testing can be essential.

## CONCLUSIONS

- Managing an animal with a potential unknown toxicant exposure is challenging and difficult.
- Obtaining a complete and accurate history, performing a thorough physical examination followed by the appropriate laboratory diagnostics, and consultation with an animal poison control center should help the practitioner make a diagnosis and formulate an appropriate treatment plan.

### Abbreviations

- 5-HT = 5-hydroxytryptamine
- ADD/ADHD = attention deficit disorder/attention-deficit/hyperactivity disorder
- GHB = gamma-hydroxybutyrate
- LSD = lysergic acid diethylamide
- MAOI = monoamine oxidase inhibitor
- MDMA = 3,4-methylenedioxymethamphetamine, commonly known as the illicit drug ecstasy
- SNRI = serotonin and norepinephrine reuptake inhibitor
- SSRI = selective serotonin reuptake inhibitor
- TCA = tricyclic antidepressant

### Suggested Reading

Brutlag AG, Puschner B. Approach to diagnosis for the toxicology case. In: Peterson ME, Talcott PA (eds) *Small Animal Toxicology*, 3rd edn. St Louis: Elsevier, 2013; pp. 45–52.

Khan SA. Investigating fatal suspected poisonings. In: Poppenga RH, Gwaltney-Brant SM (eds) *Small Animal Toxicology Essentials*. Ames: Wiley-Blackwell, 2011; pp. 71–76.

Khan SA. Differential diagnosis of common acute toxicologic versus nontoxicologic illness. *Vet Clin North Am Small Anim Pract* 2018;48(6):1069–1079.

**Authors**: Ahna G. Brutlag, DVM, MS, DABT, DABVT and Robert H. Poppenga, DVM, PhD, DABVT

**Consulting Editor**: Steven Epstein, DVM, DACVECC

# Chapter 5

# Laboratory Diagnostics for Toxicology

## INTRODUCTION

- Diagnosis of poisoning generally depends on fulfilling five major diagnostic criteria.
  - History.
  - Clinical signs.
  - Clinical laboratory evaluation.
  - Postmortem lesions.
  - Chemical analysis.
- Used properly, they are an effective combination for detecting and understanding clinical poisoning.

### Historical Information

- Knowledge of a known exposure to toxicants and the circumstances surrounding an exposure are often essential to an effective toxicological diagnosis.
- However, one must refrain from basing a diagnosis exclusively on history of exposure. The post hoc fallacy (*Post hoc ergo propter hoc*), as translated from the original Latin, admonishes "After the fact, therefore because of the fact."
- To avoid this, history is used only as a starting point in the diagnostic process.
- The presence of poisons such as rodenticides, insecticides, drugs, paints, household products, over-the-counter and prescription drugs, drugs of abuse, fertilizers, feed additives, and poisonous plants on the premises or a history of their availability or use should be determined when possible.
- It is important to ask specific questions with regard to what might be in an animal's environment rather than asking "Do you know if there are any toxic materials or products that could have/might have been accessible by your pet?" This is because pet owners do not recognize the toxicity of many materials or products that are accessible.
- The adage that the "Dosage makes the poison" means exposure alone without knowing the amount or dosage encountered is not sufficient for a diagnosis. An attempt should be made to estimate the amount or degree of exposure even if it is an overestimate; this provides a "worst-case scenario."
- The food and water supply along with the animal's environment should be examined carefully for algae, fungi, toxic plants, and foreign matter (e.g., baits or chemical spills) as well as odors or physical changes that suggest contamination. Detection of evidence of chewing on product containers is helpful in confirming exposures to toxicants.

*Blackwell's Five-Minute Veterinary Consult Clinical Companion: Small Animal Toxicology*, Third Edition.
Edited by Lynn R. Hovda, Ahna G. Brutlag, Robert H. Poppenga, and Steven E. Epstein.
© 2024 John Wiley & Sons, Inc. Published 2024 by John Wiley & Sons, Inc.

- A thorough history will lead to a more informed clinical examination and choice of diagnostic tests. Fundamental information should include patient identification and characteristics, important demographic factors about the environment, and group or individual issues for affected animals.
- Table 5.1 provides a guide for systematic evaluation of history, environment, and clinical effects.

---

**TABLE 5.1 Checklist for information collection in suspected poisoning of small animals.**

**Owner Data:**
Date: _____
Owner: _____
Manager: _____
Address: _____
Phone: _____
FAX: _____
E-mail: _____

**Health History:**
- Illness past 6 months
- Exposure to other animals last 30 days
- Vaccination history
- Medications: sprays, dips, hormones, minerals, wormers past 6 months – administered by owner or veterinarian?
- Last exam by a veterinarian

**Environmental Data:**
- Location: pasture, woods, near river or pond, confined indoors; recent location changes
- Housing: indoors, outdoors, or combination
- Approximate age of home or kennel
- Type of construction (wood frame, metal, concrete)
- Recent changes in access to trash or garbage; pesticides, flower garden, treated wood, old construction materials; recent burning of materials?
- Confined to fenced yard?
- Allowed to roam free?
- If yes, is animal always supervised?
- Businesses or commercial structures accessible?
- Other (describe): _____

**Patient Data:**
Species: _____
Breed: _____
Sex: _____
Pregnancy: _____
Weight: _____
Age: _____

**Current Clinical and Environmental History:**
- Housing: indoors/outdoors/with/without other animals
- Common feed or water if multiple animals affected?
- If a group, what is:
  – morbidity ___ mortality ___
- When first observed sick?
- How long has problem existed in the animal?
- If dead, when last seen alive and healthy?
- Any recent malicious threats; if yes, describe
- Recent pet losses at home or in neighborhood?
- Pesticide use (insecticides, rodenticides, herbicides) and specific types or names if available (ask for tags or bags to ID)
- Materials used for construction/renovation
- Services: e.g., lawn care, seeding, tree planting, fertilization, pest control
- Access to automotive products, cleaning agents, hobby materials, flower gardens, ornamental trees?
- OTC and prescription medications in the home?
- Interactions with wildlife?

**Dietary Data:**
- Diet components: dry food only, canned food only, combination? Access to snacks or table foods? Lot number or manufacturing date
- Recent changes in total diet or specific diet component(s): list any OTC or prescribed supplements
- Method of feeding: hand feeding, free choice? Is feeding supervised? Food bowl outside?
- Access to molded or spoiled food, mushrooms, bulbs, flower garden plants, indoor plants?
  o Provide common or scientific plant names if possible
- Recent changes in home/yard: painting, remodeling, pest control, weed sprays, burning trash?
- Any evidence of digging in yard or garden, evidence of damage to plants?
- Water source (flowing stream, pond, well, county or city water)

| TABLE 5.1 *Continued* | | | |
|---|---|---|---|
| **Clinical Signs** (check all that apply): | **GI Signs** | **Cardiovascular** | **Blood** |
| | Anorexia | Arrhythmia | Anemia |
| **Nervous System** | Colic | Bradycardia | Hemorrhage |
| Ataxia | Vomiting | Hypotension | Icterus |
| Salivation | Diarrhea | Tachycardia | Hemoglobinuria |
| Blindness/vision impaired/ | Melena | Other | Methemoglobinemia |
| pupil response | Constipation | | |
| Depression | Polyphagia | **Pulmonary** | **Other** |
| Excitement | | Cyanosis | Straining |
| Seizures | **Urinary – Renal** | Dyspnea | Fever |
| Cerebellar signs | Polydipsia | Hyperpnea/Tachypnea | Weakness |
| Paraparesis or tetraparesis | Polyuria | Rales | |
| Dysphonia | Hematuria | | |
| Syncope | | | |
| Other (describe): | | | |

## Clinical Signs

- Clinical signs are of prime importance to the clinician and toxicologist.
  - Both the nature of the signs and sequence of occurrence are important.
    - Did the signs begin explosively and taper off, or did they begin as mild events and worsen with time?
    - Is one body system primarily affected, or are major signs present in several systems?
- Details are often important.
  - For example, a wide range of CNS signs exists and a general description of "seizures" or "tremors" is less useful than an explicit description.
    - Are the signs a typical cranial-to-caudal epileptiform seizure?
    - Is the animal ataxic with cerebellar, vestibular, or peripheral nerve signs?
    - Are there parasympathetic signs such as vomiting, salivation, urination, diarrhea, and dyspnea?
    - Are there parasympatholytic signs such as bloat, dry mouth, mydriasis, hallucinations, or bradycardia?
  - Careful attention to changes in heart rate and rhythm can help define several cardiotoxins.
  - The attending veterinarian may see only one phase of a toxicological response, so the owner or caretaker should be queried for more information.
  - There are dangers in making a toxicological diagnosis based solely on clinical signs as there are thousands of toxic agents but only a limited range of clinical responses that can be expressed by an animal.
  - Unfortunately, in many cases an animal is found dead without any clinical signs being noted. Sudden death in an animal otherwise noted to be healthy might be a tip-off for exposure to a toxicant.

## Clinical Laboratory Evaluation

- Evaluation of clinical laboratory changes can help refine associations with specific toxicants or toxicant groups, as well as suggest potential mechanisms of action and alterations in homeostasis that need correction to save the animal.
- Some changes are very characteristic of certain toxicants, while the absence of organ damage is typical of other toxicants.

- CBC and serum chemistries are useful tools for evaluating clinical signs and identifying target organ systems and formulating a treatment plan.
- Table 5.2 provides some typical clinical chemistry and hematological changes that help define various poisons.

| TABLE 5.2 Selected clinical laboratory tests supporting toxicological diagnosis. | |
|---|---|
| **Clinical laboratory assay** | **Example toxicants** |
| Ammonia (serum) | Hepatic encephalopathy secondary to a number of hepatotoxic chemicals |
| Aplastic anemia | Phenylbutazone, chloramphenicol, gasoline, petroleum solvents, trichothecene mycotoxins |
| AST, ALT, LDH increase | Aflatoxin, blue-green algae, fumonisins, pyrrolizidine alkaloids, *Lantana* spp., amanitin-containing mushrooms, sago palm, xylitol |
| Azotemia (BUN, creatinine) | Arsenic, cadmium, antifreeze, oak, oxalate-containing plants (e.g., lilies), NSAIDs, grapes/raisins, ACE inhibitors, beta-blockers, calcium channel antagonists, mercury |
| Basophilic stippling | Lead, zinc |
| Bile acids | Aflatoxin, other hepatotoxicants (e.g., blue-green algae, amanitin-containing mushrooms, xylitol) |
| Bilirubin | Aflatoxin, zinc, many hepatotoxicants (e.g., blue-green algae, amanitin-containing mushrooms, xylitol) |
| Carboxyhemoglobin | Carbon monoxide (buildings, trailers), smoke inhalation |
| Cholinesterase | Organophosphorus/carbamate insecticides, blue-green algae, *Solanum* plants |
| CK increase | Ionophores (monensin, lasalocid), white snake root, *Cassia* spp., toxicants resulting in tremoring or seizuring (causing secondary increased CK) such as metaldehyde, tremorgenic mycotoxins, pyrethrin/pyrethroid insecticides, illicit drugs |
| Coagulopathy (PT, PTT) | Anticoagulant rodenticides, many hepatotoxicants, DIC secondary to toxicants resulting in hyperthermia (e.g., hops, amphetamines, SSRIs) |
| Crystalluria | Antifreeze, oxalate-containing plants |
| GGT increase | Aflatoxin, pyrrolizidine alkaloids, glucocorticoids, other hepatotoxicants |
| Hemolysis | Copper, garlic, onion, red maple, phenothiazine wormers, zinc |
| Hypercalcemia | Vitamin $D_3$, day-blooming jessamine, calcium supplements, calcipotriene |
| Hyperkalemia | Digitalis glycosides, oleander, many nephrotoxicants (e.g., ethylene glycol, NSAIDs, grapes, raisins, calcium oxalate-containing plants, etc.). |
| Hyperosmolarity | Antifreeze, aspirin, ethanol, propylene glycol |
| Hypocalcemia | Antifreeze, oxalate poisoning, nephrotoxicants resulting in renal secondary hyperparathyroidism |
| Hypoproteinemia | Aflatoxins, chemotherapeutics, blood loss (e.g., secondary to anticoagulant rodenticides, DIC, NSAID-induced gastric ulceration, etc.) |
| Iron (serum) and TIBC | Iron toxicosis |
| Methemoglobin | Acetaminophen, copper, nitrites, chlorates, methylene blue, smoke inhalation |
| Urinary casts | Nephrotoxicants (e.g., aminoglycosides, NSAIDs, ethylene glycol, grapes, lilies, beta-blockers, ACE inhibitors, etc.), arsenic, cadmium, mercury, oak |

## Postmortem Lesions

- Loss of one or more animals in a group or a single animal at risk provides an invaluable opportunity to increase diagnostic information by conducting a thorough postmortem examination.
  - Postmortem examinations help improve diagnosis and possible treatment for other affected animals.
  - They can also provide guidance to the owner/manager in planning ahead and eliminating risks to other animals or people.
- Necropsy and microscopic lesions may be invaluable in supporting insurance claims or actions where liability or litigation is involved.
  - Thorough examination of gastrointestinal contents can provide clues to what might have been consumed (e.g., plant fragments, pill/tablet fragments, container pieces, bait formulations).
  - Lesions are typically absent in certain toxicoses, while the presence of lesions may correlate with other toxicoses.
  - Many insecticides and drugs, strychnine and lead, among others, often cause few or very subtle lesions.
  - Ethylene glycol, microcystins, amanitin-containing mushrooms, bromethalin, anticoagulant rodenticides, and many other toxicants provide defined lesions helpful for making a diagnosis or narrowing a differential list.
  - Necropsy should include the brain (and a rabies exam) if neurological signs are present.
  - A thorough selection of samples collected at necropsy is easier and more inclusive if consistently performed. Tissue samples for toxicology should be fresh and not placed into formalin. Collecting more sample amount than is likely needed is recommended so that if initial testing is not diagnostic, further analyses can be considered.
  - Should legal or insurance claims be likely, a necropsy is usually essential. In this instance, photographs and detailed notes regarding the necropsy and premise examination should be taken and preserved.
  - Table 5.3 summarizes recommended necropsy specimens.
  - Specimens collected for possible toxicology testing can be stored refrigerated or frozen pending results from histopathological examination of formalin-fixed tissue samples or other postmortem testing.

**TABLE 5.3 Necropsy specimen collection recommended for toxicology.**

**Brain** ½ frozen, ½ formalin. *Leave midline in formalin for pathologist orientation*

**Ocular fluid** (2–4 mL) chilled or save entire eyeball to submit

**Injection site** (100 g) frozen

**Stomach and intestinal contents** (1 kg or as much as possible) frozen

**Adipose tissue** (25–50 grams) frozen

**Liver** (200 g) frozen

**Kidney** (200 g) frozen

**Urine** if present (100 mL or as much as possible) ½ chilled, ½ frozen

## Environmental/Food Sampling

- Food and environmental samples are often important for a diagnosis of intoxication. Any unusual materials noted in an animal's environment should be collected, stored in appropriate containers, and frozen for later analysis. In suspected malicious poisonings, these types of samples might be critical for case resolution.
- Many pet owners suspect that a new pet food caused an animal's illness. Food/feed items should be retained pending need for testing. In cases of suspected pet food poisonings, the Food and Drug Administration Center for Veterinary Medicine should be alerted through its reporting portal: How to Report a Pet Food Complaint | FDA
- If a plant can't be identified but is of concern, specimens can often be sent for confirmatory ID; the plant specimens need to be as complete as possible. Roots can be wrapped in wet paper towels, and speciments placed in zip-lock bags. Refrigeration is generally adequate to preserve plants for several days prior to submission.

## Chemical Analysis

- Chemical analysis is an indispensable aid in forming a toxicological diagnosis. When used properly, and in the right context, chemical analysis may be the single best diagnostic criterion.
- Limitations to chemical analysis include the following.
  - Chemical tests should not be relied upon without supporting historical, clinical data, and postmortem findings when available.
  - Time course of the intoxication, changes since death, or limitations on testing methodology can render a chemical analysis less useful or ineffective for diagnostic confirmation.
  - While there is no single test that can detect all potential toxicants, advances in analytical methodology allow for many toxicants to be detected by nontargeted screening via gas chromatography and/or high-performance liquid chromatography coupled with large chemical mass spectral databases.
  - Current analytical methodology is quite sensitive; often various chemicals are detected that are not necessarily related to noted clinical signs or lesions.
  - Identify a laboratory in advance and be familiar with its reputation and performance before rapid or critical testing is needed.
- Most laboratories welcome inquiries about appropriate sampling and test limitations.
- A good laboratory will inform you when a received sample is inadequate or the test requested is not part of their routine and approved offerings.
- For some toxicoses, chemical analysis may not be developed, or a toxic principle may be unknown, so reliance must be on clinical and pathological confirmation for your diagnosis.
- Depending on the circumstances of a particular case, detection of any amount of toxicant is sufficient to confirm exposure and sometimes intoxication. In other cases, quantification of a toxicant in a fluid or tissue sample is necessary to make a diagnosis of intoxication.

# GETTING THE MOST FROM YOUR DIAGNOSTIC EFFORT

- The principles and approaches described here give your clients a combination of your best efforts and the best value you can obtain from laboratory assistance. Not all suspected acute or chronic poisonings become a positive diagnosis.
- The approach outlined is widely accepted and provides a standard of diagnosis that should be supportable and acceptable in veterinary practice.

## Abbreviations

See Appendix 1 for a complete list.
- ACE = angiotensin-converting enzyme
- NSAID = nonsteroidal antiinflammatory drug
- SSRI = selective serotonin reuptake inhibitor

## Suggested Reading

Lohmeyer C. Taking a toxicologic history. In: Poppenga RH, Gwaltney-Brant SM (eds) *Small Animal Toxicology Essentials*. Ames: Wiley-Blackwell, 2011.

Puschner B, Brutlag AG. Approach to diagnosis for the toxicology case. In: Peterson ME, Talcott (eds) *Small Animal Toxicology*, 3rd edn. St Louis: Elsevier, 2013; pp. 45–52.

Talcott PA. Effective use of a diagnostic laboratory. In: Peterson ME, Talcott (eds) *Small Animal Toxicology*, 3rd edn. St Louis: Elsevier, 2013; pp. 125–132.

Acknowledgment: Gary D. Osweiler, DVM, PhD, DABVT

Author: Robert H. Poppenga, DVM, PhD, DABVT
Consulting Editor: Robert H. Poppenga, DVM, PhD, DABVT

# Chapter 6

# Medico-legal Considerations for Companion Animal Practitioners

## OVERVIEW

Although complaints of veterinary misconduct are infrequent, this chapter briefly touches on important areas for attention when veterinary misconduct is alleged that may lead to administrative action, civil action, or both. Administrative actions most frequently involve the state board of veterinary medicine taking enforcement action regarding a veterinarian's ability to practice. Two of the most common board complaints relate to medical record-keeping and client communication. Civil actions generally involve allegations of veterinary malpractice.

Occasionally veterinarians are asked to provide professional expertise on a case with potential civil or criminal ramifications. These cases require added attention to appropriate medical record-keeping and client communication.

We briefly discuss administrative actions, civil actions, and then animal cruelty as an example of veterinary expertise involving civil or criminal cases.

### State License Board Discipline

Clients may submit a complaint to the state veterinary medical board (VMB) which may then review the facts for violation of the state practice act. In some states the VMB may initiate its own investigation. The VMB is generally a state administrative agency empowered to *regulate* the practice of veterinary medicine as delegated in state statute and regulations. The VMB overseeing the practice of veterinary medicine serves a consumer protection function. The group consists of both veterinary professionals and members of the public. After reviewing the facts, the VMB decides whether and what disciplinary action is appropriate within the state's regulations.

### State Practice Acts

- State practice acts generally delegate authority to a state veterinary medical board to promulgate regulations to protect the public. The statutes and regulations governing the practice of veterinary medicine vary between states.
- The state practice act defines what constitutes the practice of veterinary medicine in each state.
- In many states, the practice act also defines license requirements (CE requirements); the veterinarian–client–patient relationship; details the disciplinary process for licensees; and includes requirements for reporting animal cruelty and potential related immunity provisions.

### Medical Records

- Medical records are critical to answer a variety of medico-legal questions. For example, in an alleged toxicosis, case records might be used to answer questions of whether the animal had a previous illness or was healthy, whether it was exposed to a potentially toxic dose of a toxicant, and whether the clinical signs or other adverse effects of the toxicant, if known, were

*Blackwell's Five-Minute Veterinary Consult Clinical Companion: Small Animal Toxicology*, Third Edition.
Edited by Lynn R. Hovda, Ahna G. Brutlag, Robert H. Poppenga, and Steven E. Epstein.
© 2024 John Wiley & Sons, Inc. Published 2024 by John Wiley & Sons, Inc.

observed. If the case involves a criminal matter, medical records, along with other evidence, might be used to determine whether exposure to the toxicant was accidental or intentional.

■ Many states include specific minimum requirements that must be included in a patient's medical record. See Figure 6.1 for one example of state medical record-keeping requirements.

    ● The general goals of medical record-keeping requirements are to promote standardization, accessibility, retrievability, confidentiality and integrity.

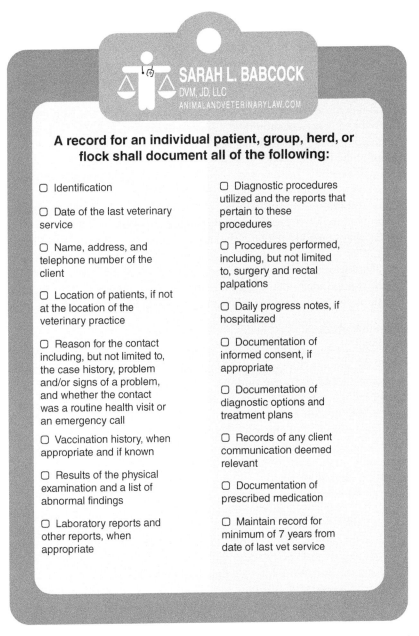

■ **Figure 6.1** Example of state record-keeping requirements to include in veterinary records for individual patients or groups of animals.

- A good medical record entry is legible, accurate, timely, objective, concise, and consistent. Ask yourself: is my record reflective of my thought processes?
- An opponent may try to create the impression that your care was negligent, or you are not credible if you depart from appropriate record-keeping standards.
- The patient history will be critical in determining a diagnosis and treatment plan so it should be reflected in the medical record, including interpretation of laboratory results.
- A complete physical examination including cardiovascular, neurological, and respiratory systems should probably be documented in the medical record, especially for cases of toxicosis.
- Items that are generally considered part of the record include radiographs; client communications (texts; video sent; pictures); imaging and reports.
- Abbreviations used in the record should be limited to those defined in the record and/or in a standard reference. Additionally, assessments such as "NSF" indicating no significant findings should not be used but rather include in the medical record the data to conclude a normal finding.
- Medical records are the property of the practice; however, the information belongs to the client and generally should be released upon client request.
- Information in the record should be considered confidential and not shared without consent of the animal owner absent a state regulatory exception.
- States will generally include requirements for how long you must retain records and how to properly dispose of them.
- Medical records should authenticate who provided the care with supporting details.
- Documentation is critical in maintaining chain of custody of collected evidence.
  - Chain of custody refers to the movement and location of real evidence from the time it is obtained to the time it is presented in court.
  - This includes documenting the date and time samples were collected and the type of storage used; identification of witnesses to sample collection; and the names of parties responsible for the samples during both collection and storage.

## Client Communication

- Client complaints often allege a veterinarian did not obtain valid consent, so a shared decision-making process did not occur. Complaints may allege lack of discussion of risks, benefits, diagnostic and treatment options, prognosis, and cost.
  - Specific failures noted in license discipline actions include lack of referral to a specialist or failure to seek a consultation; failure to provide written discharge instructions and follow-up care; not ensuring the client is aware of who is providing care; inappropriate delegations of patient diagnostics or treatment; assuming a client consent form is the same as obtaining valid, informed client consent.
- A consent form should be written in plain language, signed by the client, and the client offered the opportunity to ask questions.

## Client Confidentiality

- Veterinarians have an ethical obligation and, in about half of the states, a legal duty to maintain confidentiality of patient information.
  - As mentioned in other chapters, an owner may not be forthcoming with a patient history that involves toxic substances and authors have noted potential abuse. These confidentiality provisions may help in obtaining needed information.
  - Absent an exception (animal cruelty reporting), it is prudent for a veterinarian to consult their state practice regulations on the specific requirements for confidentiality of client communications and medical records.

- If information is released, it is wise to include a signed client consent form for the medical record absent a regulatory exception.

## Veterinary Professional Conduct

- Veterinary malpractice refers to negligence or misconduct by a veterinarian. Such allegation may be raised when a patient is injured or damaged due to an error made by a veterinarian that a reasonable veterinarian would not have done.
- For a veterinary negligence case, the acts or omissions at issue must involve matters of medical science or require special skills not ordinarily possessed by laypersons. State law helps discern which issues are deemed professional by listing those actions for which an individual must have a state-issued veterinary license or, in other words, those activities that fall under the definition of "practice of veterinary medicine" in the state.
- In a malpractice case, the burden of proof is on the plaintiff (generally the client in a civil matter and the state in a criminal matter) to present evidence that the defendant veterinarian is liable. The veterinarian's medical record and perhaps the testimony of expert witnesses are common sources of information to substantiate the treating veterinarian's quality of care.

## SPECIAL CASES REQUIRING VETERINARY EXPERTISE

### Reporting Animal Cruelty

- Veterinarians play an essential role in the recognition, investigation, and prosecution of animal cruelty. Veterinarians have an ethical and, in an increasing number of states, legal duty to report suspected cases of animal cruelty.
  - Animal cruelty laws vary from state to state but are intended to promote animal and public health, safety, and welfare.
  - Knowing how your state defines animal cruelty is threshold knowledge. For example, poisoning may be a form of animal cruelty in your state.
  - Does the detection of alcohol or drugs of abuse in a pet require reporting to anyone other than the client?
  - Some states provide immunity from liability for veterinarians participating in cruelty investigations.
  - Ensure all medical records include the minimum requirements for the state:

Specific suggestions of facts to include in the medical record when animal cruelty is suspected are: "[w]henever nonaccidental injury is suspected, the attending veterinarian should obtain a minimum database, including estimated age, an accurate body weight, and a body condition score, and should perform a complete physical examination, a thorough oral examination to establish the condition of the teeth, otoscopic and ophthalmic examinations to identify potential head trauma, radiographic examinations to rule out occult injuries, and other species-specific examinations as necessary" (Babcock and Neihsl, 2006).

### Referral or Consultation

- Veterinarians may consider consultation, referral, or both if the medico-legal aspect of the case is known at the outset.
  - Veterinarians may have an ethical duty to offer clients a referral and/or seek a consultation if the veterinarian is not comfortable providing the needed care. Recent state license disciplinary cases have included claims for failure to offer the client a referral at the onset of the examination and to document this in the medical record.

- Consultation on laboratory testing may be provided by the veterinary laboratory you use, the American Association of Veterinary Laboratory Diagnosticians (AAVLD) accredited lab in your area, or both. AAVLD accredited laboratories have experience working with state and federal agencies on cases with regulatory ramifications.
- Some 22 different veterinary specialties are now recognized in the US. Depending on the circumstances of the particular case, one or more veterinary specialists may be helpful for consultation or referral.

### Abbreviations

- VMB = Veterinary Medical Board
- AAVLD = American Association of Veterinary Laboratory Diagnosticians

### Suggested Reading

AVMA. Principles of veterinary medical ethics of the AVMA. www.avma.org/resources-tools/avma-policies/principles-veterinary-medical-ethics-avma

AVMA's Veterinary specialties website: www.avma.org/education/veterinary-specialties

Babcock SL, Neihsl A. Requirements for mandatory reporting of animal cruelty. *J Am Vet Med Assoc* 2006;229(5):685–689.

Babcock SL, Pfeiffer C. Laws and regulations concerning the confidentiality of veterinarian-client communication. *J Am Vet Med Assoc* 2006;229(3):365–369.

*Celinski v. State*, 911 S.W.2d 177 (Tex. App. 1996)

Gwaltney-Brant SM. Veterinary forensic toxicology. *Vet Pathol* 2016;53(5):1067–1077.

**Authors**: Sarah L. Babcock, DVM, JD and Ahna G. Brutlag, DVM, MS, DABT, DABVT
**Consulting Editors**: Ahna G. Brutlag, DVM, MS, DABT, DABVT and Robert H. Poppenga, DVM, PhD, DABVT

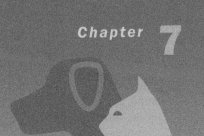

# Chapter 7

# Pet Food

## INTRODUCTION

- Since the contamination of pet foods with melamine and related compounds in 2007, there has been an increased sensitivity to pet foods as a cause of illness of an animal.
- The diagnosis of a pet food-related illness requires careful investigation and often consultation with specialists and government agencies which have regulatory oversight of pet foods, particularly the FDA's Center for Veterinary Medicine (CVM).
- Commercial pet foods are usually safe but incidents of contamination do occur as a result of natural contaminants, chemical adulteration, nutritional imbalances, and presence of infectious agents such as *Salmonella* spp. and *Listeria monocytogenes*.
  - Pet food recalls since the melamine and cyanuric acid incident have been due to the presence of aflatoxins, pentobarbital, vitamin $D_3$, and methionine.
  - The causes of some pet food-related problems have not been determined. Fanconi syndrome in dogs associated with feeding chicken jerky treats and megaesophagus in dogs associated with feeding a specific pet food product are examples of strong associations of illness with a food for which no specific toxicant has been identified.
- If a pet food adulteration is confirmed by the CVM, the agency can initiate a voluntary or, in some cases, involuntary recall.
  - Most commonly, recalls fall into one of three categories: Class I, Class II, or Class III.
    - Class I: a situation in which there is a reasonable probability that the use of, or exposure to, a violative product will cause serious adverse health consequences or death.
    - Class II: a situation in which the use of, or exposure to, a violative product may cause a temporary or medically reversible adverse health consequence or where the probability of a serious adverse health consequence is low.
    - Class III: a situation in which use of, or exposure to, a violative product is not likely to cause an adverse consequence.

### Medico-Legal Aspects

- If an adulteration is confirmed, or even strongly suspected without a toxicant being identified, there is always the possibility of subsequent legal action being taken by pet owners.
- Given this possibility, it is critical that veterinarians do thorough patient assessments and maintain complete and understandable medical records for each suspect animal.

---

*Blackwell's Five-Minute Veterinary Consult Clinical Companion: Small Animal Toxicology*, Third Edition.
Edited by Lynn R. Hovda, Ahna G. Brutlag, Robert H. Poppenga, and Steven E. Epstein.
© 2024 John Wiley & Sons, Inc. Published 2024 by John Wiley & Sons, Inc.

- In the unfortunate event of an animal's death, efforts should be made to have a complete postmortem examination conducted, preferably by a board-certified pathologist.
  - In some cases, a gross postmortem examination can be performed at the clinic with appropriate samples submitted for additional testing (e.g., histopathology, toxicologic testing). See Chapter 5, Laboratory Diagnosis for Toxicology.

## Historical Information

- Often, a pet food-related concern begins with a recent change in a pet food that coincides chronologically with the onset of a change in eating behavior or illness.
  - It can take days to weeks of the new diet for signs of a toxicosis to develop if the toxicant is present at low levels. If immediate clinical signs are present upon eating a new diet, infectious causes are often prioritized over toxicants as the cause, although they cannot be completely excluded.
  - It is important in such situations for veterinarians to take such a concern seriously but not reach conclusions until a more thorough patient assessment is conducted.
  - In many cases, a concern about a pet food turns out to be unfounded.
- In addition to obtaining information germane to any animal's illness (e.g., signalment, complete medical history, results of any clinical testing, progression of clinical signs), the following information can help to identify a potential pet food-related problem.
  - Time between feeding the food and onset of clinical signs or change in behavior.
  - Duration of feeding the food and the amount of food consumed by the pet(s).
  - Number of pets affected in the household and the number of animals given the food.
  - Food storage and handling practices.
  - Potential for other toxicant exposures.
- The FDA website has a complete list of information requested when reporting a suspected problem (www.fda.gov/animal-veterinary/report-problem/how-report-pet-food-complaint).

## Clinical Signs and Clinical Laboratory Evaluation

- It is important to try to determine organ systems affected based upon clinical signs and clinical laboratory evaluation.
  - This is critical to formulation of an appropriate differential list and subsequently helping to formulate an effective strategy for testing suspect food samples submitted to a diagnostic laboratory.
  - For example, the liver would be the primary target organ for pet food adulterated with aflatoxin, whereas the kidneys are the primary target organ in cases of melamine and cyanuric acid intoxication.
- This information is critical to the CVM in order to compare apparent disparate cases for detection of patterns of importance.
- Along with collecting samples for routine clinical evaluation, biological samples for possible toxicologic testing should be obtained and appropriately stored.

## Postmortem Lesions

- Conducting thorough postmortem examinations in the event of a death is one of the most neglected procedures in case assessment.
- Postmortem examinations can confirm a cause of death or can identify disease processes not obvious from antemortem testing.
- Ideally, postmortem examinations should be conducted by a board-certified veterinary pathologist; when this is not possible, a gross examination should be conducted by the clinician with appropriate samples collected and stored for histopathologic, toxicologic, or other diagnostic testing.

## Food Sampling and Chemical Analysis

- Retain any remaining food and store appropriately for possible toxicologic testing.
  - Dry foods can be retained in their original packaging under ambient conditions for quite some time.
  - Moist foods can be retained in their original packaging and kept refrigerated for short periods of time or frozen for extended periods of time.
  - If there is any question about how to store a particular food sample, freezing is the best option.
- It is often prudent to complete the case assessment (antemortem and/or postmortem) before submitting food samples for toxicologic testing. This often helps to determine what tests should be performed.
- A veterinary diagnostic laboratory can be consulted with regard to availability of specific targeted testing (e.g., testing for aflatoxins) or options for nontargeted testing when a specific toxicant of concern is unknown.
  - Veterinarians can consult the webpage of the American Association of Veterinary Laboratory Diagnosticians (www.aavld.org/) for its state diagnostic laboratory; if a state laboratory does not offer a full suite of testing, it can often refer veterinarians to other state laboratories or forward samples when necessary.
  - If the CVM identifies a potential pet food problem, officials there can help identify appropriate veterinary diagnostic laboratories to provide testing and, in some cases where a real concern is identified, cover the cost of testing.

## Reporting

- In order for reporting of a suspected pet food problem to be as useful as possible to the CVM, it is critical for veterinarians to be involved in the process. Veterinarians provide essential historical details and interpretation of clinical data.
- Multiple reports of illness associated with specific pet foods from a broad geographic area support a conclusion that the association is real.
- Although pet food manufacturers are required to report potential adverse effects to regulatory authorities, it is recommended that any concerns be reported first to the CVM.
- Reporting can occur through the FDA's Safety Reporting Portal or the FDA Consumer Complaint Coordinators for the state where the complaint originated (www.fda.gov/animal-veterinary/report-problem/how-report-pet-food-complaint).
- The following information is critical when reporting a suspected problem (see the FDA website for a complete list of requested information).
  - Brand name, manufacturer, product's description from the label.
  - Type of food (e.g., canned, kibble, raw, etc.) and type of product container.
  - Purchase date, location and total amount purchased.
  - Lot number and expiry date.
  - UPC barcode, product date and code.
  - Amount of food used and the amount of unused food remaining (important for possible testing).

## Suggested Reading

Bischoff K, Rumbeiha WK. Pet food recalls and pet food contaminants in small animals: an update. *Vet Clin North Am Small Anim Pract* 2018;48:917–931.

Hurley KJ, Mansfield C, VanHoutan IM. A comparative analysis of two unrelated outbreaks in Latvia and Australia of acquired idiopathic megaesophagus in dogs fed to brands of commercial dry dog foods: 398 cases (2014–2018). *J Am Vet Med Assoc* 2021;259(2):172–183.

Swirski A, Pearl DL, Berke O, O'Sullivan TL. Can North American animal poison control center call data provide early warning of outbreaks associated with contaminated pet food? Using the 2007 melamine pet food contaminant incident as a case study. *PLoS One* 2022;17(12):e0277100.

Wilson-Frank CR, Hooser SB. Investigative diagnostic toxicology and the role of the veterinarian in pet food-related outbreaks: an update. *Vet Clin North Am Small Anim Pract* 2018;48:909–915.

**Author**: Robert H. Poppenga, DVM, PhD, DABVT
**Consulting Editor**: Steven Epstein, DVM, DACVECC

# Specific Toxins and Toxicants

# Alcohols and Glycol Ethers

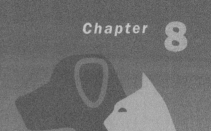

# Chapter 8

# Alcohols

## DEFINITION/OVERVIEW

- Alcohols are hydrocarbons with a hydroxyl (-OH) group.
- Methanol (wood alcohol; $CH_3OH$), ethanol (ethyl alcohol; $CH_3CH_2OH$), and isopropanol (rubbing alcohol; $(CH_3)_2CHOH$) are commonly encountered examples and are the subject of this chapter. These alcohols are found in medicinal, cleaning, automotive products, and certain fuels. Methanol is found in certain automotive windshield washer fluids.
- Ethanol has been used to treat ethylene glycol poisoning in dogs and cats.
- Exposure can occur from consumption of products containing these alcohols. Ethanol exposure also occurs from the consumption of alcoholic beverages and certain raw bread dough.
- Exposure to these alcohols most commonly results in vomiting, CNS depression, and ataxia. Management is predominantly directed at correction of dehydration and acid–base status.

## ETIOLOGY/PATHOPHYSIOLOGY

Poisonings arising from exposure to short-chain alcohols are occasionally observed in veterinary medicine. Most veterinary cases involving accidental ingestion of ethanol occur from the ingestion of alcoholic beverages, raw bread or pizza dough, fermented garbage, rotten apples, and consumer products including certain mouthwashes (up to 27% ethanol), perfumes and colognes (>50%), and hand sanitizers (>60%). Methanol and isopropyl alcohol are also found in some consumer products. Consumer products with high methanol concentrations include model engine fuels (60–80% methanol), deicers (>30%), windshield washer fluids (>50%), and varnish and stain removers (>30%). Consumer products with high isopropanol concentrations include engine water removers (>50% isopropanol), deicers (>20%), windshield-coating fluids (>50%), and certain sanitizers (>50%).

### Mechanism of Action

The neurotoxic effects of these short-chain alcohols are multifactorial. Short-term consumption depresses brain function by altering the balance between inhibitory and excitatory neurotransmission. For example, at some doses ethanol increases the function of the inhibitory neurotransmitter gamma-aminobutyric acid (GABA). These alcohols are also a direct irritant to mucous membranes and the eyes. The germicidal mechanism of action of alcohols involves denaturation of proteins and disruption of cell membranes.

Methanol is metabolized by hepatic alcohol dehydrogenase to formic acid via formaldehyde. Species with low levels of tetrahydrofolate (e.g., humans and other primates) have slower rates of formate metabolism, resulting in metabolic acidosis and blindness. Dogs and cats have higher rates of formate detoxification and do not develop these signs.

*Blackwell's Five-Minute Veterinary Consult Clinical Companion: Small Animal Toxicology*, Third Edition. Edited by Lynn R. Hovda, Ahna G. Brutlag, Robert H. Poppenga, and Steven E. Epstein. © 2024 John Wiley & Sons, Inc. Published 2024 by John Wiley & Sons, Inc.

## Pharmacokinetics – Absorption, Distribution, Metabolism, Excretion

- Short-chain alcohols can be absorbed orally, by inhalation, or by dermal exposure, with oral exposure occurring most commonly.
- Oral absorption occurs rapidly. The highest blood levels are seen after oral dosing, with lower levels after inhalation and lowest levels after dermal application.
- These alcohols rapidly distribute throughout the body and cross the blood–brain barrier and placenta. Ethanol, methanol, and isopropanol are initially metabolized by hepatic alcohol dehydrogenase to acetaldehyde, formaldehyde, and acetone, respectively. Acetaldehyde is subsequently metabolized to acetic acid, formaldehyde to formic acid, and acetone to acetic acid.
- Excretion of the parent alcohols occurs predominantly through the urine and exhalation. A fraction of the metabolites formed will be excreted in the urine.

## Toxicity

### Ethanol

- The $LD_{LO}$ intravenous route for ethanol in dogs is 1.6 mL/kg. The $LD_{LO}$ oral is 5–8 mL/kg.
- The oral $LD_{50}$ of ethanol in rats is 9 mL/kg.

### Methanol

- The oral $LD_{50}$ for methanol in dogs is reported to be 4–8 mL/kg.
- Toxic doses for methanol in canines and felines are approximately the same as for ethanol.

### Isopropanol

- The oral $LD_{50}$ for isopropanol in dogs is reported to be approximately 2 mL/kg of a 70% isopropanol solution (rubbing alcohol).
- In general, isopropanol is considered to be twice as potent a CNS depressant as ethanol.

## Systems Affected

- Nervous – CNS depression, ataxia, lethargy, sedation.
- Gastrointestinal – nausea, vomiting.
- Endocrine/metabolic – methanol: metabolic acidosis in nonhuman primates; ethanol: lactic acidosis, hypoglycemia, hypokalemia, hypomagnesemia, hypocalcemia, and hypophosphatemia have been reported in people.
- General – hypothermia.

 # SIGNALMENT/HISTORY

- Canines are more commonly reported to ingest alcohol-based products than felines.
- Younger animals tend to chew and drink articles not intended for consumption.

## Risk Factors

- Ethanol toxicosis often occurs during holiday seasons (e.g., Christmas, Easter), when pet owners may be baking desserts more frequently. Methanol toxicosis often occurs during the spring and summer, when windshield wiper fluid is more readily available in the garage.

## Historical Findings

- Ingestion witnessed by the owner; chewed product container found by the owner.
- Clinical signs including ataxia, CNS depression, and lethargy are often noted by the pet owner.

## Location and Circumstances of Poisoning

- Ethanol toxicity may occur in the kitchen, where raw bread dough is handled.
- Dogs housed in the garage may be at higher risk for ingestion.
- Chewed containers may be found in the garage or outdoor environment.

 # CLINICAL FEATURES

- CNS depression, ataxia, lethargy, and sedation.
- Hypothermia.
- Metabolic acidosis.
- Clinical signs (ataxia and CNS depression) would be expected rapidly (within an hour) if the animal ingested a toxic dose.
- Excessive gas accumulation in the gastrointestinal tract, flatulence, bloating, abdominal pain, vomiting, retching, and nausea can occur in animals ingesting fermented bread dough. The smell of ethanol may be obvious on the pet's breath.
- Isopropanol intoxications may be more prolonged compared to ethanol and methanol intoxications because the acetone metabolite is also a CNS depressant.

 # DIFFERENTIAL DIAGNOSIS

- Other toxicants with sedative and/or CNS depressant effects include the following.
  - 2-butoxyethanol.
  - Amitraz.
  - Barbiturates.
  - Benzodiazepines.
  - Ethylene glycol.
  - Macrolide antiparasitics.
  - Marijuana.
  - Other volatile alcohols.
- Primary neurological disease (e.g., inflammatory, infectious, infiltrative, etc.).
- Primary metabolic disease (e.g., hypoglycemia, hepatic encephalopathy).
- Hypoglycemia (e.g., juvenile hypoglycemia, xylitol toxicosis, hypoadrenocorticism, insulinoma, hepatic tumor, hunting dog hypoglycemia).

 # DIAGNOSTICS

### Clinical Laboratory

- A PCV/TS, blood glucose, and venous blood gas should be performed to evaluate severity of dehydration and electrolyte and acid–base status.
- In isopropanol toxicosis, an osmole gap may develop.
- Many diagnostic laboratories are capable of determining ethanol, methanol, or isopropanol levels in blood although ethanol determination is most commonly available as a routine test.
- Blood ethanol concentrations of 87–109 mmol/L (400–500 mg/dL) and above are considered severe and potentially life-threatening in people and are of similar concern in companion animals.

### Pathological Findings

- There are no specific gross or histologic lesions observed in alcohol-poisoned companion animals.

# THERAPEUTICS

## Detoxification

- Alcohols are usually absorbed very quickly from the gastrointestinal tract so the use of emetics is rarely effective. The administration of medications to cause emesis is generally not recommended because of the rapid onset of CNS depression and risk of aspiration pneumonia.
- Ethanol and other short-chain alcohols are poorly adsorbed by activated charcoal, which is therefore not recommended.
- If dermal exposure to volatile alcohols has occurred, rinse the affected area with a mild detergent shampoo and water.
- Forced diuresis is generally not effective.
- Hemodialysis may be an effective means of enhancing elimination of ethanol from the body and can therefore be beneficial in cases expected to be potentially life-threatening or associated with high morbidity.

## Antidotes and Drugs of Choice

- There are no known antidotes for ethanol or isopropanol. Antidotes used for methanol (e.g., ethanol or fomepizole) toxicosis in humans are not used with dogs and cats since blindness due to formic acid formation has not been reported in these species.
- Therapy should include careful rehydration with dextrose solution to correct hypoglycemia.
- A balanced, isotonic crystalloid IV fluid can be used in symptomatic patients to aid in correction of dehydration.
- In the presence of a severe metabolic acidosis (e.g., pH <7.0, BE ≤15 mmHg, $HCO_3$ <11 mmHg), the judicious use of sodium bicarbonate can be considered.

## Appropriate Health Care

- Hospitalization may be required to manage severe CNS depression, metabolic acidosis, and respiratory depression.
- If respiratory function is compromised, a cuffed endotracheal tube should be placed and ventilation supported mechanically as required.
- Maintaining normal body temperature is important.
- Alcohol toxicosis can result in severe CNS depression/coma, and appropriate nursing care is imperative. Patients should be kept in a padded cage and should be turned every six hours to prevent atelectasis.
- Provide respiratory support and mechanical ventilation if needed.
- Monitor temperature, heart rate, and respiratory rate.
- Monitor blood pressure and blood glucose frequently and treat appropriately.
- Ophthalmic lubrication may be necessary every six hours. Keeping the patient clean and dry is imperative.

## Precautions/Interactions

- If other substances have been coingested, initiate specific treatment for those substances, if available.

## Follow-up

- Follow-up is generally unnecessary, as patients are clinically normal once signs resolve.

## Activity

- Patients should be restricted from activity until clinical signs resolve, as ataxia and CNS depression will be apparent. Once clinical signs resolve, no exercise restriction is necessary.

## Patient Monitoring

- Acid–base monitoring is recommended in symptomatic animals.
- Blood glucose concentrations should be monitored frequently.

# COMMENTS

### Prevention/Avoidance

- Prevent access of pets to obvious or potential sources of alcohol.
- Prevention is critical. Advise clients that alcohol-containing products are potentially dangerous for their pets. Educate clients about common sources of alcohol available in the home (e.g., kitchen).
- Early treatment is also important. Clients should be taught to contact their veterinarian if an exposure has occurred or an animal is displaying unusual clinical signs.

### Expected Course and Prognosis

- Most cases involving mild signs usually resolve with close monitoring and supportive care within a 24-hour period.
- No long-term effects are expected unless brain injury secondary to prolonged respiratory depression and hypoxia has occurred.
- The prognosis is fair to guarded in cases involving metabolic acidosis, severe CNS or respiratory system depression, or aspiration pneumonia.

### Abbreviations

See Appendix 1 for a complete list.

### Suggested Reading

Keno LA, Langston CE. Treatment of accidental ethanol intoxication with hemodialysis in a dog. *J Vet Emerg Crit Care* 2011;21(4):363–368.

LaHood AJ, Kok SJ. Ethanol toxicity. StatPearls. www.ncbi.nlm.nih.gov/books/NBK557381/.

Means C. Bread dough toxicosis in dogs. *J Vet Emerg Crit Care* 2003;13(1):39–41.

Rayar P, Ratnapalan S. Pediatric ingestions of house hold products containing ethanol: a review. *Clin Pediatr* 2013;52(3):203–209.

Valentine WM. Short-chain alcohols. *Vet Clin North Am Small Anim Pract* 1990;20(2):515–523.

**Author:** David C. Dorman, DVM, PhD, DABVT, DABT
**Consulting Editor:** Robert H. Poppenga, DVM, PhD, DABVT

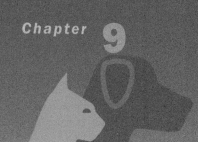

# Ethylene Glycol and Diethylene Glycol

## DEFINITION/OVERVIEW

- Ethylene glycol (EG) is often used in the manufacture of synthetic fibers and plastic bottles. Most commonly, exposure occurs in animals from ingestion of antifreeze and other automotive chemicals/fluids. EG is a clear, odorless liquid.
- Diethylene glycol (DEG) can be found in lotions, skin creams, and deodorants as well as in brake fluid, lubricants, wallpaper strippers, and heating/cooking fuel.
- EG intoxication can be successfully treated with early intervention despite a commonly grave prognosis if recognized late in the clinical course of the intoxication.
- Clinical signs of EG intoxication include CNS depression, ataxia, knuckling, nausea, vomiting, polyuria/polydipsia, and hypothermia, depending on the dose and time from ingestion.
- Ethanol or fomepizole treatments should be used as soon as the intoxication is suspected or proven. Fomepizole can be used in both dogs and cats with EG intoxication. Cats, however, require a much higher dosage.
- Hemodialysis is highly effective at removing EG and its more toxic metabolites from the patient. Like other treatments, it is best used as early as possible following exposure.
- DEG intoxication, although rare, has similar signs to EG intoxication but without oxalate crystalluria. Both reportedly have a sweet taste, which may promote significant ingestion in some animals.

## ETIOLOGY/PATHOPHYSIOLOGY

### Mechanism of Action

- EG is metabolized by alcohol dehydrogenase into many toxic metabolites. Oxalic acid is of particular note for its high toxicity. Oxalic acid binds calcium to form calcium oxalate crystals which are found in the urine and deposited in the kidneys, causing acute kidney injury (AKI) and failure. Signs of AKI include anorexia, vomiting, lethargy, polyuria with potentially rapid progression to oliguria/anuria, and polydipsia. Hypocalcemia is often found in patients with EG intoxication. Toxic metabolites (glycoaldehyde, glyoxylic acid, oxalic acid, and especially glycolic acid) contribute to a severe metabolic acidosis and a large osmolar gap.
- DEG is metabolized through an alternative pathway in the liver to a weak acid that is ultimately filtered by the kidney and does not induce calcium oxalate crystalluria. However, clinical signs can be similar to EG intoxication.

*Blackwell's Five-Minute Veterinary Consult Clinical Companion: Small Animal Toxicology*, Third Edition.
Edited by Lynn R. Hovda, Ahna G. Brutlag, Robert H. Poppenga, and Steven E. Epstein.
© 2024 John Wiley & Sons, Inc. Published 2024 by John Wiley & Sons, Inc.

## Pharmacokinetics – Absorption, Distribution, Metabolism, Excretion

- EG is rapidly absorbed from the gastrointestinal tract with quick distribution to the blood and tissues. The plasma half-life is three hours. Some EG is excreted unchanged in the urine. However, most is metabolized by alcohol dehydrogenase to glycoaldehyde and organic acids. The liver is the primary site of metabolism. The parent compound and metabolites are usually completely eliminated by the kidneys within 24–48 hours.
- DEG has very quick absorption and metabolism, often with complete excretion in 36 hours. Diglycolic acid (DGA) is the presumed nephrotoxic metabolite of DEG.

## Toxicity

- A minimum lethal dose for undiluted EG is 6.6 mL/kg in dogs and 1.5 mL/kg for cats.
- Toxicity of DEG for dogs and cats is not well defined. In adult humans, a mean estimated fatal dose is approximately 1 mL/kg of pure DEG.

## Systems Affected

- Gastrointestinal – direct irritation causes vomiting in both dogs and cats.
- Nervous – obtundation and ataxia can be related to hyperosmolality and cerebral edema.
- Metabolic – metabolic acidosis from the organic acid metabolites is common and severe.
- Renal – with EG, renal failure occurs due to renal epithelial damage from oxalate crystalluria. DGA is believed to be accumulated by renal proximal tubular cells, resulting in cellular dysfunction and cell necrosis.

 # SIGNALMENT/HISTORY

- Clinical signs are dependent upon the species, the amount of food in the stomach (slower absorption if food present), and the amount ingested. Cats are more sensitive to intoxication but are intoxicated less often, likely due to their tendency to be more discriminating than dogs when ingesting products containing EG or DEG.

## Risk Factors

- Any pet with access to EG or DEG may be at risk.
- Given the mildly sweet flavor of these products, they may be particularly palatable to dogs. Cats may be affected by grooming spilled products off their paws.

## Historical Findings

- Exposure to EG- or DEG-containing products may be suspected or witnessed in many circumstances, but this is not always the case.
- For EG, the most common exposure is from automobile radiator leakage (antifreeze) or windshield deicing agents. However, EG is found in many products in the home or garage (paint solvent, photographic developing solutions, hydraulic brake fluid, motor oil, ink, wood stains).

## Location and Circumstances of Poisoning

- Due to the sources of EG and DEG, exposure is often within the home when the animal has access to areas where there are automobiles, workshops, or storage of leaking containers of chemicals.
- Antifreeze access can be more common in cold or freezing climates. However, exposure can occur during any season as products may be stored or leak year round.
- Malicious poisoning has been reported to occur.

## CLINICAL FEATURES

- Clinical signs may be divided into three stages: acute signs, a "recovery" phase with some resolution of initial clinical signs, and ultimately oliguric/anuric renal failure.
- Acute signs (first 30 minutes to 12 hours) are mostly related to gastric irritation (nausea, vomiting) and plasma hyperosmolality (mental dullness, ataxia – sometimes reported by owners as "drunken" behavior; osmotic diuresis with resulting polyuria and polydipsia).
- After this time, dogs often appear to have recovered until the next phase of clinical signs appears. Most cats remain depressed.
- For EG, after 12–24 hours in cats and 36–72 hours in dogs, the signs are consistent with acute oliguric renal failure (anorexia, vomiting, oral ulcers, obtundation to coma). Painful, enlarged kidneys are often found on physical examination. These signs are caused by the toxic metabolites binding calcium to form oxalate nephrolithiasis that results in renal tubular epithelial damage and rapidly progressive renal failure. Anuric renal failure develops by 72–96 hours post ingestion.

 ## DIFFERENTIAL DIAGNOSIS

- Vomiting – dietary indiscretion, foreign body/obstruction, pancreatitis.
- Ataxia – ethanol, methanol, propylene glycol, xylitol, barbiturate, ivermectin, marijuana.
- High anion gap metabolic acidosis – diabetic ketoacidosis, severe lactic acidosis, other forms of renal failure and uremia.
- Acute renal failure – NSAIDs, leptospirosis, aminoglycoside antibiotics, oxalate-containing plants (lily ingestion in cats), grapes/raisins (dogs), and acute on chronic renal failure.

 ## DIAGNOSTICS

- Blood gas – to identify a high anion gap metabolic acidosis, which occurs by three hours post EG ingestion.
- Serum biochemistry – to quantitate azotemia (occurs approximately 24–48 hours after ingestion in dogs and 12 hours in cats) and electrolyte derangements (particularly hypocalcemia). Occasionally, hyperphosphatemia may be found due to presence of a phosphate rust inhibitor in some commercial antifreeze products.
- Urinalysis – to identify calcium monohydrate or dihydrate oxalate crystalluria as well as measure urine specific gravity (often isosthenuric by three hours post ingestion).
- Measured osmolality – to compare to calculated osmolality. High osmolar gaps are commonly found by one hour following EG ingestion (often the earliest clinicopathologic change). Osmole gap diminishes as EG is metabolized but calculated/measured osmolality will increase with azotemia.
- Serum EG concentration – for confirmation of the presence of the EG or its metabolites. Point-of-care tests for EG are available that provide semi-quantitative glycol concentrations; however, false positives can occur if the patient is treated with drugs with a propylene glycol vehicle (methocarbamol, diazepam, some activated charcoal products). Point-of-care tests can be relatively insensitive (do not detect serum EG concentrations <50 mg/dL). Therefore, false-negative results can occur in some cats (toxicosis may occur below this threshold) or in animals presenting several hours after exposure (once EG is metabolized).

- Wood's lamp examination of face, paws, vomitus, or urine – due to the presence of fluorescent dyes placed in some antifreeze products.
- Abdominal ultrasonography – can aid in identification of hyperechoic kidneys late in the intoxication once calcium oxalate crystals have deposited to a significant level in renal tubules.

## Pathological Findings

- Histopathology – the kidneys are the primary target for postmortem (and rarely premortem) diagnosis of EG intoxication and show proximal tubular degeneration and necrosis with intraluminal calcium oxalate crystal deposits. Calcium oxalate crystals may also be found in a wide array of other tissues. Focal hemorrhage may be seen in the gastric and intestinal mucosa, brain, and other organs. DEG causes proximal tubular cell necrosis without crystalluria.

 # THERAPEUTICS

The goal of therapy is to inhibit metabolism, to remove the parent compound and toxic metabolites, and to correct the physiological derangements of AKI.

## Detoxification

- The rapid systemic absorption of EG and DEG following ingestion often precludes effective gastrointestinal decontamination.
- Activated charcoal is not effective for the adsorption of EG.

## Drug(s) and Antidotes of Choice

- Fomepizole and ethanol act indirectly as antidotes. Fomepizole is an ADH inhibitor and ethanol is a competitive substrate with a higher affinity for ADH than EG. Both act to interrupt metabolism of EG and DEG and thus allow time for urinary excretion of unchanged parent compound.
- Either drug can be used and they are most effective when used early. The side-effects of ethanol require that the patient be hospitalized and monitored closely due to the potential for aspiration pneumonia from recumbency. Fomepizole is often preferred since it does not require such intensive nursing care. However, fomepizole is more expensive and less available than ethanol. The complete costs for each treatment and hospitalization need to be considered.
- Dogs (choose ONE of the following treatments):
  - Fomepizole: 20 mg/kg IV followed q 12 hours by 15 mg/kg IV for two doses, then 5 mg/kg IV for one dose.
  - Ethanol IV CRI: 1.3 mL of 30% ethanol/kg IV bolus followed by 0.42 mL/kg/h for 48 hours.
  - Ethanol IV boluses: 5.5 mL 20% ethanol/kg IV q 4 hours for five treatments, then q 6 hours for four treatments.
- Cats (choose ONE of the following treatments):
  - Fomepizole (off-label): 125 mg/kg IV followed q 12 hours by 31.25 mg/kg IV for three doses.
  - Ethanol IV CRI: 1.3 mL of 30% ethanol/kg IV bolus followed by 0.42 mL/kg/h for 48 hours (note: same as dogs above).
  - Ethanol IV boluses: 5 mL 20% ethanol/kg IV q 6 hours for five treatments, then q 8 hours for four treatments.

## Extracorporeal Therapy

- In areas near specialty centers skilled at hemodialysis and extracorporeal blood purification, early referral is essential for best patient outcomes only after initial steps directed at the inhibition of EG metabolism are completed by the primary care provider.

## Appropriate Health Care

Additional treatment will revolve around correcting acid–base abnormalities, electrolyte derangements, and fluid imbalances, as well as symptomatic care.

- Correct hypocalcemia:
  - Treat severe hypocalcemia (*total* less than 7 mOsm/l, *ionized* less than 0.7 mM/l or if symptomatic – muscle twitching/fasciculations, weakness) while monitoring heart rate, EKG, and respiratory rate during.
  - Dogs: calcium gluconate 10% 5–15 mg/kg (0.5–1.5 mL/kg) IV over 20 minutes to effect.
  - Cats: calcium gluconate 10% 10–15 mg/kg (1.0–1.5 mL/kg) IV over 20 minutes to effect.
- Correct severe metabolic acidosis:
  - Treat severe metabolic acidosis (pH <7.0, bicarbonate <10 mEq/L) for dogs and cats.
  - Bicarbonate replacement (mEq required = body weight (kg) × base deficit × 0.3).
  - Administer 1/3–1/2 of the calculated replacement IV over 30 minutes.
  - Recheck blood gas and consider another infusion if pH remains below 7.2 or bicarbonate <12 mEq/L.
- Correct fluid imbalances:
  - Correct dehydration – calculate isotonic fluid replacement and administer this amount IV over 4–6 hours (or longer depending on signalment and comorbidities).
  - Provide maintenance fluids – calculate hourly isotonic fluid rate and administer at this rate hourly as long as urine output continues.
  - Administer estimated abnormal ongoing losses – provide this amount extra each hour as long as polyuria, vomiting, diarrhea, or other fluid losses continue. Reevaluate every four hours.
- Additional supportive care for symptoms associated with AKI:
  - Antiemetics, gastrointestinal protectants, and phosphate binders can be used with the above treatments at the clinician's discretion.
  - Dextrose IV should be provided as needed to prevent hypoglycemia if ethanol is used.

## Precautions/Interactions

- Treatment with ethanol alters the patient's mentation and provides temporary immobilization and sedation. As such, the patient is at higher risk for aspiration pneumonia but is not necessarily sedated sufficiently to allow endotracheal intubation. Hypothermia is also a risk.
- Rare anaphylactic reactions have been reported in dogs after a second dose of fomepizole. CNS depression may be seen in cats treated with fomepizole.

## Patient Monitoring

- Skilled nursing care for the critically ill and recumbent patient must be employed while the patient is treated with ethanol due to the higher risk of aspiration.
- Frequent monitoring and detailed reassessment of patient status and treatment orders are required for these patients over several days. Important monitoring includes mentation, temperature, urine output, hydration/fluid balance, blood pressure, and recheck bloodwork.

### Diet

- Food and water should be withheld in the recumbent patient.

## COMMENTS

### Prevention/Avoidance

- Removal of the offending substances from the reach of animals is essential to prevent exposure.
- Use propylene glycol-based antifreeze products instead of EG-based products due to their lower toxicity profile.
- Clients should be educated about prevention, as well as early intervention and treatment if exposure occurs.

### Possible Complications

- Aspiration pneumonia can be a sequela.
- Hemorrhage is possible due to anticoagulation needed for hemodialysis.
- Prevention of a septic abdomen requires diligent sterile technique and hygiene in patients receiving peritoneal dialysis.

### Expected Course and Prognosis

- Prognosis for EG depends mainly on the expediency of appropriate treatment as well as amount ingested and species. Outcomes have been reported to be good to excellent for dogs treated within 5–8 hours of ingestion and for cats treated within three hours of ingestion. However, prognosis is guarded to poor for patients with a prolonged time to treatment and poor for those with oliguric renal failure.
- Chronic renal impairment can occur even for treated EG-intoxicated patients. Renal tubular damage by EG may be reversible, but complete recovery may take months and require chronic hemodialysis. For people who survive the initial syndrome, recovery of renal function is common with hemodialysis.
- Overall mortality in dogs has been reported to range from 60% to 70%, but this value is thought to be higher in cats.
- The sequelae of DEG intoxication are currently unknown.

### Synonym

- Antifreeze toxicity/poisoning.

### Abbreviations

See Appendix 1 for a complete list.
- AKI  = acute kidney injury
- DEG = diethylene glycol
- DGA = diglycolic acid

### See Also

Chapter 8 Alcohols
Chapter 10 Propylene Glycol

## Suggested Reading

Bischoff K, Mukai M. Diethylene glycol. In: Peterson M, Talcott P (eds) *Small Animal Toxicology*, 3rd edn. St Louis: Elsevier, 2013; pp. 543–546.

Connally HE, Thrall MA, Forney SD et al. Safety and efficacy of 4-methylpyrazole as treatment for suspected or confirmed EG intoxication in dogs: 107 cases (1983–1995). *J Am Vet Med Assoc* 1996;209:1880–1883.

Connally HE, Thrall MA, Hamar DW. Safety and efficacy of high-dose fomepizole compared with ethanol as therapy for EG intoxication in cats. *J Vet Emerg Crit Care* 2010;20(2):191–206.

Lewis DH, Goggs RA. Possible DEG toxicity in a dog. *Vet Rec* 2009;164:127.

Thrall MA, Connally HE, Grauer GF, Hamar DW. Ethylene glycol. In: Peterson M, Talcott P (eds) *Small Animal Toxicology*, 3rd edn. St Louis: Elsevier, 2013; pp. 551–567.

**Authors**: Kate S. Farrell, DVM, DACVECC and Karl E. Jandrey, DVM, MAS, DACVECC
**Consulting Editor**: Robert H. Poppenga, DVM, PhD, DABVT

# Chapter 10

# Propylene Glycol

## DEFINITION/OVERVIEW

- Propylene glycol (propane-1,2-diol) is an organic compound with the chemical formula $C_3H_8O_2$. Chemical structure is $CH_3CHOHCH_2OH$.
- It is miscible with water and is used as a carrier for hydrophobic compounds that are relatively insoluble in water.
- It is a colorless, odorless liquid with a wide range of consumer, pharmaceutical, food, and industrial uses.
- Propylene glycol is also used in certain brands of automotive antifreeze. It does not produce the same syndrome as ethylene glycol-based antifreeze products.
- It has been used in veterinary medicine as a source of energy for food-producing animals (cattle, sheep, goats, pigs, poultry).
- Acute clinical effects of oral exposure include ataxia and CNS depression with lactic acidosis.
- For cats, exposure can result in Heinz body anemia.

## ETIOLOGY/PATHOPHYSIOLOGY

- Propylene glycol has been classified by the US Food and Drug Administration (FDA) as generally regarded as safe (GRAS) and is approved by the agency for use as an anticaking agent, antioxidant, dough strengthener, emulsifier, flavor agent, formulation aid, humectant, processing aid, stabilizer, and thickener, among other uses. Examples of maximum levels, as served, allowed by the US FDA include 5% for alcoholic beverages, 24% for confections and frostings, and 2.5% for frozen dairy products.
- Propylene glycol is used as a vehicle for certain pharmaceutical preparations including lorazepam, diazepam, phenobarbital, and phenytoin. Some formulations intended for IV use contain >30% propylene glycol.
- Poisoning arising from exposure to propylene glycol is occasionally observed in veterinary medicine. Most veterinary cases will involve accidental ingestion of concentrated forms of propylene glycol.
- Propylene glycol poisoning in cats has also been associated with its use in moist cat food preparations. The use of propylene glycol in cat food is contraindicated.
- Household products that may contain propylene glycol can be categorized into medicinal, cosmetic, personal hygiene, or cleaning products.

*Blackwell's Five-Minute Veterinary Consult Clinical Companion: Small Animal Toxicology*, Third Edition.
Edited by Lynn R. Hovda, Ahna G. Brutlag, Robert H. Poppenga, and Steven E. Epstein.
© 2024 John Wiley & Sons, Inc. Published 2024 by John Wiley & Sons, Inc.

■ Consumer products with high propylene glycol content can include certain soaps (14–20%), leather conditioners (10–30%), stain removers (10–40%), tire sealants (45–50%), and antifreezes (>90%).

## Mechanism of Action

■ The toxicity of propylene glycol is mainly due to the parent compound and not to its metabolites.
■ Propylene glycol has an irritant effect on direct contact with eyes, mucous membranes, and possibly after prolonged contact with skin.
■ Propylene glycol causes CNS depression. The mode of action of propylene glycol neurotoxicity is poorly understood.

## Pharmacokinetics – Absorption, Distribution, Metabolism, Excretion

■ Little is known about the pharmacokinetics of propylene glycol in dogs and cats. It is expected that data derived in people can apply to these species.
■ Propylene glycol is rapidly absorbed from the gastrointestinal tract of humans with plasma maximum concentrations observed within one hour of ingestion.
■ Propylene glycol is metabolized by alcohol dehydrogenase to lactaldehyde and then by aldehyde dehydrogenase to lactate and pyruvate. The d-lactate isomer has a greater tendency to accumulate and result in an anion gap.
■ In adult humans, approximately 45% of the administered dose of propylene glycol is eliminated through the kidney. The remaining 55% is metabolized through hepatic alcohol dehydrogenase. Approximately 30% is excreted via the kidneys as a glucuronide conjugate.
■ The elimination half-life of propylene glycol is estimated to be approximately 2–5 hours in most species.

## Toxicity

■ The acute oral $LD_{50}$ for propylene glycol in rats is approximately 20 g/kg BW/kg.
■ The acute oral $LD_{50}$ for propylene glycol in dogs is approximately 22 g/kg BW/kg. Other authors report the acute $LD_{50}$ for dogs to be as low as 9 mL/kg BW.
■ Cats appear to be more sensitive and develop an anion gap with d-lactic acidosis seen at oral doses of 1600 mg/kg BW for 35 days.
■ Signs of acute toxicosis have been reported in a dog with a propylene glycol blood concentration of 1100 mg/dL.

## Systems Affected

■ Nervous – CNS depression, ataxia.
■ Gastrointestinal – nausea, vomiting.
■ Hematological – Heinz body anemia (cat).
■ Endocrine/metabolic – metabolic acidosis, hypothermia.
■ Respiratory – increased respiratory rate and effort secondary to metabolic acidosis.

# SIGNALMENT/HISTORY

■ Canines are more commonly reported to ingest propylene glycol-based products than felines.
■ Younger animals tend to chew and drink articles not intended for their consumption.

## Risk Factors

- Prolonged elimination half-lives of 10.8–30.5 hours have been reported in preterm human neonates, suggesting that younger animals are likely at greater risk.
- Some metabolites undergo glucuronidation and in cats this is quite limited, thus reducing the effective urinary excretion of these metabolites through the kidney. This results in cats being particularly sensitive to hematological changes, manifesting as Heinz body formation and a reduced lifespan of red blood cells.
- Diabetes mellitus and hyperthyroidism are reported to increase susceptibility to Heinz body anemia, potentially worsening the severity of propylene glycol toxicosis.

## Historical Findings

- Ingestion witnessed by the owner; chewed containers found by the pet owner.
- Clinical signs including ataxia, CNS depression, and lethargy are often noted by the pet owner.

## Location and Circumstances of Poisoning

- Animals housed in the garage may be at higher risk for ingestion of propylene glycol-based products.
- Iatrogenic poisonings have been suspected following repeated use of drug formulations containing propylene glycol.

 # CLINICAL FEATURES

- High-dose exposure may result in bradycardia, CNS depression, ataxia, increased anion gap, lactic acidosis, hepatic dysfunction, or kidney injury.
- Cats have been known to also develop Heinz body formation with or without anemia.
- Rarely seen effects include seizures or coma.
- Hypotension and/or cardiovascular collapse can occur.
- Polyuria and polydipsia may occur.

 # DIFFERENTIAL DIAGNOSIS

- Other toxicants with sedative and/or CNS depressant effects.
- Other agents that produce Heinz body formation with or without anemia in cats (e.g., onion, propofol, acetaminophen, benzocaine products, phenols, methylene blue, d-L methionine, vitamin $K_3$, naphthalene, zinc, and copper).
- Other toxicants that produce metabolic acidosis, including ethylene glycol.
- Primary neurological or metabolic diseases.

 # DIAGNOSTICS

## Clinical Laboratory

- A PCV/TS, blood glucose, urinalysis, and venous blood gas should be performed to evaluate severity of electrolyte and acid–base status and to rule out other diseases.
- Acute high-dose exposure might increase d-lactic acidemia.
- Heinz body formation in cats can be observed on a peripheral blood smear. Some cats develop anemia with decreased RBC count, increased reticulocyte count, and elevated mean corpuscular hemoglobin concentration.

- Some laboratories are capable of determining propylene glycol levels in gastric contents or blood.

## Pathological Findings

- There are no specific acute gross or histological lesions observed in propylene glycol-poisoned companion animals.
- Heinz body formation may be observed in cats.

# THERAPEUTICS

## Detoxification

- Propylene glycol is absorbed relatively quickly from the gastrointestinal tract. Thus the use of emetics may have limited effectiveness.
- If a large amount of gastric contents is present in a symptomatic patient, gastric lavage may need to be performed under sedation and with an inflated endotracheal tube to prevent aspiration.
- Propylene glycol is likely poorly adsorbed by activated charcoal. Therefore activated charcoal and cathartics are rarely recommended.
- If dermal exposure has occurred, rinse the affected area with a mild detergent shampoo and water.
- Forced diuresis is generally not effective.
- Hemodialysis may be an effective means of enhancing elimination of propylene glycol from the body and can therefore be beneficial in cases expected to be potentially life-threatening or associated with high morbidity.

## Drugs and Antidotes of Choice

- The efficacy of fomepizole, an alcohol dehydrogenase inhibitor, in the treatment of propylene glycol toxicosis toxicity is unclear.
- Therapy should include careful rehydration with dextrose solution to correct hypoglycemia.
- A balanced, isotonic crystalloid IV fluid can be used in symptomatic patients to aid in correction of dehydration.
- In the presence of a severe metabolic acidosis (e.g., pH <7.0, BE ≤15 mmHg, $HCO_3$ <11 mmHg), the judicious use of sodium bicarbonate can be considered.
- Ascorbic acid can be used in cats as an antioxidant. However, research with cats indicates that common antioxidants (e.g., N-acetylcysteine, d-l alpha-tocopherol, ascorbic acid) are not effective in reducing the hematological effects of propylene glycol.

## Appropriate Health Care

- Hospitalization may be required to manage severe CNS depression, metabolic acidosis, and respiratory depression.
- If respiratory function is compromised, a cuffed endotracheal tube should be placed and ventilation supported mechanically as required.
- Maintaining normal body temperature is important.
- Propylene glycol toxicosis can result in severe CNS depression/coma and appropriate nursing care is imperative. Patients should be kept in a padded cage and should be turned every six hours to prevent atelectasis.
- Provide respiratory support and mechanical ventilation if needed.
- Monitor temperature, heart rate, and respiratory rate.

- Monitor blood pressure and blood glucose frequently and treat appropriately.
- Ophthalmic lubrication may be necessary every six hours.
- Keep the patient clean and dry.

### Precautions/Interactions

- If other substances have been coingested (or injected in the case of pharmaceutical agents), initiate specific treatment for those substances, if available.

### Follow-up

- Follow-up is generally unnecessary, as patients are clinically normal once signs resolve.

### Activity

- Patients should be restricted from activity until clinical signs resolve, as ataxia and CNS depression will be apparent. Once clinical signs resolve, no exercise restriction is necessary.

 ## COMMENTS

### Prevention/Avoidance

- Prevention is critical. Advise clients that propylene glycol-containing products are potentially dangerous for their pets. Educate clients about common sources of propylene glycol available in the home (e.g., certain automotive antifreezes).
- Do not use propylene glycol as a food additive in cats.
- Early treatment is also important. Clients should be taught to contact their veterinarian if an exposure has occurred or an animal is displaying unusual clinical signs.

### Patient Monitoring

- Acid–base monitoring is recommended in symptomatic animals.
- Blood glucose concentrations should be monitored frequently.

### Expected Course and Prognosis

- Most exposures are not expected to result in clinical signs.
- Most cases involving mild signs usually resolve with close monitoring and supportive care within a 24-hour period.
- No long-term effects are expected unless brain injury secondary to prolonged respiratory depression and hypoxia has occurred.
- The prognosis can be good even in cases involving metabolic acidosis and moderate CNS depression.
- Monitor RBC morphology, which should return to normal 6–8 weeks post exposure (cats).

### Abbreviations

See Appendix 1 for a complete list.
- GRAS = generally regarded as safe

### Suggested Reading

Bauer MC, Weiss DJ, Perman V. Hematologic alterations in adult cats fed 6% or 12% propylene glycol. *Am J Vet Res* 1992;53(1):69–72.
Bischoff K. Propylene glycol. In: Peterson ME, Talcott PA (eds) *Small Animal Toxicology*. St Louis: Elsevier, 2006; pp. 996–1001.

Claus MA, Jandrey KE, Poppenga RH. Propylene glycol intoxication in a dog. *J Vet Emerg Crit Care* 2011;21:679–683.

Fowles JR, Banton MI, Pottenger LH. A toxicological review of the propylene glycols. *Crit Rev Toxicol* 2013;43(4):363–390.

Peterson J, Stadlen R, Radke J. Propylene glycol toxicity from compulsive corn starch ingestion. *Am J Emerg Med* 2022;53:286.e1–286.e3.

**Author:** David C. Dorman, DVM, PhD, DABVT, DABT
**Consulting Editor:** Robert H. Poppenga, DVM, PhD, DABVT

# Construction and Industrial Materials

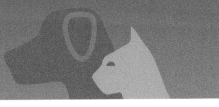

# Chapter 11

# Glues and Adhesives

## DEFINITION/OVERVIEW

- Cyanoacrylate glues or adhesives, also called instant glues, have uses in the home as well as in the medical field as tissue adhesives. Common brand names include Super Glue and Krazy Glue®.
- Dermal or GI exposure to cyanoacrylate adhesives can result in local tissue adhesions, skin irritation, and GI irritation. Adhesions and gastroenteritis are usually mild, self-limiting, and easily treated.
- Diisocyanate glues can include wood glue, construction glue, and high-strength glues. Gorilla Glue™ is a common brand name.
- Diisocyanate glue ingestion results in GI irritation and risk for foreign body obstruction due to glue expansion, often necessitating surgical intervention. Inhalation may cause airway irritation.
- Polyvinyl acetate (PVA or PVAc) glues or adhesives are typically rubbery, water-soluble glues used on paper, for crafts, and children's activities. Elmer's glue is a common brand name. Ingestion may cause minor gastroenteritis.
- Glue traps, used to trap insects and rodents, do not typically contain insecticides or rodenticides but may contain small amounts of eugenol and do not pose a systemic toxicity concern. Ingestion can be irritating to the mouth and GI tract.

## ETIOLOGY/PATHOPHYSIOLOGY

### Mechanism of Action

- On contact with the skin or mucous membranes, cyanoacrylate glue hardens and adheres to surfaces.
- Diisocyanate adhesive expands significantly in the moist environment of the GI tract. Inhalation causes irritation to the lungs.

### Toxicokinetics – Adsorption, Distribution, Metabolism, Excretion

- No significant systemic absorption occurs with the glues described in the Definition/Overview section.

### Toxicity

- Ingestion of glues described in this chapter is typically considered a nontoxic ingestion.
- Small amounts of ingested diisocyanate (as little as 0.5 oz) can result in foreign body obstruction.

---

*Blackwell's Five-Minute Veterinary Consult Clinical Companion: Small Animal Toxicology*, Third Edition. Edited by Lynn R. Hovda, Ahna G. Brutlag, Robert H. Poppenga, and Steven E. Epstein. © 2024 John Wiley & Sons, Inc. Published 2024 by John Wiley & Sons, Inc.

### Systems Affected

- Cyanoacrylate glues.
    - Gastrointestinal: gastroenteritis, oral adhesions.
    - Skin: dermal irritation, adhesions.
    - Respiratory: inhalation irritation, upper airway obstruction (rare).
    - Ophthalmic: corneal irritation, eyelid adhesions.
- Diisocyanate glues.
    - Gastrointestinal: gastroenteritis, foreign body obstruction (common).
    - Skin: dermal irritation, adhesions.
    - Respiratory: tachypnea, coughing, sneezing, airway obstruction (rare).

 # SIGNALMENT/HISTORY

### Risk Factors

- Dogs are more commonly affected than cats due to chewing behaviors. No breed or sex predilection.
- Younger animals are more commonly affected due to indiscriminate chewing.

### Historical Findings

- Pet owners frequently report a chewed product container or ingestion of material with glue on it. Glue may also be noted on the skin or teeth.
- Anorexia and vomiting are commonly reported.

### Location and Circumstances of Poisoning

- Most exposures occur in the home, garage, or work area.

 # CLINICAL FEATURES

- Cyanoacrylate.
    - Clinical signs occur within seconds to minutes of glue exposure.
    - Most common signs include glue adherence to the fur, teeth, tongue or mucous membranes and local tissue adhesions.
    - Vomiting can occur with large ingestions.
    - Oropharyngeal obstruction from glue can cause cyanosis and respiratory distress.
- Diisocyanate.
    - Clinical signs occur within 15 minutes up to 20 hours after ingestion.
    - Most common clinical signs are consistent with gastroenteritis and GI foreign body obstruction and include retching/gagging, vomiting, anorexia, abdominal pain, and abdominal distension. Dehydration can develop with prolonged clinical signs.
    - Tachypnea can be seen with inhalation of fumes or with pain secondary to GI obstruction.

 # DIFFERENTIAL DIAGNOSIS

- Cyanoacrylate.
    - Gastrointestinal signs: foreign body obstruction, gastroenteritis, pancreatitis, inflammatory bowel disease, metabolic disease.
    - Respiratory signs: upper airway obstruction, laryngeal paralysis, lower airway disease.

- Diisocyanate.
    - Gastrointestinal signs: foreign body obstruction, food bloat, gastric dilation and volvulus, gastroenteritis, pancreatitis, inflammatory bowel disease, metabolic disease.
    - Respiratory signs: asthma, bronchitis, pneumonia, pulmonary edema.

 # DIAGNOSTICS

## Clinical Pathological Findings

- CBC and chemistry: no significant changes expected.

## Other Diagnostics

- Abdominal radiographs (4–24 hours after exposure) for diisocyanate ingestion often show a mottled gas and soft tissue opacity within the stomach lumen with gastric distension often resembling food ingestion (Figure 11.1).

## Pathological Findings

- Cyanoacrylate: no specific gross or histopathological findings aside from tissue adhesions.
- Diisocyanate: gross findings include a foreign body present within the stomach. Mucosal congestion, ulceration, and laceration noted on histopathological findings.

 # THERAPEUTICS

## Detoxification

- Gastrointestinal.
    - Emesis can be performed immediately after exposure with large ingestions but is generally not recommended due to risk for esophageal and GI obstruction.

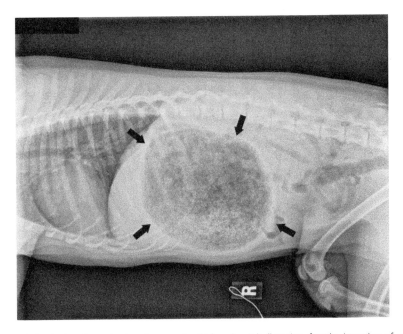

■ Figure 11.1 Abdominal radiograph of a nine-month-old female pit bull terrier after the ingestion of approximately 1.5 oz of Gorilla Glue 12 hours previously. Surgical extraction yielded a large, firm, glue obstruction, approximately 7–8 inches in diameter. Note the similarity of the glue to food or ingesta. Source: Photo courtesy of Dr Catherine A. Angle.

- Gastric lavage can be attempted but is generally not successful due to rapid expansion of diisocyanate glue.
- Activated charcoal is not recommended.
- Respiratory.
  - Oxygen therapy as needed.
  - Airway obstruction requires a sedated oral exam for glue removal.
- Ocular.
  - Irrigate for 15 minutes with eye wash or room temperature water.
  - Fluorescein stain if indicated.
  - May need sedation or anesthesia for eyelid adhesions.
- Skin.
  - Warm, soapy water or vegetable oil rubbed onto fur or teeth to loosen glue adhesions. Remove glue from fur with clippers as needed. Glue not causing morbidity does not need to be removed and will wear off with time.

## Appropriate Health Care

- Treatment of nonobstructive ingestion involves removal of glue from skin or fur and supportive care for GI symptoms. Surgery for foreign body removal is often needed for diisocyanate ingestion.
- IV fluids as needed for dehydration and postsurgical care.

## Drug(s) of Choice

- Antiemetics as needed such as maropitant 1 mg/kg SQ q 24 hours. May mask signs of foreign body obstruction but antiemetics are recommended in symptomatic patients, especially if serial radiographs are being performed.

## Precautions/Interactions

- Avoid prokinetics such as metoclopramide until a foreign body obstruction has been ruled out.

## Surgical Considerations

- Exploratory laparotomy and gastrotomy needed for dogs with evidence of a gastric obstruction.
- Postoperatively, patients should be monitored for hydration, vomiting, diarrhea, appetite, and pain. Postsurgical analgesia should be provided.

## Patient Monitoring

Recheck postsurgical patients in 10–14 days for suture/staple removal.

## Diet

Nutritional supplementation as needed postoperatively.

    **COMMENTS**

### Prevention/Avoidance

- Owners should be educated about the dangers of glue expansion and the high risk of foreign body obstruction.
- Keep pets out of areas where glues and adhesives are being used or stored.

## Possible Complications

■ Postoperative ileus and incisional dehiscence can occur.
■ Gastric rupture can occur with diisocyanate obstruction if left untreated.

## Expected Course and Prognosis

■ With mild, nonobstructive ingestion, symptoms generally resolve within 24 hours.
■ Prognosis is generally good if treated appropriately.
■ Up to 75% of patients need surgery after diisocyanate ingestion. Surgery for foreign body removal can prolong and complicate recovery.

## Synonyms

■ Cyanoacrylate glue: instant glue, Krazy Glue, Super Glue.
■ Diisocyanate glue: 4,4'-diphenyl methane diisocyanate, diphenylmethyl diisocyanate, diphenylmethane diisocyanate (MDI), methylenedi-p-phenyl diisocyanate, Gorilla Glue.

## See Also

Chapter 80 Foreign Objects

## Abbreviations

See Appendix 1 for a complete list.

### Suggested Reading

Bailey T. The expanding threat of polyurethane adhesive ingestion. *Vet Tech* 2004;25;426–428.
Fitzgerald KT, Bronstein AC. Polyurethane adhesive ingestion. *Topics Compan Anim Med* 2013;28:28–31.
Friday S, Murphy C, Lopez D, Mayhew P, Holt D. Gorilla Glue ingestion in dogs: 22 cases (2005–2019). *J Am Anim Hosp Assoc* 2021;57(3):121–127.
Horstman CL, Eubig PA, Khan SA et al. Gastric outflow obstruction after ingestion of wood glue in a dog. *J Am Anim Hosp Assoc* 2003;39:47–51.
Lubich C, Mrvos R, Krenzelok EP. Beware of canine *Gorilla glue* ingestions. *Vet Human Toxicol* 2004;46:153–154.

**Author**: Katherine L. Peterson, DVM, DACVECC, DABT
**Consulting Editor**: Ahna G. Brutlag, DVM, MS, DABT, DABVT

# Chapter 12

# Hydrocarbons

## DEFINITION/OVERVIEW

- Hydrocarbons encompass a large group of chemicals that contain hydrogen and carbon as main constituents (Figures 12.1, 12.2).
- Toxicity depends on the volatility and viscosity of the product. Examples:
  - Highly volatile: benzene, toluene, and xylene.
    - Primarily CNS signs.
  - Intermediate volatility, low to intermediate viscosity: gasoline and kerosene.
    - Either CNS or respiratory changes or both. This is the most common hydrocarbon exposure in pets.
  - Low volatility, low viscosity: mineral seal oil in furniture products.
    - Severe respiratory changes after aspiration of product directly or when vomited.

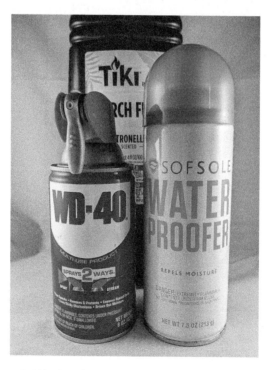

■ **Figure 12.1** Common household hydrocarbon-based products.

*Blackwell's Five-Minute Veterinary Consult Clinical Companion: Small Animal Toxicology*, Third Edition.
Edited by Lynn R. Hovda, Ahna G. Brutlag, Robert H. Poppenga, and Steven E. Epstein.
© 2024 John Wiley & Sons, Inc. Published 2024 by John Wiley & Sons, Inc.

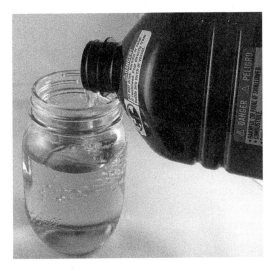

■ Figure 12.2 Demonstrating the low volatility and high viscosity nature of Tiki® Torch Oil with ingredients of white mineral oil and citronella oil.

- • Low volatility, high viscosity: Mineral oil, diesel fuel, motor oil.
  - o Lower risk for toxicity unless aspirated.
- ■ Toxicity depends on the route of exposure, the dose, and the duration of exposure.
- ■ Hydrocarbon exposure most often occurs after ingestion and may lead to gastrointestinal irritation, aspiration, and CNS depression. Less commonly reported complications include CNS excitation, dermal irritation or burns, ocular irritation or burns, cardiovascular arrhythmias. Rare renal damage, hepatic damage, and intravascular hemolysis have been reported in humans.

 ## ETIOLOGY/PATHOPHYSIOLOGY

### Mechanism of Action

- ■ Dermal: direct irritant. Dissolution of lipid membranes to impart damage, causing irritation in acute exposures, drying, and defatting in chronic exposure.
- ■ Ocular and ingestion: direct irritant.
- ■ Respiratory: intermediate and low-viscosity hydrocarbons with low surface tension carry risk for aspiration when ingested or vomited, resulting in direct toxic effects. Pneumonia and pulmonary tissue damage, pulmonary edema and/or hemorrhage may develop.
- ■ CNS: mechanism is unclear, but hypoxia may play a role. Lipophilic hydrocarbons may dissolve nerve cell membranes and disrupt cell function.
- ■ Cardiovascular: mechanism is unclear, and this outcome is rare in dogs and cats. Hydrocarbons can lead to myocardial sensitization to catecholamines and consequent arrhythmias.
- ■ Systemic effects after exposure to hydrocarbons are otherwise uncommon. Rare renal damage, liver damage, and hemolysis are reported in humans.

### Toxicokinetics – Adsorption, Distribution, Metabolism, Excretion

- ■ Wide variety of compounds with variable ADME. In general:
- ■ Absorption:
  - • Ingestion: poorly absorbed.
  - • Dermal: poorly absorbed from healthy skin.
  - • Inhalation/aspiration: vapors rapidly absorbed.

- Distribution: aliphatic hydrocarbons may preferentially distribute to fatty tissues.
- Metabolism:
  - Hepatic: oxidation by CYP450 and conjugation to water-soluble compounds.
    - May either activate or detoxify hydrocarbons.
- Excretion:
  - Primary: renal.
  - Secondary: exhalation, hepatobiliary.

## Toxicity

- Wide variety of compounds with variable toxicity.
- Oral $LD_{50}$ in rat models shows a wide variability between specific agents.
  - Gasoline: 13 600 mg/kg.
  - Kerosene: 15 000 mg/kg.
  - Mineral spirits: >5000 mg/kg.

## Systems Affected

- Gastrointestinal: vomiting or diarrhea. Vomiting will increase aspiration risk.
- Respiratory: respiratory irritation with subsequent coughing and tachypnea. Aspiration pneumonia and pneumonitis with subsequent hypoxemia and pulmonary edema may occur.
- Nervous: inhalation of vapors may cause CNS depression or agitation, ataxia, tremors, and rare seizures. Aspiration and subsequent hypoxemia may also lead to depression.
- Cardiovascular: inhalation can cause nonspecific arrhythmias (e.g., VPCs) and cardiac sensitization. Compounds that more profoundly affect the CNS will also lead to more significant cardiac abnormalities.
- Skin/exocrine: mild to moderate dermal irritation. Chronic exposure may lead to drying and defatting. Rare caustic injury may occur.
- Ophthalmic: ocular irritation, rarely ulceration.
- Renal/urologic: chronic exposure may rarely lead to acute renal failure.
- Hepatobiliary: chronic exposure may rarely lead to nonspecific liver injury.
- Heme/lymphatic/immune: rare intravascular hemolysis,

 # SIGNALMENT/HISTORY

## Risk Factors

- Pediatrics, geriatrics, and those animals with concurrent disease are at increased risk.

## Location and Circumstances of Poisoning

- Frequently found with spilled material or containers that have been chewed.
- Animals may be left in a poorly ventilated area following a spill of a volatile hydrocarbon.
- Animals with saturated fur coats may continue to inhale or groom and ingest the product.

 # CLINICAL FEATURES

- Dependent on route of exposure.
- The fur/coat and breath may smell strongly of the hydrocarbon.
- Oral exposure: mucosal irritation, salivation, vomiting, diarrhea, poor appetite. Vomiting may lead to aspiration. Rarely HGE and caustic injury. Onset of GI signs is 1–4 hours with a duration of 24–48 hours.

- Inhalation exposure: CNS depression or agitation, ataxia, coughing, wheezing, gagging, and tachypnea. Monitor for aspiration pneumonia – onset of respiratory changes: 1–24 hours with a duration of 3–10 days. CNS signs resolve quickly after patient is moved to fresh air and bathed. Cardiac arrhythmias may occur after inhalation.
- Dermal exposure: erythema, dermatitis, thermal injury from hot oils and tars.
- Ocular exposure: injected sclera, conjunctival irritation, blepharospasm, lacrimation, pawing at the face. Corneal ulceration is rare.
- Hyperthermia may be noted in cases of aspiration pneumonia.

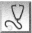

# DIFFERENTIAL DIAGNOSIS

- Primary or infectious respiratory disease.
- Primary GI disease including gastroenteritis, ingestion of other GI irritants such as plants, cleaning products, foreign material, essential oils, etc.
- Primary dermal disease, atopic dermatitis, hypersensitivity, external parasites, exposure to other irritants such as household cleaners.
- Intoxications: CNS depressants, hepatotoxins (e.g., acetaminophen, xylitol, cycad/sago palm), renal toxins (e.g., ibuprofen, grapes/raisins, ethylene glycol).

# DIAGNOSTICS

## Clinical Pathological Findings

- CBC: leukocytosis +/- a left shift indicative of pneumonia. Rare hemolytic anemia.
- Chemistry profile: BUN, creatinine, ALT, AST, ALP elevations possible in chronic exposures. Mild elevations in BUN, creatinine, and total protein may occur secondary to dehydration.
- Urinalysis – urine specific gravity alterations dependent on hydration and renal status.

## Other Diagnostics

- Radiographs – right middle or multilobular pneumonia consistent with aspiration or pulmonary edema in severe cases. Changes may be delayed up to 8–24 hours.
- ECG – nonspecific tachyarrhythmia.

## Pathological Findings

- Pulmonary edema, pulmonary hemorrhage, and damage to the pulmonary epithelium and surfactant layers may be noted. Rarely reports of renal cell degeneration or fatty changes to the liver.

# THERAPEUTICS

- Efforts focused on decontamination, symptomatic, and supportive care.
- Critically ill patients may require aggressive support with oxygen or a ventilator, stringent monitoring and treatment of cardiac arrhythmias. Once stabilized, transfer to a referral center should be considered.

## Detoxification

- Dermal:
  - Bathe with a nonmedicated degreasing shampoo or hand dishwashing soap. Several baths may be necessary.

- Clip the fur to remove thick or dried products such as tar/asphalt. The use of solvents is not recommended.
- Ocular:
  - Irrigate eyes, including beneath the third eyelid/nictitans.
  - Elizabethan collar to prevent self-trauma.
- Ingestion:
  - Rinse the oral cavity for 15 minutes.
  - Emesis and gastric lavage: **contraindicated** due to risk of aspiration.
  - Activated charcoal: **contraindicated**. It will not bind to hydrocarbons and may increase the risk for aspiration.

## Appropriate Health Care

- Ocular.
  - Fluorescein stain, slit lamp examination.
  - Topical medication as needed.
- Dermal.
  - Mild irritation: vitamin E oil, skin protectants, topical antibiotic if needed.
  - Moderate-to-severe dermatitis: topical steroids.
  - Severe dermal compromise (burns and blistering): wound care, antibiotics, and analgesics.
- Oral exposures.
  - Oral exam for rare injury.
  - Antiemetics:
    - Maropitant 1 mg/kg SQ or IV q 24 hours.
    - Ondansetron 0.1–0.5 mg/kg IV q 8 hours.
    - Gastroprotectants:
      Omeprazole 1 mg/kg PO q 12 hours.
      Famotidine 1 mg/kg PO, SQ, IM, or IV q 12 hours.
      Sucralfate: 0.5–1 g/dog (not mg/kg) PO q 8 hours.
    - GI support diet × 5–7 days.
  - If rare oral injury is noted, endoscopy may be needed to evaluate the extent of injury. Consider broad-spectrum antibiotics, analgesics, and nutritional support.
  - Animals exhibiting respiratory distress after ingestion or inhalation of hydrocarbons will require hospitalization and aggressive care.
  - Prophylactic use of antibiotics and steroids is generally not recommended.
- Inhalation/respiratory exposure.
  - Thoracic radiographs to determine the extent of pulmonary injury in symptomatic animals. Radiographic changes may be delayed 8–24 hours.
  - Supplemental oxygen or mechanical ventilation.
  - Blood gas analysis in severely affected cases.
  - Beta-2-agonists such as albuterol may be needed for bronchodilation.
  - Nebulization.
  - Use of antibiotics for aspiration pneumonia is controversial.
- Cardiac signs.
  - Low-stimulus environment.
  - Beta-blockers for ventricular dysrhythmias.
    - Propranolol 0.02–0.06 mg/kg IV slowly.
    - Esmolol 0.25–0.5 mg/kg followed by 10–200 mcg/kg/min CRI.
  - Use of epinephrine is reserved for resuscitation needs only, as it may precipitate arrhythmias.

- Renal impairment.
  - IV fluids: 2–3 times maintenance × 48 hours or until azotemia resolves.
- Hepatobiliary disease.
  - Hepatoprotectants.
    - S-adenosyl-methionine (SAMe): 17–20 mg/kg PO q 24 hours.
    - Silymarin/milk thistle: 20–50 mg/kg PO q 24 hours.
      Consider commercial combination products dosed by body weight according to manufacturer instructions (e.g. Denamarin®).
    - N-acetylcysteine (NAC) in severe cases. Dilute to 5% solution, loading dose 140–280 mg/kg IV through a 0.2 micron filter or PO followed by 70 mg/kg IV or PO q 6 hours for 48–96 hours.

## Antidote

None.

## Precautions/Interactions

- Emesis induction, gastric lavage, and activated charcoal are contraindicated due to risk of aspiration.
- Use sympathomimetic agents cautiously if arrhythmias are detected due to sensitization of the myocardium.

## Alternative Drugs

- If clinical signs are mild, symptomatic outpatient care is appropriate. This may include ocular/oral irrigation, bathing, antiemetics and gastrointestinal support, and subcutaneous fluids. The patient should be reevaluated if progressive signs or respiratory changes are noted.

## Patient Monitoring

- Owners should monitor closely for gastrointestinal signs and subsequent respiratory signs for 12–24 hours.
- If aspiration pneumonia occurs, intermittent monitoring of CBC and thoracic radiographs may be warranted until the patient has recovered.

## Diet

- A gastrointestinal diet may be considered as needed.

      # COMMENTS

### Prevention/Avoidance

- Products should be used in a well-ventilated area, appropriate personal protection worn, and pets should be kept away from these areas until space is fully ventilated.
- Store products in secure areas that limit accessibility and in the labeled original containers with tight, child-proof seals.

### Expected Course and Prognosis

- Course and prognosis depend on the type of exposure and the severity of signs.
- Animals remaining free of respiratory problems for 12–24 hours following exposure carry a good prognosis.
- Moderate-to-high morbidity, low mortality rate.

## See Also

Chapter 87 Essential Oils and Liquid Potpourri
Chapter 95 Phenols and Pine Oils

## Suggested Reading

Bates N. Risks from exposure to petroleum distillates in pets. *Compan Anim* 2016;21(12):706–711.

Dorman DC. Petroleum distillates and turpentine. *Vet Clin North Am Sm Anim Pract* 1990;20(2):505–513.

Lifshitz M, Sofer S, Gorodischer R. Hydrocarbon poisoning in children: a 5-year retrospective study. *Wilderness Environ Med* 2003;14(2):78–82.

Murphy LA, Gwaltney-Brant SM, Albretsen JC, Wismer TA. Toxicologic agents of concern for search-and-rescue dogs responding to urban disasters. *J Am Vet Med Assoc* 2003;222(3):296–304.

Young BC, Strom AM, Prittie JE, Barton LJ. Toxic pneumonitis caused by inhalation of hydrocarbon water-proofing spray in two dogs. *J Am Vet Med Assoc* 2007;231(1):74–78.

## Acknowledgments

The author and editors acknowledge the prior contributions of Stephen H. LeMaster, PharmD, MPH, who authored this topic in a previous edition.

**Author**: Holly Hommerding, DVM, DABT, DABVT
**Consulting Editor**: Ahna G. Brutlag, DVM, MS, DABT, DABVT

# Chapter 13

# Hydrofluoric Acid

## DEFINITION/OVERVIEW

- Hydrofluoric acid (HF) is an inorganic weak acid used in glass etching, metal polishing, rust removers, automotive cleaning products (e.g., wheel cleaners), aluminum brighteners, and industrial metal cleaners and degreasers.
- Unlike most acids which cause immediate pain and superficial burns without systemic acidosis, HF penetrates deep into tissue, disassociates into hydrogen and free fluoride ions, and can result in serious systemic intoxication.
- Free fluoride ions bind to calcium and magnesium to form insoluble complexes that precipitate in tissue, leading to serious burns to the eyes, skin, and GI tract as well as systemic effects including hypocalcemia, cardiac abnormalities, and death.
- Any product containing HF should be considered potentially toxic.

## ETIOLOGY/PATHOPHYSIOLOGY

### Mechanism of Action

- HF penetrates deep into tissue layers and dissociates into hydrogen and fluoride ions.
- Free fluoride ions bind to calcium and, to a lesser extent, magnesium to form insoluble complexes that precipitate in tissue, leading to pain, necrosis, and bone decalcification.
- Severe hypocalcemia and hypomagnesemia (less common), with resulting potassium efflux and hyperkalemia, may cause myocardial irritability and dysrhythmias.
- Fluoride ions also bind and inhibit multiple enzyme systems, including acetylcholinesterase, adenyl cyclase, and Na-K ATPase, which results in excessive cholinergic stimulation and potassium efflux.

### Toxicokinetics – Adsorption, Distribution, Metabolism, Excretion

- HF is highly lipophilic and readily absorbed via any route of exposure. Systemic absorption occurs readily from the stomach because of its acidic environment.
- Fluoride volume of distribution is 0.5–0.7 L/kg.
- Fluoride is not metabolized and is excreted by the kidney, with a small percentage (5–10%) excreted in the feces.
- Fluoride elimination half-life is 2–9 hours.

### Toxicity

- Corrosive to skin and mucous membranes, especially with concentrations >5%.
  - Systemic toxicosis is possible from dermal exposures with low to moderately concentrated products (i.e., even <10% can be harmful).

*Blackwell's Five-Minute Veterinary Consult Clinical Companion: Small Animal Toxicology*, Third Edition. Edited by Lynn R. Hovda, Ahna G. Brutlag, Robert H. Poppenga, and Steven E. Epstein. © 2024 John Wiley & Sons, Inc. Published 2024 by John Wiley & Sons, Inc.

- Electrolyte imbalance, dysrhythmias, and death have been reported in human adult following ingestion of 2–3 oz of 6–8% HF.
- In a 10 kg child, the MTD is 50 mg.
- Deep penetration of fluoride ions into the anterior chamber structures of the eye can cause stromal corneal edema, sloughing, and conjunctival ischemia.
- $LC_{50}$ (inhalation):
  - Rat: 1276 ppm/1 hour.
  - Guinea pig: 4327 ppm/15 minutes.
  - Monkey: 1774 ppm/1 hour.

## Systems Affected

- Dermatological – severe and potentially delayed pain, erythema, edema, and necrosis.
- Gastrointestinal – nausea, vomiting, diarrhea, esophagitis, gastritis (may be hemorrhagic), dysphagia, corrosive burns throughout GI tract.
- Ocular – pain, corneal burns, necrosis, and opacification. Conjunctivitis may persist for several months.
- Respiratory – nasal irritation, mucosal inflammation, cough, dyspnea, bronchospasm, chemical pneumonitis, pulmonary edema (often hemorrhagic), and chemical burns to the upper airways can also occur (onset may be delayed).
- Cardiovascular – QTc prolongation, Torsade de Pointes, dysrhythmias, and cardiac arrest.
- Electrolyte and acid–base – hypocalcemia, hyperkalemia, hypomagnesemia, and metabolic acidosis.
- Bone – decalcification and dissolution.
- Neuromuscular – anxiety, confusion, seizures, paresthesia, paralysis, and tetany from hypocalcemia and hyperkalemia.

 # SIGNALMENT/HISTORY

### Historical Findings

- Exposure to rust removers, automotive cleaning products, or other products containing HF.
- Clinical signs following topical exposure are often delayed. As a result, HF exposure in animals may not be reported until toxicosis is severe.

### Location and Circumstances of Poisoning

- The most common household products are rust removers. Cases reported to Pet Poison Helpline often involve dogs drinking from toilets or bathtubs where HF-containing rust removers were used.
- HF is more commonly used in industrial settings: car wash/auto detailing (wheels/tire cleaners); etching and cleaning silicone, glass, metal, stone and porcelain; enameling and galvanizing; gasoline production; oil wells; aluminum production.

 # CLINICAL FEATURES

- Ingestion: signs may begin within 1–2 hours and include oral irritation, vomiting, hypersalivation, anorexia, dysphagia, +/- pain (may be delayed). Ultimately, expect ulcerations and necrosis. May see signs associated with increased bronchial secretions secondary to cholinergic stimulation.
- Dermal exposure: pain and erythema may be delayed:
  - Up to 24 hours if HF concentration is <20%.
  - Up to 8 hours if HF concentration is between 20% and 50%.
  - No delay if HF concentration is >50%.

- Ocular: immediate or delayed pain (concentration dependent), irritation, conjunctival injection, corneal abrasion/ulceration.
- As toxicosis progresses, may see evidence of pain and whitish erosive or ulcerative lesions (calcium precipitates) at the sites of tissue contact. Severe cases may show signs of hypocalcemic tetany, weakness, and collapse (secondary to cardiac arrhythmias).
- In dog studies, death following HF exposure was often the result of delayed sudden cardiovascular collapse with ventricular fibrillation.

# DIFFERENTIAL DIAGNOSIS

- Intoxications: aspirin, tricyclic antidepressants, beta-blockers, calcium channel blockers or other fluoride-containing products may result in some similarities such as metabolic acidosis or hypocalcemia but they will **not** have accompanying tissue damage or severe pain.
- Corrosive injury from other products (acids, alkaline agents, etc.) will **not** have concurrent hypocalcemia.

# DIAGNOSTICS

## Clinical Pathological Findings

- Serum biochemistry and ionized calcium – hypocalcemia and hyperkalemia; potential hypomagnesemia, azotemia.
- Blood gases – metabolic acidosis.
- Urinalysis – hematuria and proteinuria indicate renal dysfunction.

## Other Diagnostics

- ECG – QTc prolongation, peaked T-waves/arrhythmias, or dysrhythmias.
- Endoscopic evaluation within 12 hours to evaluate for esophageal/gastric ulceration, especially if exposed to concentrated HF. Lesion development may be delayed up to 24 hours in burns with HF concentrations <20%.
- Thoracic radiographs to evaluate for pneumonitis or pulmonary edema.
- Urine or serum fluoride results would likely not return within a clinically relevant timeframe.

## Pathological Findings

- Necropsy may reveal GI erosion, hemorrhagic pulmonary edema and/or burns to the pulmonary tract; severe, deep necrotic tissue damage; corneal erosion, necrosis.

# THERAPEUTICS

## Detoxification

- Ensure all veterinary caregivers wear appropriate PPE.
- Dermal – immediately/at home, irrigate with copious amounts of lukewarm water for at least 30 minutes. Bathe with hand dish washing detergent if needed. Rub 2.5% calcium gluconate or carbonate gel to affected area for 15–30 minutes, reapplying q 15–30 minutes. Gel will turn white as it binds fluoride ions. Rub into affected area and reapply new gel every 15 minutes until pain subsides/white discoloration ceases. Reapply 4–6 times daily for four days.
  - If calcium gluconate gel is unavailable, it can be made by mixing 25 mL of 10% Ca gluconate with 75 mL sterile water-soluble lubricant.

- Ingestion – do **not** induce vomiting (due to corrosivity) or give activated charcoal. Immediately/at home, administer a calcium- (preferred) or magnesium-containing product such as milk (1 oz/10 lb), chewable calcium carbonate tablets (1–2 tab/15 lb), or milk of magnesia (5 mL/15 lb). If a large volume of HF was ingested, consider removal via a nasogastric tube if within one hour of exposure and lavage with 10% calcium gluconate solution.
- Ocular – immediately/at home, irrigate with water, eye wash, or saline for 15 minutes (calcium solutions have not been shown to be more effective than saline for ocular irrigation). Topical ophthalmic anesthetic solutions may be used during this process. Continue irrigation until ocular pH is normal (check with litmus paper). Excessive irrigation may result in worse outcome. Obtain ophthalmology consultation.
- Inhalation – immediately administer humidified oxygen and assist with ventilation as needed. Administer 2.5% calcium gluconate by nebulizer.

### Appropriate Health Care

- Asymptomatic patients with minimal exposure to <5% HF solutions should be decontaminated, have baseline electrolytes measured, and observed in hospital for at least six hours. Administer GI protectants (see Drugs of Choice) and recheck electrolytes q 4–6 hours.
- Animals with unknown or larger exposures to dilute HF or any with exposure to concentrations >5% HF should be hospitalized for 24 hours minimum. Perform treatments as indicated above.

### Antidote

- None.

### Drug(s) of Choice

- Fluid therapy with IV crystalloids to maintain perfusion and correct losses.
- If systemic intoxication (hypocalcemia) is suspected and patient is severely affected, administer initial doses of calcium while waiting for labs to return.
  - Calcium **gluconate** 10% (0.5–1.5 **mL**/kg) IV over 20–30 minutes while monitoring ECG, followed by 0.25-0.35 **mL**/kg/h CRI.
  - Calcium **chloride** 10% (0.2–0.6 **mL**/kg) preferred over calcium gluconate due to a greater concentration of calcium *if* given using a central line. Tissue injury secondary to drug extravasation of calcium chloride can be significant if using a peripheral catheter.
- Hyperkalemia >7.5 mEq/L requires emergency treatment and may be irreversible.
  - Regular insulin (0.1–0.5 IU/kg) with dextrose (2 g/unit insulin) diluted IV *and/or*
  - Sodium bicarbonate: 1–2 mEq/kg IV over 30 min.
- Arrhythmias – amiodarone (for potassium channel blockade) and correction of hypocalcemia, hypomagnesemia, and hyperkalemia. Avoid agents that may increase the QTc interval (e.g., propranolol and certain calcium channel blockers).
- Hypomagnesemia should be treated with IV magnesium chloride (preferred) CRI (0.75–1.0 mEq/kg/day).
- GI support.
  - Antiemetics as needed. Example: maropitant 1 mg/kg SQ or IV (slow) q 24 hours.
  - $H_2$ blockers, proton pump inhibitors (injectable therapy may be used while hospitalized if patient is NPO). Examples:
    - Famotidine (0.5–1 mg/kg PO q 12 hours × 7–10 days).
    - Omeprazole (1-1.5 mg/kg PO q 24 hours × 7–10 days).
  - Sucralfate: 0.25–1 g PO q 8–12 hours for 7–10 days.
- Provide adequate analgesia using opioids or analgesics. Avoid NSAIDs if the GI tract is compromised.

## Precautions/Interactions

- Do not perform ocular irrigation more than once since this has been shown to increase corneal damage.
- Intradermal and subcutaneous administration of 10% calcium chloride solution is damaging to tissues and should be avoided.

## Alternative Drugs

- Epsom salts (magnesium sulfate), Mylanta® (magnesium hydroxide), calcium acetate soaks, and iodine preparations are additional topical detoxification options.
- A 0.5 mL/cm² subcutaneous infiltration of 5% calcium gluconate solution is an option if pain continues for >30 minutes after applying calcium gluconate gel, but should be avoided in the extremities.
- Oral or IV corticosteroids and inhaled beta-2-agonists may help control bronchospasms.

## Extracorporeal Therapy

- Hemodialysis may be considered as a last-line option to remove fluoride anions in critical cases of systemic toxicosis or to treat hyperkalemia.

## Surgical Considerations

- In cases of severe dermal necrosis with refractory hypocalcemia, surgical debridement of affected skin region(s) may be necessary or amputation as a last resort.

## Patient Monitoring

- The animal should be given frequent opportunities to urinate to help excrete fluoride ions if catheterization is not feasible.
- Frequent blood pressure and continuous cardiac monitoring are recommended during hospitalization and for up to 48 hours post exposure. QTc prolongation commonly precedes dysrhythmias and indicates the presence of hypocalcemia.
- Monitor respiratory function for up to 72 hours after inhalation of HF.
- Serum electrolyte levels (especially iCa or serum Ca) should be obtained every 30–60 minutes in cases of systemic toxicosis or large dermal exposures.
- Animals with well-controlled pain, normal electrolyte levels and ECG readings, and insignificant burns can be sent home after six or more hours.

 **COMMENTS**

### Prevention/Avoidance

Prevent access to HF-containing products in the home, particularly while cleaning.

### Possible Complications

- Esophageal and GI strictures.
- Scarring.
- Ocular damage, changes in vision, and blindness.
- Pulmonary edema and chronic lung disease.
- Hypocalcemia induced by systemic HF toxicosis can lead to coagulation abnormalities and hemorrhage.

## Expected Course and Prognosis

- Prognosis depends on HF concentration, route and duration of exposure, and quantity exposed to or ingested.
- Single, small exposures are linked to good prognosis with low risk of long-term effects.
- Larger, multiple, or more severe exposures may require up to 72 hours of monitoring with potential systemic and long-term effects.

## Synonyms

Fluohydric acid, hydrogen fluoride, fluoric acid solution, hexafluorosilicic acid, hydrofluoride solution.

## See Also

Chapter 89 Acids
Chapter 24 Calcium Channel Blockers
Chapter 107 Fluoride

## Abbreviations

- HF = hydrofluoric acid
- $LC_{50}$ = median lethal concentration

## Suggested Reading

Bajraktarova-Valjakova E, Korunoska-Stevkovska V, Georgieva S et al. Hydrofluoric acid: burns and systemic toxicity, protective measures, immediate and hospital medical treatment. *Open Access Maced J Med Sci* 2018;6(11):2257–2269.

Centers for Disease Control and Prevention. Hydrogen fluoride (as F). 2014. www.cdc.gov/niosh/idlh/7664393.html

National Toxicology Program. *Pharmacokinetics and Concentrations of Fluoride Measured in Tissue, Blood, Urine, or Bone.* National Toxicology Program, Research Triangle Park. www.ncbi.nlm.nih.gov/books/NBK552757/

Schwerin DL, Hatcher JD. *Hydrofluoric Acid Burns.* 2022. www.ncbi.nlm.nih.gov/books/NBK441829/

Su MK. Hydrofluoric acid and fluorides. In: Nelson L, Howland M, Lewin N et al. (eds) *Goldfrank's Toxicologic Emergencies,* 11th edn. McGraw Hill, New York, 2019.

**Authors:** Anna Folska, PharmD and Ahna G. Brutlag, DVM, MS, DABT, DABVT
**Consulting Editor:** Ahna G. Brutlag, DVM, MS, DABT, DABVT

# Drugs: Human Prescription

# Chapter 14

# 5-Fluorouracil

## DEFINITION/OVERVIEW

5-Fluorouracil (5-FU) is an antineoplastic medication.

- 5-FU is available as a 1% or 5% topical cream, but is also available as a 1%, 2%, and 5% topical solution, and a 50 mg/mL solution for injection.
- 5-FU exposures should be treated aggressively and carry a guarded prognosis if neurologic signs are present. Direct ingestion of the cream is more likely to be severe than if the cream is licked off treated skin.
- 5-FU can cause severe GI upset, seizures, pulmonary edema, cardiac arrhythmias, and bone marrow suppression.
- The onset of seizures can occur rapidly or be delayed up to 26 hours post exposure.
- Seizures can be difficult to control and refractory to typical antiepileptics.
- Bone marrow suppression can be seen 5–30 days post exposure.

## ETIOLOGY/PATHOPHYSIOLOGY

### Mechanism of Action

- 5-fluorouracil is an antimetabolite, antineoplastic medication. It has been proposed that two metabolites, a-fluoro-b-alanine (FBAL) and fluoroacetic acid, are responsible for neurotoxicity seen with 5-FU in dogs and suspected in cats. Experimentally, administration of either of these metabolites resulted in lamellar splitting of the myelin sheaths in nerve cells, leading to vacuolization of the myelin.
- Additionally, fluoroacetic acid is metabolized to fluorocitrate which has been proposed to cause toxicity by inhibiting the tricarboxylic acid cycle, subsequently blocking the gamma-aminobutyric acid (GABA) shunt. This is thought to result in low levels of GABA in the brain, causing seizures.
- Rapidly growing cells, such as those in the bone marrow and intestinal crypts, absorb fluorouracil rapidly, resulting in severe GI upset and bone marrow aplasia due to cytotoxicity. 5-FU also has several active metabolites, such as 5-fluorouridine-5'-triphosphate which is slower to cross cell membranes than fluorouracil, resulting in delayed clearance in the bone marrow.

### Pharmacokinetics or Toxicokinetics – Absorption, Distribution, Metabolism, Excretion

#### Absorption

- Systemic absorption is about 6% when applied dermally (human).
- Oral absorption is erratic.

*Blackwell's Five-Minute Veterinary Consult Clinical Companion: Small Animal Toxicology*, Third Edition. Edited by Lynn R. Hovda, Ahna G. Brutlag, Robert H. Poppenga, and Steven E. Epstein.
© 2024 John Wiley & Sons, Inc. Published 2024 by John Wiley & Sons, Inc.

### Distribution

- Volume of distribution is 25 L/kg (human).
- Distributes into intestinal mucosa, bone marrow, liver.
- Crosses the blood–brain barrier and placenta.

### Metabolism

- Metabolized in the liver to several active metabolites.

### Excretion

- Within six hours, 7–20% is excreted unchanged in the urine.
- Expired as carbon dioxide.
- Minor excretion in bile.

## Toxicity

- $LD_{50}$ (oral in a rat) 115 mg/kg.
- $LD_{50}$ (oral in dog) 30 mg/kg.
- $LD_{50}$ (oral in rabbit) 18.9 mg/kg.
- Dose of concern is questionable but proposed to be 5.5 mg/kg (dog).
- Margin of safety is very narrow.
- The no observed adverse effect level, the lowest observed adverse effect level, and minimum lethal dose are all very close, so any exposure warrants monitoring.

## Systems Affected

- Gastrointestinal – affects rapidly dividing cells, such as those in the intestinal crypts. Results in vomiting, diarrhea, desquamation and sloughing of the GI tract, and stomatitis.
- Nervous – low GABA levels and splitting and vacuolization of myelin, resulting in seizures, ataxia, tremors, depression, disorientation, head tremors.
- Hepatobiliary – can cause increased liver enzymes.
- Respiratory – pulmonary edema due to multiple mechanisms.
- Cardiovascular – myocardial ischemia and cardiac arrhythmias, potentially from coronary vasospasm.
- Hemic/lymphatic/immune – bone marrow suppression.
- Reproductive – crosses the placenta and is teratogenic and embryotoxic.
- Skin/exocrine – delayed alopecia, typically reversible.

 ## SIGNALMENT/HISTORY

## Risk Factors

- Living in areas of high human UV exposure (mountains, large bodies of water), as owners in these areas have increased use of topical 5-FU.
- Underlying renal or hepatic dysfunction may slow elimination.
- Poodles, poodle mixes, and other breeds with continuous hair growth are at increased risk of developing alopecia, though alopecia occurs in other breeds.

## Historical Findings

- Owners will typically report an exposure to 5-FU.
- Vomiting often seen, rarely with cream present in vomitus.
- Owners may report seizure-like activity at home.

### Location and Circumstances of Poisoning

- Most commonly, pets will chew into a tube of ointment that has been left within reach.
- Sometimes, pet owners will report that their pets have licked it off treated human skin, applicators or fabric with residue, or chewed an IV line being used for at-home infusion.
- Rarely, accidental overdose as a part of a chemotherapy regimen.

 # CLINICAL FEATURES

- Onset of gastrointestinal signs is 10 minutes to five hours post exposure.
- Onset of seizures is 30 minutes to 26 hours post exposure. The time to onset of seizures does not seem to correlate with their severity or prognosis for the patient.
- Clinical signs often noted are vomiting, diarrhea (often with blood), seizures, ataxia, tremors, depression, disorientation, vocalization, pain, hypothermia, hyperthermia, agitation, hyperesthesia, absent menace response, coma, head tremors, and pulmonary edema.
- Leukopenia, neutropenia, thrombocytopenia, anemia, increased liver enzymes, and metabolic acidosis are also often noted on blood work.

 # DIFFERENTIAL DIAGNOSIS

- Sodium fluoroacetate (1080) toxicosis will present with similar clinical signs due to similar mechanism of action. Clinical signs with 1080 are peracute.
- Zinc phosphide toxicosis will also present with GI upset and seizures. However, the seizures will often respond to traditional antiepileptics.
- Metaldehyde toxicosis will often present with GI upset and seizures. Metaldehyde toxicosis can be differentiated from 5-FU by prominent generalized muscle tremors and presence of bait in the vomitus or stool.
- Bromethalin toxicosis will often present with GI upset and seizures. Bromethalin toxicosis can be differentiated from 5-FU by additional neurologic signs, such as paresis, ataxia, weakness, and decerebrate posture, as well as presence of bait in the vomitus or stool.
- Strychnine toxicosis can also present with seizures that are severe and difficult to control. However, strychnine will typically show tetany, severe hyperesthesia, and opisthotonos.

 # DIAGNOSTICS

### Clinical Pathological Findings

- CBC with differential.
  - Baseline, recheck at 12 and 24 hours for neutropenia and then q 24–72 hours for two weeks for bone marrow suppression in normal animals or until return to normal in patients with bone marrow suppression present (may take up to 30 days).
- Serum biochemistry.
  - Baseline, recheck PRN.
  - Increased liver enzymes can be measured but are typically mild. Fulminant hepatic failure is not expected.
  - Increased creatine kinase may be seen with seizures.
- Acid–base status.
  - Check PRN. Metabolic acidosis can be seen with hyperlactatemia, especially if seizures are severe or difficult to control.

## Other Diagnostics

Serum 5-FU levels are not clinically relevant due to rapid redistribution.

## Pathological Findings

Hemorrhagic colitis, gastric and intestinal ulceration, desquamation of the GI tract, stomatitis, myocardial ischemia, pulmonary edema, congestion of the lungs, liver, thymus, kidney, and small intestine, myelin splitting and secondary vacuole formation in the cerebrum.

 **THERAPEUTICS**

## Detoxification

- Oral exposures.
  - Emesis is not recommended, due to potential for rapid onset of seizures.
  - Activated charcoal with a cathartic, if less than one hour post exposure and pet is asymptomatic.

## Appropriate Health Care

- Hospitalize and monitor for the onset of seizures for at least 26 hours, even if asymptomatic.
- IV fluids: fluid diuresis is recommended to maintain hydration and promote elimination; reduce or discontinue if pulmonary edema is observed.

## Antidote

Vistonuridine (uridine triacetate) is used in human medicine as an antidote. Its use has not been reported in veterinary medicine. Vistonuridine is now available at some human pharmacies, and its use could be considered though efficacy is unknown. Vistonuridine must be given prior to the onset of neurologic signs.

## Drug(s) of Choice

- Antiepileptics.
  - Note: seizures can be very difficult to control.
  - Levetiracetam 30–60 mg/kg IV. Considered drug of choice.
  - Phenobarbital 4–24 mg/kg IV titrated in 4 mg/kg increments to effect.
  - Inhalant anesthesia (isoflurane, sevoflurane, etc.).
  - Propofol CRI 0.05–0.4 mg/kg/minute.
- GI protectants.
  - Sucralfate slurry 1g PO q 8 hours for large dogs; 0.5 g PO TID for small dogs and cats.
  - Omeprazole 1 mg/kg PO q 12 hours.
  - Pantoprazole 1 mg/kg IV q 12 hours.
- Antiemetics.
  - Maropitant 1 mg/kg IV, 2.0 PO q 24 hours.
  - Ondansetron 0.1–1.0 mg/kg PO or slow IV q 12 hours.
- Antidiarrheals:
  - Probiotics and bland diet.
- Colony stimulating factors.
  - Filgrastim (Neupogen®) 4–6 mcg/kg SQ for neutropenia.
- Pain control.
  - Opioids: buprenorphine 0.005–0.02 mg/kg IM, IV, transmucosal q 6–12 hours.

### Precautions/Interactions

- Metronidazole – reduces clearance and increases serum concentrations of 5-FU and all signs of toxicity.
- Hydrochlorothiazide – increases risk of myelosuppression.
- Leucovorin – increases risk of myelosuppression and GI toxicity.
- Cimetidine – increases peak plasma concentrations of fluorouracil.
- NSAIDs – can increase GI upset and irritation.
- Benzodiazepines—not contraindicated, but often not effective for the control of seizures, due to low levels of GABA in the brain.

### Extracorporeal Therapy

- Due to rapid cellular uptake of 5-FU, extracorporeal elimination is generally not considered to be effective.

### Surgical Considerations

- Patients may have delayed healing time and increased risk of infection due to leukopenia. Excessive bleeding may be a concern due to thrombocytopenia.

### Patient Monitoring

- Monitor ECG, body temperature, pulse, and blood pressure.
- Respiratory effort and lung sounds should be monitored for indications of pulmonary edema.
- Monitor blood gases ($PCO_2$) in heavily sedated or anesthetized animals if possible.

### Diet

- Bland, soft diet should be started once tolerated and seizure are controlled.

## COMMENTS

### Prevention/Avoidance

Pets should be kept away from 5-FU. Spills should be cleaned up promptly with pets in another room. Dogs and cats should be prevented from licking human skin treated with 5-FU or from ingesting materials used to apply 5-FU (especially cotton-tipped applicators in the trash).

### Possible Complications

Increased susceptibility to infection is possible in animals with myelosuppression.

### Expected Course and Prognosis

- GI upset typically, but not always, precedes seizures.
- Seizures can be delayed and onset may take up to 26 hours post exposure.
- Suppression of one or more cell lines can be noted. Leukopenia and thrombocytopenia are more commonly decreased at day 5–7. Anemia is typically noted around day 9. The nadir for all cell types is typically noted at 9–14 days. Resolution is expected by 30 days post exposure.
- Prognosis is guarded to poor once clinical signs occur.
- One study showed that 30% of symptomatic dogs died or were euthanized.

### Synonyms

Efudex®, Adrucil®, Carac®, Fluoroplex®, Tolak®, 5-FU.

## See Also

Chapter 125 Sodium Monofluoroacetate (Compound 1080)

## Abbreviations

- 5-FU = 5-Fluorouracil
- TCA cycle = tricarboxylic acid cycle
- GABA = gamma-aminobutyric acid

## Suggested Reading

Immelman LM, Goodman IH, Keller N. Transient chemotherapy-induced alopecia after successful reversal of 5-fluorouracil myelosuppression and neurotoxicosis in a 9-month-old dog. *Aust Vet J* 2022;100(6):236–242.

Sayre RS, Barr JW, Bailey EM. Accidental and experimentally induced 5-fluorouracil toxicity in dogs. *J Vet Emerg Crit Care* 2012;22:545–549.

Yashimata K, Yada H, Ariyoshi T. Neurotoxic effects of fluoro-alanine and fluoroacetic acid on dogs. *J Toxic Sci* 2004;29:155–166.

**Author**: Laura Stern, DVM, DABVT

**Consulting Editor**: Steven E. Epstein, DVM, DACVECC

# Chapter 15

# Amphetamines

## DEFINITION/OVERVIEW

- Amphetamines can be either prescription medications for ADHD or weight loss (Adderall® [dextroamphetamine, amphetamine aspartate, dextroamphetamine sulfate, amphetamine sulfate], Concerta® [methylphenidate], Dexedrine® [dextroamphetamine sulfate], Focalin® [dexmethylphenidate], Ritalin® [methylphenidate], Vyvanse® [lisdexamfetamine]) or illegal drugs (methamphetamine, ecstasy).
- Intoxication stimulates the CNS and cardiovascular systems.

## ETIOLOGY/PATHOPHYSIOLOGY

- Amphetamines are sympathomimetic amines. They cause stimulation of the CNS and cardiovascular systems leading to stimulatory signs (agitation, tachycardia, tremors, seizures).
- Amphetamine intoxication in animals is not uncommon, especially in households with ADHD children.
- Animals may also be given the wrong medication by mistake.

### Mechanism of Action

- Amphetamines are stimulants of the CNS and cardiovascular system. They stimulate the medullary respiratory center and reticular activating system.
- Amphetamines increase the concentration of catecholamines at nerve endings by increasing their release and inhibiting their reuptake and metabolism.
- There is also an increase in the presynaptic release of serotonin.

### Pharmacokinetics or Toxicokinetics – Adsorption, Distribution, Metabolism, Excretion

- Amphetamines are quickly absorbed orally.
- Signs can begin within minutes (methamphetamine) or may be delayed for several hours (extended-release formulations). If signs have been present for a while, hyperthermia and myoglobinuria may be noted.
- High lipid solubility leads to high concentrations in the liver, kidneys, and lungs.
- They cross the blood–brain barrier.
- Metabolism is minimal, and most are excreted as the parent compound.
- Amphetamines are eliminated in the urine. Urinary elimination is pH dependent. The half-life varies from seven to 34 hours (shorter with acidic urine).

*Blackwell's Five-Minute Veterinary Consult Clinical Companion: Small Animal Toxicology*, Third Edition. Edited by Lynn R. Hovda, Ahna G. Brutlag, Robert H. Poppenga, and Steven E. Epstein. © 2024 John Wiley & Sons, Inc. Published 2024 by John Wiley & Sons, Inc.

## Toxicity

- The oral lethal dose in dogs for most amphetamines ranges from 10 to 23 mg/kg. Signs can be seen as low as 1 mg/kg.

## Systems Affected

- Nervous – stimulation resulting in agitation, tremors, or seizures.
- Cardiovascular – stimulation resulting in tachycardia and hypertension.
- Respiratory – stimulation resulting in tachypnea.
- Gastrointestinal – stimulation resulting in vomiting, hypersalivation, and diarrhea.
- Ophthalmic – mydriasis.

 # SIGNALMENT/HISTORY

### Risk Factors

- All species and breeds can be affected.
- Greater risk if ADHD medications are in the household.

### Historical Findings

- Owners may have evidence of exposure to amphetamines.
- Owners often report agitation (running around), tremors (shaking), and tachycardia (heart racing).

### Location and Circumstances of Poisoning

- Patient may be exposed at home if prescription or illicit medications are present.
- Drug enforcement animals may be exposed while working.

 # CLINICAL FEATURES

- Agitation, tachycardia, panting, tremors, hyperthermia, seizures, and/or death.

 # DIFFERENTIAL DIAGNOSIS

- Other stimulants, including methylxanthines (caffeine, theobromine, theophylline), nicotine, hops, and serotonergic medications.

 # DIAGNOSTICS

### Clinical Pathological Findings

- Blood gas – metabolic acidosis.
- Urinalysis – myoglobinuria secondary to rhabdomyolysis.
- Biochemistry – elevated creatinine kinase, blood urea nitrogen and creatinine, and hypoglycemia are possible.

### Other Diagnostics

- Illicit drug urine test: amphetamines will show up positive on amphetamine and/or methamphetamine tests, although these tests have not been validated in animals.
- Amphetamines can be detected in urine or stomach contents by human hospital laboratories or veterinary diagnostic laboratories.

## Pathological Findings

- There are no specific histopathological lesions consistent with this toxicosis.

 **THERAPEUTICS**

- Treatment is aimed at controlling life-threatening CNS and cardiovascular signs.
- Protect kidneys from rhabdomyolysis.

### Detoxification

- Emesis if <15 minutes and asymptomatic.
- Gastric lavage if large amounts of pills have been ingested.
- Activated charcoal to reduce absorption if ingestion is over a lethal dose.
- Acidifying urine to 4.5–5.5 pH with either ammonium chloride (100–200 mg/kg/day PO divided QID) or ascorbic acid (20–30 mg/kg PO, SQ, IM or IV) to enhance elimination.

### Appropriate Health Care

- Most animals will need hospitalization for monitoring of body temperature, respirations, and heart rate.
- Monitor blood pressure.
- Monitor acid–base status.
- ECG for arrhythmias.

### Drug(s) of Choice

- IV fluids to help regulate body temperature and to protect kidneys from myoglobinuria.
- Agitation.
    - Phenothiazine.
        - Acepromazine 0.01–0.10 mg/kg IV or IM, titrate to effect as needed.
    - Cyproheptadine.
        - Dogs: 1.1 mg/kg PO or rectally; serotonin antagonist.
        - Cats: 2–4 mg total dose per cat.
- Tachycardia.
    - Beta-blockers.
        - Propranolol 0.02–0.06 mg/kg IV q 8 hours PRN.
        - Esmolol 0.1 mg/kg loading dose then 10–200 mcg/kg/min IV CRI titrated to effect.
- Tremors.
    - Methocarbamol 50–100 mg/kg IV, titrate up as needed with maximum dose of 330 mg/kg/day.
- Seizures.
    - Levetiracetam 30–60 mg/kg IV PRN.
    - Barbiturates to effect.
        - Phenobarbital 3–4 mg/kg IV.

### Precautions/Interactions

- Benzodiazepines can increase the dysphoria and lead to increased morbidity. They are not recommended for use in amphetamine toxicosis.
- Sodium bicarbonate alkalinizes the urine, causing increased renal tubular reabsorption of amphetamines.
- Avoid serotonergic medications (tramadol, trazodone) as they can increase agitation.

### Alternative Drugs

- Seizures –inhalant anesthetics (isoflurane, sevoflurane), propofol CRI.

### Patient Monitoring

- Temperature, BP, HR should be monitored hourly (consider continuous temperature monitoring); interval can be increased as patient responds to care.
- Minimize sensory stimuli.
- Monitor urine color, hourly at first and then less often if the animal remains clinically normal.

### Diet

- No diet change is needed, except NPO during severe CNS signs.

## COMMENTS

- Treatment in most cases is very rewarding.
- These animals tend to require large doses of phenothiazines to control their clinical signs.

### Prevention/Avoidance

- Keep all medications out of the reach of pets.
- Do not store human and animal drugs in the same area to decrease medication errors.

### Possible Complications

- DIC secondary to severe hyperthermia (rare).
- Rhabdomyolysis and secondary renal failure (rare).

### Expected Course and Prognosis

- If CNS and cardiac signs can be controlled, prognosis is good.
- Animals with preexisting cardiac disease may be more at risk for developing severe signs and fatal arrhythmias.
- Signs may last up to 72 hours with extended-release products.
- No long-term problems are expected in most cases.

### See Also

Chapter 36 Club Drugs (MDMA, GHB, Flunitrazepam, Bath Salts)
Chapter 40 Methamphetamine
Chapter 32 SSRI and SNRI Antidepressants

### Suggested Reading

Crecraft C. Prittie J, Mastrocco A. Hypoglycemia and presumptive rhabdomyolysis secondary to lisdexamfetamine toxicosis in 3 cats. *J Vet Emerg Crit Care* 2022;32(1):113–118.
Genovese DW, Gwaltney-Brant SM, Slater MR. Methylphenidate toxicosis in dogs: 128 cases (2001–2008). *J Am Vet Med Assoc* 2010;237(12):1438–1443.
Stern LA, Schell M. Management of attention-deficit disorder and attention-deficit/hyperactivity disorder drug intoxication in dogs and cats: an update. *Vet Clin North Am Small Anim Pract* 2018;48(6): 959–968.

**Author:** Tina Wismer, DVM, MS, DABVT, DABT
**Consulting Editor:** Steven E. Epstein, DVM, DACVECC

# Chapter 16

# Angiotensin-Converting Enzyme Inhibitors

## DEFINITION/OVERVIEW

- Angiotensin-converting enzyme inhibitors (ACEIs) are prescription medications used to treat cardiovascular disease (primarily congestive heart failure), systemic hypertension, and some renal diseases.
- Adverse effects include hypotension, gastrointestinal disturbances, hyperkalemia, and acute kidney injury (AKI).
- In most patients, the effects of an ACEI overdose are mild, and no specific treatment is required.
- Patients with moderate to severe hypotension require close monitoring, administration of intravenous fluids, and vasoactive support.
- Administration of naloxone has been described in people with severe refractory hypotension.

## ETIOLOGY/PATHOPHYSIOLOGY

### Mechanism of Action

- The renin-angiotensin-aldosterone system (RAAS) regulates fluid volume and blood pressure via release of angiotensin II (AngII) and aldosterone.
- The RAAS serves an important homeostatic function in health. However, chronic and inappropriate RAAS activation in cardiovascular and renal disease leads to hypertension, tissue remodeling, inflammation, and fibrosis.
- ACEIs suppress the RAAS by inhibiting ACE-mediated conversion of angiotensin I to AngII.
- Beneficial effects of RAAS suppression include reduced blood pressure, reduction of AngII-induced mesangial cell proliferation, and renal vasodilation with reduction in proteinuria.
- Toxic effects of ACEIs are directly related to their pharmacologic effects. AngII is a potent vasoconstrictor and increases sympathetic drive. It stimulates aldosterone secretion as well as thirst, water retention, and tubular sodium reabsorption which increase extracellular fluid volume. Blockade of these effects causes vasodilation and loss of sodium and water.

### Pharmacokinetics or Toxicokinetics – Adsorption, Distribution, Metabolism, Excretion

- Commonly prescribed ACEIs in cats and dogs are benazepril and enalapril. However, many other ACEIs are available, including captopril, cilazapril, fosinopril, imidapril, lisinopril, moexipril, perindopril, quinapril, ramipril, trandolapril, and zofenopril.
- All the ACEIs except captopril and lisinopril are prodrugs that must be metabolized to their active form (e.g., benazepril is converted to benazeprilat).

---

*Blackwell's Five-Minute Veterinary Consult Clinical Companion: Small Animal Toxicology*, Third Edition. Edited by Lynn R. Hovda, Ahna G. Brutlag, Robert H. Poppenga, and Steven E. Epstein. © 2024 John Wiley & Sons, Inc. Published 2024 by John Wiley & Sons, Inc.

- ACEIs have two elimination phases with initial clearance of free drug and subsequent release of tissue-bound drug.
- Benazepril.
  - Dogs: peak concentration occurs at 75 minutes with a duration of effect up to 30 hours. Terminal half-life is approximately 19 hours. Benazepril is 85% protein bound and undergoes both hepatic (55%) and renal (45%) excretion.
  - Cats: peak concentration at two hours with a terminal half-life of 16–23 hours. Excretion is renal (15%) and hepatic (85%).
- Captopril.
  - Dogs: half-life is approximately 2.8 hours with a duration of effect of around four hours. Captopril is 40% protein bound and more than 95% is renally excreted.
- Enalapril.
  - Dogs: onset of action is 4–6 hours with a duration of action of 12–14 hours. Approximately 95% of metabolite enalaprilat is renally excreted.
- Imidapril.
  - Dogs: peak concentrations occur in around five hours with an elimination half-life of at least 10 hours. The metabolite imidaprilat is moderately protein bound.
- Lisinopril.
  - Dogs: peak concentrations at around four hours with a duration of action of 24 hours.
- Ramipril.
  - Dogs: effects may last for 24 hours.
  - Cats: half-life is around 20 hours.

## Toxicity

- Benazepril.
  - Dogs: therapeutic dose 0.25–1 mg/kg PO q 12–24 h.
  - Cats: therapeutic dose 0.25–0.5 mg/kg PO q 12–24 h.
  - Toxicity: reduced red blood cell counts occurred in cats given 10 mg/kg/day and dogs receiving 150 mg/kg/day for 12 months. A 200-fold overdose was tolerated in dogs.
- Enalapril.
  - Dogs: therapeutic dose 0.25–2 mg/kg PO q 12–24 h.
  - Cats: therapeutic dose 0.25–0.5 mg/kg PO q 12–24 h.
  - Toxicity: administration of 200 mg/kg was reported to be lethal in dogs, but 100 mg/kg was not. No adverse effects were noted in dogs given 15 mg/kg/day for up to one year.
- Captopril.
  - Dogs: therapeutic dose 0.5–2 mg/kg PO q 8 h.
  - Cats: therapeutic dose 3.125–6.25 mg PO q 8–12 h.
  - Toxicity: doses >6.6 mg/kg q 8 h may lead to AKI in dogs. A 1.5 g/kg dose in dogs caused vomiting and hypotension.
- Imidapril.
  - Dogs: therapeutic dose 0.25 mg/kg PO q 12–24 h.
  - Toxicity: no signs in cats administered 0.5 mg/kg/day PO for three months. Doses up to 5 mg/kg are tolerated in dogs.
- Lisinopril.
  - Dogs: therapeutic dose 0.5 mg/kg PO q 12–24 h.
  - Cats: therapeutic dose 0.25–0.5 mg/kg PO q 24 h.

- Toxicity: in dogs, doses below 20 mg/kg may cause vomiting while 27 mg/kg may lead to hypotension. Hypotension developed in 1/218 cats given 4.9 mg/kg.
- Ramipril.
  - Dogs and cats: therapeutic dose 0.125–0.25 mg/kg PO q 24 h.
  - Toxicity: doses up to 1 g/kg induced mild gastrointestinal signs in dogs.

## Systems Affected

- Gastrointestinal – anorexia, vomiting, and diarrhea.
- Cardiovascular – hypotension secondary to excessive vasodilation.
  - May lead to compensatory tachycardia.
  - Rarely leads to bradycardia (thought to result from loss of sympathetic stimulation by AngII and/or discontinuation of AngII-mediated vagal inhibition).
- Renal/urologic – AKI secondary to loss of AngII-mediated renal autoregulation and reduction in glomerular filtration rate.
- Endocrine/metabolic – hyperkalemia secondary to reduced aldosterone levels.
- Reported in people.
  - Respiratory – coughing and angioedema due to accumulation of bradykinin (which is usually degraded by ACE); may progress to upper airway obstruction.
  - Hemic/lymphatic/immune – skin rashes, agranulocytosis, anemia, neutropenia, thrombocytopenia.
  - Hepatobiliary – cholestatic hepatotoxicity.

# SIGNALMENT/HISTORY

## Risk Factors

- No apparent breed or sex predilection.
- Patients with heart failure, salt depletion, hepatic dysfunction, and/or renal disease may be more vulnerable to toxicity.
- ACEIs may be given in combination with angiotensin receptor blockers (ARBs), calcium channel blockers, and/or spironolactone.
  - Dual RAAS blockade with ACEIs and ARBs may increase the risk for hypotension, hyperkalemia, and AKI.
  - Combined ACEI and dihydropyridone overdose in people leads to increased rates of hypotension and bradycardia.
  - Concurrent spironolactone administration may increase the risk of hyperkalemia.

## Historical Findings

- Lethargy and vomiting are commonly reported clinical signs.

## Location and Circumstances of Poisoning

- Patients may gain access at home as ACEIs are prescribed to both people and animals.
- Iatrogenic toxicity in the clinic is possible.

# CLINICAL FEATURES

- Weakness, syncope and/or ataxia.
- Hypotension +/– compensatory tachycardia (rarely bradycardia).

# DIFFERENTIAL DIAGNOSIS

- Hypotension may be caused by primary cardiac disease (e.g., arrhythmias, reduced systolic function), decreased preload (e.g., hypovolemia, hypoadrenocorticism), decreased vascular tone (e.g., anaphylaxis, sepsis) or decreased venous return (e.g., cardiac tamponade). History, physical exam, ECG, point-of-care ultrasound, and bloodwork will help to differentiate these causes.
- Other drugs/toxins leading to hypotension include ARBs, beta-blockers, and calcium channel blockers.

 # DIAGNOSTICS

- Blood ACEI levels are not readily available and do not correlate well with clinical effects in people.
- Blood pressure – hypotension.
- Serum chemistry and electrolytes – may see hyponatremia, hyperkalemia, and/or azotemia (hepatotoxicity is also reported in people).
- Complete blood count – anemia and neutropenia are possible.

 # THERAPEUTICS

### Detoxification

- Induce emesis in asymptomatic animals presented within two hours of ingestion.
- Consider gastric lavage if recent/massive ingestion and induction of emesis deemed inappropriate.
- Activated charcoal should be given if recent (e.g., within two hours) and/or large dose ingestion and no contraindications.

### Appropriate Health Care

- Patients may be monitored at home following small overdoses (<5× therapeutic dose).
- In-hospital monitoring of asymptomatic patients for six hours has been recommended in human medicine following larger dose ingestion as hypotension develops by around five hours irrespective of which ACEI has been ingested.
- Hypotension is treated initially with intravascular volume expansion using a balanced crystalloid solution. Care must be taken to avoid fluid overload, particularly in patients with cardiovascular and/or renal disease.
- Vasopressor administration may be required in patients with persistent hypotension (MAP <60 mmHg).
- Monitoring of perfusion parameters, hydration status, urine output, blood pressure, heart rate, electrolytes, and renal parameters is recommended. AKI may not become evident for several hours or more and the risk is increased following periods of hypotension.

### Antidote

- Theoretically, AngII would be the ideal antidote for ACEI-induced hypotension, but pharmaceutical preparations are not readily available.

### Drug(s) of Choice

- Intravenous fluids – use a balanced crystalloid, e.g., Lactated Ringer's solution.
  - Bolus 20 mL/kg (dog) or 10 mL/kg (cat) as needed to address volume-responsive hypotension.
  - Care must be taken to avoid fluid overload.

- Vasopressors if persistent hypotension with direct blood pressure and ECG monitoring to maintain MAP >60 mmHg. Vasopressors should not be administered via a peripheral vessel for more than 1–2 hours due to the risk of ischemic injury.
  - Dogs: norepinephrine 0.05–1.0 mcg/kg/min IV CRI.
  - Cats: dopamine 5–20 mcg/kg/min IV CRI.
- In some people with ACEI-induced hypotension refractory to vasopressors, naloxone has proven effective. This is because ACEIs promote endorphin-mediated hypotensive effects. Naloxone has relatively limited adverse effects and its use could be considered in cases of severe ACEI toxicity.
- Antiemetics as needed to help control gastrointestinal signs.
  - Ondansetron 0.25–0.5 mg/kg IV q 8–12 h.
  - Maropitant 1 mg/kg IV/SQ q 24 h.

## Precautions/Interactions

- Antihistamines, diuretics, other antihypertensives, and alpha-2 adrenergic agonists may exacerbate ACEI-induced hypotension.
- Concurrent NSAIDs could increase the risk for nephrotoxicity.
- Potassium supplements and spironolactone may increase the risk of hyperkalemia.

## Extracorporeal Therapy

- The dialyzability of different ACEIs varies widely in people.
- Captopril, enalapril, lisinopril, and perindopril can be removed by hemodialysis due to their low protein binding and relatively small volume of distribution.
- Hemoperfusion and/or therapeutic plasma exchange could be considered for severe overdose of more highly protein-bound ACEIs such as ramipril and fosinopril.
- However, major adverse effects are rare in ACEI overdose and extracorporeal therapy is seldom necessary.

## Patient Monitoring

- Perfusion parameters and hydration status should be reassessed every four hours following initial stabilization.
- Blood pressure should be monitored intermittently (every four hours).
- In vasopressor-dependent patients, continuous and direct blood pressure and ECG monitoring is recommended.
- Serum chemistry (including renal parameters) every 24 hours.

 **COMMENTS**

### Expected Course and Prognosis

- Prognosis is excellent in most cases.
- Based on human guidelines, asymptomatic patients may be discharged from the hospital after six hours.
- If a patient has been symptomatic or hypotensive, they should be monitored for at least 24 hours.
- Vasopressors can usually be weaned and discontinued within 12 hours.
- If significant hypotension is documented, patients should be observed for 36 hours as hypotensive episodes have recurred up to 36 hours post ingestion in people.

## Abbreviations

- ACEI = angiotensin-converting enzyme inhibitor
- AKI = acute kidney injury
- AngII = angiotensin II
- ARB = angiotensin receptor blocker
- MAP = mean arterial pressure

## Suggested Reading

Hamlin RL, Nakayama T. Comparison of some pharmacokinetic parameters of 5 angiotensin-converting enzyme inhibitors in normal beagles. *J Vet Intern Med* 1998;12(2):93–95.

Hayashi SA. Angiotensin blockers and ACE inhibitors. In: Olson KR (ed.) *Poisoning & Drug Overdose*, 6th edn. McGraw-Hill, New York, 2012.

Lucas C, Christie GA, Waring WS. Rapid onset of haemodynamic effects after angiotensin converting enzyme-inhibitor overdose: implications for initial patient triage. *Emerg Med J* 2006;23(11):854–857.

Plumb DC. *Plumb's Veterinary Drug Handbook*, 9th edn. Stockholm, Wisconsin: Pharma Vet Inc., 2018.

Robert M, De Bels D, Chaumont M, Honoré PM, Gottignies P. Angiotensin converting enzyme inhibitor intoxication: naloxone to the rescue? Naloxone for ACE inhibitor intoxication. *Am J Emerg Med* 2019;37(6):1217.e1–1217.e2.

**Author**: Helen S. Philp, BVMS, DACVECC

**Consulting Editor**: Steven E. Epstein, DVM, DACVECC

# Chapter 17

# Antiseizure Medications (Lamotrigine, Phenobarbital, Others)

## DEFINITION/OVERVIEW

- Antiseizure/anticonvulsant medications act by a variety of mechanisms to control seizures in both human and veterinary patients.
- Many drugs available for human epileptics are unavailable or unused in veterinary patients. Due to their minimal use, toxic effects are difficult to predict and are not well described.
- Anticonvulsant toxicosis may produce general clinical signs, but specific drugs also produce unique toxicity profiles.

## ETIOLOGY/PATHOPHYSIOLOGY

### Mechanism of Action

- Anticonvulsants exert their effects via a variety of mechanisms (Table 17.1) and many of these drugs have multiple mechanisms of action.
- The most common mechanisms include:
  - GABA potentiation (e.g., phenobarbitol, imepitoin, KBr).
  - Sodium channel blockers (e.g., phenytoin, lamotrigine).
  - Calcium channel blockers (e.g., zonisamide).
  - Other mechanisms (e.g., levetiracetam).

### Pharmacokinetics or Toxicokinetics – Adsorption, Distribution, Metabolism, Excretion

- All anticonvulsants are generally rapidly and well absorbed from the gastrointestinal tract, but interpatient variability is likely.
- In general, the volume of distribution is low.
- Many undergo hepatic metabolism and renal excretion (Table 17.1).
- Extended-release formulations will significantly prolong drug half-life.

### Toxicity

- There is limited information on doses of anticonvulsants that will cause clinical signs in dogs and cats and often the dose ingested is unknown.
- The toxic dose and $LD_{50}$ vary by drug and species, and in many cases are unavailable for dogs and cats (Table 17.1).

### Systems Affected

- Neuromuscular – ataxia, paraparesis, anisocoria, mydriasis, nystagmus, sedation, CNS depression, hyperexcitability, seizures, loss of gag reflex, coma.

*Blackwell's Five-Minute Veterinary Consult Clinical Companion: Small Animal Toxicology*, Third Edition. Edited by Lynn R. Hovda, Ahna G. Brutlag, Robert H. Poppenga, and Steven E. Epstein. © 2024 John Wiley & Sons, Inc. Published 2024 by John Wiley & Sons, Inc.

**TABLE 17.1 Select antiseizure medication mechanisms and toxic principles.**

| Drug | Drug class/additional mechanisms | Half-life (hours)* | Metabolism/ excretion | Drug specific toxicity |
|---|---|---|---|---|
| Carbamazine | Na and Ca channel blocker, anticholinergic effects | 0.5–1.5 (dogs) | Hepatic/renal | Cardiotoxicity Anticholinergic signs |
| Felbamate | Na and Ca channel blocker, GABA potentiation, NMDA antagonism | 4–6 (dogs) | Hepatic/renal | Hepatotoxicity KCS Blood dyscrasias |
| Imepitoin | GABA potentiation, partial benzodiazepine agonist | 1.5–2 (dogs) | Hepatic/fecal | None known |
| Lacosamide | Na channel blocker | 13 (humans) | Hepatic/renal | Cardiotoxicity |
| Lamotrigine | Phenyltriazine/ Na, Ca, and K channel blocker, SSRI | 24–30 (humans) | Hepatic/renal | Cardiotoxicity Rhabdomyolysis Serotonin syndrome |
| Oxcarbazine | Na and Ca channel blocker | 4 (dogs) | Hepatic/renal | Cardiotoxicity Hyponatremia |
| Phenobarbital | Barbiturate, GABA potentiation | 50–125 (dogs), 34–43 (cats) | Hepatic/renal | Hepatotoxicity Bone marrow suppression Coagulopathy Pancreatitis |
| Phenytoin | Class Ib antiarrhythmic (Na channel blockade) | 2–8 (dogs), 42–108 (cats) | Hepatic/renal | Insulin and ADH inhibition Bradyarrhythmias Dogs – hepatotoxicity Cats – dermal atrophy syndrome, thrombocytopenia |
| Potassium bromide (KBr) | Halide salt, GABA potentiation | 15–45 **days**˙ (dogs) | None/renal | Bromism Pancreatitis Panniculitis Cats – respiratory disease |
| Topiramate | Na and Ca channel blocker, GABA potentiation | 2-4 (dogs) | None/renal | Glaucoma Acid–base disturbances |
| Valproic acid | Succinate semialdehyde dehydrogenase inhibitor, GABA potentiation | 1.5–2.8 (dogs), longer in cats | Hepatic/renal | Hepatotoxicity Hyperammonemia Pancreatitis L-carnitine deficiency Delayed cerebral edema Coagulopathy Acid–base disturbances |
| Zonisamide | Na and Ca channel blocker, GABA potentiation | 15 (dogs), 33 (cats) | Renal | Hepatotoxicity Blood dyscrasias Acid–base disturbances |

- Respiratory – hypoventilation, respiratory arrest.
- Gastrointestinal – anorexia, hypersalivation, vomiting, diarrhea, pancreatitis.
- Hepatobiliary – liver enzyme elevation/hepatotoxicity.
- Cardiovascular – hypotension, bradycardia, AV block, supraventricular and ventricular tachyarrhythmias.
- Hematologic – blood dyscrasias, coagulopathy.
- Metabolic – hypothermia, acid-base disturbances.

# SIGNALMENT/HISTORY

- No specific species, age, or breed predilections.
- Iatrogenic overdose is possible in patients on anticonvulsants in the hospital.

## Risk Factors

- Owner or patient on anticonvulsants regularly and patient has access to medication in the home.
- Renal or liver insufficiency may worsen or prolong toxicity.

## Historical Findings

- Owner observed ingestion, chewed or open pill bottle.
- Neurologic signs may be appreciated by owner.
- Known iatrogenic overdose.

# CLINICAL FEATURES

- The most common clinical signs are neurologic in origin (ataxia, seizures, hyperexcitability, sedation, coma, respiratory depression) followed by gastrointestinal (anorexia, hypersalivation, vomiting, diarrhea).
- Hemodynamic instability, hypotension, hypothermia, and shock are also possible with any anticonvulsant toxicity.
- Other clinical signs are species, drug, and dose dependent. Due to limited experience with certain drugs in small animals, some adverse effects listed are reported in humans and may not be valid in dogs and cats.
  - Phenobarbital – liver enzyme elevations/hepatotoxicity, bone marrow suppression, coagulopathy, pancreatitis, pseudolymphoma.
  - KBr.
    - Dogs: bromism (includes standard neurologic signs plus can include myoclonus, megaesophagus, upper and lower motor neuron paresis, muscle pain), pancreatitis, panniculitis.
    - Cats: cough, dyspnea (eosinophilic airway inflammation).
  - Valproic acid – liver enzyme elevations/hepatotoxicity, pancreatitis, hyperammonemia, delayed cerebral edema, L-carnitine deficiency and cardiomyopathy, coagulopathy (thrombocytopenia/thrombocytopathia), dermatologic (rash, alopecia).
  - Topiramate – acute myopia and glaucoma.
    - Cats: renal tubular acidosis and neutropenia reported.
  - Phenytoin – insulin and ADH inhibition, bradyarrhythmias.
    - Dogs: hepatotoxicity, blood dyscrasia (myelofibrosis) reported.
    - Cats: dermal atrophy syndrome, thrombocytopenia .
  - Lamotrigine – ventricular and tachyarrhythmias, rhabdomyolysis, serotonin syndrome.
  - Felbamate – hepatotoxicity, KCS, tremors/limb rigidity, blood dyscrasias.
  - Lacosamide – arrhythmias.
  - Carbamazine – anticholinergic effects (ileus), arrhythmias.
  - Oxcarbazine – tachyarrhythmias, hyponatremia.
  - Zonisamide – liver enzyme elevations, blood dyscrasias (neutropenia), renal tubular acidosis.
  - Levetiracetam has a wide margin of safety and minimal to no known toxic effects beyond mild neurologic effects (sedation, mild ataxia) and mild GI signs (nausea, hypersalivation, vomiting, inappetence). Extremely high doses may cause respiratory depression.

# DIFFERENTIAL DIAGNOSIS

- Any toxin that causes neurologic signs, especially CNS depression or agitation.
- CNS disease – infectious or inflammatory encephalopathies, traumatic brain injury.
- Hepatic encephalopathy.

# DIAGNOSTICS

## Clinical Pathological Findings

- Venous blood gases analysis: hypercapnia.
- Phenobarbital.
  - Anemia, neutropenia, and thrombocytopenia possible.
  - Liver enzyme elevations, liver failure.
  - Prolonged coagulation times.
- Valproic acid.
  - Thrombocytopenia/thrombocytopathia, leukopenia, anemia.
  - Elevated liver enzymes .
  - High anion gap metabolic acidosis, hypernatremia, hypocalcemia.
- Topiramate: hyperchloremic metabolic acidosis.
- Phenytoin.
  - Thrombocytopenia in cats.
  - Liver enzyme elevations, hyperglycemia.
  - Hypernatremia.
- Lamotrigine: creatine kinase elevations.
- Felbamate.
  - Leukopenia, thrombocytopenia.
  - Liver enzyme elevations.
- Oxcarbazine: hyponatremia.
- Zonisamide.
  - Neutropenia.
  - Liver enzyme elevations.
  - Hyperchloremic metabolic acidosis.
- Serum drug concentration can be measured if available, but do not necessarily correlate to clinical signs.

## Other Diagnostic Findings

- Abdominal ultrasound may show evidence of pancreatitis.
- Electrocardiogram should be evaluated for evidence of arrhythmias.

# THERAPEUTICS

- Therapeutic objectives include intensive stabilization, monitoring and nursing care, and symptomatic treatment. Detoxification and enhanced drug elimination can be implemented when possible.

## Detoxification

- Emesis induction is unlikely to be of benefit due to rapid absorption of most anticonvulsants. If the ingestion was recent and the patient is not clinical (neurologically inappropriate), emesis can be attempted.

■ Intubation and gastric lavage can be considered if a large dose was ingested, or clinical signs preclude emesis induction.

■ Activated charcoal administration may be beneficial in cases of phenobarbital, valproic acid, topiramate, phenytoin, lamotrigine, carbamazine, oxcarbazine, and zonisamide. If drug undergoes enterohepatic recirculation, multiple doses may be indicated.

### Appropriate Health Care

■ If known ingestion or clinical signs are present, hospitalization should be recommended.

■ IV fluids and vasopressors as needed to treat hypotension and promote renal perfusion.

■ Provide heat support where necessary.

■ If excessive sedation and loss of gag reflex, endotracheal intubation may be required.

■ Mechanical ventilation may be indicated in cases of severe hypercapnia.

■ Recumbent patient care (patient rotation, bladder expression, oral and ocular care) is crucial to avoid additional complications including aspiration pneumonia, sores, and ocular ulcers.

### Drug(s) of Choice

■ Anticonvulsant specific treatments.
  • KBr.
    o IV fluid of choice is 0.9% NaCl as its high chloride concentration washes out bromide.
    o Furosemide (2 mg/kg IV) can also aid in urinary excretion of KBr.
  • Imepitoin – flumazenil (0.01 mg/kg IV) may partially reverse effects; repeat PRN if improvement noted post administration.
  • Valproic acid.
    o Carbapenems (meropenem 8–25 mg/kg SQ or IV q 8–12 h) inhibits aceylpeptide hydrolase which may prevent reabsorption of valproic acid metabolites from GI tract.
    o Naloxone (0.04 mg/kg IV, IM, SQ) may partially reverse effects; repeat PRN if improvement noted post administration.
    o L-carnitine supplementation may improve metabolic abnormalities. 50–200 mg/kg PO q 8–12 h in dogs, 250–500 **mg/cat/day** PO in cats.

■ Sodium bicarbonate is indicated for ventricular arrhythmias caused by anticonvulsants that have sodium channel blocker properties (phenytoin, lamotrigine, topiramate, lacosamide, carbamazine, oxcarbazine, zonisamide).
  • Sodium bicarbonate can also be employed to enhance elimination of certain anticonvulsants via alkalization of the urine (phenobarbital, topiramate, lamotrigine).
  • 8.4% sodium bicarbonate can be given over 30 minutes at 1–2 mEq/kg diluted with sterile water.

■ Treat seizures with benzodiazepines.
  • Diazepam 0.5–1.0 mg/kg IV PRN.
  • Midazolam 0.25–0.5 mg/kg IV PRN.
  • Consider levetiracetam 20–30 mg/kg IV q 8 h.

### Alternative Drugs

■ Intralipid emulsion may be considered in cases of anticonvulsants which are lipid soluble such as phenobarbital, phenytoin, lamotrigine, and carbamazine. A CRI of 0.25 mL/kg/min for 30–60 minutes can be used. If lipemia is not present in 4–6 hours, then it may be repeated if clinical signs are still severe.

## Precautions/Interactions

- For anticonvulsants with SSRI properties, drugs that can cause additive serotonergic affects (tramadol, trazodone) should be avoided.
- Anticonvulsants that affect cytochrome P450 isoenzymes (phenobarbital, phenytoin, carbamazine, felbamate, topiramate) can affect the hepatic metabolism of other drugs. Alternatively, drugs that inhibit cytochrome P450 isoenzymes can slow the metabolism of certain anticonvulsants.
- Intralipid emulsion administration may sequester additional lipophilic drugs other than the target anticonvulsant.

## Extracorporeal Therapy

- Anticonvulsants that may be amenable to extracorporeal therapy include phenobarbital, valproic acid, topiramate, phenytoin, lamotrigine, lacosamide, carbamazine, and zonisamide.

## Patient Monitoring

- Patient vital signs (heart rate, respiratory rate, temperature, and blood pressure) and neurologic status should be carefully monitored.
- Continuous ECG should be used if cardiotoxic anticonvulsant was ingested or if arrhythmias are present.
- Monitor patient pulse oximetry and/or carbon dioxide levels for indications of hypoxemia and hypoventilation.
- Thoracic radiographs to assess for aspiration pneumonia.

 **COMMENTS**

## Prevention/Avoidance

- Pet owners should be advised regarding the risks of anticonvulsant toxicity and keep medications out of reach of pets.

## Possible Complications

- Aspiration pneumonia secondary to sedation/loss of gag reflex and recumbency is a common complication.
- Lasting neurologic deficits or abnormalities are possible.
- Cardiotoxicity and subsequent arrhythmias can result in sudden death. Prolonged antiarrhythmic drugs may be indicated based on persistence of arrhythmias.

## Expected Course and Prognosis

- The expected course of clinical signs is variable with drug and dose ingested and may be prolonged with higher dose ingestions and extended-release formulations.
- Although highly variable and dependent on manifestation of toxicity, the overall prognosis for anticonvulsant toxicosis is guarded with prolonged supportive care.

## See Also

Chapter 20 Benzodiazepines

## Abbreviations

- GABA = gamma-aminobutyric acid
- KBr = potassium bromide

## Suggested Reading

Charalambous M, Shivapour SK, Brodbelt DC, Volk HA. Antiepileptic drugs' tolerability and safety – a systematic review and meta-analysis of adverse effects in dogs. *BMC Vet Res* 2016;12:79.

**Author**: Alicia Mastrocco, DVM, DACVECC
**Consulting Editor**: Steven E. Epstein, DVM, DACVECC

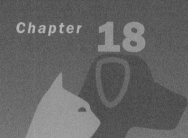

# Chapter 18

# Atypical Antipsychotics (Abilify® and Others)

## DEFINITION/OVERVIEW

- Atypical antipsychotics are a relatively new class of drugs for use in human medicine. May also be known as second-generation antipsychotics.
- Included are aripiprazole (Abilify®), asenapine (Saphris®), clozapine (Clozaril®), olanzapine (Zyprexa®), paliperidone (Invega®), quetiapine (Seroquel®), risperidone (Risperdal®), and ziprasidone (Geodon®).
- While these medications are commonly used in psychiatric disorders in humans, there is no current labeled use for them in veterinary medicine. Several of them have been used off-label in a limited manner for canine aggression.
- CNS depression or sedation, gastrointestinal disturbances (vomiting), hypotension, and tachycardia are the most common clinical signs noted in a toxicosis.

## ETIOLOGY/PATHOPHYSIOLOGY

### Mechanism of Action

- The exact mechanism of action of the atypical antipsychotics is unknown, but it is postulated that they are primarily antagonists at serotonin ($5\text{-}HT_2$) and dopamine ($D_2$) receptors. Aripiprazole is the exception; it is considered a partial agonist at dopamine ($D_2$) and serotonin $5\text{-}HT_{2(1A)}$ receptors and an antagonist at serotonin $5\text{-}HT_{2(2A)}$ receptors.
- Many of the atypical antipsychotics exhibit varying degrees of antagonism at alpha-1- adrenergic and histamine ($H_1$) receptors, which explains why they may cause orthostatic hypotension and somnolence, respectively.
- Risperidone, quetiapine, and paliperidone exhibit antagonism at alpha-2-adrenergic receptors.
- Quetiapine and olanzapine exhibit antagonism at muscarinic receptors and may cause anticholinergic signs.

### Pharmacokinetics or Toxicokinetics – Adsorption, Distribution, Metabolism, Excretion

- Based primarily on human literature; very little animal information is available.
- All the atypical antipsychotics have good oral absorption.
- All undergo varying degrees of hepatic metabolism, some through the CYP450 isoenzymes.
- All the atypical antipsychotics are excreted in the urine either as unchanged drug or as metabolites. Forced diuresis or hemodialysis is unlikely to be beneficial as these drugs generally are highly protein bound and/or have a large volume of distribution.

*Blackwell's Five-Minute Veterinary Consult Clinical Companion: Small Animal Toxicology*, Third Edition.
Edited by Lynn R. Hovda, Ahna G. Brutlag, Robert H. Poppenga, and Steven E. Epstein.
© 2024 John Wiley & Sons, Inc. Published 2024 by John Wiley & Sons, Inc.

- Risperidone (dog).
  - Oral absorption – rapid and extensive.
  - Oral bioavailability 80–100%.
  - Peak plasma parent compound 80 minutes; active metabolite 18 hours.
  - Protein-binding parent compound 92%; active metabolite 80%.

## Toxicity

- Toxic doses in animals are not well established
- Risperidone.
  - Oral $LD_{50}$ in dogs is 14–24 mg/kg.
  - Studies in the literature have revealed that animals should be able to survive a total dose of at least 5 mg with supportive care.
- Ziprasidone.
  - Oral $LD_{50}$ in dogs is 2000 mg/kg.

## Systems Affected

- Gastrointestinal – vomiting, diarrhea, hypersalivation.
- Nervous – sedation, depression, ataxia, disorientation, agitation, anxiety, hyperesthesia
- Cardiovascular – hypotension, tachycardia.
- Neuromuscular – tremors or seizures.
- Respiratory – depression.

 # SIGNALMENT/HISTORY

- All breeds or veterinary species can be affected.

## Risk Factors

- Animals with the following underlying conditions are at risk.
  - Seizure disorders.
  - Cardiovascular disease.
  - Pregnant or nursing.
  - Patients with significant renal impairment may have reduced drug clearance.

## Historical Findings

- Witnessed ingestion or administration.
- Discovery of chewed prescription bottle or pill-minder.
- The owner may find the animal vomiting, depressed, or agitated or not acting themselves.

## Location and Circumstances of Poisoning

- Exposures generally occur in the home due to unsecured medications or accidental administration.

 # CLINICAL FEATURES

- The most common signs are vomiting, CNS depression, hypotension, and tachycardia.
- Other signs, occurring less often and which may be drug dependent, include the development of ataxia, agitation, anxiety, hyperactivity, diarrhea, tremors, seizures, and possible arrhythmias.

# DIFFERENTIAL DIAGNOSIS

- CNS depressants – benzodiazepines, phenothiazines, barbiturates, marijuana, ivermectin, antidepressants, muscle relaxants.
- Cardiovascular drugs – ACE inhibitors, beta-blockers, calcium channel blockers.

# DIAGNOSTICS

## Clinical Pathological Findings

- Biochemistry – check for preexisting disease that may affect elimination of the drug.
- Electrolytes – hyponatremia, hypokalemia.

## Other Diagnostics

- Blood pressure.
- ECG.
- In severe cases, 24/7 intensive care monitoring will be warranted.

## Pathological Findings

- No specific gross or histopathological findings.

# THERAPEUTICS

- The goals of treatment are to prevent absorption, address neurological and cardiovascular status, and provide supportive care.

## Detoxification

- Induce emesis if ingestion occurred within the past 30–60 minutes and the dog is asymptomatic.
- If emesis was not induced at home, perform in DVM's office within 60 minutes of ingestion.
  - Note: risperidone and olanzapine may reduce the effectiveness of dopamine agonists such as apomorphine and ropinirole.
- Activated charcoal with a cathartic may be given for one dose. Generally, most beneficial when given within 60 minutes of ingestion.
- Multidose activated charcoal without a cathartic may be considered when significant ingestion of sustained-release formulations has occurred. Multiple doses of activated charcoal should be given eight hours apart for no more than 48 hours.

## Appropriate Health Care

- If clinical signs are present, hospitalize until asymptomatic, generally about 12–24 hours.
- Maintain hydration and monitor for hypernatremia if using multiple-dose activated charcoal.
- Monitor vitals including blood pressure and mental status.

## Drug(s) of Choice

- IV fluids to improve renal perfusion and correct hypotension.
- Vasopressor agents only after hydration is optimized and when hypotension does not respond to IV fluids. Use of norepinephrine and phenylephrine may be preferred over

epinephrine or dopamine due to their beta-adrenergic effects worsening hypotension in the face of drug-induced alpha blockade.
  - Norepinephrine 0.05–0.3 mcg/kg/min IV CRI.
  - Phenylephrine 1–3 mcg/kg/min IV CRI.
- Agitation and CNS stimulation.
  - Diazepam 0.5–1 mg/kg IV.
  - Midazolam 0.1–0.3 mg/kg SC, IM, IV.
  - Phenobarbital 3–5 mg/kg IV PRN.
- Extrapyramidal syndrome.
  - Diphenhydramine 2–4 mg/kg IM or PO.

## Precautions/Interactions

- In humans, there are many potential drug interactions. While many of them are theoretical and focus on concern for worsening QT interval (not commonly noted in veterinary patients with atypical antipsychotic toxicoses), they include several common medications used in veterinary medicine. These include but are not limited to sodium channel-blocking or potassium-blocking antiarrhythmics, TCAs, dolasetron, ondansetron, phenothiazine tranquilizers, cisapride, ketoconazole, itraconazole, sulfamethoxazole trimethoprim, and metronidazole.
- Both atypical antipsychotics and cyproheptadine are antagonists at the serotonin 5-HT$_{2A}$ receptor. Therefore, cyproheptadine is unlikely to be helpful in treating atypical antipsychotic toxicoses.
- For those drugs that are metabolized via hepatic CYP450 isoenzymes, there may be interactions with drugs that affect CYP450 (phenobarbital).
- There is some controversy about whether true neuroleptic malignant syndrome, found in human beings and other species, occurs in dogs and cats. Some veterinarians agree, some disagree.
- Do not induce vomiting in symptomatic animals.

## Alternate Drugs

- Intravenous lipid emulsion (ILE) may be considered in severe cases as at least some of the atypical antipsychotics are lipid soluble.
  - ILE 20% emulsion: 0.25 mL/kg/min (15 mL/kg/h) IV for 30–60 minutes.
  - Can consider repeating the dose if lipemia is absent in 4–6 hours, and the patient is still symptomatic.

## Extracorporeal Therapy

- For drugs with high protein binding, therapeutic plasma exchange may be of benefit if clinical signs are severe.

## Patient Monitoring

- Observation may be required for as long as 24 hours.
- Patients should be normal for 4–6 hours after any therapeutic intervention before discharge.

## Diet

- Animal may return to normal diet at discharge or may be given several days of bland diet if GI irritation is persistent.

## COMMENTS

### Prevention/Avoidance

- Store medications in locked or difficult-to-reach cabinets.
- Keep purses and full shopping bags off the floor and away from easy-to-reach places.
- Do not leave medications on countertops that may be accessible to a pet.
- Store human and veterinary medications separately to avoid mix-ups.

### Possible Complications

- Rhabdomyolysis if seizures or tremors occur and are left untreated.

### Expected Course and Prognosis

- Clinical signs typically develop within one hour but may take up to several hours.
- Signs resolve in 12–24 hours but may be prolonged when sustained-release products have been ingested.
- Prognosis for recovery is excellent, especially with early treatment. Appropriately treated animals rarely die after ingestion of atypical antipsychotics.

### Synonyms

Aripiprazole (Abilify®), asenapine (Saphris®), clozapine (Clozaril®), olanzapine (Zyprexa®), paliperidone (Invega®), quetiapine (Seroquel®), risperidone (Risperdal®), and ziprasidone (Geodon®).

### Abbreviations

See Appendix 1 for a complete list.

### Suggested Reading

Ader M, Kim SP, Catalano KJ et al. Metabolic dysregulation with atypical antipsychotics occurs in the absence of underlying disease: a placebo-controlled study of olanzapine and risperidone in dogs. *Diabetes* 2005;54(3):862–871.

Depoortere R, Barret-Gevoz C, Bardin L et al. Apomorphine-induced emesis in dogs: differential sensitivity to established and novel dopamine D2/5HT(1A) antipsychotic compounds. *Eur J Pharmacol* 2008;597:1–3.

Juurlink D. Antipsychotics. In: Flomenbaum NE, Goldfrank LR, Hoffman RS et al. (eds) *Goldfrank's Toxicologic Emergencies*, 8th edn. New York: McGraw-Hill, 2006; pp. 1039–1051.

**Author**: Kirsten Waratuke, DVM, DABT, DABVT
**Consulting Editor**: Steven E. Epstein, DVM, DACVECC

# Chapter 19

# Baclofen

## DEFINITION/OVERVIEW

- Baclofen (gamma-amino-beta-[p-chlorophenyl]-butyric acid) is a centrally acting skeletal muscle relaxant that mimics gama-aminobutyric acid (GABA) within the spinal cord and brain.
- It is used primarily in people to alleviate muscle spasticity and pain associated with multiple sclerosis, cerebral palsy, and spinal cord disorders.
- Baclofen has also been used extra-label in dogs to treat urinary retention by reducing urethral sphincter tone. However, it is used uncommonly in dogs given its narrow margin of safety and is not recommended in cats.
- In dogs and cats with baclofen toxicosis, the CNS is the most common body system affected, but clinical signs can also involve the respiratory, GI, CV, and urinary systems. The most life-threatening signs include refractory seizures, coma, respiratory depression, and respiratory arrest.

## ETIOLOGY/PATHOPHYSIOLOGY

### Mechanism of Action

- The mechanism of action of baclofen is not completely understood, but it is believed to reduce afferent reflex activity in the spinal cord, causing decreased muscle tone and spasticity.
- Baclofen is a selective agonist of $GABA_B$ receptors in the spinal cord and brain. Binding of the drug to $GABA_B$ receptors reduces calcium influx into presynaptic nerve terminals, thereby preventing release of excitatory neurotransmitters (glutamate, aspartate, and substance P) by primary afferent neurons. $GABA_B$ agonism also results in opening of selective $K^+$ channels and hyperpolarization of the neuronal membrane, and an increase in inhibitory neuronal signals in postsynaptic neurons.
- The mechanism for baclofen-induced seizures is also not entirely understood but may result from reduced GABA release from presynaptic neurons, causing excessive postsynaptic nerve firing.
- At therapeutic doses, baclofen crosses the blood–brain barrier in small amounts. However, in overdoses significant concentrations can be reached in the CSF, contributing to signs such as coma and respiratory depression.

### Pharmacokinetics or Toxicokinetics – Absorption, Distribution, Metabolism, Excretion

- Baclofen is rapidly and completely absorbed from the GIT, although absorption may be prolonged over several hours in cases of overdoses or large volume of gastric contents.

---

*Blackwell's Five-Minute Veterinary Consult Clinical Companion: Small Animal Toxicology*, Third Edition.
Edited by Lynn R. Hovda, Ahna G. Brutlag, Robert H. Poppenga, and Steven E. Epstein.
© 2024 John Wiley & Sons, Inc. Published 2024 by John Wiley & Sons, Inc.

- Peak plasma concentration of baclofen is within 2–3 hours. Plasma half-life is 2–6 hours, though this can increase significantly with overdoses.
- Baclofen has a moderate volume of distribution and low protein binding (30%).
- Approximately 70–85% of the drug is eliminated unchanged in the urine via the kidneys. The remainder undergoes deamination in the liver to an inactive product and is excreted in the bile. Some deamination occurs in the renal tubules.

## Toxicity

- There is no current established toxic dose of baclofen in dogs or cats.
- The oral $LD_{50}$ has been reported to be 145 mg/kg in rats and 200 mg/kg in mice, but clinical effects are noted at significantly lower doses in dogs and cats.
- In dogs, the lowest dose of ingested baclofen reported to cause clinical signs (CNS depression, dyspnea, hypothermia) was 0.7 mg/kg in one study. The lowest dose at which death was reported was 2.3 mg/kg.
- Of two cats with a known baclofen dose, ingested quantities were 1.7 mg/kg and 14.7 mg/kg. Both developed clinical signs; the latter died two hours after exposure.
- As wide ranges are reported to be toxic in dogs and cats, all ingestions should be considered potentially clinically relevant.

## Systems Affected

- Nervous – CNS depression, ataxia, vocalization, agitation, disorientation, blindness, nystagmus, miosis, mydriasis, tremors, seizures, coma.
- Respiratory – tachypnea, dyspnea, respiratory depression or hypoventilation, pulmonary edema, respiratory arrest.
- Gastrointestinal – vomiting, hypersalivation, anorexia, diarrhea, regurgitation.
- Cardiovascular – bradycardia, tachycardia, arrhythmias, hypotension, hypertension.
- Renal/urological – urinary incontinence.
- Endocrine/metabolic – hypothermia, hyperthermia.

 # SIGNALMENT/HISTORY

### Risk Factors

- Dogs and cats have a greater risk for exposure and ingestion if they live in households with baclofen.

### Historical Findings

- A history of ingestion coupled with suggestive clinical signs is helpful for diagnostic purposes. History of ingestion may include evidence of a chewed bottle, witnessed ingestion, or inadvertent/accidental administration by a pet owner.

 # CLINICAL FEATURES

- Onset of clinical signs may be rapid (30–60 minutes) or delayed (several hours) following acute ingestion. In dogs, onset of signs has been reported to be as early as 15 minutes or as late as seven hours after exposure.
- CNS signs occur in most animals. CNS depression, lethargy, vocalization/agitation, and ataxia are common. Coma, generalized flaccid paralysis, and seizures can be life threatening and may necessitate intubation and mechanical ventilation.

- GI signs occur frequently, while respiratory, cardiovascular, and urinary signs are less common. Respiratory depression and hypoventilation secondary to paralysis of the diaphragm and intercostal muscles can also be life-threatening and require mechanical ventilation.
- Because baclofen is cleared slowly from the CNS, clinical signs can continue after serum baclofen concentration has normalized. The duration of signs has been reported to vary from several hours to several days.

 # DIFFERENTIAL DIAGNOSIS

- Neuromuscular disease such as lower motor neuron disease (e.g., botulism, polyradiculoneuritis, tick paralysis, myasthenia gravis).
- Intracranial causes of brain disease (e.g., infectious, inflammatory, neoplastic).
- Primary metabolic disease (e.g., renal, hepatic, hypoadrenocorticism, hypoglycemia, electrolyte abnormalities).
- Other toxicants (e.g., benzodiazepines, opioids, barbiturates, SSRIs, TCAs, illicit drugs).

 # DIAGNOSTICS

## Clinical Pathological and Other Diagnostic Findings

- Serum baclofen concentrations can be determined in specialized laboratories, but turnaround times may be delayed, and serum concentrations may be normal despite clinical signs.
- Oxygenation may be assessed using arterial blood gas analysis or pulse oximetry.
- Ventilation may be evaluated using arterial blood gas analysis, venous blood gas analysis (in cardiovascularly stable patients), or $ETCO_2$ monitoring.
- Thoracic radiographs are useful to detect aspiration pneumonia.
- CBC and biochemistry can be used to assess systemic health or evaluate for other differentials, but there are no findings specific to baclofen intoxication.

 # THERAPEUTICS

## Detoxification

- Induce emesis as soon as possible if recent ingestion and asymptomatic.
- Consider gastric lavage if known large quantities were ingested and emesis is unproductive or not possible.
- Administer one dose of activated charcoal with a cathartic (baclofen does not undergo enterohepatic circulation).
- Enhance elimination with IV fluid diuresis.

## Appropriate Health Care

- The majority of therapy is symptomatic and supportive care – medical therapy for seizures and other signs that arise, recumbent care, temperature control, repeated assessment of airway protection, and respiratory support as needed.
- Intravenous crystalloids are recommended to address volume or hydration deficits, maintenance needs, and ongoing excessive losses as needed.
- Additional considerations to reduce the effects of baclofen include intravenous lipid emulsion therapy and hemodialysis/hemoperfusion (see below).
- Severe hypoventilation or hypoxemia may warrant intubation and mechanical ventilation.

## Drug(s) of Choice

- Intravenous lipid emulsion therapy can be utilized to reduce the effects of lipophilic toxins. Complications associated with ILE can include hyperlipidemia, corneal lipidosis, hemolysis, acute respiratory distress, cardiovascular dysfunction, AKI, and coagulopathy.
  - ILE 20% emulsion: 0.25 mL/kg/min (15 mL/kg/h) IV for 30–60 minutes.
  - Can consider repeating the dose if lipemia is absent, and the patient is still symptomatic.
- For seizure control, benzodiazepines are the primary treatment option. If there are refractory seizures, anesthesia with propofol may be required.
  - Diazepam 0.25–0.5 mg/kg IV.
  - Midazolam 0.1–0.5 mg/kg IV, can follow with CRI of 0.1–0.3 mg/kg/h IV if needed.
  - Propofol 1–4 mg/kg IV slow bolus, followed by CRI of 0.05–0.4 mg/kg/min IV.
- To alleviate agitation, one of the following sedatives can be considered.
  - Acepromazine 0.01–0.04 mg/kg IV, SQ, IM q 4–6 hours PRN.
  - Diazepam 0.1–0.25 mg/kg IV to effect PRN.
  - Midazolam 0.1–0.25 mg/kg IV to effect PRN.
- To reduce vocalization or disorientation, cyproheptadine hydrochloride (serotonergic antagonist) can be considered.
  - Dogs: 1.1 mg/kg PO or rectally (crushed and mixed with saline) q 4–6 hours PRN.
  - Cats: 2–4 mg total dose PO or rectally q 4–6 hours PRN.
- For bradycardia, atropine can be considered.
  - Atropine 0.01-0.04 mg/kg IV.
- Anti-nausea medication can be administered as needed.

## Alternative Drugs

- Flumazenil has been used in people with baclofen toxicosis and in experimental rats with variable results. The drug can potentially precipitate seizures.
  - Flumazenil 0.01 mg/kg IV to effect.

## Extracorporeal Therapy

- Hemodialysis and hemoperfusion have shown some success in veterinary case reports in shortening the serum elimination half-life of baclofen, reducing clinical signs, and decreasing hospitalization and recovery time. Baclofen's low molecular weight, low protein binding, and moderate volume of distribution suggest it is potentially suitable for removal by hemodialysis.

## Patient Monitoring

- Minimum requirements include regular monitoring of vitals and recheck physical and neurologic examinations.
- Depending on the severity of critical illness, intensive monitoring may be required and may include continuous ECG, pulse oximetry, capnography, blood pressures, blood gas monitoring, and temperature probe.
- Patients that are recumbent or intubated require meticulous attention to eye care, oral care, airway management, cleaning, and rotation/passive range of motion.

 **COMMENTS**

### Prevention/Avoidance

- Client education and prevention of access to baclofen are essential.

## Possible Complications

■ Aspiration pneumonia is a common and potentially severe complication. Patients are prone to this complication given a frequent combination of altered mentation, seizures, vomiting, and paralysis of respiratory muscles.

## Expected Course and Prognosis

■ Prognosis will vary significantly based on quantity ingested, expediency of appropriate treatment, and development of complications. Prognosis is likely to be good with early, appropriate care but may be guarded to poor with extended time to veterinary care, large ingestion, and development of seizures or aspiration pneumonia.

■ In one retrospective study of baclofen ingestion, 84% (57/68) of dogs with a known outcome survived. The amount of baclofen ingested was significantly lower in dogs that survived (median 4.2 mg/kg, range 0.61–61 mg/kg) compared to nonsurvivors (median 14 mg/kg, range 2.3–52.3 mg/kg).

■ In the same retrospective study, two out of three cats with known status survived.

■ Hospitalization up to 5–7 days may be required for full recovery depending on severity. No residual CNS or other effects are expected.

## See Also

Chapter 20 Benzodiazepines
Chapter 32 SSRI and SNRI Antidepressants
Chapter 31 Opiates and Opioids

## Abbreviations

■ AKI = acute kidney injury
■ $ETCO_2$ = end-tidal carbon dioxide
■ GABA = gamma-aminobutyric acid

## Suggested Reading

Fox CM, Daly ML. Successful treatment of severe baclofen toxicosis initially refractory to conventional treatment. *Clin Case Rep* 2016;5(1):44–50.

Gabba L, Iannucci C, Vigani A. Hemodialysis as emergency treatment of a severe baclofen intoxication in a 3 kg dog. *Vet Med Sci* 2023;9:43–46.

Hoffman L, Londoño LA, Martinez J. Management of severe baclofen toxicosis using hemodialysis in conjunction with mechanical ventilation in a cat with chronic kidney disease. *JFMS Open Rep* 2021;7(2):20551169211033770.

Khorzad R, Lee JA, Wheelan M et al. Baclofen toxicosis in dogs and cats: 145 cases (2004–2010). *J Am Vet Med Assoc* 2012;241(8):1059–1064.

Wismer T. Baclofen overdose in dogs. *Vet Med* 2004;99:406–408.

**Author:** Kate S. Farrell, DVM, DACVECC
**Consulting Editor:** Steven E. Epstein, DVM, DACVECC

# Chapter 20

# Benzodiazepines

## DEFINITION/OVERVIEW

- Several benzodiazepines are commonly used in veterinary medicine – diazepam (Valium®), midazolam (Versed®), alprazolam (Xanax®), and zolazepam found in combination with tiletamine, a dissociative agent (Telazol®).
- Many other benzodiazepines are used in human medicine (see Table 20.1).
- Benzodiazepines are used as tranquilizing sedatives. They act as anxiolytics, muscle relaxants, and anticonvulsants.
- Benzodiazepines have a wide margin of safety.
- Common clinical signs of overdose are related to the CNS and include confusion, ataxia, and depression, but paradoxical reactions including agitation and aggression can be seen.

## ETIOLOGY/PATHOPHYSIOLOGY

### Mechanism of Action

- Benzodiazepines interact with the benzodiazepine receptors that modulate gamma-aminobutyric acid (GABA), an inhibitory neurotransmitter.
- Chronic oral use of diazepam in cats can result in fulminant hepatic failure through an unknown mechanism. Toxicity may relate to the cat's inherent deficiency in glucuronide conjugation and glutathione detoxification of reactive intermediates.

### Pharmacokinetics or Toxicokinetics – Absorption, Distribution, Metabolism, Excretion

- Well absorbed orally.
- All are highly protein bound and lipid soluble.
- Peak plasma levels generally occur between 30 and 120 minutes.
- Widely distributed to brain, liver, and spleen; poorly to fat and muscle.
- Metabolized in liver to active and inactive metabolites.
- Half-life elimination of diazepam (cat) after IV dosing – 5.46 hours.
- Half-life elimination of nordiazepam (active diazepam metabolite) (cat) after IV dosing – 21.3 hours.
- Conjugated with glucuronide and excreted in urine.
- Duration of action is specific for each benzodiazepine compound.

*Blackwell's Five-Minute Veterinary Consult Clinical Companion: Small Animal Toxicology*, Third Edition. Edited by Lynn R. Hovda, Ahna G. Brutlag, Robert H. Poppenga, and Steven E. Epstein. © 2024 John Wiley & Sons, Inc. Published 2024 by John Wiley & Sons, Inc.

**TABLE 20.1** Benzodiazepine drugs currently on the market.

| Generic name | Trade name | Peak plasma level in hours (human data) | T½ in hours (human data) | Speed of onset |
|---|---|---|---|---|
| Alprazolam | Xanax® | 1–2 | 6.3–26.9 | Intermediate |
| Chlordiazepoxide | Librium® | 0.5–4 | 5–30 | Intermediate |
| Clonazepam | Klonopin® | 1–2 | 18–50 | Intermediate |
| Clorazepate | Tranxene® | 1–2 | 40–50 | Fast |
| Diazepam | Valium® | 0.5–2 | 20–80 | Very fast |
| Estazolam | Prosom® | 2 | 8–28 | Fast |
| Flurazepam | Dalmane® | 0.5–1 | 2–3 | Fast |
| Lorazepam | Ativan® | 2–4 | 10–20 | Intermediate |
| Midazolam | Versed® | 0.28–0.83 | 2.2–6.8 | Very fast |
| Oxazepam | Serax® | 2–4 | 5–20 | Slow |
| Quazepam | Doral® | 1–2 | 41 | Fast |
| Temazepam | Restoril® | 1.6–2 | 3.5–18.4 | Fast |
| Triazolam | Halcion® | 1–2 | 1.5–5.5 | Fast |

## Toxicity

- Overdose as a single exposure is rarely life-threatening in healthy animals.
- Generally, oral diazepam overdoses of >20 mg/kg are considered significant. Other more potent benzodiazepines are proportionately more toxic.
- Chronic exposure of more than one dose of diazepam may be life-threatening in the cat.

## Systems Affected

- Nervous – CNS depression, dysphoria, ataxia, excitement, aggression.
- Respiratory – respiratory depression.
- Cardiovascular – bradycardia, hypotension.
- Endocrine/metabolic – hypothermia from sedation.
- Hepatic – fulminant hepatic necrosis (cats only); appears as anorexia, lethargy, vomiting, dehydration, hypothermia, icterus, increased liver enzymes, coagulopathy, hypoglycemia.

# SIGNALMENT/HISTORY

### Risk Factors

- Any age or breed of dog or cat can be affected.
- Overdose usually occurs due to iatrogenic administration of an improper dose or ingestion of medication.
- Benzodiazepines present in the household may pose an increased risk of exposure to pets.
- Pediatric, geriatric, or debilitated patients with underlying metabolic disease may have prolonged duration of effects from toxicosis, or even from therapeutic dosing.
- Cats given oral, chronic diazepam for behavior modification treatment may develop acute fulminant hepatic necrosis.

### Historical Findings

- Witnessed exposure by pet owner.
- Pet owner may find chewed pill vial or suspect missing pill.
- Clinical symptoms of ataxia, sedation, agitation, and dysphoria may be noted by the pet owner.

 CLINICAL FEATURES

- Common clinical signs include CNS depression, ataxia, confusion, disorientation, agitation, and aggression.
- As ingested dose increases, risks for hypotension, hypothermia, coma, and seizures occur.
- In approximately 40–50% of cases, paradoxical stimulation and excitation occur in both dogs and cats.

 DIFFERENTIAL DIAGNOSIS

- Primary metabolic disease (hepatic encephalopathy, hypoglycemia).
- Primary neurological disease.
- Toxicants.
    - Sedation.
        - Alcohols and glycols (e.g., ethanol, methanol, ethylene glycol).
        - Barbiturates.
        - Marijuana.
        - Opioids.
        - Phenothiazines.
    - Agitation.
        - Amphetamines.
        - Antidepressants (serotonin syndrome).
        - Cocaine.
        - Pseudoephedrine.

 DIAGNOSTICS

- Baseline CBC, chemistry, UA to evaluate underlying metabolic disease.
- The Quick Screen Pro Multi Drug Screening Test is a human testing kit that has been validated by GC/MS for use in animals. It may provide a rapid and accurate diagnosis if the drug is present in high enough concentrations and the time frame is appropriate.
- Urine or serum can be submitted specifically for GC/MS or LC/MS, but the results will take several days to be returned and will only indicate exposure.
- In cats suspected of having acute hepatic necrosis, a coagulation panel should be done to evaluate PT/aPTT.
- Blood gas monitoring may be indicated when severe clinical signs are present to monitor for respiratory depression.

### Pathological Findings

- No histological changes are expected in acute overdoses.
- Histology of the feline liver shows severe, acute to subacute, lobular to massive hepatic necrosis.

**THERAPEUTICS**

- For exposures of <20 mg/kg PO diazepam or equivalent for other benzodiazepines, many animals can be monitored at home. Animals should be confined to areas where they cannot injure themselves, e.g., by falling down stairs.
- Treatment consists of general supportive measures, early decontamination, and if necessary, administration of the reversal agent flumazenil.

### Detoxification

- Emesis with extreme caution due to rapid onset of signs.
- One dose of activated charcoal with a cathartic for large ingestions although an increased risk of aspiration should be considered.

### Appropriate Health Care

- Monitor body temperature and blood pressure; support appropriately with warming methods and IV fluid therapy. Monitor for severe CNS or respiratory depression; if indicated, consider the use of flumazenil.
- Cats suffering from hepatic failure due to oral diazepam need medical treatment.

### Antidote

- Flumazenil is the specific antidote for benzodiazepine overdose but should be used only in cases where CNS depression or agitation is severe. Flumazenil rapidly reverses the sedative and muscle relaxant effects of the benzodiazepine agonists. Effects are usually seen within five minutes. Seizures have been associated with the use of flumazenil.
  - Dose: flumazenil 0.01 mg/kg IV to effect, repeat PRN. If a long-acting benzodiazepine has been ingested, repeated doses of flumazenil may be necessary, due to its short duration of action (1–2 hours).

### Drug(s) of Choice

- IV fluids as needed to treat hypotension, maintain perfusion, and correct dehydration. A balanced crystalloid should be used.
- If the animal is experiencing paradoxical stimulation (e.g., agitation, aggression), treatment with additional benzodiazepines (e.g., diazepam) is contraindicated. An alternative sedative or anxiolytic should be used.
  - Acepromazine 0.01–0.1 mg/kg, IV, SQ, IM PRN.
  - Dexmedetomidine 1–3 mcg/kg IV PRN.

### Precautions/Interactions

- Diazepam is not water soluble, and the parenteral formula contains 40% propylene glycol and 10% ethanol. It is very irritating, painful, and poorly absorbed when given IM. Excessive propylene glycol exposure in cats may cause Heinz body formation.

 **COMMENTS**

### Prevention/Avoidance

- Owners should be informed about the risks of benzodiazepines in pets, and keep them out of reach, particularly in the bedroom (sleep aid medication placed on bedroom table).
- Owners should be advised not to use their own medicines to treat their pets and to keep them out of the reach of pets.

## Patient Monitoring

- While hospitalized, excessively sedate patients should have blood pressure, ECG, TPR, and ventilatory status closely monitored.

## Expected Course and Prognosis

- Once decontaminated, animals generally only need to be monitored for 4–8 hours. If no clinical signs develop, the patient can be monitored at home. If signs develop, they should be monitored until clinical signs have resolved (typically 8–24 hours depending on the drug involved).
- In those animals experiencing a single overdose exposure, the prognosis is excellent.
- In those cats experiencing idiosyncratic hepatic failure due to repeated doses of oral diazepam, the prognosis is poor to guarded. Based on this, oral chronic use of benzodiazepines should be avoided in cats.

## See Also

Chapter 9 Ethylene Glycol and Diethylene Glycol
Chapter 31 Opiates and Opioids
Chapter 30 Nonbenzodiazepine Sleep Aids

## Abbreviations

See appendix 1

## Suggested Reading

Center SA, Elston TH, Rowland PH et al. Fulminant hepatic failure associated with oral administration of diazepam in 11 cats. *J Am Vet Med Assoc* 1996;209:618–625.
Lemke KA. Anticholinergics and sedatives. In: Tranquilli WJ, Thurmon JC, Grimm KA (eds) *Lumb & Jones Veterinary Anesthesia and Analgesia*, 4th edn. Ames: Blackwell, 2007; pp. 203–239.
Malouin A, Boiler M. Sedatives, muscle relaxants, and opioids toxicity. In: Silverstein DC, Hopper K (eds) *Small Animal Critical Care Medicine*. St Louis: Elsevier, 2009; pp. 350–356.

**Author**: Eric Dunayer, MS, VMD, DABT, DABVT
**Consulting Editor**: Steven E. Epstein, DVM, DACVECC

# Beta-2 Receptor Agonists (Albuterol and Others)

# Chapter 21

## DEFINITION/OVERVIEW

- Beta-2 receptor agonists such as albuterol (salbutamol), formoterol, clenbuterol and terbutaline are used as bronchodilators in human and veterinary medicine in the management of asthma and chronic obstructive pulmonary disease (COPD).
- They are available as tablets, oral solutions, as powders and solutions for inhalers, and pressurized metered-dose inhalers.
- Most cases in pets involve dogs chewing and piercing an albuterol inhaler.
- Common signs include tachycardia, tachypnea, vomiting, lethargy, panting, hypokalemia, and tremors.

## ETIOLOGY/PATHOPHYSIOLOGY

### Mechanism of Action

- Activation of beta-2 receptors stimulates the adenylyl cyclase-cyclic adenosine monophosphate (cAMP) system resulting in decreased intracellular calcium concentration, increased membrane potassium conductance and inhibition of myosin phosphorylation. This leads to relaxation of bronchial, vascular, and uterine smooth muscle.
- Selectivity for beta-2-adrenergic receptors is diminished at high doses, causing activation of beta-1-adrenergic receptors resulting in cardiovascular stimulation.
- Increased heart rate can occur as a reflex response to systemic hypotension resulting from beta-2 receptor agonist-induced peripheral and coronary vasodilation or activation of beta-1-adrenergic receptors.
- Hypokalemia occurs due to cAMP-mediated stimulation of the $Na^+/K^+$ adenosine triphosphate (ATP) pump causing transcellular shifts. The decrease in serum potassium is transient and total body potassium does not decrease.
- Complications of hypokalemia include muscle hyperpolarization which can cause arrhythmias, muscle weakness and flaccid paralysis.

### Pharmacokinetics or Toxicokinetics – Adsorption, Distribution, Metabolism, Excretion

- Beta-2 receptor agonists are rapidly and well absorbed. Effects can occur within minutes of inhalation and 30 minutes of ingestion but may take up to four hours with ingestion.
- These drugs are widely distributed and cross the blood–brain barrier and placenta, to varying degrees.
- Both unchanged parent drug and hepatic metabolites are excreted.

---

*Blackwell's Five-Minute Veterinary Consult Clinical Companion: Small Animal Toxicology*, Third Edition.
Edited by Lynn R. Hovda, Ahna G. Brutlag, Robert H. Poppenga, and Steven E. Epstein.
© 2024 John Wiley & Sons, Inc. Published 2024 by John Wiley & Sons, Inc.

- The majority of the absorbed dose is excreted renally (70–80%) with less excreted in the feces. With formoterol, however, approximately half is excreted renally and half in the feces.
- Albuterol has an oral half-life of approximately three hours in dogs (5–7 hours for sustained-release preparations). The oral half-life of formoterol is 4–6 hours in dogs.

## Toxicity

- The dose is usually unknown in pets that have punctured an inhaler, but most develop clinical signs of toxicosis and require immediate veterinary evaluation.
- Clinical signs are expected in cats and dogs that ingest >0.1 mg/kg of an oral formulation of albuterol.
- Dose-dependent effects have been reported in dogs with oral clenbuterol doses of >3 mcg/kg.
- In dogs the oral $LD_{50}$ of terbutaline is 1000–2000 mg/kg and the minimum lethal oral dose of formoterol is 3000 mg/kg.

## Systems Affected

- Cardiovascular.
  - Excessive beta-2-adrenergic stimulation can cause peripheral vasodilation, hypotension, and reflex tachycardia.
  - Excessive beta-1-adrenergic stimulation results in severe tachycardia and a mild increase in blood pressure.
  - Hypokalemia-induced ECG changes and cardiovascular collapse are rare.
  - Myocardial hypoxia may lead to arrhythmias (VPCs, ventricular tachycardia, etc.).
  - Rarely, chordae tendineae rupture may occur leading to pulmonary edema.
- Endocrine/metabolic.
  - Hypokalemia.
  - Transient hyperglycemia.
  - Rarely, hypophosphatemia.
- Gastrointestinal.
  - Vomiting, polydipsia, inappetence, hypersalivation, and oral inflammation.
  - Possible foreign body ingestion if broken pieces of inhaler are swallowed.
- Neuromuscular/musculoskeletal.
  - Tremors and ataxia may occur due to excessive stimulation of skeletal muscle.
  - Weakness and lethargy occur due to catecholamine depletion in prolonged/untreated toxicosis, pronounced hypokalemia, and poor cardiac output.
  - Severe hypokalemia may result in respiratory muscle paralysis.
  - Rarely rhabdomyolysis.
- Nervous.
  - Excessive beta-adrenergic stimulation in the brain may lead to anxiety, restlessness, apprehension, hyperesthesia, agitation, and rarely, seizures.
- Ophthalmic.
  - Dilated pupils, scleral injection, conjunctival hyperemia, and ocular inflammation.
- Renal/urologic.
  - Rarely, pigmenturia and acute kidney injury secondary to rhabdomyolysis.
- Respiratory.
  - Beta-adrenergic stimulation results in bronchodilation, panting, and tachypnea.
  - Respiratory alkalosis is possible.
- Skin/exocrine.
  - Occasional facial inflammation following puncture of a pressurized inhaler.

# SIGNALMENT/HISTORY

- No sex or breed predilections have been identified, although greyhounds may be more susceptible to developing rhabdomyolysis secondary to beta-2 adrenoreceptor toxicosis due to their heavily muscled body condition.
- No genetic risks of toxicosis.
- Most cases of beta-2 receptor agonist toxicosis occur in dogs.
- Cases of beta-2 receptor agonist toxicosis in cats are uncommon and more likely to occur due to a medication error.

## Risk Factors

- Animals with underlying cardiovascular disease are at greater risk of complications from beta-2 receptor agonist toxicosis.
- Exposure in pregnancy may cause maternal and fetal tachycardia and hyperglycemia and inhibit uterine contractions in late pregnancy.

## Historical Findings

- Owners may report apparent distress, panting, racing, or pounding heart, shaking, weakness, vomiting, bloodshot eyes, and restlessness or hyperactivity.
- History may also include evidence of exposure with a pierced/punctured inhaler (owners may report the sound of the pressurized gas escaping when the inhaler was punctured). Evidence of spilled oral solution or chewed tablet packaging may be found.

## Location and Circumstances of Poisoning

- Exposure typically occurs in unattended household pets with access to medications.

 # CLINICAL FEATURES

- Signs can occur within a few minutes of accidental exposure to an inhaler. Effects may occur within a few hours of ingestion of immediate-release oral preparations or 5–7 hours with extended-release formulations.
- Physical examination may reveal a distressed animal with apprehension, agitation, hyperactivity, restlessness, panting, tachypnea, weakness, tachycardia (and possibly arrhythmias), changes in pulse quality (weak, deficits), tremors, hyperthermia, mild vomiting, scleral injection, and/or conjunctivitis.

 # DIFFERENTIAL DIAGNOSIS

- Vasoconstrictive shock.
- Intoxications.
  - Methylxanthines (e.g., chocolate, caffeine).
  - CNS stimulants (e.g., amphetamines and related drugs, cocaine, sympathomimetic drugs).
  - Metaldehyde.
  - Hops.
  - Tremorgenic mycotoxicosis.

**DIAGNOSTICS**

### Clinical Pathological Findings

- On biochemistry, hypokalemia and hypophosphatemia may be present. In patients given aggressive potassium supplementation, rebound hyperkalemia is possible. Mild hyper- or hypoglycemia may occur. AST and CK may be elevated due to tremors.

### Other Diagnostics

- Continuous ECG and intermittent blood pressure and heart rate monitoring.
- Thoracic radiographs if known cardiac or respiratory disease if indicated (based on auscultation) and/or if dyspneic.

### Pathological Findings

- Rupture of chordae tendineae and pulmonary edema are possible.
- Histopathological evidence of myocardial necrosis and fibrosis, or rhabdomyolysis affecting cardiac and skeletal muscle tissue.

 **THERAPEUTICS**

### Detoxification

- Induction of emesis is indicated if a toxic dose has been ingested, the animal is asymptomatic, and it is within 30 minutes of ingestion of immediate-release tablets or a solution. An emetic may be worthwhile up to 3–4 hours following ingestion of extended-release tablets.
- A single dose of activated charcoal can be given within 30 minutes of an immediate-release tablets or a solution or 3–4 hours after ingestion of extended-release tablets.

### Appropriate Health Care

- All animals that have punctured an inhaler should be evaluated by a veterinarian. Cases involving tablets or solutions should be assessed on an individual basis.
- Patients should be hospitalized until the heart rate and rhythm (ECG), CNS status, and electrolytes normalize.
- Intravenous crystalloids are recommended for hypotension.
- Monitor TPR, heart rhythm, blood pressure, and CNS status.
- Monitor electrolytes, particularly potassium and phosphorus, on presentation, in the presence of ECG changes, during fluid therapy, and in recovery.
- Mechanical ventilation may be required in patients with respiratory paralysis.

### Drug(s) of Choice

- A beta-blocker is recommended for tachycardia (HR >160 bpm in large dogs or >180–200 bpm in small dogs).
  - Propranolol 0.02 mg/kg IV as a nonselective beta-1 and beta-2 receptor antagonist may be of benefit; however, the half-life may be longer than inhaled albuterol.
  - Esmolol 0.1–0.5 mg/kg by slow IV and then a CRI of 10–200 mcg/kg/min to maintain heart rate.
- A benzodiazepine may be given for CNS stimulation, tremors.
  - Diazepam 0.5–1 mg/kg IV to effect.
  - Midazolam 0.1–0.3 mg/kg IV or IM to effect.

- Supplementation if the potassium continues to fall despite a beta-blocker or if the concentration is <2.5 mEq/L (2.5 mmol/L). Give in IV fluids, at a starting rate not exceeding 0.5 mEq/kg/h (0.5 mmol/kg/h).
- Lidocaine for arrhythmias despite beta-blocker administration and potassium supplementation/correction (2 mg/kg slowly IV, bolus followed by 25–80 mcg/kg/min IV CRI).
- Hypophosphatemia usually resolves without intervention. In severe cases (serum phosphorus <1 mg/dL), intravenous supplementation may be necessary (0.06–0.18 mmol/kg of potassium phosphate IV over 6 h, adjust according to response).

### Precautions/Interactions

- Caution with aggressive fluid therapy in patients with hypertension or significant arrhythmias.
- Caution with loop diuretics as these will exacerbate hypokalemia.

### Alternative Drugs

- An oral beta-blocker can be used if an intravenous formulation is not available.
  - Propranolol 0.1–0.2 mg/kg PO q 8 hours (dogs); 2.5–10 mg (total) PO q 8 hours (cats).
  - Metoprolol 0.4–1 mg/kg PO q 8–12 hours (dogs); 2–15 mg (total) PO q 8 hours (cats).
  - Atenolol 0.25–1.5 mg/kg PO q 12 hours (dogs); 6.25 mg (total) PO q 12 hours (cats).

### Patient Monitoring

- Continuous ECG and intermittent blood pressure monitoring.
- Close monitoring of CNS and neuromuscular status.
- Monitoring of serum potassium and phosphorus concentration.
- Regular examination of the oral cavity for up to 24 hours if a pressurized metered-dose inhaler was pierced.

 **COMMENTS**

### Prevention/Avoidance

- Beta-2 receptor agonist medicines, particularly asthma inhalers, should be stored away from pets. Even apparently empty inhalers can cause toxicosis if pierced and the contents inhaled.

### Possible Complications

- Aggressive potassium supplementation can result in rebound hyperkalemia in recovery.
- Potential for catecholamine depletion and prolonged weakness.
- Potential for myocardial necrosis/fibrosis.
- Persistent arrhythmias for up to two months have been reported.
- Rhabdomyolysis and acute kidney injury have been reported in a greyhound that punctured an albuterol inhaler.
- Thermal injury to the oral cavity resulting in airway compromise can occur from puncturing a metered-dose inhaler.

### Expected Course and Prognosis

- Recovery usually occurs within 12–24 hours, sometimes 48 hours.
- Prognosis is excellent with prompt treatment in a healthy animal.
- Cardiac sequelae are rare.

## See Also

Chapter 25 Cocaine
Chapter 71 Chocolate and caffeine
Chapter 36 Club drugs
Chapter 40 Methamphetamine
Chapter 41 Miscellaneous hallucinogens/dissociatives

## Abbreviations

- ATP = adenosine triphosphate
- CNS = central nervous system
- COPD = chronic obstructive pulmonary disease
- cAMP = cyclic adenosine monophosphate
- ECG = electrocardiogram
- VPC = ventricular premature contractions

## Suggested Reading

Crouchley J, Bates N. Retrospective evaluation of acute salbutamol (albuterol) exposure in dogs: 501 cases. *J Vet Emerg Crit Care* 2022;32(4):500–506.

Granfone M, Walker JM. Acute nontraumatic rhabdomyolysis in a Greyhound after albuterol toxicosis. *J Vet Emerg Crit Care* 2021;31(6):818–822.

Mackenzie SD, Blois S, Hayes G, Vince AR. Oral thermal injury associated with puncture of a salbutamol metered-dose inhaler in a dog. *J Vet Emerg Crit Care* 2012;22(4):494–497.

Matos M, Jenni S, Fischer N, Bienz H, Glaus T. [Myocardial damage and paroxysmal ventricular tachycardia in a dog after albuterol intoxication]. *Schweiz Arch Tierheilkd* 2012;154(7):302–305.

Meroni ER, Khorzad R, Bracker K, Sinnott-Stutzman V. Retrospective evaluation of albuterol inhalant exposure in dogs: 36 cases (2007–2017). *J Vet Emerg Crit Care* 2021;31(1):86–93.

**Author**: Nicola Bates, BSc (Brunel), BSc (Open), MSc, MA, SRCS
**Consulting Editor**: Steven E. Epstein, DVM, DACVECC

# Chapter 22

# Beta Receptor Antagonists (Beta-blockers)

## DEFINITION/OVERVIEW

- Beta receptor antagonists (also referred to as beta-adrenergic antagonists or "beta-blockers") are class II antiarrhythmics. In humans, beta-blockers are commonly used to treat systemic hypertension, coronary artery disease, tachyarrhythmias, migraine headaches, benign essential tremors, anxiety, hyperthyroidism, and glaucoma (topical ophthalmic preparations). Beta-blockers are used in animals to treat hypertrophic cardiomyopathy in cats and tachyarrhythmias, systemic hypertension, and glaucoma in cats and dogs.
- This class of drugs has a narrow margin of safety and can cause clinical consequences such as bradycardia, hypotension, hypoglycemia, hyperkalemia, ischemic kidney injury, seizures, and death.
- There is no single antidote or treatment strategy for beta-blocker overdoses. The majority of evidence is low quality, and no single treatment can be recommended over another. Management involves supportive care for hypotension and bradycardia and can include IV fluids, atropine, calcium, intravenous lipid emulsion, high-dose insulin and dextrose therapy, glucagon, and catecholamines.

## ETIOLOGY/PATHOPHYSIOLOGY

### Mechanism of Action

- Beta-adrenergic antagonists work primarily by competitively antagonizing the effects of catecholamines at the beta-adrenergic receptors.
- Negative inotropic and chronotropic actions include decreased sinus HR, slowed AV nodal conduction, diminished cardiac output at rest and during exercise, decreased myocardial oxygen demand, and reduced BP.
- Beta-1 receptors are primarily located in the heart, eye, adipose tissue, and kidney. Cardiovascular effects of beta-1 receptor blockade include bradycardia and decreased contractility.
- Beta-2 receptors are found in bronchial smooth muscle, the gastrointestinal tract, pancreas, liver, skeletal muscle, blood vessels (e.g., coronary, hepatic and skeletal arteries) and heart. Blockade of beta-2 receptors may result in bronchoconstriction or bronchospasm and peripheral vasodilation resulting in hypotension.
- Beta-2-adrenergic stimulation increases insulin release, but also causes pancreatic glucagon secretion and upregulates hepatic glycogenolysis and gluconeogenesis causing a net increase in glucose. Beta-blockers can impair the ability of patients to compensate for hypoglycemia.

*Blackwell's Five-Minute Veterinary Consult Clinical Companion: Small Animal Toxicology*, Third Edition.
Edited by Lynn R. Hovda, Ahna G. Brutlag, Robert H. Poppenga, and Steven E. Epstein.
© 2024 John Wiley & Sons, Inc. Published 2024 by John Wiley & Sons, Inc.

- Beta-2-adrenergic antagonism inhibits catecholamine-mediated uptake of potassium by skeletal muscle. Beta-blockers may cause slight elevations in serum potassium concentrations.

## Pharmacokinetics or Toxicokinetics – Absorption, Distribution, Metabolism, Excretion

- See Table 22.1 for human information.
- Limited data in dogs and cats.
  - Absorption – oral dosing results in rapid absorption for most drugs.
  - Atenolol – beta-1-selective receptor antagonist; at higher dosages beta-2-blockade can occur.
    - Absorption – oral bioavailability in cats up to 90%.
    - Distribution – low protein-binding characteristics (5–15%); water soluble.
    - Metabolism – minimal hepatic biotransformation.
    - Excretion – 40–50% excreted unchanged in the urine; remainder excreted unchanged in the feces. Reported half-lives: dogs 3.2 hours; cats 3.7 hours.
  - Carvedilol – nonselective, beta receptor antagonist with selective alpha-1-adrenergic blocking activity.
    - Absorption – oral bioavailability 3–23%; peak concentrations occur about one hour post oral dose in cats; Vd in dogs ~1.4 L/kg.
    - Excretion – elimination half-life was 100 minutes in dogs after oral dosing and ~4.5 hours in cats.
  - Esmolol – ultra-short-acting beta-1-selective antagonist.
    - Absorption – IV injection results in steady-state blood level 5 minutes after bolus; 20–30 minutes after start of CRI.
    - Distribution – rapidly and widely distributed throughout the body.
    - Metabolism – rapidly metabolized in the blood by esterases.
    - Excretion – terminal half-life is about 10 minutes; duration of action after discontinuing CRI is about 20 minutes in the dog.
  - Metoprolol – beta-1-selective receptor antagonist; at higher dosages beta-2-blockade can occur.
    - Absorption – rapidly and completely absorbed. Large first-pass effect with reduced bioavailability.
    - Distribution – low protein binding of 5–15%.
    - Metabolism – liver.
    - Excretion – primarily excreted in the urine; half-life in dogs is 1.6 hours; cats 1.3 hours.
  - Propranolol – nonselective; blocks both beta-1 and beta-2 receptors.
    - Absorption – rapid first-pass effect through the liver reduces systemic bioavailability to approximately 2–27% in dogs.
    - Metabolism – liver.
    - Excretion – <1% is excreted unchanged into the urine. Half-life in dogs has been reported to range from 0.77 to 2 hours.
  - Sotalol – nonselective beta receptor antagonist and Class III antiarrhythmic agent (potassium channel blocker). The beta-blocking activity of sotalol is about 30% that of propranolol.
    - Absorption – food may reduce the bioavailability.
    - Distribution – low lipid solubility; virtually no protein binding.
    - Elimination – primarily renal; most of the drug is excreted unchanged. Dogs' half-life is 5 hours.

**TABLE 22.1 Human pharmacokinetic information for beta receptor antagonist drugs.**

| | Adrenergic blocking activity | Partial agonist activity (ISA) | Membrane stabilizing activity | Vasodilating property | Lipid solubility | Protein binding | Oral bioavailability | Half-life (h) | Metabolism | Volume of distribution (L/kg) |
|---|---|---|---|---|---|---|---|---|---|---|
| Acebutolol | Beta-1 | Yes | Yes | No | Low | 25% | 40% | 2–4 | Hepatic/renal | 1.2 |
| Betaxolol (ophthalmic and tabs) | Beta-1 | No | Yes | Yes (calcium channel blockade) | Low | 50% | 80–90% | 14–22 | Hepatic/renal | NA |
| Bisoprolol | Beta-1 | No | No | No | Low | 30% | 80% | 9–12 | Hepatic/renal | NA |
| Bucindolol | Beta-1, beta-2 | beta-2 agonism | | Yes (beta-2 agonism) | Moderate | | 30% | 8 ± 4.5 | Hepatic | NA |
| Carteolol (ophthalmic) | Beta-1, beta-2 | Yes | No | Yes (beta-2 agonism and nitric oxide mediated) | Low | 30% | 85% | 5–6 | Renal | NA |
| Celiprolol | Alpha-2, beta-1 | Beta-2 agonism | | Yes (beta-2 agonism) | Low | 22–24% | 30–70% | 5 | Hepatic | NA |
| Labetalol | Alpha-1, beta-1, beta-2 | No | Low | Yes (alpha-1 antagonism) | Moderate | 50% | 20–33% | 4–8 | Hepatic | 9 |
| Levobunolol (ophthalmic) | Beta-1, beta-2 | No | No | No | NA | NA | NA | 6 | NA | NA |
| Metipranolol (ophthalmic) | Beta-1, beta-2 | No | No | No | NA | NA | NA | 3–4 | NA | NA |
| Nadolol | Beta-1, beta-2 | No | No | No | Low | 20–30% | 30–35% | 10–24 | Renal | 2 |
| Nebivolol | Beta-1 | No | No | Yes (nitric oxide mediated?) | Moderate | 98% | 12–96% | 8–32 | Hepatic | 10–40 |
| Oxprenolol | Beta-1, beta-2 | Yes | Yes | No | Moderate | 80% | 20–70% | 1–3 | Hepatic | 1.3 |
| Penbutolol | Beta-1, beta-2 | Yes | No | No | High | 90% | ~100% | 5 | Hepatic/renal | NA |
| Pindolol | Beta-1, beta-2 | Yes | Low | No | Moderate | 50% | 75–90% | 3–4 | Hepatic/renal | 2 |
| Timolol (ophthalmic) | Beta-1, beta-2 | No | No | No | Moderate | 60% | 75% | 3–5 | Hepatic/renal | 2 |

## Toxicity

- Limited published toxicity/overdose information in dogs and cats.
- Anecdotally, doses >2 times the published dose may cause clinical signs.
- Atenolol – therapeutic dose: dogs 0.25–1.5 mg/kg PO q 12 hours; cats 6.25–12.5 mg total dose PO q 12 hours.
- Carvedilol – therapeutic dose: dogs 0.15–0.2 mg/kg PO twice daily initially with slow titration upwards towards a dose of 1.11 mg/kg twice daily.
- Esmolol – therapeutic dose (dogs and cats): initial loading dose of 0.05–0.5 mg/kg (50–500 mcg/kg) administered IV as slow bolus over 2–5 minutes, then followed by a CRI of 10–200 mcg/kg/minute. $LD_{50}$ in dogs is approximately 32 mg/kg IV. Dogs receiving doses of 3 mg/kg/minute for 1 hour showed clinical signs.
- Metoprolol – therapeutic dose: dogs 0.2–1 mg/kg PO q 12–24 hours, slowly titrated upwards every 2–3 weeks with a maximum of 6.6 mg/kg q 8 hours; XR formulation 0.4–1 mg/kg PO q 24 hours, cats 2–15 mg total dose per cat PO q 8 hours.
- Propranolol – therapeutic dose: dogs 0.02 mg/kg IV slowly over 2–3 minutes (up to a maximum of 0.1 mg/kg). Oral dose: 0.1–0.2 mg/kg initially PO q 8 hours, up to a maximum of 1.5 mg/kg q 8 hours; cats 0.02 mg/kg IV slowly over 2–3 minutes (up to a maximum of 0.1 mg/kg). Oral dose: 2.5 mg (up to 10 mg) total dose per cat q 8–12 hours.
- Sotalol – therapeutic dose: dogs and cats 1–3 mg/kg PO q 12 hours.

## Systems Affected

- Cardiovascular – bradycardia, hypotension.
- Nervous – decreased mental status, seizures.
- Endocrine/metabolic – hypoglycemia, hyperkalemia, metabolic acidosis secondary to hypotension, and decreased perfusion.
- Renal – azotemia secondary to hypoperfusion.
- Respiratory – bronchospasm.

 # SIGNALMENT/HISTORY

## Risk Factors

- Animals with preexisting heart condition or bradyarrhythmia are at increased risk for toxicosis.
- Animals with underlying reactive airway disease may experience severe bronchospasm as a consequence of beta-2-mediated bronchodilation blockade.
- Beta-2 receptor antagonists may impair the ability of hypoglycemic patients to compensate.

## Historical Findings

- Clinical signs may include:
  - weakness.
  - collapse.
  - bradycardia.
  - altered mentation.
  - seizures.

## Location and Circumstances of Poisoning

- Poisoning may occur in the home if the owner or patient is on beta receptor antagonist(s).
- Iatrogenic toxicity may occur in the clinic, especially with IV administration.

## CLINICAL FEATURES

Onset of clinical signs will vary depending on the specific drug and formulation. In general, clinical signs will be noted within 2–8 hours after exposure with immediate-release formulations.

- Bradycardia.
- Decreased pulse quality due to hypotension/cardiogenic shock.
- Seizures.
- Respiratory compromise/bronchospasm.
- Altered mental status/coma.

 ## DIFFERENTIAL DIAGNOSIS

- Calcium channel blocker overdose.
- Cardiac disease with secondary arrhythmias.
- Other cardiovascular agent overdose (e.g., clonidine, digoxin toxicosis).
- Sick sinus syndrome.
- Atrioventricular nodal disease.
- Baclofen, opiate/opioid, alpha-2-agonist or other sedative toxicosis.
- Cholinergic drug toxicosis.

 ## DIAGNOSTICS

### Clinical Pathological Findings

- Biochemistry.
    - Hypoglycemia, hyperkalemia, azotemia, elevated liver enzymes.

### Other Diagnostics

- ECG – sinus bradycardia, first-, second-, and third-degree heart block, prolongation of the PR and QT interval or QRS complex.
- Echocardiogram – myocardial depression with negative inotropy.

 ## THERAPEUTICS

### Detoxification

- Emesis can be performed in asymptomatic animals, typically within 1–2 hours after ingestion.
- Consider gastric lavage with altered mental status or large tablet ingestion.
- Activated charcoal with a cathartic at 1–2 g/kg can be administered within 2 hours after exposure; repeat doses without a cathartic can be considered for sustained- or extended-release formulations.
- Whole-bowel irrigation (GoLytely®) can be performed for large ingestion of sustained- or extended-release formulations.

### Appropriate Health Care

- Titrated incremental volume resuscitation with IV crystalloid fluids for hypotension. May be ineffective in patients with bradycardia. Care should be taken to prevent fluid overload in animals with cardiogenic shock.

- Continuous ECG monitoring for assessment of conduction abnormalities.
- Frequent BP monitoring (indirect or direct) for development of hypotension.
- Central line placement – beneficial for frequent BG monitoring.
- Airway protection and ventilatory support as needed for decreased mental status, respiratory depression, or seizure activity.

### Drug(s) of Choice

- No specific antidote is available. Evidence in human and animal studies is low quality and confounded by the use of multiple overlapping treatments.
- Atropine
  - May be used to treat sinus bradycardia or as a pretreatment for any therapies that may increase vagal tone (e.g., induction of emesis, orogastric lavage).
  - Atropine dose 0.02–0.04 mg/kg IV.
  - Bradycardia is frequently resistant to atropine.
- Calcium
  - Used for hypotension and increased efficacy of high-dose insulin (HDI) therapy.
  - Calcium gluconate 10% (0.5–1.5 mL/kg) can be given as a slow IV bolus over 5–10 minutes. A CRI with doses up to 0.5–1.5 mL/kg/h can be initiated after the bolus and titrated as needed to maintain its effect. ECG should be monitored for bradycardia or worsening of conduction blockade.
  - Calcium chloride 10% (0.15–0.50 mL/kg). Tissue injury secondary to drug extravasation of calcium chloride can be significant. Therefore, calcium gluconate is preferred if a central line cannot be established.
  - Monitor serum ionized calcium with the goal of maintaining ionized calcium at approximately 1.5–2.0 times the normal range.
- Intravenous lipid emulsion (ILE)
  - Therapeutic option for lipid-soluble beta receptor antagonists.
  - 1.5 mL/kg IV fast bolus (if cardiac arrest) followed by 0.25 mL/kg/min IV for 30–60 minutes. If not in cardiac arrest, 0.25 mL/kg/min for 30–60 minutes IV.
    - If the patient is still experiencing severe clinical signs and the plasma is not lipemic, this dose can be repeated in 4–6 hours.
  - If BP continues to drop, may increase infusion up to 0.5 mL/kg/min.
- High-dose insulin therapy/dextrose infusion
  - Also referred to as hyperinsulinemia-euglycemia therapy.
  - Exact mechanism by which HDI works is unknown, but it is thought to improve cardiac inotropy and improve perfusion by increasing cardiac output.
  - Appears to promote the uptake and utilization of carbohydrates as an energy source in cardiac myocytes.
  - May increase intracellular calcium concentrations in myocardial cells, enhancing cardiac contractility and cardiac output.
  - Recommended dose.
    - Check blood glucose (BG) concentration first. Administer 0.5 mL/kg of 50% dextrose if BG is <100 mg/dL in dogs or <200 mg/dL in cats.
    - Regular insulin: 1 U/kg IV bolus followed by 1 U/kg/h IV CRI. May increase infusion by 0.5–1 U/kg/h every 30 minutes up to a maximum of 10 U/kg/h. **NOTE** this is 10 times the dose used in diabetic ketoacidosis treatment.
    - Administer dextrose (5–25%) to maintain euglycemia. Typically, 2 grams of dextrose is needed for each unit insulin administered. Concentrated dextrose

infusions (>7.5%) should be administered through a central line due to hyperosmolarity.

- o Example: A 10 kg dog is started on 1U/kg/h of insulin. This is accomplished by adding 25 U/kg of regular insulin to a 250 mL bag of 0.9% saline and run at 10 mL/h. The patient is receiving 10 units/h of insulin, so 20 grams of dextrose is given over that hour (e.g., 80 mL/h of a 25% dextrose solution).
- o Monitor BG every 10 minutes while titrating the insulin dose, then every 30–60 minutes once infusion dose is stabilized.
- o Monitor serum potassium hourly and supplement if below 3 mmol/L.
- o When signs of beta receptor antagonist toxicosis have resolved, decrease insulin by 1–2 units/kg/h. Dextrose administration will likely need to be continued for up to 24 hours after the insulin infusion has been stopped.
- Glucagon
  - Traditionally used as a treatment for beta receptor antagonist toxicosis in conjunction with other therapies.
  - Glucagon has a positive inotropic, chronotropic, and dromotropic effect on myocardial cells via stimulation of adenyl cyclase.
  - Dose at 0.05–0.2 mg/kg slow IV bolus; an increase in HR should be noted within a few minutes of the initial bolus. A second bolus can be administered if there is no positive effect in HR or BP after 10–15 minutes. If there is no response after the second bolus, glucagon therapy in unlikely to be of benefit. If a positive response is noted, the bolus should be followed by a CRI of glucagon at 0.05–0.10 mg/kg/h. Tachyphylaxis may occur with prolonged treatment.
  - Adverse effects of glucagon: nausea, vomiting, transient hyperglycemia. Pretreat with antiemetic.
- Catecholamines
  - Catecholamines such as dopamine, dobutamine, norepinephrine, epinephrine, phenylephrine, and isoproterenol may be required to manage hypotension in conjunction with other therapies when hypotension has not responded to other therapies. Adrenergic agents can be titrated downward once the patient responds to concomitant therapies.
  - The choice of catecholamine should treat the cardiovascular deficit(s) of the patient. Using drugs that have selective beta or alpha agonist activity or combining agents may be logical in patients hemodynamically compromised from decreased inotropy, chronotropy, and/or vasodilation.

## Precautions/Interactions

- Animals taking other antiarrhythmics such as calcium channel blockers or digoxin may be at increased risk for bradyarrhythmias to develop.

## Extracorporeal Therapy

- Hemodialysis may remove water-soluble beta receptor antagonist (e.g., atenolol, esmolol, sotalol, acebutolol, nadolol).

## Patient Monitoring

- ECG – continuous ECG to monitor for HR or conduction abnormalities.
- BP – continuous or intermittent monitoring should be performed.
- BG and electrolytes should be monitored frequently as therapies are titrated.
- Kidney values should be monitored once daily.

## COMMENTS

### Prevention/Avoidance

- Owners should keep pet medications separate from their own to avoid accidental dosing of human beta receptor antagonists.
- Advise clients on the correct dosing to avoid inadvertent overdoses.

### Possible Complications

- Acute kidney injury can develop with persistent hypoperfusion.

### Expected Course and Prognosis

- Degree and length of clinical signs will be variable depending on class, dose, and formulation (immediate versus extended release).
- Prognosis is typically good with early intervention but guarded to poor if unresponsive to therapy and coma develops.

### See Also

Chapter 24 Calcium Channel Blockers

### Abbreviations

- AV = atrioventricular
- BG = blood glucose
- BP = blood pressure
- HDI = high-dose insulin
- HR = heart rate
- Vd = volume of distribution

### Suggested Reading

Brubacher JR. β-adrenergic antagonists. In: Nelson LS, Lewin NA, Howland MA et al. (eds) *Goldfrank's Toxicological Emergencies*, 9th edn. New York: McGraw-Hill, 2011; pp. 896–909.

Kerns W. Management of beta-adrenergic blocker and calcium channel antagonist toxicity. *Emerg Med Clin North Am* 2007;25:309–331.

Malouin A, King LG. Calcium channel and beta-blocker drug overdoses. In: Silverstein DC, Hopper K (eds) *Small Animal Critical Care Medicine*. St Louis: Saunders, 2009; pp. 357–362.

Plumb DC. *Plumb's Veterinary Drug Handbook*, 9th edn. Ames: Wiley-Blackwell, 2018.

Rotella, J, Greene SL, Koutsogiannis Z et al. Treatment of beta-blocker poisoning: a systematic review. *Clin Toxicol* 2020;58(10):943–983.

**Author:** Sarah Musulin, DVM, DACVECC
**Consulting Editor:** Steven E. Epstein, DVM, DACVECC

# Chapter 23

# Calcipotriene/Calcipotriol

## DEFINITION/OVERVIEW

- Calcipotriene/calcipotriol is a synthetic analog of calcitriol, the most active metabolite of cholecalciferol (vitamin $D_3$).
- Calcipotriene is formulated into topical aerosol foams, creams, ointments, and scalp solutions used to treat human psoriasis; trade names include Dovonex®, Sorilux®, and Talconex®; some products also contain potent glucocorticoids such as betamethasone and clobetasol.
- Calcipotriene (0.005%; 50 mcg/g) is marketed in 30, 60, and 100 gram tubes and 60 and 120 gram aerosol cans.
- Ingestion of even small amounts may result in severe clinical signs in pets.

## ETIOLOGY/PATHOPHYSIOLOGY

### Mechanism of Action

- Calcipotriene has effects similar to cholecalciferol, causing significant elevations in serum calcium and phosphorus levels.
- Untreated, these levels quickly lead to mineralization of soft tissues, including heart, lungs, blood vessels, kidneys, and gastrointestinal tract. Acute kidney injury (AKI) is the most common clinical manifestation.

### Pharmacokinetics or Toxicokinetics – Adsorption, Distribution, Metabolism, Excretion

- Pharmacokinetic information on calcipotriene in domestic species is lacking.
- In humans, approximately 5–6% of topically applied calcipotriene is systemically absorbed within a few hours.
- Rapidly and well absorbed orally.
- Enterohepatic circulation occurs.
- Significant storage in fat and muscle tissue with slow release is thought to result in a long half-life.

### Toxicity

- Calcipotriene is highly toxic to dogs and cats.
- The minimum acute toxic dose in dogs is 10 mcg calcipotriene/kg body weight (BW) and the acute minimum lethal dose is 65 mcg/kg BW. Some references list 1.8–3.6 mcg/kg BW as potentially toxic to dogs.
- Dogs administered 3.6 mcg/kg/day for one week developed AKI along with increases in serum calcium, phosphorus, BUN, and creatinine.

---

*Blackwell's Five-Minute Veterinary Consult Clinical Companion: Small Animal Toxicology*, Third Edition.
Edited by Lynn R. Hovda, Ahna G. Brutlag, Robert H. Poppenga, and Steven E. Epstein.
© 2024 John Wiley & Sons, Inc. Published 2024 by John Wiley & Sons, Inc.

## Systems Affected

- Endocrine/metabolic – hypercalcemia, hyperphosphatemia, other electrolyte imbalances secondary to AKI.
- Gastrointestinal – full range of signs including anorexia, vomiting, hypersalivation, constipation, diarrhea, melena, hematemesis, abdominal pain, oropharyngeal erosions.
- Renal/urological – hypercalcemic nephropathy and AKI.
- Cardiovascular – bradycardia, arrhythmias.
- Nervous – decreased neural responsiveness, weakness.
- Musculoskeletal – decreased muscle responsiveness.

# SIGNALMENT/HISTORY

## Risk Factors

- All breeds and ages of cats and dogs are susceptible; cats and dogs under six months of age may be more susceptible.
- Diagnosis is based on history of ingestion, clinical signs, and characteristic laboratory alterations.

## Historical Findings

- Clients should be queried regarding the presence of topical antipsoriasis medication in the home in patients presenting with hypercalcemia of unknown origin.

## Location and Circumstances of Poisoning

- Pets are most often exposed at home through licking of treated human skin (especially cats) or chewing/licking of product containers or discarded gloves, swabs, or other items used to apply medication.

# CLINICAL FEATURES

- Initial signs include vomiting, depression, anorexia, diarrhea, and polyuria within 24 hours of ingestion followed by development of AKI.

# DIFFERENTIAL DIAGNOSIS

- Acute or chronic kidney injury.
- Hypercalcemia of malignancy or inflammatory disease.
- Hypoadrenocorticism.
- Idiopathic hypercalcemia of cats.
- Juvenile hypercalcemia.
- Primary hyperparathyroidism.
- Toxicants: ethylene glycol, grape/raisin toxicosis, other vitamin D products (cholecalciferol rodenticides, high-dose vitamin D supplements).

# DIAGNOSTICS

## Clinical Pathological Findings

- There is no specific laboratory test for calcipotriol/calcipotriene.
- Monitor renal blood values and urinalysis.

- Ionized and total hypercalcemia, hyperphosphatemia, elevated BUN, elevated serum creatinine, and hypercalcemic nephropathy occur between 18 and 72 hours after ingestion.
- Soft tissue mineralization can occur when serum calcium (mg/dL) × serum phosphorus (mg/dL) ≥60 in mature animals or ≥70 in growing, immature animals. Toxicosis is serious when the serum calcium is greater than 12.5 mg/dL, serum phosphorus levels are over 7 mg/dL, and hyposthenuria is documented.
- Neutrophilia may occur, although the cause is unknown.

### Other Diagnostics

- Radiographs or ultrasound may show metastatic mineralization of renal, gastrointestinal, respiratory, or cardiovascular tissues.

### Pathological Findings

- Grossly, mineralization of the renal tubules, large arteries, gastrointestinal wall, and other soft tissues; hemorrhage and ulceration of gastric mucosa.
- Histologically, renal tubular degeneration and necrosis +/– widespread mineralization in a variety of tissues including gastrointestinal mucosa/submucosa, renal tubules and basement membranes, large arteries, myocardium (especially atria), and lung.

 ## THERAPEUTICS

### Detoxification

- Early emesis or gastric lavage.
- In cases where a calcipotriene product has been licked, rinse the mouth well for 10–15 minutes.
- Activated charcoal with a cathartic initially, followed by activated charcoal without a cathartic q 8 hours for 1–2 days if GI motility is normal; monitor electrolytes for hypernatremia due to activated charcoal-induced fluid shifts.
- Cholestyramine (0.3–1 g/kg q 8 hours for four days) may aid in inhibiting calcipotriene absorption from GI tract and preventing enterohepatic recirculation; separate from activated charcoal administration by at least four hours.
- Although no studies exist to show efficacy, the use of 20% intravenous lipid emulsion (0.25–0.5 mL/kg/min IV CRI over 30–60 minutes; repeat in 6–12 hours if serum shows no signs of lipemia) may be helpful if administered early in the course of the intoxication; ILE will not remove excess vitamin D that has been stored in the liver or lipid.

### Appropriate Health Care

- Obtain baseline serum chemistries, including calcium, phosphorus, BUN, creatinine, and liver enzymes; monitor urinalysis and urine specific gravity.
- If serum calcium and phosphorus are normal, repeat lab work (at minimum: calcium, phosphorus, BUN, creatinine) in 12 hours. If levels are still within normal limits, repeat the lab work daily for four days. If normal at that time, no further treatment necessary.
- In dogs, anorexia is a fairly consistent indication of elevating serum calcium levels; have owners monitor appetite closely and bring in for repeated lab work if any degree of anorexia develops in first four days.
- If serum calcium and/or phosphorus are elevated, initiate fluid therapy and continue to monitor blood work as above; phosphorus tends to elevate before calcium.
- If at any time the serum calcium exceeds 12.5 mg/dL, or if the serum calcium × serum phosphorus exceeds 60 (adults) or 70 (growing, immature animals), increase IV fluid rates and begin aggressive medical therapy as indicated later in this chapter.

- Monitor urine output for oliguria or anuria. If urine output is at or less than 0.5 mL/kg/h, consider other options.
- Monitor blood pressure and treat accordingly.

## Antidote

- No specific antidote is available for calcipotriene toxicity.

## Drug(s) of Choice

- Bisphosphonates to inhibit bone reabsorption and minimize hypercalcemia.
- Pamidronate disodium (0.3–2 mg/kg IV diluted in 0.9% NaCl infused over two hours) is the most widely used, although zoledronate (0.1–0.25 mg/kg diluted in 45–100 mL 0.9% NaCl infused over 30 minutes) has been successfully used in cholecalciferol toxicosis.
  - Expect serum calcium and phosphorus levels to decrease in 24–48 hours.
  - Once serum calcium and phosphorus levels have declined to acceptable range, wean off medication and fluids to avoid development of hypocalcemia.
  - If levels decrease and then rebound, a second dose may be needed in 5–7 days. Anecdotally, extremely large ingestions have needed redosing in just 3–4 days.
- Aggressive 0.9% NaCl IV diuresis at 2–3 times maintenance until calcium levels decrease.
- If urine output decreases in the face of adequate hydration, one or both of the following may be used.
  - Furosemide at 1–2 mg/kg bolus IV.
  - Mannitol at 1–2 g/kg IV slowly over 20–30 minutes.
- To increase calcium excretion in patients with good urine output.
  - Furosemide 0.25–0.5 mg/kg/h IV CRI or 2.5–4.5 mg/kg PO TID.
  - Dexamethasone 0.2 mg/kg IV q 12 hours or prednisone 2–3 mg/kg PO BID.
- Phosphate binders may help maintain the calcium × phosphorus product at less than 60 or 70.
- Aluminum hydroxide 2–10 mL PO if eating q 6 hours if phosphorus levels are high.
- Antiemetics as needed for persistent vomiting.
  - Dolasetron 0.5–1.0 mg/kg IV q 24 hours.
  - Maropitant 1 mg/kg IV, SQ q 24 hours, not labeled for cats.
  - Ondansetron 0.1–1.0 mg/kg IV q 8–12 hours.
- GI protectants.
  - Omeprazole 0.5–1 mg/kg PO q 24 hours.
  - Pantoprazole 1 mg/kg IV q 24 hours
  - Sucralfate 0.25–1 g PO TID × 5–7 days if evidence of active ulcer disease.

## Precautions/Interactions

- Thiazide diuretics are contraindicated as they decrease clearance of calcium.
- Calcitonin should be used cautiously in combination with bisphosphonates and then only in refractory cases, as combined use may increase risk of soft tissue mineralization.
- Excessive doses of bisphosphonates or failure to wean off fluids and medications following normalization of serum calcium can result in hypocalcemia. Treatment with calcium carbonate, or in severe cases IV calcium gluconate, may be needed.

## Alternative Drugs

- Salmon calcitonin (Calcimar®, Micalcin®) at 4–7 IU/kg SQ q 8–12 hours; less desirable than bisphosphonates due to inconsistencies in efficacy, availability issues, and development of resistance after several days of treatment.

## Patient Monitoring

- Following normalization of serum levels, recheck calcium and phosphorus levels every third day as needed, then weekly for 3–4 weeks. Calcium and phosphorus levels should be evaluated in all exposed animals regardless of amount ingested.
- Monitor for evidence of GI ulceration secondary to uremia or soft tissue mineralization.
- Monitor appetite for anorexia, which is a fairly consistent indicator of rising calcium levels in dogs.

## Diet

- Low-calcium diet during times of hypercalcemia.

 ## COMMENTS

### Prevention/Avoidance

- Medications and waste cans use to dispose of packaging or other items that may have contacted calcipotriene-containing medication should be kept well out reach of pets.
- Do not allow the pet to lick skin where calcipotriene-containing products have been applied.

### Possible Complications

- Cardiac insufficiency and chronic kidney disease secondary to myocardial mineralization.
- Death from acute arrhythmia secondary to cardiac mineralization may occur weeks after presumed recovery.

### Expected Course and Prognosis

- The prognosis is good if serum calcium × serum phosphorus is <60 (mature animals) or <70 (growing, immature animals) and treatment is provided in a timely manner.
- The prognosis is much more guarded if the serum calcium × serum phosphorus is ≥60 (mature animals) or ≥70 (growing, immature animals) and prolonged for even a few days, as the risk of soft tissue mineralization is high.

### See Also

Chapter 124 Cholecalciferol

### Abbreviations

See Appendix 1 for a complete list

### Suggested Reading

Hostutler R, Chew DJ, Jaeger JQ et al. Uses and effectiveness of pamidronate disodium for treatment of dogs and cats with hypercalcemia. *J Vet Intern Med* 2005;19(1):29–33.
Rumbeiha WK. Cholecalciferol. In: Peterson ME, Talcott PA (eds) *Small Animal Toxicology*, 3rd edn. St Louis: Elsevier, 2013; pp. 489–498.
Saedi N, Horn R, Muffoletto A et al. Death of a dog caused by calcipotriene toxicity. *J Am Acad Dermatol* 2007;56(4):712–713.
Schenk A, Lux C, Lane J et al. Evaluation of zoledronate as a treatment for hypercalcemia in four dogs. *J Am Anim Hosp Assoc* 2018;54:3546–04.
Torley D, Drummond A, Bilsland DJ. Calcipotriol toxicity in dogs. *Br J Dermatol* 2002;147(6):1270.

**Author**: Sharon Gwaltney-Brant DVM, PhD, DABVT, DABT
**Consulting Editor**: Steven E. Epstein, DVM, DACVECC

# Chapter 24

# Calcium Channel Blockers

## DEFINITION/OVERVIEW

- Calcium channel blockers (CCBs) are commonly used in human and veterinary medicine for the management of systemic hypertension, cardiac disease (including hypertrophic cardiomyopathy and tachyarrhythmias), and potentially acute kidney injury.
- There are three classes of CCB, and they differ in their specificity for cardiac and vascular tissues (Table 24.1).
- CCBs commonly cause hypotension, tachycardia or bradycardia, weakness, and vomiting.
- CCB toxicosis can result from therapeutic use or accidental ingestion of calcium channel blocking medications.

## ETIOLOGY/PATHOPHYSIOLOGY

### Mechanism of Action

- CCBs inhibit the slow L-type voltage-sensitive calcium channels found in the heart, vascular smooth muscle, skeletal muscle, pancreas, lung, and other tissues, thus inhibiting intracellular membrane transport of calcium, causing the following:
  - Reduced AV nodal conduction.
  - Direct depressant effect on the sinus node.
  - Reduced excitation-contraction coupling of cardiac muscle and reduced cardiac inotropy.
  - Reduced calcium-induced calcium release from the sarcoplasmic reticulum, leading to reduced vascular tone and vasodilation.
- CCBs reduce insulin release from pancreatic beta cells and decrease mitochondrial calcium, leading to hyperglycemia and lactate accumulation.
- Pulmonary edema may develop due to selective dilation of afferent vessels in the capillary network, resulting in increased transcapillary pressure. There may also be drug-induced pulmonary capillary permeability changes to the alveolar membrane contributing to edema.

### Pharmacokinetics or Toxicokinetics – Absorption, Distribution, Metabolism, Excretion

The pharmacokinetics of the different CCBs vary depending on the class of CCB, the species involved, and the formulation of drug, such as immediate-release (IR) versus extended-release (ER) formulations.
- Verapamil.
  - Absorption – 90% absorption, poor bioavailability (10–23%). IR formulations reach peak concentrations in 1–2 hours while ER formulations reach peak concentrations in 7–11 hours.

*Blackwell's Five-Minute Veterinary Consult Clinical Companion: Small Animal Toxicology*, Third Edition. Edited by Lynn R. Hovda, Ahna G. Brutlag, Robert H. Poppenga, and Steven E. Epstein. © 2024 John Wiley & Sons, Inc. Published 2024 by John Wiley & Sons, Inc.

**TABLE 24.1 Relative effects of the three classes of calcium channel blockers (phenylalkylamines, benzothiazepines, and dihydropyridines) on cardiac automaticity, conduction, contractility, and vascular tone.**

| Class | Drugs | Automaticity | Conduction | Contractility | Vessel tone |
|---|---|---|---|---|---|
| Phenylalkylamine | Verapamil | +++ | +++ | +++ | +++ |
| Benzothiazepine | Diltiazem | ++++ | +++ | + | ++ |
| Dihydropyridine | Amlodipine<br>Nifedipine<br>Nisoldipine<br>Nimodipine<br>Nicardipine<br>Felodipine<br>Isradipine<br>Clevidipine | + | 0 | + | ++++ |

*Note:* Plus signs signify an increasing response, with more plus signs denoting a more inhibitory response. The zero denotes no response.

- Distribution – 90% protein bound. Distributes to the placenta and milk.
- Metabolism - extensive first-pass metabolism. Metabolized in the liver in dogs.
- Elimination – in dogs, primarily excreted in the bile with an elimination half-life of 1.8–3.8 hours.
■ Diltiazem.
- Absorption – rapidly absorbed.
  ○ Dogs – poor bioavailability (17–24%).
  ○ Cats – high bioavailability (36% for ER formulations, 71% for IR formulations).
  ○ IR formulations reach peak concentrations in 0.5–0.75 hours while ER formulations reach peak concentrations in 5.7 hours.
- Distribution – widely distributed through most tissues. 70–75% protein bound (dogs).
- Metabolism – extensive first-pass metabolism. Metabolized in the liver and undergoes enterohepatic recirculation in dogs.
- Excretion – metabolites are primarily excreted in the bile and feces with an elimination half-life of 2–4 hours in dogs and 1.8-6.8 hours in cats.
■ Amlodipine.
- Absorption – high bioavailability (90%). Peak concentrations are reached in 6–12 hours.
- Distribution – highly protein bound.
- Metabolism – liver.
- Excretion – primarily excreted in the urine with an elimination half-life of 30–60 hours.

## Toxicity

Clinical signs are possible at therapeutic dosages, particularly in animals with cardiac disease.

## Systems Affected

■ Cardiovascular – hypotension, tachycardia, bradycardia, AV blockade (first-, second-, or third-degree).
■ Endocrine/metabolic – hyperglycemia, hypoinsulinemia, hyponatremia, hypokalemia.
■ Gastrointestinal – vomiting, ileus.
■ Respiratory – pulmonary edema.

- Renal – acute kidney injury due to hypoperfusion.
- Nervous – lethargy, tremors, seizures.
- Musculoskeletal – weakness.
- Hematological – platelet aggregation inhibition (rare).

# SIGNALMENT/HISTORY

## Risk Factors

- No breed or sex predilections.
- Coadministration with other cardiac medications.
- Liver dysfunction – results in higher serum concentrations and delayed metabolism of the drug.

## Historical Findings

- Known dosing error.
- Ingestion of the owner's medications by the pet.
- Acute onset of vomiting, weakness, or lethargy.

# CLINICAL FEATURES

- Hypotension.
- Tachycardia.
- Bradycardia.
- Vomiting.
- Weakness.
- Depressed mentation.
- Respiratory distress.
- Pulmonary crackles.
- Edema.

# DIFFERENTIAL DIAGNOSIS

- Toxicants.
  - Alpha-2-adrenergic agonists.
  - Beta-adrenergic antagonists.
  - Cardiac glycoside-containing plants.
  - Digoxin.
  - Type 1a antiarrhythmics (procainamide, quinidine).
- Cardiac disease.
  - Sick sinus syndrome.
  - AV block.
- Hyperkalemia resulting in atrial standstill.

# DIAGNOSTICS

## Clinical Pathological Findings

- Biochemistry.
  - Hypokalemia.
  - Hyponatremia (due to CCB-induced natriuresis).

- Hyperglycemia (due to suppressed insulin release from pancreatic beta cells).
- Elevated blood urea nitrogen and creatinine.
■ Ionized calcium/total calcium expected to remain normal.
■ Blood gas analysis.
  - Hyperlactatemia.
  - Metabolic acidosis.

## Other Diagnostics

■ Blood pressure: hypotension.
■ ECG: sinus bradycardia, AV block, AV dissociation, junctional escape rhythms, idioventricular arrhythmias, or asystole.
■ Radiographs (if respiratory signs are seen): pulmonary edema.
■ Serum drug concentrations for CCBs are not clinically useful.

## Pathological Findings

■ Edema.
■ Pleural effusion.

 # THERAPEUTICS

## Detoxification

■ Emesis within two hours of exposure if the pet is asymptomatic.
■ Gastric lavage may be considered with recent (less than two hours) exposure to a large quantity of pills.
■ Activated charcoal (1 g/kg PO) with a cathartic such as sorbitol orally within four hours for diltiazem or verapamil exposure, within 12 hours for amlodipine exposure. With large exposures or exposures to ER formulations, activated charcoal can be repeated in 4–6 hours.

## Appropriate Health Care

■ Intravenous fluid therapy: balanced electrolyte solution should be used as needed to maintain hydration and support cardiovascular function and perfusion. If hypotensive, consider a fluid bolus of 20–30 mL/kg in dogs or 10–15 mL/kg in cats. Because of the risk for impaired cardiac function and pulmonary edema, care should be taken to avoid fluid overload.
■ Close blood pressure monitoring for hypotension.
  - For 24 hours with exposure to any form of amlodipine or ER formulations of other CCBs.
  - For 12 hours with exposure to IR medications except amlodipine.
■ Continuous ECG monitoring for assessment of conduction abnormalities.
■ Temporary transvenous pacing has been used to increase heart rate and cardiac output when other therapies have failed.

## Drug(s) of Choice

■ Calcium infusion.
  - First line of therapy for symptomatic animals. Increases calcium available for the intracellular calcium influx needed to maintain vascular smooth muscle function and cardiac contractility.
    - Calcium gluconate (10% solution): 0.5–1.5 mL/kg slowly IV over five minutes or as a CRI of 0.05 mL/kg/h, titrated to effect. Monitor ECG and discontinue if bradycardia worsens or there is worsening of conduction blockade.

- o Calcium chloride (10% solution): 0.1–0.5 mL/kg slowly may be used, but can cause tissue necrosis with extravasation and should be given through a central line.
- High-dose insulin therapy/dextrose infusion.
  - First line of therapy recommended in humans.
  - Thought to improve cardiac inotropy, promote the update and utilization of carbohydrates as an energy source, and increase intracellular calcium to enhance cardiac contractility and cardiac output.
  - Recommended dose.
    - o Check blood glucose (BG) concentration first. Administer 0.5 mL/kg of 50% dextrose if BG is <100 mg/dL in dogs or <200 mg/dL in cats.
    - o Regular insulin: 1 U/kg IV bolus followed by 1 U/kg/h IV CRI. May increase infusion by 0.5–1 U/kg/h every 30 minutes up to a maximum of 10 U/kg/h. **NOTE** This is 10 times the dose used in diabetic ketoacidosis treatment.
  - Administer dextrose (5–25%) to maintain euglycemia. Typically, 2 grams of dextrose is needed for each unit of insulin administered. Concentrated dextrose infusions (> 7.5%) should be administered through a central line due to hyperosmolarity.
    - o Example: A 10 kg dog is started on 1U/kg/h of insulin. This is accomplished by adding 25 U/kg of regular insulin to a 250 mL bag of 0.9% saline and run at 10 mL/h. The patient is receiving 10 units/h of insulin, so 20 grams of dextrose is given over that hour (e.g., 80 mL/h of a 25% dextrose solution).
    - o Monitor BG every 10 minutes while titrating the insulin dose, then every 30–60 minutes once infusion dose is stabilized.
    - o Monitor serum potassium hourly and supplement if below 3 mmol/L.
    - o When signs of CCB toxicosis have resolved, decrease insulin by 1–2 U/kg/h. Glucose administration will likely need to be continued for up to 24 hours after insulin is stopped.
- Intravenous fat emulsion.
  - Thought to act as a lipid shuttle to sequester the CCB and shuttle it to sites of metabolism (Chapter 1).
  - Increases free fatty acid availability for myocardium energy substrate, activates myocyte calcium channels to increase calcium influx, and increases nitric oxide and B-ketoacids to stimulate insulin secretion.
    - o 20% solution: 1.5 mL/kg IV over one minute if cardiac arrest, then CRI of 0.25 mL/kg/min for 30–60 minutes. If not in cardiac arrest, bolus is not needed.
    - o May be repeated in four hours if poor response and serum is not lipemic.
- Atropine: for bradycardia, AV blockade: 0.02–0.04 mg/kg IV.
- Edema can occur peripherally or in the lungs (noncardiogenic pulmonary edema).
  - Furosemide: 1–2 mg/kg IV PRN; can consider CRI of 0.2 mg/kg/h.

## Precautions/Interventions

- Aggressive IV fluid use can contribute to the development of edema.

## Alternative Drugs

- Vasopressors (often ineffective for CCB-induced hypotension, consider if hypotension persists).
  - Norepinephrine: 0.05–0.1 mcg/kg/minute IV CRI titrated up to a maximum rate of 1–2 mcg/kg/minute IV CRI.

- Dopamine: 5–20 mcg/kg/minute IV CRI, if norepinephrine is not available.
- Dobutamine: 2–15 mcg/kg/minute IV CRI.

## Patient Monitoring

- Continuous or intermittent blood pressure monitoring.
- Continuous or intermittent ECG monitoring.
- Monitor electrolytes q 12 hours.
- Renal values should be monitored daily.

 # COMMENTS

### Prevention/Avoidance

- Store medications out of reach of pets and keep animal medications separate from human ones.

### Possible Complications

- Acute kidney injury secondary to persistent hypoperfusion.
- Respiratory failure secondary to pulmonary edema.

### Expected Course and Prognosis

- Signs are expected within 12 (IR formulations) to 24 hours (amlodipine or ER formulations) and may last 2–4 days.
- Prognosis is often good with early intervention, but guarded to poor if unresponsive to therapy or presentation to the hospital is delayed.

### Synonyms

- Calcium channel antagonist.

### See Also

Chapter 22 Beta-receptor Agonists (Beta-blockers)

### Abbreviations

- CCB = calcium channel blocker
- AV = atrioventricular
- IR = immediate release
- ER = extended release
- CRI = continuous rate infusion

### Suggested Reading

Hayes CL. An update on calcium channel blocker toxicity in dogs and cats. *Vet Clin North Am Small Anim Pract* 2018;48(6):943–957.

St-Onge M, Anseeuw K, Cantrell FL et al. Experts consensus recommendations for the management of calcium channel blocker poisoning in adults. *Crit Care Med J* 2017;45(3):e306–315.

Maton BL, Simmons EE, Lee JA et al. The use of high-dose insulin therapy and intravenous lipid emulsion to treat severe, refractory diltiazem toxicosis in a dog. *J Vet Emerg Crit Care* 2013;23:321–327.

Syring RS, Costello MF. Temporary transvenous pacing in a dog with diltiazem intoxication. *J Vet Emerg Crit Care* 2008;18:75–80.

Tinsman AE, Bellis TJ. Hyperinsulinemia/euglycemia and intravenous lipid emulsion therapy for the management of severe amlodipine toxicosis in a cat. *Clin Case Rep* 2021;9:e05175.

## Acknowledgment

The author acknowledges the prior contributions of Katherine L. Peterson, DVM, DACVECC, Kristin M Engebretsen, PharmD, DABAT, and Rebecca S. Syring, DVM, DACVECC, who authored this topic in the previous edition.

**Author**: Cristine L. Hayes, DVM, DABT, DABVT
**Consulting Editor**: Steven E. Epstein, DVM, DACVECC

# Chapter 25

# Colchicine

## DEFINITION/OVERVIEW

- Colchicine is an alkaloid which is derived from *Colchicum autumnale* (autumn crocus, meadow saffron) and *Gloriosa superba* (glory lily). All animals and humans are susceptible to poisoning, with the highest concentration of the alkaloid occurring in the flowers and seeds.
- Colchicine is used as a drug in human and veterinary medicine for treatment of various conditions, including acute gouty arthritis, pericarditis, amyloidosis in familial Mediterranean fever, familial shar-pei fever, condyloma acuminata, and neutrophilic dermatoses and to prevent hepatic and renal fibrosis in dogs.
- Intoxication in small animals is commonly due to accidental ingestion of human medications or overdose.
- Off-label use of colchicine to prevent fibrosis following glaucoma drainage device placement, stent placement in trachea, to prevent stricture formation in urethra and in the treatment of some types of neoplasia.

## ETIOLOGY/PATHOPHYSIOLOGY

- Colchicine intoxication has been reported in dogs and has an acute presentation. Usually caused by ingestion of human drugs or overdose.
- Colchicine has a narrow margin of safety with intoxications occurring at 10 times the recommended dose or higher.
- It interferes with microtubule function, inhibiting mitosis. The gastrointestinal tract and bone marrow aplasia are most sensitive endpoints; however, it causes multiple organ failure including cardiovascular collapse, depressed respiration, and hypertension, among other findings.

### Mechanism of Action

- Colchicine is a potent inhibitor of cellular mitosis, by binding to intracellular tubulin which stops their polymerization into microtubules.
- Various cellular functions are inhibited by microtubule deficiency, including mitosis, degranulation, chemotaxis, and inflammatory signaling pathways.
- Prevention of fibroblast proliferation and collagen synthesis reduction.
- Direct toxic effect on muscle, myocardial cells, peripheral nervous system, and liver.
- Respiratory center depression, constriction of blood vessels and causes hypertension by central vasomotor stimulation.

*Blackwell's Five-Minute Veterinary Consult Clinical Companion: Small Animal Toxicology*, Third Edition.
Edited by Lynn R. Hovda, Ahna G. Brutlag, Robert H. Poppenga, and Steven E. Epstein.
© 2024 John Wiley & Sons, Inc. Published 2024 by John Wiley & Sons, Inc.

## Pharmacokinetics or Toxicokinetics – Adsorption, Distribution, Metabolism, Excretion

- Colchicine is rapidly absorbed orally, time to peak concentration 0.5–2.0 h.
- It has a large volume of distribution.
- It accumulates in liver, kidneys, spleen, gastrointestinal mucosa, and leukocytes.
- Eliminated predominantly through bile (80%) but also through urine (20%).
- Long half-life of elimination of 20–40 h.
- Enterohepatic recirculation causes prolonged effect in body. A single acute dose is eliminated over a period of 10 days or longer in dogs.

## Toxicity

- In dogs, oral therapeutic dose is 0.03 mg/kg/day.
- Ten times this dosage (0.3 mg/kg/day) caused intoxication in dogs within a few hours. Early diagnosis and aggressive supportive therapy proved critical.
- Fatal ingestion of 0.5–3.6 mg/kg colchicine in dog reported.

## Systems Affected

- Gastrointestinal: abdominal pain, severe salivation, vomiting, and hemorrhagic diarrhea.
- Cardiovascular: cardiotoxic.
- Hepatobiliary: liver failure.
- Renal: acute kidney injury.
- Musculoskeletal: weakness and collapse.
- Nervous: seizures.

 # SIGNALMENT/HISTORY

## Risk Factors

- Narrow therapeutic margin.
- Risk of toxicosis increases with hepatic or renal insufficiency and concurrent drugs which affect colchicine metabolism.
- Patients with gastrointestinal, kidney disease, and cardiac dysfunction.
- Older patients, pregnancy.
- Pets with colchicine in household as a therapeutic medication.

## Historical Findings

- Vomiting, diarrhea, lethargy.

## Location and Circumstances of Poisoning

- Can occur anywhere as common cause of poisoning is drug overdose.
- Households with humans or animals under treatment with colchicine.

 # CLINICAL FEATURES

- Depression, hypothermia, dehydration, signs of shock.
- Elevated protein concentration and red blood cells in the urine worsening to hematuria and hematochezia.
- Gastrointestinal symptoms, myocardial and hepatic injury, hypoproteinemia, dehydration.

- Within 24 h after ingestion, phase I indicating mucosal damage in the gastrointestinal tract with pain, vomiting, diarrhea, and GI hemorrhage.
- After 1–7 days of exposure, phase II with metabolic acidosis, shock, myelosuppression, renal and hepatic failure, and respiratory depression indicating multiple organ damage.
- Phase III, 7–21 days after ingestion: most mortality occurs during this period and bone marrow hematopoietic recovery and resolution of organ damage indicate better prognosis.

# DIFFERENTIAL DIAGNOSIS

- Gastrointestinal symptoms similar to vitamin D toxicosis, anticoagulant rodenticides, 5-fluorouracil, arsenic poisoning.

# DIAGNOSTICS

- Colchicine plasma concentration can be measured, but this test is not readily available.
- Complete blood count.
  - Increased hematocrit and plasma protein with dehydration.
  - Pancytopenia from bone marrow suppression is possible.
- Serum biochemistry.
  - Elevated liver enzymes or azotemia.
- Urinalysis.
  - Isosthenuria, hematuria.

# THERAPEUTICS

## Detoxification
- Emesis is indicated.
- Activated charcoal via nasogastric tube is effective at removing the toxin before absorption.
- Reducing absorption and removal from the gastrointestinal system early provide better results.

## Appropriate Health Care
- For patients with dehydration and GI symptoms, intravenous fluids with isotonic crystalloids are indicated.
- Antiemetics.
  - Maropitant 1 mg/kg IV, SQ q 24 h for vomiting and nausea.
  - Ondansetron 0.5–1.0 mg/kg IV, SQ q 8–12 h.
- Use of N-acetylcysteine improves cellular damage caused by oxidative stress induced by colchicine.

## Drug(s) of Choice
- Colchicine-specific Fab fragment antibodies. Experimental. Restore tubulin activity by releasing colchicine for excretion.
- Engineered lipocalin (Lcn2) to complex colchicine and aid in removal.

## Precautions/Interactions
- Medications causing bone marrow suppression like immunosuppressants, chloramphenicol, antineoplastics interact with colchicine.

- Literature citing human cases also mention macrolide antibiotics, fluoroquinolones, antifungals, statins, digoxin, antiarrhythmics, angiotensin-converting enzyme inhibitors.
- CYP3A4 inhibitors and P-glycoprotein inhibitors are reported to increase toxicity of colchicine.

 ## COMMENTS

### Expected Course and Prognosis

- Prognosis is guarded to fair depending on the dose ingested and clinical signs present due to the ability of toxin to cause multiple organ damage.

### Suggested Reading

Goodman IH. Survival of a dog with accidental colchicine overdose. *J Vet Emerg Crit Care* 2020;30:74–80.
Slobodnick A, Shah B, Pillinger MH, Krasnokutsky S. Colchicine: old and new. *Am J Med* 2015;128(5):461–470.
Wagenaar Z Accidental colchicine poisoning in a dog. *Can Vet J* 2004;45(1):55–57.
Wu J, Liu Z. Progress in the management of acute colchicine poisoning in adults. *Intern Emerg Med* 2022;17:2069–2081.

**Authors**: Deepa Ashwarya Kuttappan, DVM, PhD, DABT and Wilson K. Rumbeiha DVM, PhD, DABT, DABVT
**Consulting Editor**: Steven E. Epstein, DVM, DACVECC

# Chapter 26

# Cyclosporine A

## DEFINITION/OVERVIEW

- Cyclosporine is a cyclic lipophilic polypeptide macrolide used as a potent immunosuppressive and immunomodulatory drug.
- It is most commonly used in dogs to manage a variety of chronic inflammatory and immune-mediated diseases including canine atopic dermatitis, sebaceous adentitis, anal furunculosis, inflammatory bowel disease, immune-mediated hemolytic anemia, and immune-mediated thrombocytopenia.
- It is less commonly used in cats, with reported uses including chronic allergic dermatitis, pemphigus complex, pure red cell aplasia, and feline stomatitis.
- The margin of safety in both acute and chronic overdosing is wide, with adverse effects usually consisting of mild gastrointestinal distress (diarrhea, vomiting, inappetence).
- Two commercially available forms of oral dosing of the medication exist for humans.
  - Vegetable oil-based formulation (Sandimmune®).
  - Microemulsified formulation (Neoral®).
- There is one veterinary product, Atopica®, which is identical to Neoral.

## ETIOLOGY/PATHOPHYSIOLOGY

### Mechanism of Action

- Both antiinflammatory and antipruritic effects.
- Calcineurin inhibitor; preferentially suppresses T-lymphocyte activation.
  - Inhibits the antigen-presenting function of the skin immune system.
  - Blocks recruitment and activation of eosinophils, keratinocytic production of cytokines, Langerhans cell function, mast cell degranulation and release of histamine and proinflammatory cytokines.

### Pharmacokinetics or Toxicokinetics – Adsorption, Distribution, Metabolism, Excretion

- Absorption.
  - Primarily absorbed in the intestine by passive diffusion.
    - Absorption of the vegetable oil-based form in humans and dogs is dependent on biliary secretion.
    - Absorption of the microemulsified form is not dependent on bile secretion. Oral bioavailablility is 35% in dogs, 25–29% in cats, and <5% in rabbits and guinea pigs. Coadministration of food in dogs decreases bioavailablility.

*Blackwell's Five-Minute Veterinary Consult Clinical Companion: Small Animal Toxicology*, Third Edition.
Edited by Lynn R. Hovda, Ahna G. Brutlag, Robert H. Poppenga, and Steven E. Epstein.
© 2024 John Wiley & Sons, Inc. Published 2024 by John Wiley & Sons, Inc.

- Well absorbed into corneal and conjunctival epithelium.
- Poorly absorbed through keratinized skin.
■ Distribution.
  - Lipophilic – large volume of distribution; cyclosporine is distributed widely in skin and adipose tissue, liver, fat, and blood cells.
■ Metabolism.
  - Metabolized primarily in the liver (cytochrome P450), and to a lesser extent in the intestine and kidney.
    ○ Dogs metabolize at 2–3 times greater capacity than humans, rabbits, and rats.
  - Approximately 30 metabolites of cyclosporine are formed by sulfation, hydroxylation, and demethylation.
■ Elimination.
  - Primarily biliary, with minimal renal excretion.
  - Dogs: elimination half-life is 5–12 hours.
  - Cats: elimination half-life varies (6.8–40 hours).

## Toxicity

■ Wide margin of safety for both acute and chronic overdosing.
■ Adverse effects increase with increased dose and duration of administration.
■ Long-term exposure to cyclosporine is associated with increased incidence of malignant neoplasia.

## Systems Affected

■ Gastrointestinal – gastroenteritis.
■ Skin/exocrine – rare pruritus, gingival hyperplasia, other dermatoses.
■ Hepatobiliary – rare hepatocellular injury.
■ Renal/urologic – rare kidney injury.
■ Hemic/lymphatic/immune – rare lymphoid system hematological compromise.

 # SIGNALMENT/HISTORY

■ Any species may be affected.

## Risk Factors

■ Not approved for use in breeding, pregnant or nursing animals – fetotoxic and embryotoxic in rats and rabbits.
■ Caution if preexisting renal or hepatic compromise.
■ Caution in animals <6 months of age and <1.8 kg body weight (safety and efficacy unknown).
■ Dogs with the MDR1/ABCB1 genetic mutation may be at increased risk for immunosuppression.

## Historical Findings

Most commonly reported clinical signs include inappetence, vomiting, and diarrhea.

## Location and Circumstances of Poisoning

Overdose is usually secondary to iatrogenic administration or inappropriate ingestion by pet.

# CLINICAL FEATURES

- Common clinical signs include gastrointestinal distress (vomiting, diarrhea, inappetence).
- As ingested dose increases, reported uncommon or rare effects include dermal pruritus, hepatotoxicity, thromboembolism, secondary opportunistic infection, renal dysfunction (in already compromised humans and rats), changes in blood pressure, diabetes mellitus (dog), bone marrow suppression, flaring of latent viral infections (cats).

# DIFFERENTIAL DIAGNOSIS

- Other gastrointestinal diseases.
- Other toxicants causing mild gastrointestinal signs.

# DIAGNOSTICS

### Clinical Pathological Findings

- CBC and serum biochemistry abnormalities are largely extrapolated from human medicine and may be useful as baseline.

### Other Diagnostics

- Abdominal radiographs may be useful to rule out other causes of gastrointestinal disease.

# THERAPEUTICS

### Detoxification

- Emesis induction with acute ingestions.
- Single dose of activated charcoal.

### Appropriate Health Care

- Cases with mild GI upset can often be treated as outpatients.
- More severe overdoses may require hospitalization, bloodwork monitoring, and aggressive supportive care.

### Antidote

- No specific antidote is available.

### Drug(s) of Choice

- Judicious IV fluid use, maintaining hydration and blood pressure as needed.
- Antiemetics if vomiting is severe or persistent.
  - Maropitant 1 mg/kg IV or SQ q 24 hours.
  - Ondansetron 0.1–0.3 mg/kg IV or SQ q 6–12 hours.

### Precautions/Interactions

- Toxicity may be enhanced in animals concurrently ingesting the following drugs: acetazolamide, allopurinol, amlodipine, azithromycin, azole antifungals, bromocriptine, calcium channel blockers, carvedilol, cimetidine, chloramphenicol, ciprofloxacin/enrofloxacin, cisapride, clarithromycin, clopidogrel, colchicine, corticosteroids, danazol, digoxin, estrogens, fluvoxamine, glipizide/glyburide, grapefruit juice/grapefruit juice powder, imipenem, losartan, valsartan, medroxyprogesterone, metoclopramide, metronidazole, omeprazole, sertraline, tinidazole, vitamin E.

### Extracorporeal Therapy

- Combining hemodialysis with charcoal hemoperfusion has been shown to significantly reduce blood cyclosporine concentrations following acute overdose.
- Case reports suggest therapeutic plasma exchange or red blood cell exchange may have a benefit.

### Patient Monitoring

- Baseline CBC, biochemistry profile, and blood pressure.

### Diet

- Temporary fasting followed by a bland diet for patients exhibiting gastrointestinal signs.

 ## COMMENTS

### Prevention/Avoidance

- Owners should be educated about keeping oral medications out of reach of pets.

### Possible Complications

- Severe signs and complications are rare.

### Expected Course and Prognosis

- Generally excellent prognosis with control of presenting signs (usually only gastrointestinal).
- In rare cases of organ dysfunction (renal) or bone marrow disorders, prognosis may be more guarded.

### Synonyms

Tacrolimus (a related calcineurin inhibitor).

### Suggested Reading

Colombo S, Sartori R. Ciclosporin and the cat: current understanding and review of clinical use. *J Feline Med Surg* 2018;20(3):244–255.

Forsythe P, Paterson S. Cyclosporine 10 years on: indications and efficacy. *Vet Rec Focus* 2014; March:13–21.

Kovalik M, Thoday K, van den Broek A. The use of cyclosporine A in veterinary dermatology. *Vet J* 2012;193:317–325.

Roberts E, VanLare K A, Strehlau G et al. Safety, tolerability, and pharmacokinetics of 6-month daily dosing of an oral formulation of cyclosporine (ATOPICA for cats©) in cats. *J Vet Pharm Ther* 2013;37:161–168.

Segev G, Cowgill LD. Treatment of acute kidney injury associated with cyclosporine overdose in a dog using hemodialysis and charcoal hemoperfusion. *J Vet Emerg Crit Care* 2018;28(2):163–167.

Vivano K. Update on immunosuppressive therapies for dogs and cats. *Vet Clin North Am Small Anim Pract* 2013;43:1152–1153.

**Authors:** Julie Schildt, DVM, DACVECC and David R. Brown, PhD
**Consulting Editor:** Steven E. Epstein, DVM, DACVECC

# Diuretics

# Chapter 27

## DEFINITION/OVERVIEW

- Diuretic toxicosis is generally confined to plasma volume depletion, with consequent hypoperfusion of critical organs, mainly the kidneys, and electrolyte abnormalities.
- Rehydration is normally sufficient to correct acute diuretic overdosing.

## ETIOLOGY/PATHOPHYSIOLOGY

- Diuretics are primarily used in management of congestive heart failure in veterinary medicine. More recently, potassium-sparing diuretics have been used in combination with chemotherapeutics in canine osteosarcoma therapy (amiloride) and primary hyperaldosteronism in cats (spironolactone).
- Aggressive administration can result in a volume-responsive acute kidney injury (AKI) and if renal perfusion pressure drops sufficiently or is prolonged, an intrinsic AKI may occur (rare).
- Less common complications include electrolyte depletion or excess such as hypokalemia, hypomagnesemia, and hyperkalemia (diuretic dependent).

### Mechanism of Action

- All diuretics commonly used in veterinary medicine affect electrolyte transfer (and water) across the nephron.
  - Diuretics work in specific sites along the renal tubule; locations vary based on diuretic type.
- See Table 27.1 for the mechanism and site of action of most known diuretics.

### Pharmacokinetics or Toxicokinetics – Absorption, Distribution, Metabolism, Excretion

- Furosemide.
  - Administered parenterally or orally.
  - Onset and duration of action – onset of action is within 30 minutes, and duration of action is approximately six hours. Little data exists for cats, but cats generally require lower doses than dogs for comparable degrees of CHF, suggesting an increased sensitivity to furosemide.
  - Absorption – fairly rapid rate of absorption with oral bioavailability of 77% in dogs.

*Blackwell's Five-Minute Veterinary Consult Clinical Companion: Small Animal Toxicology*, Third Edition. Edited by Lynn R. Hovda, Ahna G. Brutlag, Robert H. Poppenga, and Steven E. Epstein.
© 2024 John Wiley & Sons, Inc. Published 2024 by John Wiley & Sons, Inc.

**TABLE 27.1** Mechanism of action of various diuretics. Diuretics of veterinary importance are highlighted in bold. Dashes signify that there is no renal location of action.

| Classification | Examples | Mechanism | Location |
|---|---|---|---|
| No specific classification | Ethanol<br>Water | Inhibit antidiuretic hormone secretion | – |
| Acidifying salts | $CaCl_2$<br>$NH_4Cl$ | | – |
| Aquaretics | Goldenrod<br>Juniper | Increase plasma volume | – |
| Xanthines | Caffeine<br>Theophylline | Inhibit reabsorption of $Na^+$, increase GFR | Proximal tubule |
| Osmotic diuretics | Glucose (especially in uncontrolled diabetes),<br>**mannitol** | Promote osmotic diuresis | Proximal tubule, descending limb |
| Na-H exchange antagonists | **Dopamine** | Promote $Na^+$ excretion, increase GFR | Proximal tubule |
| Carbonic anhydrase inhibitors | **Acetazolamide**<br>Dorzolamide | Inhibit $H^+$ secretion, resultant promotion of $Na^+$ and $K^+$ excretion | Proximal tubule |
| Loop diuretics | Bumetanide<br>Ethacrynic acid<br>**Furosemide**<br>**Torsemide** | Inhibit the Na-K-2Cl transporter | Loop of Henle |
| Thiazides | Bendroflumethiazide<br>**Hydrochlorothiazide** | Inhibit reabsorption by $Na^+/Cl^-$ symporter | Distal convoluted tubules |
| Arginine vasopressin receptor 2 antagonists ("vaptans") | Amphotericin B<br>Lithium citrate<br>Tolvaptan | Inhibit antidiuretic hormone binding | Collecting duct |
| Potassium-sparing diuretics | **Amiloride, spironolactone**<br>Triamterene<br>Potassium Canrenoate | Inhibition of $Na^+/K^+$ exchanger. Spironolactone inhibits aldosterone action. Amiloride inhibits epithelial sodium channels | Cortical collecting ducts |
| Renal outer medullary potassium channel (ROMK) inhibitor | MK-7145, MK-8153<br>(still in development) | Inhibition of $Na^+$ reabsorption by inhibiting delivery of potassium to supply the $Na^+/K^+/2Cl^-$ cotransporter | Thick ascending loop of Henle and cortical collecting duct |

- Distribution – large volume of distribution, with 90% protein binding.
- Metabolism – approximately 10% hepatic metabolism.
- Excretion – 60–90% renal excretion, with the remaining in feces and bile, amount dependent on route of administration.
- Elimination half-life – 1–1.5 hours.
- Oral disintegrating film has successfully been developed for ease in administration of furosemide, not yet marketed.

- Hydrochlorothiazide.
  - Administered orally.
  - Onset and duration of action – in dogs, onset of action is within two hours, with peak plasma concentrations at 2.4 hours. Effects last approximately 12 hours. No data available for cats.
  - Absorption – occurs in the proximal part of the intestine. In humans, approximately 60–80% is absorbed.
  - Distribution – predominantly confined to extracellular space and kidneys, with 40% protein binding.
  - Metabolism – no appreciable metabolism.
  - Excretion – renally excreted in the urine, unchanged, with 61% being eliminated at 24 hours.
  - Elimination half-life – approximately six hours in the dog.
- Spironolactone.
  - Administered orally.
  - Onset and duration of action – diuretic action takes several days to reach its effect and lasts for several days after cessation.
  - Absorption – rate of absorption is rapid with a variable oral bioavailability of 50% at fasting and up to 90% with a meal.
  - Distribution – large volume of distribution, with 90% protein binding.
  - Metabolism – occurs in liver and kidney, extent is unknown.
  - Excretion – 70% renal excretion, with the remaining in feces and bile.
  - Elimination half-life – 20 hours for the active metabolite canrenone.
- Torsemide.
  - Administered orally.
  - Onset and duration of action – onset of diuretic effects is within one hour in dogs and 2–4 hours in cats.
  - Absorption – rapid absorption of 30 minutes to one hour in dogs, with oral bioavailability of 80–100% in both dogs and cats, up to 98% in dogs, when fed.
  - Distribution – large volume of distribution with 98% protein binding.
  - Metabolism – partially metabolized with majority eliminated unchanged in dogs.
  - Excetion – predominant renal excetion, with 60–61% excreted unchanged in the urine of dogs, unknown in cats.
  - Elimination half-life – 6–10 hours in dogs, 13 hours in cats.

## Toxicity

- Diuretics have a fairly wide margin of safety.
  - The oral $LD_{50}$ of furosemide in dogs is >1000 mg/kg.
  - Dehydration and electrolyte imbalances are the most common result of toxicity.
  - Most acute diuretic intoxications do not cause primary nephrotoxicity, but may be seen with chronic overdosing.

## Systems Affected (Table 27.2)

- Cardiovascular – arrhythmias, hypoperfusion.
- Endocrine/metabolic – electrolyte disturbances.
- Gastrointestinal – vomiting, anorexia secondary to azotemia/uremia.
- Musculoskeletal – weakness due to hypokalemia, hypomagnesemia.
- Skin/exocrine – pruritic excoriative dermatitis with spironolactone in cats.

**TABLE 27.2 Adverse effects and clinical signs associated with diuretics.**

| Adverse effect | Diuretics | Clinical signs |
| --- | --- | --- |
| Hypovolemia | Loop diuretics, thiazides | Polydipsia, polyuria, hypotension, azotemia/uremia, oliguric acute renal failure |
| Hypokalemia | Loop diuretics, thiazides | Muscle weakness, arrhythmias |
| Hyperkalemia | Spironolactone | Arrhythmias |
| Hyponatremia | Thiazides Furosemide Torsemide | Potentially CNS signs if severe hyponatremia. Not clinically reported in small animals |
| Metabolic alkalosis | Loop diuretics Thiazides | Common, but rarely a clinical problem |
| Hypercalcemia | Thiazides | Only a problem if administered to hypercalcemic patients |
| Hyperuricemia | Thiazides Loop diuretics | Uric acid retention (Dalmatians) |
| Ototoxicity | Furosemide Torsemide | Only at supraphysiological doses or used in patients with hyponatremia or severe renal impairment |
| Dermatopathy | Spironolactone | Excoriative dermatopathy in cats |

# SIGNALMENT/HISTORY

### Risk Factors

- There are no specific breed or species predispositions to diuretic intoxication.
- Patients with cardiac disease, especially output failure, severe renal impairment, anorexia, and hypodipsia can have an increase in drug effects.

### Historical Findings

- Vomiting, anorexia, polyuria/polydipsia, anuria, depression, and weakness are the most common presenting signs of diuretic toxicosis.

### Location and Circumstances of Poisoning

- May be due to continued and/or inappropriate administration in patients with CHF, or other diseases necessitating diuretic use.
- Many poisonings occur due to ingestion of human medication in the house.

# CLINICAL FEATURES

- Depression, weakness, lethargy.
- Dehydration.
- Vomiting if severely uremic.

# DIFFERENTIAL DIAGNOSIS

- Allergic dermatopathy in cats administered spironolactone.
- Gastroenteritis (vomiting).

- Toxicants.
  - Digoxin.
  - Other toxins that can cause primary kidney injury (e.g., NSAIDs, raisins, vitamin $D_3$/ cholecalciferol, *Lilium* sp. and *Hemerocallis* sp. in cats, soluble oxalate crystal containing plants).
- Primary acute kidney injury.
- Primary hyperaldosteronism.
- Diabetes insipidus.
- Hyperthyroidism.

# DIAGNOSTICS

## Clinical Pathological Findings

- General biochemical analysis should be sufficient to identify dehydration or electrolyte imbalances and any renal concerns.

## Other Diagnostics

- Electrocardiography for possible arrhythmias.

# THERAPEUTICS

- Correct dehydration.

## Detoxification

- Early emesis followed by activated charcoal with cathartic in acute and severe overdose situations.

## Appropriate Health Care

- Care should be taken when rehydrating patients that have severe cardiac disease to avoid volume overloading.
- Hourly monitoring of the patient's respiratory rate and effort can help determine if fluid therapy is precipitating CHF recurrence.

## Drug(s) of Choice

- Intravenous fluid administration will assist with increasing plasma volume and result in increased diuresis and drug excretion.
  - Electrolyte administration may be required in some cases, especially with severe hypokalemia.

## Precautions/Interactions

- Aminoglycosides should be used cautiously with furosemide therapy.
- Furosemide can increase the potential for aminoglycoside ototoxicity and nephrotoxicity.
- Clinically relevant hyperkalemia is extremely unlikely with potassium-sparing diuretics, even if coadministered with ACE inhibitors.
- Hypokalemia/hypomagnesemia is more likely with coadministration of loop and thiazide diuretics.

- Furosemide can increase the toxicity of digoxin due to hypokalemia and hypomagnesemia.
- Spironolactone can increase digoxin half-life, resulting in increased digoxin concentrations.
- Amiloride has been shown to have synergistic action with doxorubicin to potentiate apoptosis of canine osteosarcoma cells.

## Alternative Drugs

- If intravenous fluid therapy is not available, increasing oral fluid intake should be encouraged.

## Patient Monitoring

- Monitor urine output.
- Recheck BUN/creatinine 24–48 hours after initial treatment of toxicosis.
- Monitor electrolytes every 4–6 hours until hydration status and electrolyte abnormalities have returned to normal.
- Monitor body weight and PCV to assess correction of hydration deficits.
- Monitor respiratory rate and effort.

## Diet

- In cases of chronic hypokalemia, a high-potassium supplement can help minimize recurrence.

 **COMMENTS**

### Prevention/Avoidance

- Use caution when administering diuretics and the lowest effective dose should be administered.
- Extra vigilance is required when combining diuretics, as the risk of dehydration increases.

### Possible Complications

- Clients should be advised to watch for changes in appetite, thirst, or urination while the patient is receiving diuretics. If the patient becomes anorexic or hypodipsic, then the diuretic administration should be suspended, and the veterinarian consulted.
- Continued administration of diuretics in anorexic or adipsic patients substantially increases the risk of severe dehydration. Consumption of commercial pet food generally provides sufficient electrolytes to avoid electrolyte depletion.

### Expected Course and Prognosis

- Treatment of dehydration due to diuretics is generally straightforward, and if done carefully in heart disease patients, usually results in complete resolution of clinical signs within a few days.

### Synonyms

Water pill.

### See Also

## Suggested Reading

Furosemide: www.rxlist.com/lasix-drug.htm

Torsemide: www.rxlist.com/demadex-drug.htm

Koh SK, Jeong JW, Choi SI et al. Pharmacokinetics and diuretic effect of furosemide after single intravenous, oral tablet, and newly developed oral disintegrating film administration in healthy beagle dogs. *BMC Vet Res* 2021;17:295.

Packham L. In dogs with congestive heart failure, is torsemide superior to furosemide as a first line diuretic treatment? *Vet Evid* 2020;5:4.

Poon AC, Inkol JM, Luu AK, Mutsaers AJ. Effects of the potassium-sparing diuretic amiloride on chemotherapy response in canine osteosarcoma cells. *J Vet Intern Med* 2019;33:800–811.

**Author:** Renee D. Schmid, DVM, DABT, DABVT

**Consulting Editor:** Steven E. Epstein, DVM, DACVECC

# Chapter 28

# Estrogen and Progesterone

## DEFINITION/OVERVIEW

- Estrogen and synthetic estrogens are used for a variety of conditions including mismating, urinary incontinence, estrus induction, pseudopregnancy, prostatic hypertrophy, perianal adenomas, and testicular neoplasms.
- Estrogen and progesterone are commonly used in people as hormone replacement therapy, contraception, and a wide variety of other underlying conditions.
- Estrogen toxicity is mainly due to bone marrow suppression and death occurs due to complications of hemorrhage and infection.
- Progesterone toxicity is not well described in animals.

## ETIOLOGY/PATHOPHYSIOLOGY

### Mechanism of Action

- Estrogens and progesterones are steroid compounds, which are normally produced by the ovaries but may also be synthesized by the testicles, adrenal cortex, and placenta.
- Estrogens are necessary for many physiologic processes including:
  - Growth and development of the female reproductive tract.
  - Mammary gland growth.
  - Estrous cycle.
  - Uterine health and contraction.
- Estrogens are myelotoxic secondary to the production of myelopoiesis-inhibitory factor by thymic stromal cells.
  - The effects of estrogen on the hematopoietic system occurs in three stages with acute ingestion or chronic administration.
    - Stage 1: 0–13 days; increased platelet number followed by severe thrombocytopenia.
    - Stage 2: 13–20 days; bone marrow granulocyte hyperplasia characterized by leukocytosis with a left shift.
    - Stage 3: 21–45 days; bone marrow recovery or aplasia (dose dependent).
- Progesterone toxicity may result in changes in reproductive organs, similar to the effects of estrogen, but no toxic effects have been noted in the liver, kidney, or bone marrow.

### Pharmacokinetics or Toxicokinetics – Absorption, Distribution, Metabolism, Excretion

- All estrogens administered or consumed chronically in high doses are toxic.
- Both natural and synthetic compounds have been reported to be toxic.
- Estrogens are available in oral and parenteral forms.

*Blackwell's Five-Minute Veterinary Consult Clinical Companion: Small Animal Toxicology*, Third Edition.
Edited by Lynn R. Hovda, Ahna G. Brutlag, Robert H. Poppenga, and Steven E. Epstein.
© 2024 John Wiley & Sons, Inc. Published 2024 by John Wiley & Sons, Inc.

- Injectable forms are often in 2 mg/mL of 4 mg/mL preparations and can be given intramuscularly.
- Progesterone is marketed for horses and available in oral preparations.
- Estrogen is well absorbed through the intestinal tract.
- Estrogen and progesterone are metabolized by the liver and excreted in the liver and bile.

## Toxicity

- The bone marrow is the primary target site of toxicity result in bone marrow destruction.
- The mechanism is unclear but suspected due to direct inhibition of stem cells.
- During the first three weeks of toxicity, a leukocytosis predominates.
- Approximately three weeks following acute ingestion, pancytopenia is most often noted.
- Doses below 0.1 mg/kg/day rarely cause mortality in dogs and cats.
- At doses of 2–4 mg/kg/day, animals tend to survive an average of 25–75 days and doses of 4–10 mg/kg/day had average survivals of 10–25 days.
- Doses >30 mg/kg resulted in death within 24 hours.

## Systems Affected

- Bone marrow.
  - Osteosclerosis with partial/complete occlusion of the medullary cavitary.
  - Bone marrow hypocellularity.
- Reproductive system.
  - Vaginal cornification.
  - Uterine hypertrophy.
  - Cystic hyperplasia.
  - Pyometra.
  - Feminization.
- Endocrine glands.
  - Suppressed follicular development.
  - Pituitary enlargement.
  - Adrenal cortical hyperplasia/hypertrophy.
- Liver.
  - Vacuolization.
  - Fatty infiltration.
  - Necrosis.
  - Liver damage in dogs is inconsistently reported regarding severity and incidence and is not noted in a clearly dose-dependent manner.
  - Cats appear to be more sensitive to hepatic consequences than dogs and hepatic lesions may be the primary cause of death.
- Skin.
  - Alopecia characterized by bilaterally symmetrical hair loss beginning in the perineal and inguinal region that may progress to the abdomen, thorax, flanks, and proximal extremities.

 # SIGNALMENT/HISTORY

### Risk Factors

- Dogs and cats are both susceptible to toxicity, but cats are noted to be more sensitive.
- Intact animals are at increased risk due to predisposition for testicular or ovarian neoplasia.
- Increased risk associated with household exposure to topical hormone replacement therapy.
- Increased risk associated with prescribed medications, including diethylstilbestrol which is a prescribed synthetic estrogen used to treat urinary continence in female dogs, induction of estrus or treatment of male dogs with benign prostatic hypertrophy.

- The response of the bone marrow to estrogen varies in individual dogs, which does not seem to be dependent on breed, nutrition, or route of administration.
- Bone marrow response does appear to correlate with age, type of estrogen used, total dose, and physical condition of the animal.

## Historical Findings

- Non-specific signs.
  - Anorexia.
  - Depression.
  - Weakness.
  - Exercise intolerance.
  - Collapse.

## Location and Circumstances of Poisoning

- Toxicity may be secondary to:
  - Inadvertent ingestion.
  - Chronic administration of prescribed medications.
  - Testicular tumors.
    - Interstitial.
    - Sertoli cell tumor.
  - Ovarian granulosa cell tumors.

 CLINICAL FEATURES

- Pallor.
- Petechiation.
- Mucosal hemorrhage.
  - Epistaxis.
  - Vaginal bleeding.
  - Gastrointestinal bleeding/melena.
  - Hematuria.
- Dyspnea.
- Edema.
- Mammary hypertrophy/feminization.
- Irregular/persistent estrous cycles.
- Gynecomastia.
- Vaginal discharge.
- Alopecia.

 DIFFERENTIAL DIAGNOSES

- Hematologic dyscrasias.
  - Sulfadiazine toxicity.
  - 5-Fluorouracil toxicity.
  - Phenylbutazone toxicity.
  - Ehrlichiosis.
  - Neoplasia.
  - Immune-mediated disease.
  - Osteosclerosis.
  - Myelofibrosis.

- Alopecia.
  - Congenital alopecia.
  - Color dilution alopecia.
  - Follicular dysplasia.
  - Hypothyroidism.
  - Hypercortisolism.
  - Alopecia X.

 # DIAGNOSTICS

## Clinical Pathological Findings

- Complete blood count.
  - Leukocytosis in early phases.
  - Leukopenia.
  - Anemia – non-regenerative.
  - Thrombocytopenia.
- Biochemistry.
  - Increased ALP/ALT.
  - Hyperbilirubinemia.

## Other Diagnostics

- Thorough history including medications in the household.
- Bone marrow aspirate/biopsy.
  - Bone marrow hypocellularity/hypoplasia/aplasia.
- Skin biopsy.
  - Epidermal atrophy.
  - Orthokeratotic hyperkeratosis.
  - Basal melanosis.
  - Small sebaceous glands.

## Pathological Findings

- Necropsy findings include:
  - Splenomegaly with hypoplastic germinal centers.
  - Reduction in ovarian/testicular size.
  - Enlarged uterus/prostate.
  - Lymphocyte depletion.
  - Hepatic amyloidosis/lipidosis.

 # THERAPEUTICS

- Therapeutic intervention is often dependent on the underlying etiology and stage of toxicity.
- Treatment is aimed at:
  - Correction of anemia/thrombocytopenia.
  - Treatment/prevention of infection.
  - Stimulation of remaining bone marrow.

## Detoxification

- Induction of emesis should be performed with known acute oral ingestion.
- Administration of one dose of activated charcoal with acute ingestions may reduce absorption.

## Appropriate Health Care

- Patients with ingestion should seek veterinary care.
- Obtain a baseline CBC and biochemistry panel.
- Correction of anemia and thrombocytopenia via blood transfusions including packed red blood cell or whole blood transfusions may be needed.
  - Multiple transfusions may be needed over the course of treatment.
- Administration of broad-spectrum antimicrobials in patients with <2000 neutrophils/mcl may be indicated.
- Stimulation of bone marrow/neutrophil production.
  - Lithium has been reported to stimulate neutrophil and other hematopoietic cell lines and has been reported to be successful in estrogen-induced bone marrow hypoplasia in a dog.
  - Androgen therapy has been used in humans to stimulate bone marrow recovery.

## Drugs(s) of Choice

- Drugs of choice include the following.
  - Transfusion therapy to manage anemia and thrombocytopenia.
    - Packed red blood cell transfusion as needed for clinical anemia.
    - Whole blood transfusion as needed for clinical anemia with hemorrhage from thrombocytopenia.
  - Broad-spectrum antibiotics should be used in patients with leukopenia and concern for secondary infection.
    - Ampicillin/sulbactam 30 mg/kg IV q 8 hours.
    - Amoxicillin/clavulanic acid 13.75 mg/kg PO q 12 hours.

## Precautions/Interactions

- Patients with bone marrow suppression are often significantly immunosuppressed, so appropriate barrier precautions should be utilized.
- Gloves should be worn by all personnel when handling patients.
- Aseptic technique is essential during all procedures with patients with immunosuppression (catheter placement, etc.).

## Alternative Drugs

- Lithium carbonate 1 mg/kg PO q 12 hours has been successfully used in a case report of bone marrow hypoplasia secondary to estrogen toxicity.

## Surgical Considerations

- In cases of estrogen-producing tumors (testicular or ovarian), surgical removal of the source is recommended and may be curative.

## Patient Monitoring

- Patients should be monitored closely during hospitalization, including:
  - Temperature.
  - Heart rate.
  - Respiratory rate.
  - Mucous membranes.
  - Capillary refill time.
  - Packed cell volume/total protein.
- Complete blood cell count monitoring should be performed weekly once discharged from hospital, more frequently if any clinical concerns are noted.

- At-home monitoring for:
  - Systemic illness.
    - ○ Lethargy.
    - ○ Anorexia.
    - ○ Vomiting.
    - ○ Diarrhea.
    - ○ Hematuria/hematochezia.
    - ○ Epistaxis.
    - ○ Hemorrhage.

 **COMMENTS**

### Prevention/Avoidance

- Prevention is aimed at reducing contact with estrogen/progesterone-containing products, specifically those used to treat people.
- Spay/neuter should be considered to reduce the risk of developing testicular and ovarian tumors.

### Possible Complications

- Major complications associated with estrogen/progesterone toxicity include secondary infections due to immunosuppression.

### Expected Course and Prognosis

- Cases of estrogen toxicity resulting in bone marrow suppression often end in either death or prolonged recovery.

### Synonyms

Hormone replacement therapy toxicity.

### See Also

Chapter 14 5-Fluorouracil

### Suggested Reading

Berger DJ, Lewis TP, Schick AE, Miller RI, Loeffler DG. Canine alopecia secondary to human topical hormone replacement therapy in six dogs. *J Am Anim Hosp Assoc* 2015;51(2):136–142.

Hall EJ. Use of lithium for treatment of estrogen-induced bone marrow hypoplasia in a dog. *J Am Vet Med Assoc* 1992;200(6):814–816.

Hart JE. Endocrine pathology of estrogens: species differences. *Pharmacol Ther* 1990;47(2):203–218.

Hillesheim HG, Hoffmann H, Güttner J, Oettel M. Toxicity of the progestagen STS 557 compared to levonorgestrel in beagles after oral administration for 6 months. *Arch Toxicol* 1982;5(Suppl.):221–224.

Plumb DC. Diethylstilbestrol. In: *Plumb's Veterinary Drugs*. https://app.plumbs.com/drug-monograph/vTu5mODx1yPROD.

Sontas HB, Dokuzeylu B, Turna O, Ekici H. Estrogen-induced myelotoxicity in dogs: q review. *Can Vet J* 2009;50(10):1054–1058.

Weiss DJ, Tvedten H. Erythrocyte disorders. In: Willard M, Tvedten H (eds) *Small Animal Clinical Diagnosis by Laboratory Methods*, 5th edn. St Louis: Elsevier, 2004; pp. 38–62.

**Author:** Rebecca A.L. Walton, DVM, DACVECC
**Consulting Editor:** Steven E. Epstein, DVM, DACVECC

# Chapter 29

# Gabapentin

## DEFINITION/OVERVIEW

- Gabapentin is a water-soluble white to off-white crystalline solid typically formulated as capsules, tablets or oral solution.
- Clinical uses include adjunctive anticonvulsive therapy in dogs, control of some types of chronic and perioperative pain in dogs and cats, and to reduce handling stress in cats.
- The prevalence of gabapentin toxicosis in dogs and cats has not been published.

## ETIOLOGY/PATHOPHYSIOLOGY

### Mechanism of Action

- Gabapentin is believed to produce pain relief by acting on ascending and descending spinal pain pathways.
- It decreases neurotransmitter release in presynaptic spinal neurons due to selective inhibition of voltage-gated calcium channels containing the alpha-2-delta-1 subunit.
- It activates descending inhibitory spinal noradrenergic signaling secondary to decreasing presynaptic neuronal gamma-aminobutyric acid (GABA) release and increasing astrocytic glutamate release in the locus coeruleus.
- The mechanism underlying its anticonvulsant and calming effects is unknown.

### Pharmacokinetics or Toxicokinetics – Absorption, Distribution, Metabolism, Excretion

### Absorption

- Approximately 80–95% of an oral dose reaches the systemic circulation in dogs and cats.
- Transdermal absorption is likely poor in cats.
- Maximal plasma concentrations are achieved within two hours of an oral dose in dogs and cats. In dogs, plasma protein binding is very low (<3%).
- Repeated administration does not alter gabapentin pharmacokinetics in dogs and cats.

### Metabolism

- Approximately 40% is biotransformed to N-methyl-gabapentin before renal excretion while the remaining 60% is excreted unchanged.

### Excretion

- Elimination half-life after oral administration is approximately 2–4 hours in dogs and cats.
- In dogs, up to 32% of an oral dose is eliminated in the feces. Approximately 40% is biotransformed to N-methyl-gabapentin before renal excretion while the remaining 60% is excreted unchanged. Elimination of the metabolite is slower than the parent drug. Although no

*Blackwell's Five-Minute Veterinary Consult Clinical Companion: Small Animal Toxicology*, Third Edition.
Edited by Lynn R. Hovda, Ahna G. Brutlag, Robert H. Poppenga, and Steven E. Epstein.
© 2024 John Wiley & Sons, Inc. Published 2024 by John Wiley & Sons, Inc.

similar data can be found for cats, chronic kidney disease in cats is associated with higher gabapentin serum concentrations that also positively correlates with serum creatinine values compared to healthy cats.

## Toxicity

- No gabapentin acute or chronic toxicologic studies can be found specifically in dogs and cats.
- In dogs, life-threatening adverse effects are exceptionally unlikely with therapeutic doses as high as 500 mg/kg/day.
- The most commonly reported acute adverse effects in dogs and cats include depression of the central nervous system (sedation), decreased activity, ataxia, muscle tremors, and weakness.
- Developmental toxicity (increased fetal skeletal and visceral abnormalities and increased embryofetal mortality) might occur with the use of gabapentin in pregnant animals based on studies in pregnant mice, rats, and rabbits.
- In a two-year carcinogenesis study, rats treated with supratherapeutic doses of gabapentin had increased incidence of pancreatic acinar cell adenoma and carcinoma.
- Human patients receiving gabapentin concurrently with other respiratory depressant drugs such as opioids have increased risk of serious respiratory depression.
- Oral solutions formulated for humans may contain xylitol, a sugar alcohol that can be toxic to dogs (increased insulin secretion, hypoglycemia, vomiting, weakness, depression, hypokalemia, seizures, liver injury). Xylitol does not appear to be toxic to cats.

## Systems Affected

- Central nervous system – decreased mentation.
- Musculoskeletal system – tremors, ataxia.
- Reproductive – developmental toxicity.
- Respiratory – depression in humans.
- Pancreas – pancreatitis.

 # SIGNALMENT/HISTORY

## Risk Factors

- Patients being medicated with gabapentin could be considered at risk, although risk of life-threatening adverse effects is unlikely at therapeutic doses as high as 500 mg/kg/day.
- Risk of respiratory depression in patients receiving other respiratory depressant medications is a possibility, although specific data for dogs and cats are not available.
- Gabapentin therapy during pregnancy may increase risk of fetal abnormalities.
- Pets living in households with family members prescribed with gabapentin could be at risk of inadvertent exposure.

 # CLINICAL FEATURES

- Increased sedation, decreased activity, muscle tremors, ataxia, weakness, coma.
- In dogs, ingestion of xylitol-containing formulation might cause vomiting, weakness, signs of hepatic encephalopathy (depression, seizures, coma), and icterus.

 # DIFFERENTIAL DIAGNOSIS

- Any condition associated with changes in mentation status and neuromuscular function.

# DIAGNOSTICS

### Clinical Pathological Findings

- There are no reported clinical pathological findings related specifically to gabapentin toxicity in dogs and cats.
- In dogs exposed to xylitol-containing formulations, possible findings include hypoglycemia, hypokalemia, and other changes suggestive of liver injury/failure (hyperbilirubinemia, increased serum activity of liver enzymes, increased prothrombin and activated partial thromboplastin time, thrombocytopenia, hypoalbuminemia).

# THERAPEUTICS

- Patient monitoring (mentation status, cardiorespiratory function, urine production, plasma glucose and electrolytes, etc.) and supportive care (fluid and electrolyte therapy, glucose therapy, oxygen therapy, blood pressure support, nursing care) aimed at stabilizing underlying clinical features and clinical pathological findings.
- There is no known antagonist for gabapentin.
- Dose requirement of sedative or anesthetic drugs might be reduced in patients receiving gabapentin.

# COMMENTS

- No toxicological studies in dogs and cats could be found at the time of this writing. Reported adverse effects in clinical studies include sedation, decreased activity, ataxia, muscle tremors, and weakness.
- Some gabapentin effects (e.g, sedation) can be considered desirable or undesirable depending on the setting and therapeutic goal.
- Based on available literature, risk of acute toxicity of gabapentin can be considered relatively low in patients receiving therapeutic doses.

### Suggested Reading

Adrian D, Papich MG, Baynes R, Stafford E, Lascelles B. The pharmacokinetics of gabapentin in cats. *J Vet Intern Med* 2018;32:1996–2002.

Davis LV, Hellyer P, Downing R, Kogan L. Retrospective study of 240 dogs receiving gabapentin for chronic pain relief. *J Vet Med Res* 2020:7(4):1194.

Guedes AGP, Meadows JM, Pypendop BH, Johnson EG, Zaffarano B. Assessment of the effects of gabapentin on activity levels and owner-perceived mobility impairment and quality of life in osteoarthritic geriatric cats. *J Am Vet Med Assoc* 2018:253:579–585.

Pankratz KE, Ferris KK, Griffith EH, Sherman BL. Use of single-dose oral gabapentin to attenuate fear responses in cage-trap confined community cats: a double-blind, placebo-controlled field trial. *J Feline Med Surg* 2018;10(6):535–543.

Peck C. The adverse effect profile of gabapentin in dogs: a retrospective questionnaire study. Degree project in veterinary medicine, Swedish University of Agricultural Sciences, 2018.

**Author**: Alonso G.P. Guedes DVM, MS, PhD, DACVAA
**Consulting Editor**: Steven E. Epstein, DVM, DACVECC

# Chapter 30

# Nonbenzodiazepine Sleep Aids

## DEFINITION/OVERVIEW

- Three nonbenzodiazepine (NBZD) sleep aids are commonly prescribed in human medicine – eszopiclone (Lunesta®), zaleplon (Sonata®), and zolpidem (Ambien®).
- They have a similar mechanism of action to benzodiazepines (BZD) but are chemically distinct from them.
- NBZD sleep aids are used for induction of sleep in people.
- Common clinical signs of overdose are related to the CNS and include agitation, ataxia, and depression.

## ETIOLOGY/PATHOPHYSIOLOGY

### Mechanism of Action

- NBZD sleep aids interact with the type 1 benzodiazepine receptors that modulate GABA, an inhibitory neurotransmitter. They have strong hypnotic, i.e., sleep-inducing, properties but unlike benzodiazepines, do not have strong antianxiety or anticonvulsive effects.

### Pharmacokinetics or Toxicokinetics – Absorption, Distribution, Metabolism, Excretion

- NBZDs are well absorbed orally.
- Depending on the compound, they are moderately (eszopiclone, zaleplon) to highly (zolpidem) protein bound.
- Peak plasma levels generally occur between 60 and 90 minutes.
- Metabolized in liver to mainly inactive or less active metabolites.
- Half-life elimination in humans ranges from one to six hours depending on drug.
- Mainly excreted in urine.

### Toxicity

- Overdose as a single exposure is rarely life-threatening in healthy animals.
- Lower doses generally cause CNS depression while higher doses may cause CNS excitation (paradoxical reaction).
- Eszopiclone: dosages of >0.37 mg/kg were associated with signs.
- Zaleplon.
  - In dogs, dosages >0.11 mg/kg have been associated with restlessness and hyperactivity.
  - In cats, dosages of >1.25 mg/kg caused paradoxical reactions.

*Blackwell's Five-Minute Veterinary Consult Clinical Companion: Small Animal Toxicology*, Third Edition.
Edited by Lynn R. Hovda, Ahna G. Brutlag, Robert H. Poppenga, and Steven E. Epstein.
© 2024 John Wiley & Sons, Inc. Published 2024 by John Wiley & Sons, Inc.

- Zolpidem.
  - In dogs, dosages >0.2 mg/kg cause mild sedation while those >0.6 cause paradoxical reactions.
  - Paradoxical reactions were seen in cats with dosages of >0.34 mg/kg.

## Systems Affected

- Nervous – CNS depression, dysphoria, ataxia, excitement, aggression.
- Respiratory – respiratory depression.
- Cardiovascular – bradycardia, hypotension.
- Endocrine/metabolic – hypothermia.

 # SIGNALMENT/HISTORY

- Any age or breed of dog or cat can be affected.
- Smaller animals are more prone to paradoxical reactions due to higher dosages received.
- Overdose usually occurs due to accidental ingestion of owner's medication.

## Risk Factors

- NBZD sleep aids present in the household may pose an increased risk of exposure to pets.
- Pediatric, geriatric, or debilitated patients with underlying metabolic disease may have prolonged duration of effects from toxicosis.

## Historical Findings

- Witnessed exposure by pet owner.
- Pet owner may find chewed pill vial or discover that a pill is missing.
- Clinical symptoms of ataxia, sedation, agitation, and dysphoria may be noted by the pet owner.

 # CLINICAL FEATURES

- Common clinical signs include CNS depression, ataxia, confusion, and disorientation.
- As ingested dose increases, risks for paradoxical reactions, hypotension, hypothermia, coma, and seizures occur.
- In approximately 50% of cases, paradoxical stimulation and excitation occur in both dogs and cats.

 # DIFFERENTIAL DIAGNOSIS

- Primary metabolic disease (e.g., hepatic encephalopathy, hypoglycemia).
- Primary neurological disease.
- Toxicants.
  - Sedation.
    - Alcohols and glycols (e.g., ethanol, methanol, ethylene glycol).
    - Barbiturates.
    - Marijuana.
    - Opiates and opioids.
    - Phenothiazines.
  - Agitation.
    - Amphetamines.
    - Antidepressants (serotonin syndrome).

- o Cocaine.
- o Pseudoephedrine.

# DIAGNOSTICS

- While not routinely available, urine or serum can be submitted specifically for GC/MS or LC/MS, but the results will take several days to be returned and will only indicate exposure.
- Blood gas monitoring may be indicated in patients with severe clinical signs to monitor for respiratory depression.

## Pathological Findings

- No specific findings are expected.

# THERAPEUTICS

## Detoxification

- Emesis with extreme caution due to rapid onset of signs.
- One dose of activated charcoal with a cathartic for large ingestions although risk of aspiration must be considered.

## Appropriate Health Care

- If clinical signs exist at the time of presentation, the patient should be hospitalized.
- Body temperature and blood pressure should be monitored.
- IV fluid therapy and general nursing care should be provided.
- Monitor for severe CNS or respiratory depression; if indicated, consider the use of flumazenil.

## Antidote

- Flumazenil is the specific antidote for benzodiazepine overdose and has been shown to be useful in NBZD sleep aid exposure. It should be used only in cases where CNS depression or agitation is severe. Flumazenil rapidly reverses the sedative effects of the NBZDs. Effects are usually seen within five minutes. Seizures have been associated with the use of flumazenil.
- Dose: flumazenil 0.01 mg/kg IV to effect, repeat PRN. Repeated doses of flumazenil may be necessary, due to its short duration of action (1–2 hours).

## Drug(s) of Choice

- IV fluids as needed to treat hypotension, maintain perfusion, and correct dehydration. A balanced crystalloid should be used.
- If the animal is experiencing paradoxical stimulation (e.g., agitation, aggression), treatment with benzodiazepines (e.g., diazepam) is contraindicated. An alternative sedative or anxiolytic should be used.
    - Acepromazine 0.01–0.1 mg/kg, IV, SQ, IM PRN.
    - Dexmedetomidine 1–3 mcg/kg IV PRN.

## Precautions/Interactions

- Coingestion of sedative or stimulants may intensify signs.

## Patient Monitoring

- While hospitalized, excessively sedated patients should have blood pressure, ECG, TPR, and ventilatory status closely monitored.

# COMMENTS

### Prevention/Avoidance

- Owners should be informed about the risks of NBZD sleep aids in pets, and keep them out of reach, particularly in the bedroom (e.g., tablet placed on bedroom table prior to ingestion).

### Expected Course and Prognosis

- Once decontaminated, animals generally only need to be monitored for 2–4 hours.
  - If no clinical signs develop, the patient can be monitored at home.
  - If signs develop, they should be monitored until clinical signs have resolved (typically 12–24 hours depending on the drug involved).
- In those animals experiencing a single overdose exposure, the prognosis is excellent.

### See Also

Chapter 20 Benzodiazepines
Chapter 9 Ethylene Glycol and Diethylene Glycol
Chapter 31 Opiates and Opioids

### Abbreviations

- BZD = benzodiazepine
- NBZD = nonbenzodiazepine

### Suggested Reading

Lancaster AR, Lee JA, Hovda LR et al. Sleep aid toxicosis in dogs: 317 cases (2004–2010). *J Vet Emerg Crit Care* 2011;21(6):658–665.

Richardson JA, Gwaltney-Brant SM, Albertsen JC et al. Clinical syndrome associated with zolpidem ingestion in dogs: 33 cases (January 1998–July 2000). *J Vet Intern Med* 2002;16:208–210.

**Author**: Eric Dunayer, MS, VMD, DABT, DABVT
**Consulting Editor**: Steven E. Epstein, DVM, DACVECC

# Chapter 31

# Opiates and Opioids

## DEFINITION/OVERVIEW

- Opiates and opioids are often referred to as "opioids."
  - Opiates: naturally occurring substances (e.g., morphine).
  - Opioids: lab-manufactured compounds derived from morphine.
    - Semisynthetic (e.g., hydromorphone).
    - Synthetic (e.g., fentanyl).
- Many different prescription opioids are commercially available (Table 31.1).
- Simbadol® is a high-concentration formulation of buprenorphine (1.8 mg/mL) labeled for SQ injection in cats.
- Zorbium® is a buprenorphine long-acting transdermal solution labeled for cats and supplied in single use dose applicator tubes (20 mg/mL).

## ETIOLOGY/PATHOPHYSIOLOGY

### Mechanism of Action

- Opioids interacts with opioid receptors throughout the body.
  - Brain, spinal cord, primary sensory neurons, chemoreceptor trigger zone, gastrointestinal tract, synovium, urinary tract, uterus, immune cells, peripheral chemo and baroreceptors, airways and lungs mechanoreceptors.
  - Distribution varies with species.
- Different opioid receptors exist.
  - Mu/MOR, kappa/KOR, delta/KOR.
  - They produce different effects once activated by the proper agonist.
- Opioids have different affinity and intrinsic activity at opioid receptors (Table 31.1).
  - Full agonist: produces a dose-dependent effect until maximum receptor activation.
  - Partial agonist: produces partial receptor activation with dose-dependent effect with maximum effect less than a full agonist.
  - Full antagonist: affinity but no activity at opioid receptors. Generally used as reversal agents (inhibits binding of and displaces previously bound agonist).
  - Mixed agonist-antagonist: affinity at all opioid receptors with activity at only some.
- The effect of each drug and patients' response vary depending on the drug's affinity and intrinsic activity at opioid receptors, drug's pharmacokinetic profile, receptors distribution and genetic variations, differences in patient's pharmacodynamics/pharmacokinetics.

---

*Blackwell's Five-Minute Veterinary Consult Clinical Companion: Small Animal Toxicology*, Third Edition.
Edited by Lynn R. Hovda, Ahna G. Brutlag, Robert H. Poppenga, and Steven E. Epstein.
© 2024 John Wiley & Sons, Inc. Published 2024 by John Wiley & Sons, Inc.

| TABLE 31.1 Prescription opioids. | | | |
|---|---|---|---|
| Drug name | Opioid receptor activity | Route of administration | LD$_{50}$ |
| Alfentanil | MOR agonist | IV | >20 mg/kg (dogs) |
| Buprenorphine | Partial MOR and DOR agonist, KOR antagonist | IM, IV, OTM, transdermal, epidural, intranasal | 79 mg/kg (dogs) |
| Buprenorphine + naloxone | | | |
| Butorphanol | MOR antagonist to partial agonist, KOR agonist | IM, IV, SQ, nasal spray | 10 mg/kg (dogs) |
| Carfentanil | MOR agonist | IM, PO (if specially prepared) | |
| Codeine | MOR and DOR agonist | PO – many combination formulations with acetaminophen for pain and dextromethorphan or guaifenesin for cough | 98 mg/kg IV (dogs) |
| Diprenorphine | KOR and MOR antagonist, DOR partial agonist –reverses etorphine and carfentanil | IM, IV | |
| Etorphine | MOR, KOR, DOR agonist | IM | |
| Fentanyl | MOR agonist, DOR and KOR partial agonist | IM, IV, transdermal, PO (lollipop/lozenge), buccal (soluble film/tablet), epidural | 14 mg/kg IV (dogs) |
| Heroin | MOR, KOR, DOR agonist | Illicit drug | |
| Hydrocodone Hydrocodone + acetaminophen Hydrocodone + ibuprofen Hydrocodone + aspirin | MOR agonist, DOR and KOR partial agonist | PO – only available as a combination product in the USA | |
| Hydromorphone | MOR and DOR agonist, KOR partial agonist | IM, IV, SQ, PO, rectal suppository | |
| Loperamide | Act on receptors in myenteric plexus of large intestine, no CNS effects | PO | |
| Meperidine | MOR and DOR agonist | IM, IV, SQ, PO | 68 mg/kg (dogs); 30 mg/kg in cats has been known to cause seizures |
| Methadone | MOR agonist, DOR and KOR partial agonist | IM, IV, SQ, PO, OTM, epidural | 29 mg/kg IV (dogs) |

**TABLE 31.1** *Continued*

| Drug name | Opioid receptor activity | Route of administration | LD$_{50}$ |
|---|---|---|---|
| Morphine | MOR agonist, DOR and KOR partial agonist | IM, IV, SQ, PO, rectal suppository, epidural | 110–175 mg/kg IV (dogs); 210 mg/kg SQ (dogs); 40 mg/kg SQ (cats) |
| Nalbuphine | MOR and KOR partial agonist | IM, IV | 140 mg/kg (dogs) |
| Naloxone Naloxone + buprenorphine Naloxone + pentazocine | Antagonist | IV, IM, SQ Talwin® NX is PO only | |
| Naltrexone Naltrexone + morphine sulfate | Antagonist (duration twice as long as naloxone) | IM, PO | |
| Oxycodone Oxycodone + acetaminophen Oxycodone + aspirin Oxycodone + ibuprofen | MOR agonist | PO | |
| Oxymorphone | MOR agonist, DOR and KOR partial agonist | IM, IV, SQ, PO | |
| Pentazocine Pentazocine + naloxone Pentazocine + acetaminophen | MOR antagonist or partial agonist, KOR agonist | IM, IV, SQ Talwin® NX and Talacen® are PO only | |
| Remifentanil | MOR agonist | IV | |
| Sufentanil | MOR agonist | IV, epidural, sublingual tablet | 14 mg/kg (dogs) |
| Tapentadol | MOR partial agonist, DOR and KOR partial agonist | PO | |
| Thiafentanil | MOR agonist | IM | |
| Tramadol | MOR partial agonist | PO | 40–100 mg/kg (dogs) |

MOR, mu opioid receptor; KOR, kappa opioid receptor; DOR, delta opioid receptor.

## Pharmacokinetics or Toxicokinetics – Adsorption, Distribution, Metabolism, Excretion

- Opioids are well absorbed by all routes.
  - Absorption of SQ buprenorphine at standard dose can be erratic.
- Poor bioavailability PO (about 25%), due to extensive first-pass metabolism, and less predictable effect.
- Low bioavailability oral transmucosal (OTM) (about 20–40%).
- Simbadol® shows biphasic rapid and slow absorption from the SQ route (0.24 mg/kg cats; 0.12 mg/kg dogs) and an approximate 24-hour duration in cats.

- Fentanyl patch: there is interindividual and intraindividual variation in fentanyl absorption.
- Zorbium has slow absorption kinetics with extended plasma buprenorphine concentrations and duration for up to 96 hours.
- Distribution.
  - High lipid solubility, easily cross BBB and placenta.
  - Small amounts of opioids distribute into the milk.
- Extensive hepatic metabolism (hydrolysis, oxidation, N-dealkylation).
  - Remifentanil: hydrolyzed by plasma esterase.
  - Morphine: metabolized to active metabolite morphine-6-glucuronide.
    - Dogs and cats produce little amount.
  - Meperidine: metabolized to normeperidine (proconvulsant).
- Renal elimination.
- Some biliary excretion via feces.
- Neonates may have an underdeveloped hepatic function and decreased opioid metabolism.
- Geriatric and animals with impaired liver and renal function, inadequate metabolism and excretion can occur.

## Toxicity

- See Table 31.1 for $LD_{50}$.
- Zorbium and Simbadol were well tolerated at doses five times the labeled dose in cats, with side-effects typical of opioids administration.

## Systems Affected

- Varies with opioids and species involved.
- Respiratory: depression.
- CNS: depression or excitation.
- Cardiovascular: bradycardia.
- Gastrointestinal.
  - Reduced GI motility with constipation.
  - Emesis or antiemetic.
- Ophthalmic: miosis (dogs)/mydriasis (cats), nystagmus.
- Renal: antidiuretic, urinary retention.
- Thermoregulation: hypothermia or hyperthermia (cats).
- Endocrine/metabolic: weak serotonin reuptake inhibition (meperidine, methadone, tapentadol, tramadol).

 # SIGNALMENT/HISTORY

### Risk Factor

- Police, airport and other narcotic dogs in active service are at a greater risk of exposure.
- Age.
  - Neonates and pediatric animals may have an incomplete BBB and show more severe signs.
- Loperamide should be used with caution in dogs with the ATP-binding cassette polymorphism (collies, Shetland sheepdogs, old English sheepdogs, other herding type dogs).
- Meperidine, methadone, tapentadol, tramadol are weak serotonin reuptake inhibitors: best not to use with TCAs, SSRIs, or MAOIs as this may lead to serotonin syndrome.

- Fentanyl and oxycodone: often reported to be associated with serotonin syndrome in people, and might affect the serotonergic system via a different mechanism.
- Prolonged and increased sedation was observed in dogs treated with ketoconazole prior to morphine administration.

### Historical Findings

- Discovery of a chewed pill bottle, fentanyl patch or lollipops, or the loss of a fentanyl patch that the animal has chewed off.

### Location and Circumstances of Poisoning

- Usually through iatrogenic dose miscalculation or accidental ingestion of an oral product, patch, or human use product.
  - Discarded fentanyl patches worn for three days by humans still retain 24–84% of the original amount of fentanyl.

# CLINICAL FEATURES

- Nervous.
  - Euphoria to dysphoria, vocalization, disorientation, agitation, excitement, hyperresponsiveness to sensory stimuli, increased locomotor activity (cats).
  - Sedation, lethargy, ataxia, weakness, recumbency, frank stupor, seizures, coma, death.
- Respiratory: slow, shallow, irregular breathing, $CO_2$ retention with possible respiratory arrest.
  - Panting may be seen in dogs due to thermoregulatory dysfunction.
- Gastrointestinal: hypersalivation, nausea, vomiting, defecation, decreased GI motility, constipation, decreased gag response.
- Renal/urological: urinary retention, antidiuresis or diuresis.
- Cardiovascular: bradycardia, hypertension, hypotension.
- Ophthalmic: miosis (dogs), mydriasis (cats), nystagmus.
- Thermoregulation: hypothermia, hyperthermia (cats).

# DIFFERENTIAL DIAGNOSIS

- Primary neurological disease (e.g., infectious, inflammatory, neoplastic, etc.).
- Primary metabolic disease (e.g., renal, hepatic, hepatic encephalopathy, hypoglycemia, hypoadrenocorticism).
- Drugs/toxicants.
  - Amitraz.
  - Amphetamines/methylphenidate/methamphetamine/methylenedioxymethamphetamine.
  - Barbiturates.
  - Benzodiazepines.
  - Cannabinoids.
  - Cocaine.
  - Ethylene glycol.
  - Metaldehyde.
  - Strychnine.
- Toxicities resulting in bradycardia.
  - Alpha-2-agonist drugs.
  - Beta-blockers.
  - Calcium channel blockers.

# DIAGNOSTICS

## Clinical Pathological Findings

- Opioids can be detected from urine or serum at human hospitals or laboratory via GC/MS or LC/MS. Results might take several days and will not provide information rapidly enough to guide therapy.
- Quick Screen Pro Multi Drug Screening Test: human testing kit validated by GC/MS for use in animals. It may provide a rapid and accurate diagnosis if the drug is present in high enough concentrations and the time frame is appropriate.
- Blood gas analysis to evaluate oxygenation and ventilation.

# THERAPEUTICS

## Detoxification

- After recent ingestion, if the animal is alert, vomiting should be induced followed by activated charcoal with a cathartic for one dose.
- Gastric lavage if large doses ingested.
- Decontamination, even several hours post ingestion, is often effective due to decreased GI motility.
- Removal of ingested fentanyl patches via endoscopy or surgery.
- For working dogs, decontaminate both the dog and the tack (dry blot, dry rub, and soap bath). Wash mouth and eyes (keep head down to avoid aspiration of liquids).
    - Use PPE as people are sensitive to the depressant effects of opioids.

## Appropriate Health Care

- Monitor closely for signs of respiratory depression. If respiratory depression leads to hypoxemia and hypercarbia, oxygen therapy, intubation and mechanical ventilation may be required. Intubation will also protect the airway from possible aspiration of gastric contents.
- Close patient monitoring of heart rate, blood pressure, body temperature, and ventilation.
- In body temperatures >105.5°F, active cooling may be required.
- Monitor for normal urination.

## Antidote

- Naloxone is the antidote of choice.
    - 0.01–0.02 mg/kg IM, IV, SQ, is often enough but doses up to 0.04 mg/kg may be required.
    - Naloxone lasts 30–60 minutes, so repeat doses may be necessary. A continuous IV infusion 0.004–0.008 mg/kg/h can be used.
    - Rapid reversal IV with high dosages can precipitate acute reactions of severe pain, excitement, profound stress. The associated sympathetic stimulation can lead to tachycardia, hypertension, pulmonary edema, and cardiac arrhythmia. Naloxone can elicit convulsions due to some GABA antagonist actions although this is usually not a clinical consideration.
    - Intranasal naloxone (Narcan®, 4 mg fixed-dose naloxone atomizer) is well and quickly absorbed (Figure 31.1). Repeat q10 min until effect is seen.
        - Limited studies in dogs and cats.

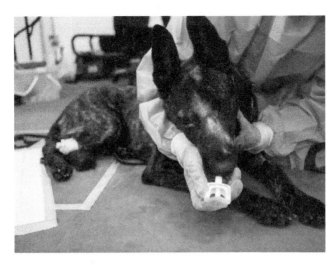

■ **Figure 31.1** A fentanyl sedated dog receiving intranasal naloxone. Source: Courtesy of Jennifer L. Essler and Tracy Darling.

## Drug(s) of Choice

■ Anticholinergic to treat vagally mediated bradycardia.
  • Atropine (0.01–0.04 mg/kg) or glycopyrrolate (0.005–0.02 mg/kg) IV, IM, SQ.
■ Midazolam 0.2–0.4 mg/kg IV or IM if seizures.
■ Sedation might be required with severe excitatory signs.
  • Dexmedetomidine 0.001–0.01 mg/kg IV, IM.
■ Serotonin receptor antagonists if serotonin toxicity.
  • Chlorpromazine 0.2–0.5 mg/kg IV, IM, SQ q 6 hours.
  • Cyproheptadine 1.1 mg/kg dogs and 2–4 mg/kg cats PO q 4–6 hours.

## Precautions/Interactions

■ Buprenorphine is not reliably reversible due to its high affinity for the MOR receptor.
■ Simbadol and Zorbium may require reversal for up to multiple days.

## Alternative Drugs

■ Butorphanol 0.02–0.2 mg/kg IV can be used to partially reverse MOR agonists.
■ Naltrexone: opioid antagonist with duration of action twice that of naloxone.
  • Often used to reverse ultrapotent opioids: 100 mg of naltrexone per 1 mg of carfentanil, typically one-quarter IV and the remainder SQ.
  • In cats, hourly administration of 0.6 mg/kg IV antagonizes behavioral and antinociceptive effects of a high dose of remifentanil.

## Surgical Considerations

■ Remove ingested fentanyl patches or lollipops via endoscopy or surgery.

## Patient Monitoring

■ Monitor TPR, respiration, and blood pressure frequently.
■ Pulse oximetry and arterial/venous blood gas analysis to evaluate oxygenation and ventilation.

**COMMENTS**

### Prevention/Avoidance

- Keep all controlled medications out of reach of pets.
- Monitor pets with fentanyl patch and adopt preventive measures (e.g., e-collar, bandage, tape) to prevent ingestion. Seek immediate veterinary attention if the patch is missing and cannot be found.

### Possible Complications

- Aspiration pneumonia.

### Expected Course and Prognosis

- Good prognosis if the respiratory and cardiovascular function is maintained; guarded prognosis if seizures develop.

### See Also

Chapter 42 Opiates and Opioids (Illicit)
Chapter 20 Benzodiazepines
Chapter 30 Nonbenzodiazepine Sleep Aids

### Abbreviations

- BBB = blood–brain barrier
- DOR = delta opioid receptor
- KOR = kappa opioid receptor
- MOR = mu opioid receptor

### Suggested Reading

Essler JL, Smith P, Berger D *et al*. A randomized cross-over trial comparing the effect of intramuscular versus intranasal naloxone reversal of intravenous fentanyl on odor detection in working dogs. *Animals* 2019;9(6):385.

KuKanich B, Wiese AJ. Opioids. In: Grimm KA, Lamont L, Tranquilli W et al. (eds) *Veterinary Anesthesia and Analgesia*, 5th edn. Ames: Wiley-Blackwell, 2015; pp. 207–226.

KuKanich B, Papich MG. Opioid analgesic drugs. In: Riviere JE, Papich MG (eds) *Veterinary Pharmacology and Therapeutics*, 10th edn. Ames: Wiley-Blackwell, 2018; pp. 281–323.

McMichael MA, Singletary M, Akingbemi BT. Toxidromes for working dogs. *Front Vet* 2022;9(July):1–12.

Teitler JB. Evaluation of a human on-site urine multidrug test for emergency use with dogs. J Am Anim Hosp Assoc 2009;45(2):59–66.

**Author**: Alessia Cenani, DVM, MS, DACVAA, CVA
**Consulting Editor**: Steven E. Epstein, DVM, DACVECC

# Chapter 32

# SSRI and SNRI Antidepressants

## DEFINITION/OVERVIEW

- Toxicosis secondary to the overdose of a selective serotonin reuptake inhibitor (SSRI), serotonin norepinephrine reuptake inhibitor (SNRI), or coingestion of two types of serotonergic drugs.
- SSRIs include citalopram (Celexa®), escitalopram (Lexapro®), fluoxetine (Prozac®), fluvoxamine (Luvox®), paroxetine (Paxil®), sertraline (Zoloft®), vilazodone (Viibryd®), vortioxetine (Brintellix®). Most SSRIs are used as antidepressants.
- SNRIs include desvenlafaxine (Pristiq®), duloxetine (Cymbalta®), levomilnacipran (Fetzima®), milnacipran (Ixel®, Savella®), sibutramine (Meridia®, Reductil®) and venlafaxine (Effexor®). SNRIs are used to treat depression, chronic pain, generalized anxiety disorder, fibromyalgia, and obesity.

## ETIOLOGY/PATHOPHYSIOLOGY

- SSRIs inhibit reuptake of serotonin, a neurotransmitter involved in aggression, anxiety, appetite, depression, migraine, pain, and sleep.
- Excessive stimulation of serotonin receptors leads to serotonin syndrome. Serotonin syndrome is characterized in humans as a combination of symptoms that include at least three of the following: myoclonus, mental aberration, agitation, hyperreflexia, tremors, diarrhea, ataxia, or hyperthermia.
- SNRIs inhibit the reuptake of both serotonin and norepinephrine. Norepinephrine (noradrenaline) acts as both a hormone and neurotransmitter. It is involved in the sympathetic system and can increase blood pressure and heart rate.
- Serotonin syndrome can occur along with cardiovascular signs (tachycardia, hypertension).

### Mechanism of Action

- SSRIs: highly selective reuptake inhibitors of serotonin at the presynaptic membrane with little to no effect on other neurotransmitters.
- SNRIs: potent inhibitors of neuronal serotonin and norepinephrine reuptake.

### Pharmacokinetics or Toxicokinetics – Adsorption, Distribution, Metabolism, Excretion

- Most forms are well absorbed from the GI tract.
- Onset of signs can be within 1–2 hours for immediate-release products and up to eight hours for extended/sustained-release products.

---

*Blackwell's Five-Minute Veterinary Consult Clinical Companion: Small Animal Toxicology*, Third Edition.
Edited by Lynn R. Hovda, Ahna G. Brutlag, Robert H. Poppenga, and Steven E. Epstein.
© 2024 John Wiley & Sons, Inc. Published 2024 by John Wiley & Sons, Inc.

- Peak effects will vary depending on the formulation (immediate vs sustained/extended release).
- Most SSRIs and SNRIs are highly protein bound.
- Most undergo hepatic metabolism.
- Excretion may be renal or fecal.

## Toxicity

- Toxic dosage varies widely among commonly available SSRIs and SNRIs and is not well defined in veterinary medicine.

## Systems Affected

- Cardiovascular – increased vascular tone (hypertension), increased heart rate, and stroke volume (tachycardia).
- Gastrointestinal – increased smooth muscle contractility (vomiting, diarrhea).
- Nervous – stimulation (agitation, restlessness, seizures) and altered mental status (vocalization, disorientation).
- Neuromuscular – autonomic dysfunction (hyperactivity) and neuromuscular hyperactivity (hyperreflexia, myoclonus, tremors).
- Ophthalmic –mydriasis.
- Respiratory – increased bronchial smooth muscle contraction.

 # SIGNALMENT/HISTORY

### Risk Factors

- All species, breeds, ages, and sexes can be affected.
- There is an increased risk if humans or animals in the household are on these medications.

### Historical Findings

- Agitation or lethargy.
- Dilated pupils.
- Vomiting.
- Tremors.
- Hypersalivation.
- Diarrhea.
- Seizures.
- Nystagmus.

### Location and Circumstances of Poisoning

- Most poisonings occur within the home.
- Animals may be given the wrong medication by mistake or may have access to prescription medications.

 # CLINICAL FEATURES

- Agitation.
- Ataxia.
- Mydriasis.
- Tremors.
- Vomiting.
- Disorientation.

- Hyperthermia.
- Vocalization.
- Depression.
- Tachycardia.
- Hypotension.
- Diarrhea.
- Blindness.
- Seizures.
- Hypersalivation.
- Death.

# DIFFERENTIAL DIAGNOSIS

- Toxicological: TCAs, MAOIs, 5-HTP, metaldehyde, lead, ethylene glycol, hops, anticholinergics, antihistamines, amphetamines.
- Nontoxicological: meningitis (e.g., rabies, canine distemper), neoplasia, heat stroke, malignant hyperthermia.

# DIAGNOSTICS

- There are no diagnostic tests to confirm serotonin syndrome.
- Testing for individual SSRIs/SNRIs can be performed, but the tests are not clinically useful.

## Clinical Pathological Findings

- Biochemistry: elevated creatinine kinase can be seen in tremoring/seizing patients with subsequent elevated blood urea nitrogen and creatinine.
- Blood gas: metabolic acidosis and hyperlactatemia may be seen.
- Pigmenturia secondary to rhabdomyolysis from tremors can be seen.

## Pathological Findings

- No pathological changes are expected.

# THERAPEUTICS

## Detoxification

- Emesis (if asymptomatic and recent ingestion) or gastric lavage (if large number of pills ingested).
- Activated charcoal with cathartic (if severe signs are expected).

## Appropriate Health Care

- Most patients will need to be hospitalized for monitoring of temperature, HR, and BP.
- Minimize sensory stimuli.
- Monitor acid–base status if tremors or seizures.
- ECG for arrhythmias.
- IV fluids to help regulate body temperature and blood pressure and to protect kidneys from myoglobinuria secondary to rhabdomyolysis.

## Antidote

Some medications can decrease serotonin (e.g., cyproheptadine), but there is no specific antidote.

## Drug(s) of Choice

- Agitation.
  - Phenothiazine.
    - Acepromazine 0.01–0.05 mg/kg IV or IM, titrate to effect as needed.
  - Cyproheptadine.
    - Dogs: 1.1 mg/kg PO or rectally; serotonin antagonist.
    - Cats: 2–4 mg total dose per cat.
- Tachycardia.
  - Beta-blockers.
    - Propranolol 0.02–0.06 mg/kg IV.
    - Esmolol 0.1 mg/kg loading dose then 10–200 mcg/kg/min IV CRI titrated to effect.
- Tremors.
  - Methocarbamol 50–100 mg/kg IV, titrate up as needed.
- Seizures.
  - Benzodiazepines.
    - Diazepam 0.5–2 mg/kg IV PRN.
    - Midazolam 0.3-0.5 mg/kg IV PRN.
  - Barbiturates to effect.
    - Phenobarbital 3–4 mg/kg IV PRN.
  - Levetiracetam 30–60 mg/kg IV PRN.

## Precautions/Interactions

- Any drug that may affect serotonin levels or that is metabolized via CYP enzymes in the liver may lead to drug–drug interactions.
- Avoid using trazodone, tramadol, TCAs, cimetidine, amiodarone, and class 1C antiarrhythmics (propafenone, flecainide). Use of these can worsen clinical signs of serotonin syndrome.

## Alternative Drugs

- Seizure control: inhalant anesthetics (isoflurane, sevoflurane), propofol CRI.
- Intralipid emulsion may be considered in cases where SSRI/SNRI are lipid soluble. 1.5 mL/kg IV fast bolus (if cardiac arrest or near arrest) then CRI of 0.25 mL/kg/min for 30–60 minutes can be used. If lipemia is not present in 4–6 hours, then it may be repeated if clinical signs are still severe.

## Patient Monitoring

- Monitor HR, BP, and temperature. This should be hourly (consider continuous temperature) and the interval may be increased depending on the clinical signs.
- Evaluate urine color for potential myoglobinuria development.

## Diet

- No diet change is needed, except NPO during severe CNS signs.

 **COMMENTS**

- Treatment in most cases is very rewarding.
- Note: venlafaxine will give a false positive for PCP on many urine drug screens.

## Prevention/Avoidance

■ Keep all medications out of the reach of pets.

■ Do not store human and animal drugs in the same area to decrease medication errors.

## Possible Complications

■ No long-term problems are expected in most cases.

■ DIC secondary to severe hyperthermia (rare).

■ Rhabdomyolysis and secondary renal failure (rare).

## Expected Course and Prognosis

■ If CNS and cardiac signs can be controlled, prognosis is good.

■ Signs may last up to 72 hours with extended-release products.

## Synonyms

Serotonin syndrome.

## See Also

Chapter 36 Club Drugs (MDMA, GHB, Flunitrazepam, and Bath Salts)
Chapter 40 Methamphetamine

## Abbreviations

■ MAOI = monoamine oxidase inhibitor

■ PCP = phencyclidine (angel dust)

## Suggested Reading

Fitzgerald KT, Bronstein AC. Selective serotonin reuptake inhibitor exposure. *Top Comp Anim Med* 2013;28(1):13–17.

Mohammad-Zadeh LF, Moses L, Gwaltney-Brant SM. Serotonin: a review. *J Vet Pharmacol Ther* 2008;31(3):187–199.

**Author**: Tina Wismer, DVM, MS, DABVT, DABT
**Consulting Editor**: Steven E. Epstein, DVM, DACVECC

# Chapter 33

# Tacrolimus

## DEFINITION/OVERVIEW

- Tacrolimus is a macrolide antibiotic immunosuppressant produced by *Streptomyces tsukubaensis* that is used to manage immune-mediated disorders and prevent graft-versus-host disease in transplant patients.
- Tacrolimus is formulated as capsules (0.5 mg, 1 mg, 5 mg), ointments (0.03%, 0.1%), and injectable solutions (5 mg/mL). Aqueous ophthalmic solutions are frequently compounded for veterinary use.

## ETIOLOGY/PATHOPHYSIOLOGY

### Mechanism of Action

- The immunosuppressive activity of tacrolimus is thought to be due to inhibition of calcineurin which blocks T-lymphocyte activation, thus impeding cell-mediated immunity.
- The mechanisms of the toxic effects of tacrolimus, including intussusception in dogs, are not known.

### Pharmacokinetics or Toxicokinetics – Adsorption, Distribution, Metabolism, Excretion

- There is minimal systemic absorption following topical (epidermal) application and slight absorption following ocular administration.
- Oral bioavailability of tacrolimus is 9% in dogs. Bioavailability varies considerably among species. Presence of food reduces the rate and extent of absorption.
- Tacrolimus is 99% protein bound, primarily to red blood cells. It is highly lipophilic and distributes widely throughout body.
- Peak plasma levels occur in 0.7 hours in cats and 1.4 hours in dogs.
- Some species (e.g., pig, rat) have significant first-pass metabolism that occurs in the intestine and/or liver.
- Metabolized in liver by demethylation and hydroxylation.
- Excreted primarily in bile; little in urine.
- Undergoes enterohepatic recirculation.
- Half-life of tacrolimus is 10.3 hours in dogs and 20.5 hours in cats.

### Toxicity

- Anecdotal reports from animal poison control centers indicate that clinical signs in dogs (vomiting and diarrhea +/– blood) may be seen at 0.08 mg/kg PO and deaths have occurred at 3.89 mg/kg PO.

---

*Blackwell's Five-Minute Veterinary Consult Clinical Companion: Small Animal Toxicology*, Third Edition.
Edited by Lynn R. Hovda, Ahna G. Brutlag, Robert H. Poppenga, and Steven E. Epstein.
© 2024 John Wiley & Sons, Inc. Published 2024 by John Wiley & Sons, Inc.

- In a two-week oral toxicity study of tacrolimus in dogs, 0.32 mg/kg resulted in significant vomiting, while 1 mg/kg resulted in colonic intussusception; dogs were precluded from further toxicity studies due to these adverse effects.
- In canine transplant studies, doses of tacrolimus of >0.15 mg/kg/day IM have been associated with toxicosis, predominantly the development of intestinal intussusception, in 25–75% of treated dogs.
- Doses >2 mg/kg/day PO resulted in degenerative changes in pancreas, liver, and kidney.
- Although necrotizing vasculitis was identified in dogs in one study, when the study was unblinded it was determined that vasculitis had occurred in both control and treated dogs with equal frequency, so necrotizing vasculitis was not considered to be a result of tacrolimus therapy.
- Toxic effects in cats have not been described. Cats receiving tacrolimus at 0.375 mg/kg q 12 hours for 14 days following renal transplantation did not develop signs that could confidently be attributed to tacrolimus administration.
- While some rabbit breeds appear to tolerate tacrolimus at 1 mg/kg/day, Dutch-Belted rabbits developed toxicosis at dosages >0.08 mg/kg/day IM.

## Systems Affected

- Gastrointestinal – vomiting, diarrhea, increased intestinal gas, gastrointestinal hemorrhage, intussusception, pancreatic degeneration, hepatocellular degeneration.
- CNS – lethargy, anorexia, convulsions.
- Renal/urological – renal proximal tubular degeneration, acute kidney injury.
- Cardiovascular – cardiac hypertrophy.
- Respiratory – pulmonary edema, dyspnea.

 # SIGNALMENT/HISTORY

### Risk Factors

- All ages, sexes, and breeds of dogs are susceptible following ingestion of tacrolimus; topical and ocular application of tacrolimus to dogs do not appear to pose risk of toxicosis.
- Cats appear to be more resistant than dogs to toxicosis.
- Dutch-Belted rabbits are much more susceptible than other rabbit breeds.

### Historical Findings

- History of ingestion of tacrolimus capsules, ointments, or solutions by dogs.

### Location and Circumstances of Poisoning

- Most exposures happen at home via accidental ingestion of capsules, ointments, or solutions.

 # CLINICAL FEATURES

- In dogs, initial vomiting after ingestion may be severe and may be accompanied by lethargy, anorexia, and diarrhea; development of further GI signs, including abdominal discomfort, increased intestinal gas, and intussusception, may occur within 3–6 days following exposure.

- In rabbits: anorexia, convulsions, pulmonary edema, heart failure, renal failure, and death occurred within one week of initiation of tacrolimus daily therapy; similar signs were reported in acute overdosing of rabbits with tacrolimus.

# DIFFERENTIAL DIAGNOSIS

- Dogs: infectious/inflammatory gastroenteritis, GI foreign body obstruction, GI neoplasia, gastric dilation/volvulus.
- Rabbits: primary cardiac disease, infectious/inflammatory encephalitis, primary CNS disease, primary renal disease.

# DIAGNOSTICS

## Clinical Pathological Findings

- Tacrolimus blood levels can be measured to confirm exposure, but turnaround time makes usefulness for diagnosis of emergency cases questionable.

## Other Diagnostics

- Radiography to evaluate gastrointestinal tract for intussusception. Note that evidence of GI abnormality may not be apparent for several days following exposure.

## Pathological Findings

- Dogs: intussusception, gastrointestinal hemorrhage, renal tubular degeneration, centrilobular hepatocellular degeneration, pancreatic acinar cell degeneration.
- Rabbits: pleural effusion, pulmonary edema, myocarditis, myocardial necrosis, proximal renal tubular necrosis.

# THERAPEUTICS

- The goals of treatment are to minimize absorption, manage clinical signs and monitor for complications (e.g., intussusception, renal injury).

## Detoxification

- If ingestion was recent and patient is asymptomatic, emesis may be induced. Induction of emesis is contraindicated in rabbits.
- If patient has already vomited, manage vomiting and consider a dose of activated charcoal if it can be given without risk of aspiration.

## Appropriate Health Care

- If vomiting is protracted, consider antiemetic therapy +/- GI protectants.
- For rabbits, convulsions may be treated with standard anticonvulsants.
- IV fluid therapy to maintain hydration and provide cardiovascular support as needed.

## Antidote

- There is no specific antidote for tacrolimus.

## Drug(s) of Choice

- Antiemetics.
  - Dolasetron 0.5–1.0 mg/kg IV q 24 hours.
  - Maropitant 1 mg/kg IV, SC q 24 hours.
  - Ondansetron 0.1–1.0 mg/kg SC, IV q 8–12 hours.

- GI protectants.
  - Omeprazole 0.5–1 mg/kg PO q 24 hours.
  - Pantoprazole 1.0 mg/kg IV q 24 hours
  - Sucralfate 0.25–1 g PO q 8 hours × 5–7 days if evidence of active ulcer disease.
- Anticonvulsants.
  - Diazepam 0.25–0.5 mg/kg, IV to effect PRN.
  - Midazolam 0.1–0.3 mg/kg IV to effect.
  - Phenobarbital 2–4 mg/kg, IV to effect PRN.

## Precautions/Interactions

- Avoid drugs that directly alter intestinal motility.

## Extracorporeal Therapy

- Therapeutic plasma exchange does not remove tacrolimus as it is primarily bound in red blood cells when in circulation.

## Surgical Considerations

- Surgical reduction of intussusception may be required.

## Patient Monitoring

- Dogs: monitor for abdominal discomfort, abdominal distension, anorexia, or other signs that might suggest development of intussusception.
- Rabbits: monitor for evidence of cardiovascular or renal dysfunction.

## Diet

- Dietary alterations as needed for GI irritation (bland diet, NPO, etc.).

 **COMMENTS**

### Prevention/Avoidance

- Secure medications where they cannot be accessed by pets.
- Never apply/administer human medications to pets without consultation with a veterinarian.
- Minimize/discourage licking of site of topical application of tacrolimus.

### Possible Complications

- Dogs: intestinal intussusception may occur 2–6 days following oral exposure to tacrolimus.

### Expected Course and Prognosis

- Most dogs with tacrolimus toxicosis respond to antiemetics and fully recover within 24 hours.
- Some dogs develop abdominal pain with increased intestinal gas 2–6 days following initial tacrolimus exposure.
- Less commonly, intestinal intussusception may occur 2–6 days following exposure.

### Abbreviations

See Appendix 1 for a complete list.

## Suggested Reading

Berdoulay A, English RV, Nadelstein B. Effect of topical 0.02% tacrolimus aqueous suspension on tear production in dogs with keratoconjunctivitis sicca. *Vet Ophthalmol* 2005;8(4):225–232.

Chung TH, Ryu M-H, Kim DY, Yoon HY, Hwang CY. Topical tacrolimus (FK506) for the treatment of feline idiopathic facial dermatitis. *Austral Vet J* 2009;87(10):417–420.

Giessler GA, Gades NM, Friedrich PF, Bishop AT. Severe tacrolimus toxicity in rabbits. *Exp Clin Transplant* 2007;5(1):590–595.

**Author:** Sharon Gwaltney-Brant DVM, PhD, DABVT, DABT
**Consulting Editor:** Steven E. Epstein, DVM, DACVECC

# Chapter 34

# Thyroid Hormones (T3 and T4)

## DEFINITION/OVERVIEW

- Hypothyroidism is a common endocrine disease in both humans and dogs, and rarely a sequela in cats after radioiodine therapy for feline hyperthyroidism. Due to the presence of thyroid supplementation in many homes, the opportunity for excessive ingestions is fairly high.
- Thyroid supplementation is available in synthetic forms of T3 (liothyronine) and T4 (levothyroxine), as well as natural T3/T4 combinations (desiccated).
- While thyrotoxicosis likely occurs frequently, there is a wide margin of safety with supplementations and the development of significant effects is rare due to the animal's ability to clear thyroid hormes effectively and efficiently.

## ETIOLOGY/PATHOPHYSIOLOGY

### Mechanism of Action

- Thyroid supplementation is used to replace naturally occurring and circulating thyroid hormones, triiodothyronine (naturally occurring T3) and thyroxine (naturally occurring T4).
- Thyroid hormone acts through specific ligand–receptor interactions with the nucleus, mitochondria, and plasma membrane for numerous cellular processes in most tissues throughout the body.
- High amounts of thyroid hormone may cause changes to the cardiovascular and neurological systems, with effects generally being mild and short-lived.

### Pharmacokinetics or Toxicokinetics – Absorption, Distribution, Metabolism, Excretion

- Absorption – levothyroxine is absorbed in the small intestine. Bioavailability is increased in fasting animals.
- Distribution – levothyroxine is widely distributed throughout the body with highest concentrations in liver and kidney. A small amount of enterohepatic recirculation occurs.
- Metabolism – levothyroxine is deiodinated (45% of T4 and 70% of T3) in peripheral tissues to more active T3 and then further conjugated in the liver. Alternate pathways of metabolism are also available, including renal metabolism.
- Excretion – approximately 30% is excreted in the feces, with the remaining excreted in urine and bile. Less than 15% of T4 excreted in bile is reabsorbed from the intestinal tract during enterohepatic recirculation.
- Peak plasma level.
  - T4: 4–12 hours.
  - T3: 2–5 hours.

*Blackwell's Five-Minute Veterinary Consult Clinical Companion: Small Animal Toxicology*, Third Edition.
Edited by Lynn R. Hovda, Ahna G. Brutlag, Robert H. Poppenga, and Steven E. Epstein.
© 2024 John Wiley & Sons, Inc. Published 2024 by John Wiley & Sons, Inc.

- Half-life.
  - T4: 8–16 hours.
  - T3: 5–6 hours.

## Toxicity

- Thyroid hormones are minimally toxic to dogs and cats.
- Pets become exposed by ingesting an excessive amount of their own or their owner's oral medication.
- The minimum suggested toxic dose is approximately 1–1.5 mg/kg in healthy dogs following acute exposure.
- Data collected from calls for over 500 thyroid hormone ingestions through Pet Poison Helpline indicate little concern for ingestions less than 1.4 mg/kg.
- Chronic dosing studies show no significant effects when levothyroxine is given up to 10× the therapeutic dosing of 0.022 mg/kg for six months.
- Geriatric animals or those with underlying renal, cardiac or hepatic disease may see effects at lower doses.
- Ingested doses of T3 or desiccated thyroid must be converted to a levothyroxine (T4) equivalent.
  - One grain (65 mg) of desiccated thyroid contains approximately 0.1 mg/kg levothyroxine.
  - Liothyronine (T3) is considered to be four times as potent as levothyroxine, so its dose should be multiplied by four.

## Systems Affected

- Cardiovascular – tachycardia (HR >160 bpm), hypertension, bradycardia, arrhythmias.
- Gastrointestinal – vomiting, diarrhea, hypersalivation.
- Nervous – agitation, irritability, hyperactivity, tremors, seizures.
- Renal – polyuria/polydipsia.
- Respiratory – panting.
- Thermoregulatory – pyrexia.

 # SIGNALMENT/HISTORY

- While there is no breed or age predisposition, animals that are affected with other illnesses are at greater risk of developing symptomatic toxicosis at lower doses.

## Risk Factors

- There are no specific breed or species predispositions to thyroid hormone intoxication.
- Patients with cardiac disease, especially output failure, severe hepatic or renal impairment, can have an increase in drug effects.

## Historical Findings

- Vomiting, agitation, tachycardia, polyuria/polydipsia, and panting are the most common presenting signs of thyroid hormone toxicosis.

## Location and Circumstances of Poisoning

- May be due to continued and/or inappropriate administration in hypothyroid patients.
- Many poisonings occur due to ingestion of medication in the house.

**CLINICAL FEATURES**

- The majority of thyroid poisoning patients remain asymptomatic due to its wide margin of safety.
- Animals that do become symptomatic will have clinical signs within the first few hours of ingestion.
- The most common clinical signs in symptomatic patients are agitation, irritability, and hyperactivity, with tachycardia seen less frequently.
- Clinical signs may persist for up to 24 hours in symptomatic animals.

 **DIFFERENTIAL DIAGNOSIS**

- Toxicants.
  - Amphetamine/methamphetamine/methylphenidate.
  - Caffeine/theobromine.
  - SSRI intoxication.
- Primary hyperthyroidism.

 **DIAGNOSTICS**

### Clinical Pathological Findings

- CBC and biochemistry profile to evaluate hydration status and overall health, particularly in older patients.
- T3 and/or T4 may be evaluated in significant ingestions. Elevations to T3 may occur within three hours of ingestion and T4 elevations within nine hours. However, this is rarely necessary with acute intoxications.

### Other Diagnostics

- Electrocardiography may be beneficial to evaluate possible arrhythmias if severe and persistent tachycardia is present.

### Pathological Findings

- Histopathological findings reported in rabbits, cats, and humans.
  - Mild acute toxicosis reveals reversible changes to the CNS, consistent with hemodynamic disturbances with vascular wall permeability.
- Severe, life-threatening toxicosis reveals irreversible lesions primarily in the cerebral cortex, corpus striatum, cerebellum, and infundibular and tuberal nuclei of the hypothalamus.

 **THERAPEUTICS**

- The goal of treatment is to perform early decontamination to minimize the occurrence of clinical signs.
- In symptomatic patients, care should be taken to minimize the severity of clinical signs.

### Detoxification

- Early emesis, within one hour of ingestion ideally, followed by one dose of AC with a cathartic.
  - While there is a small amount of enterohepatic recirculation, the risks of giving multiple doses of AC, such as aspiration pneumonia and hypernatremia, outweigh the benefit of a second dose.

## Appropriate Health Care

- For healthy dogs with ingestions <1–1.5 mg/kg, no further therapy should be needed after decontamination.
  - Pet owners can monitor animals at home and if no clinical signs greater than mild agitation occur, hospitalization is rarely needed.
- For dogs with >1.5 mg/kg ingestions, or those with underlying disease, hospitalization with close monitoring is required.
- Monitor heart rate and blood pressure for tachy- or bradycardia and hypertension.
Monitor body temperature and institute cooling measures, as needed.

## Antidote

- No specific antidote is available for thyroid hormone toxicity.

## Drug(s) of Choice

- IV fluids to help with hydration and aid in small amount of urinary excretion.
- Antiemetics as needed for vomiting.
  - Dolasetron mesylate 0.6 mg/kg IV, SQ, PO q 24 hours.
  - Maropitant 1 mg/kg SQ q 24 hours.
  - Metoclopramide 0.2–0.5 mg/kg IV, SQ or PO q 8 hours.
  - Ondansetron 0.1–1.0 mg/kg IV q 8–12 hours.
- Methocarbamol 55–220 mg/kg IV if tremors develop.
- Sedation with acepromazine 0.01–0.05 mg/kg SQ, IM or IV, or butorphanol 0.2–0.4 mg/kg SQ or IM if agitation and/or tachycardia develops.
- Beta-blockers should be used only if persistent tachycardia (>180 bpm) is present and unresponsive to sedation.

## Precautions/Interactions

- Overly aggressive fluid replacement can precipitate CHF in patients with severe heart disease.

## Alternative Drugs

- If injectable sedation is not available, oral acepromazine may be administered if patient's neurological state is appropriate to receive oral medication.
- If injectable methocarbamol is not available, oral tablets may be crushed, mixed with saline and given as a rectal slurry if oral administration is contraindicated due to neurological signs.

## Extracorporeal Therapy

- Therapeutic plasma exchange is effective in humans with severe thyrotoxicosis. While the need for use in animals would be rare, it is an acceptable consideration in patients with severe toxicosis whre clinical signs are refractory to general supportive care.

## Patient Monitoring

- Heart rate and blood pressure should be evaluated throughout hospitalization.
  - Monitor body temperature.
- Symptomatic patients should remain hospitalized until clinical signs have resolved, and no further medical intervention is needed.
- If T3 or T4 levels are monitored, T3 concentrations should be monitored every 2–3 days and are expected to return to normal within 3–6 days. T4 concentrations should be monitored every 4–5 days and are expected to return to normal within 15–36 days.

COMMENTS

## Prevention/Avoidance

- Owners should be educated on the importance of keeping medication out of reach of pets, especially with the added appeal of flavored, chewable tablets.

## Possible Complications

- Clients should be advised to watch for changes in behavior, appetite, thirst, or urination while the patient is receiving thyroid hormone supplementation. If the patient develops clinical signs, then the thyroid hormone administration should be suspended and a veterinarian consulted.
  - Continued administration of thyroid hormone supplementation in symptomatic animals increases the risk of toxicosis.
- Clients should be advised to avoid compounded thyroid hormone supplementation that contains xylitol.

## Expected Course and Prognosis

- Thyrotoxicosis has a good to excellent prognosis, even in the symptomatic patient.
- While severe clinical signs such as seizures and cardiovascular abnormalities are possible, their occurrence is rare.

## Abbreviations

- AC = activated charcoal
- T3 = triiodothyronine
- T4 = thyroxine

## Suggested Reading

Builes-Montano CE, Rodrigues-Arrieta LA, Roman-Gonzalez A et. al. Therapeutic plasmapheresis for the treatment of thyrotoxicosis: a retrospective multi-center study. *J Clin Apher* 2021;36:759–765.

Ferguson DC. Thyroid hormones and antithyroid drugs. In: Rivere JE, Papich M (eds) *Veterinary Pharmacology and Therapeutics*, 10th edn. Ames: Wiley-Blackwell, 2017; pp. 691–728.

Hare JE, Morrow CK, Caldwell J, Lloyd WE. Safety of orally administered, USP-compliant levothyroxine sodium tablets in dogs. *J Vet Pharmacol Ther* 2018;41:254–265.

Reinker LN, Lee JA, Hovda LR et al. Summary of thyroid hormone ingestion: a review of 593 cases (2004–2010). Pet Poison Helpline internal document.

Rosendale M. Hypothyroid medications. In: Plumlee, KH (ed.) *Clinical Veterinary Toxicology*. St Louis: Mosby, 2004; pp. 320–322.

**Author:** Renee D. Schmid, DVM, DABT, DABVT
**Consulting Editor:** Steven E. Epstein, DVM, DACVECC

# Drugs: Illicit and Recreational

# Chapter 35

# Cannabidiol (CBD)

## DEFINITION/OVERVIEW

- The *Cannabis* plant is one of the oldest cultivated plants in history. It contains more than 120 phytocannabinoids, including THC and CBD, and over 445 phytochemicals (terpenoids, flavonoids, sterols).
- Touted for its antioxidative, anti-inflammatory, and antinecrotic effects with potential benefits in a myriad of human disease processes, cannabidiol (CBD) has been most widely studied in the management of osteoarthritis and seizures in dogs. CBD has also been suggested to aid in managing anxiety, dermatologic conditions, cancer, and other conditions in veterinary patients. (Figure 35.1)
- The use of phytocannabinoids has increased greatly worldwide. With the federal legalization of low-THC concentration *Cannabis sativa* (hemp) in the 2018 Agricultural Improvement Act (Farm Bill), the use of CBD products has soared.
    - Cannabidiolic acid or CBDA produced in the plant is decarboxylated through cooking, heating, or drying to CBD.
    - Hemp contains 0.3% THC or less. CBD content varies from 0.3% to 4.2%. Selective breeding may result in higher concentrations.
    - *Cannabis* plants have recently been bred for higher intoxicating properties, resulting in declining CBD and increasing THC concentrations.

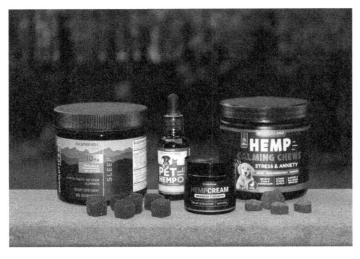

■ Figure 35.1 Some of the many CBD products marketed for humans and animals. Source: Courtesy of Lynn R. Hovda (book author).

*Blackwell's Five-Minute Veterinary Consult Clinical Companion: Small Animal Toxicology*, Third Edition. Edited by Lynn R. Hovda, Ahna G. Brutlag, Robert H. Poppenga, and Steven E. Epstein.

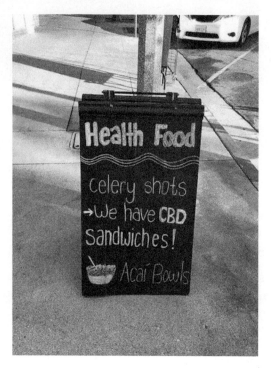

■ **Figure 35.2** Unregulated use of CBD. Source: Courtesy of Dr Rick Arthur, California.

■ Most CBD products remain unapproved by the FDA. There is no current regulatory oversight (Figure 35.2).
  • Product quality analysis indicates poorly manufactured products may contain inaccurate CBD content to label claims and can inadvertently contain THC, synthetic cannabinoids, and heavy metals including lead.
■ Epidiolex®, a cannabidiol product, was approved by the FDA in 2018, with expanded approval in 2020, to aid in the management of drug-resistant seizures in children over one year old. This remains the only FDA-approved cannabidiol product as of February 2023.

# ETIOLOGY/PATHOPHYSIOLOGY

## Mechanism of Action

■ The endocannabinoid system (ECS) is integral to both embryonic development and physiologic maintenance in mature animals. Naturally occurring endocannabinoids interact with cannabinoid receptors (CB1 and CB2) in cell membranes to inhibit neurotransmitter release.
  • The ECS displays extensive cross-reactivity with other receptor systems, including opiate, NMDA, GABA, muscarinic acetylcholine, 5-HT serotonin, dopamine, and MDR1 receptors.
■ CBD is a non-intoxicating exogenous phytocannabinoid acting on or indirectly influencing a vast array of receptors in the body.
  • CB receptors.
    ○ Partial agonist to the CB2 receptor: influences inflammation and pain.
    ○ Antagonist to the CB1 receptor: either antagonizing or potentiating the effects of THC depending on the temporal relation and ratio of the doses.

- Receptor cross-reactivity.
  - o Agonist of transient receptor potential cation channels (TRPV1 and 2) or vanilloid receptors: influencing pain pathways, inflammation, and vasodilation.
  - o Inhibits adenosine uptake: influencing neuroprotection and inflammation.
  - o Blocks uptake and hydrolysis of the endocannabinoid anandamide.
  - o Acts on 5HT1a and glycine receptors, downregulates cyclooxygenase expression, regulates intracellular calcium, and acts on dopamine and opiate receptors.
- Evidence indicates that whole plant-derived CBD is more effective than synthesized or highly purified CBD. This is likely due to synergistic effects with other cannabinoids and phytochemicals.
- Central effects: antipsychotic, anxiolytic, antihyperalgesic, anticonvulsant, neuroprotective, antinausea.
- Peripheral effects: antiinflammatory, ocular.

## Pharmacokinetics

- Absorption.
  - Dermal – minimal.
  - Ingestion.
    - o Bioavailability: 13–19%, may be higher with oral oil-based products compared to food or treats. Extensive first-pass metabolism, species, and product formulation may affect bioavailability.
    - o $T_{max}$: 1–2 hours.
    - o $C_{max}$ in cats may be one-fifth that of dogs.
- Distribution – highly lipophilic, rapid tissue distribution.
- Metabolism.
  - Primary: hepatic by hydroxylation, oxidation, and carboxylation with glucuronidation via CYP450.
    - o Metabolites vary between species.
  - Secondary: brain, intestines, lungs via alternate cytochrome pathways.
- Excretion.
  - Primary: feces.
  - Secondary: urine.
  - Half-life (2–20 mg/kg oral dosing with oil-based product): 2–4 hours.

## Toxicity

- Oral exposures are well tolerated.
  - NOAEL – not established.
  - Dogs: single oral doses up to 62 mg/kg caused mild gastrointestinal signs.
    - o Chronic oral dosing at 2 mg/kg PO q 12 h: transient ALP elevations, mild hypocalcemia, and mild hypoproteinemia. Laboratory changes were without clinical consequence. ALP elevations are suspected to be secondary to CBD induction of CYP450 enzymes.
  - Cats: single oral doses up to 80 mg/kg caused no CBD-associated adverse events. Lip smacking, head shaking, and hypersalivation noted immediately after dosing were attributed to distaste for the oil-based carrier.
    - o Chronic oral dosing of 2 mg/kg/day caused transient ALT elevation in one cat that abated after product cessation. Notably, an unrelated study also documented transient ALT elevations in one cat receiving an oil-based placebo.

- Intravenous dosing in Rhesus monkeys – IV $LD_{50}$: 250 mg/kg. Oral doses equivalent to 20–50× this dose would be needed to lead to severe intoxication.
  - IV doses of 150–300 mg/kg caused tremors, sedation, and prostration. Doses of 250–300 mg/kg precipitated convulsions, cardiopulmonary arrest, and death. These signs would not be expected in therapeutic use or acute oral overdose in pets.

## Systems Affected

- Approximately half of the CBD overdose exposure cases reported to PPH from 2018–2023 were asymptomatic.
- Oral overdoses may cause gastrointestinal signs.
- Neurological and other nongastrointestinal signs are anticipated to be related to poorly manufactured products inadvertently adulterated with THC or synthetic cannabinoids.
- Gastrointestinal – diarrhea, vomiting, hypersalivation.
- Nervous – lethargy/depression, ataxia, trembling, hyperesthesia, agitation, lateral recumbency.
- Ophthalmic – mydriasis.
- Renal/urological – urinary incontinence.

 **SIGNALMENT/HISTORY**

### Risk Factors

- Pets with known liver disease or gastrointestinal sensitivities.
- Indiscriminate eaters.
- MDR1 mutation – ECS interacts with the MDR1 receptors and may impart some degree of sensitivity to phytocannabinoids in these patients. This interaction is taken into consideration with therapeutic use of CBD, but the clinical consequences of phytocannabinoid overdose in these patients has not yet been evaluated.

### Historical Findings

- Owners may report missing or chewed product with an asymptomatic patient or those with gastrointestinal signs.
- Inadvertently adulterated or contaminated products may exhibit signs more consistent with marijuana or THC intoxication.

### Location and Circumstances of Poisoning

- The legalization of low-concentration THC *Cannabis* in the 2018 Farm Act led to a significant increase in the number of CBD products available across the country.
- In the absence of FDA regulation and regulatory oversight, product quality can vary significantly, and some CBD products may be inadvertently adulterated with THC or synthetic cannabinoids. This can result in psychotropic effects and more significant intoxications.

 **CLINICAL FEATURES**

- Gastrointestinal distress.
- If poor-quality contaminated product is ingested, clinical signs may be more consistent with those of THC.

 **DIFFERENTIAL DIAGNOSIS**

- Dietary indiscretion.
- Foreign body obstruction.

- Other gastrointestinal irritant ingestion: low-toxicity profile multipurpose cleaners, insecticides, herbicides, plants, fertilizers, poorly digestible objects, etc.
- In the event of neurological signs more consistent with THC exposure secondary to poor-quality product.

 # DIAGNOSTICS

- Liver profile monitoring may be warranted in large overdose or chronic exposures.
- Liquid chromatography-mass spectrometry of urine can confirm exposure, but is rarely indicated.

## Clinical Pathological Findings

- ALP elevation, especially with chronic dosing.
- ALT elevation rarely documented in the cat, especially with chronic dosing.
- ALT and AST elevations have been reported in humans with Epidiolex®.

## Pathological Findings

- Acute exposure-specific changes are not expected.

 # THERAPEUTICS

## Detoxification

- Emesis not recommended in oil-based product ingestion due to risk for aspiration. Indicated within 1–2 hours of ingestion of very large-volume chew or food-based products.
- Activated charcoal, though effective, generally not indicated due to wide margin of safety of CBD.

## Appropriate Health Care

- Asymptomatic patients may be monitored at home.
- Symptomatic patients may be managed supportively as for gastroenteritis: fluid support, antiemetics, digestive diets, antidiarrheals as needed.
- Symptomatic patients with signs more consistent to THC exposure may be managed supportively as per Chapter 39.

## Drug(s) of Choice

- Fluid therapy – SQ or IV depending on hydration status.
- Maropitant 1 mg/kg SQ or IV q 24 hours.
- Probiotics, antidiarrheals, and gastrointestinal support if needed and as based on clinician preferences.

## Precautions/Interactions

- CBD is a potent inhibitor of CYP450, and drugs that are metabolized through this enzymatic pathway may have altered metabolism and/or kinetics.
  - Anticonvulsants.
    - Phenobarbital – recent studies have indicated concomitant use does not affect the pharmacokinetic profile. Dose adjustments may not be necessary despite historical concerns and considerations.
    - CBD did not affect serum levels of zonisamide, phenobarbital, or bromide when given concomitantly. Adverse events such as ataxia were not significantly different from placebo.

- Proton pump inhibitors – concomitant use may increase CBD concentrations.
- Opiates – synergistic, may require dose reduction.
- Benzodiazepines – concomitant interaction at GABA receptors may potentiate effects, may require dose reduction.
- Propofol – concentrations may increase with CBD use, may require dose adjustment.

■ THC may be antagonistic or synergistic. Outcome may depend on the THC:CBD ratio and administration of the cannabinoids in temporal relation to one another.

### Extracorporeal Therapy

Generally not indicated.

### Patient Monitoring

Generally not indicated unless signs more consistent with THC exposure are noted due to poor product quality.

### Diet

Gastrointestinal support diet as needed.

 ## COMMENTS

■ Common exposures: pet treats, human and pet oral oils/tinctures/capsules, topical creams/lotions, human foods, vaping liquid.
- Consider coingestions: THC, chocolate, raisins, macadamia nuts, xylitol.

■ Disparity in labeling claims, inaccurate quantities of CBD, unlabeled THC or synthetic cannabinoid content, and heavy metal contamination have been well documented.
- Product quality is best confirmed with a Certificate of Analysis or COA completed through a third-party laboratory on the final marketed product. The COA, if completed, is available for each lot number through the manufacturer.

### Prevention/Avoidance

■ Products should be stored in areas without pet access.

### Possible Complications

■ Rare aspiration pneumonia with oil-based products.

### Expected Course and Prognosis

■ Prognosis is excellent.
■ Recovery in 12–24 hours.

### Synonyms

CBD, cannabidiol.

### See Also

Chapter 39 Marijuana (THC)
Chapter 44 Synthetic Cannabinoids

### Abbreviations

See Appendix 1 for a complete list.
■ CBD = cannabidiol
■ CBDA = cannabidiolic acid

- ECS = endocannabinoid system
- FDA = Food and Drug Administration
- GABA = gamma-aminobutyric acid
- MDR1 = multidrug resistance 1
- NMDA = N-methyl-D-aspartate
- THC = tetrahydrocannabinol

## Suggested Reading

Cital S, Kramer K, Hughston L et al. *Cannabis Therapy in Veterinary Medicine: A Complete Guide.* Cham: Springer International Publishing, 2021.

Machado Bergamaschi M, Costa Queiroz H, Waldo Zuardi R et al. Safety and side effects of cannabidiol, a Cannabis sativa constituent. *Curr Drug Saf* 2011;6(4):237–249.

McGrath S, Bartner LR, Rao S et al. A report of adverse effects associated with the administration of cannabidiol in healthy dogs. *Vet Med* 2018;1:6–8.

Rozental AJ, Gustafson DL, Kusick BR et al. Pharmacokinetics of escalating single-dose administration of cannabidiol to cats. *J Vet Pharmacol Ther* 2023;46(1):25–33.

Vaughn D, Kulpa J, Paulionis L. Preliminary investigation of the safety of escalating cannabinoid doses in healthy dogs. *Front Vet Sci* 2020;7:51.

**Author**: Holly Hommerding, DVM, DABT, DABVT
**Consulting Editor**: Lynn R. Hovda, RPh, DVM, MS, DACVIM

# Club Drugs (MDMA, GHB, Flunitrazepam, Bath Salts)

## DEFINITION/OVERVIEW

- Toxicosis is caused by ingestion of designer drugs: MDMA (3,4-methylenedioxy-methamphet amine) (Figure 36.1), synthetic cathinones (methylone, mephedrone [4-methylmethcathinone], MDPV [methylenedioxypyrovalerone], etc.) sold as "Bath Salts," GHB (gamma-hydroxybutyric acid), and flunitrazepam (brand names Rohypnol® or Narcozep®).
- Club drugs often contain other active compounds and/or are coingested with other drugs (including other club drugs) or ethanol.
- MDMA and Bath Salts are DEA Schedule I controlled substances.
- GHB is a DEA Schedule I controlled substance, but GHB approved in the salt form (sodium oxybate) is available for medical use and is a DEA Schedule III controlled substance.
- Flunitrazepam is a DEA Schedule IV controlled substance.
- Animal cases generally include accidental exposure, but can also be due to intentional sharing of drugs or malicious poisoning.

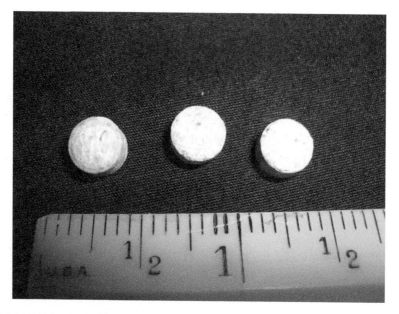

■ Figure 36.1 MDMA (ecstasy) tablets. Source: Courtesy of Ahna G. Brutlag.

*Blackwell's Five-Minute Veterinary Consult Clinical Companion: Small Animal Toxicology*, Third Edition.
Edited by Lynn R. Hovda, Ahna G. Brutlag, Robert H. Poppenga, and Steven E. Epstein.
© 2024 John Wiley & Sons, Inc. Published 2024 by John Wiley & Sons, Inc.

# ETIOLOGY/PATHOPHYSIOLOGY

- The incidence of club drug toxicosis is unknown and probably underreported due to the clandestine nature of the chemicals.
- Club or party drugs are most commonly used by young adults at all-night dance parties (raves or trances), dance clubs, and bars to increase energy, enhance mood, decrease inhibition, increase libido, and increase euphoria, but they can also be used maliciously for sedation, disorientation, and anterograde amnesia.

## Mechanism of Action

- MDMA.
  - Sympathomimetic effect.
  - Increases the release of serotonin, dopamine, and norepinephrine.
  - Blocks reuptake of serotonin.
  - Inhibits monoamine oxidase (MAO).
- Bath Salts (wide variety of synthetic cathinones) – sympathomimetic effect.
  - Increase the release of neurotransmitters – primary type of neurotransmitter varies by compound.
  - Inhibit monoamine uptake transporters.
- GHB.
  - Precursor and metabolite of the neurotransmitter GABA and, as it is naturally found in the body, acts on its own receptors.
  - May have ability to release GABA, glutamate, and dopamine.
- Flunitrazepam (benzodiazepine drug).
  - Binds to GABA receptors to affect chloride ion channels and decrease neuronal transmission.
  - May act on GABA-mediated regulation of release of monoamine neurotransmitters.

## Pharmacokinetics

- All drugs.
  - Readily and rapidly absorbed from GI tract and via insufflation.
  - Clinical signs noted within 30–45 minutes.
- MDMA.
  - Crosses blood–brain barrier.
  - Metabolized by the liver.
  - Excreted by the kidneys.
  - Duration of clinical signs 6–8 hours.
- Bath Salts.
  - Metabolism varies by compound.
  - Excreted in the urine.
  - Duration of clinical signs is usually a few hours, but can linger for days.
- GHB.
  - Highly lipophilic.
  - Distributed across blood–brain barrier and through body.
  - Rapidly metabolized and excreted as carbon dioxide through respiratory system.
  - Resolution of clinical signs is generally within seven hours.
- Flunitrazepam.
  - Widely distributed due to lipophilicity.
  - Metabolized by the liver into two active compounds.

- Excreted by the kidneys.
- Clinical signs may last 8–12 hours.

## Toxicity

- MDMA.
  - 3 mg/kg results in hyperactivity and mydriasis.
  - 9 mg/kg results in hypersalivation and circling behavior.
  - 15 mg/kg results in clinical signs and death.
- Bath Salts – difficult to measure as most contain multiple and varying compounds.
- GHB – doses exceeding 50 mg/kg have been associated with death.
- Flunitrazepam – extent of toxicosis is a direct continuation of side-effects.

## Systems Affected

- Cardiovascular.
- Hepatobiliary.
- Nervous.
- Neuromuscular.
- Renal/urological.
- Respiratory.

 **SIGNALMENT/HISTORY**

### Risk Factors

- No species/breed/sex predilections exist, but dogs may be more affected due to indiscriminate eating.
- Environmental risk factors include:
  - Animals in household with access to club drugs.
  - Police dogs or other drug-sniffing dogs.

### Historical Findings

- Clients often reluctant to give illegal drug exposure history.
- Access to drugs:
  - Personal use, possibly young people in home.
  - Guest or party in home.
  - Drug-sniffing working dog.

### Location and Circumstances of Poisoning

- Cases occur anywhere these drugs are available.

 **CLINICAL FEATURES**

- MDMA and Bath Salts.
  - CNS – hyperactivity, agitation, euphoria, confusion, hallucinations, tremors, seizures, serotonin syndrome (MDMA).
  - Cardiovascular – tachycardia, other cardiac arrhythmias.
  - Respiratory – tachypnea.
  - Ophthalmic – mydriasis.
  - Gastrointestinal – vomiting, hypersalivation.

- Other – hyperthermia.
- Kidney failure has been reported secondary to hyperthermia and rhabdomyolysis.
- Liver failure has been reported due to MDMA exposure.
- Death.
- GHB and flunitrazepam.
  - CNS – sedation, lethargy, confusion, loss of consciousness/coma, memory inhibition, tremors (GHB), seizures (GHB).
  - Neuromuscular – hypotonia, muscle relaxation.
  - Cardiovascular – bradycardia, other changes in heart rate may be noted.
  - Respiratory – respiratory depression.
  - Other – hypothermia.

# DIFFERENTIAL DIAGNOSIS

- MDMA and Bath Salts.
  - Other stimulant drugs.
    - Amphetamines and methamphetamines.
    - Diet pills and muscle/body building supplements.
    - Decongestants.
    - Other illicit drugs – cocaine.
  - Other toxic causes of neurologic and cardiovascular stimulation (including tremors/seizures).
    - Methylxanthines including caffeine and theobromine.
    - Tremorgenic mycotoxins (Penitrem A).
    - Rodenticides (strychnine, bromethalin, zinc phosphate).
    - Insecticides (metaldehyde, pyrethroids).
- GHB and flunitrazepam.
  - Other CNS depressant drugs.
    - Other benzodiazepines.
    - Baclofen.
    - Barbiturates.
    - Opioids.
  - Other toxic causes of neurologic depression.
    - Marijuana/cannabis.
    - Ethanol.
  - Other disease processes that can result in CNS changes.
    - Thrombogenic event.
    - Neoplasia.
    - Meningitis or meningoencephalitis.
    - Hepatoencephalopathy.

# DIAGNOSTICS

## Clinical Pathology Findings

- Chemistry.
  - MDMA – hyponatremia, hepatic failure.
  - Bath Salts – hyponatremia, elevated creatinine kinase, electrolyte abnormalities, renal failure.

### Other Diagnostics

- ECG.
  - Monitor for cardiac arrhythmias.
- Diagnostic for drug detection.
  - GHB is metabolized too quickly to be detected by testing and is naturally present in the body.
  - Urine may be sent to a human hospital for toxicological screen to detect MDMA and, in some cases, flunitrazepam and Bath Salts.
  - Over-the-counter urine multidrug test kits can be used; however, interpretation should be combined with clinical suspicion.
    - Tests are not designed for veterinary species although the Quick Screen Pro Multi Drug Screening Test has been validated by GC/MS for use in animals for benzodiazepines and amphetamines/methamphetamines.
    - Despite validation, false positives due to cross-reactivity can make testing challenging.
    - Club drugs are often adulterated by other compounds.

### Pathological Findings (MDMA)

- Gross findings include icterus; petechial and ecchymotic hemorrhage; dark, tarry material in the stomach (postmortem); and liver damage (postmortem).
- Histopathological findings include hepatic necrosis and evidence of generalized hemorrhagic disease.

 **THERAPEUTICS**

### Detoxification

- Often not recommended/contraindicated due to delay in presentation and presence of clinical signs.
- None for inhalation/insufflation.
- Asymptomatic patient with recent (<30 minutes) and large ingestion.
  - Induce emesis.
  - Administer single dose of activated charcoal with cathartic.
- Sedated and intubated patient (cuffed endotracheal tube) with recent and large ingestion.
  - Gastric lavage.
  - Administer single dose of activated charcoal with cathartic.

### Appropriate Health Care

- Symptomatic and supportive care.
- IV crystalloids as needed to maintain blood pressure.
- Antiemetic to prevent aspiration.
  - Maropitant 1 mg/kg SQ, IV q 24 hours.
  - Ondansetron 0.5–1 mg/kg IV q 12 hours for dogs; 0.1–1 mg/kg IV, SC, IM q 6–12 hours for cats.
- Maintain good temperature.
  - Hyperthermia (MDMA and Bath Salts) – provide active cooling if needed; stop at 103–103.5 °F.
  - Hypothermia (GHB, flunitrazepam) – provide active warming if needed.
- Maintain adequate airway – monitor respiration and $SpO_2$.
  - Intubate and ventilate if needed (GHB and flunitrazepam).

- Monitor mentation.
  - Avoid additional CNS stimulation (MDMA and Bath Salts) – keep patient in dark, quiet area.
  - Observe for signs of excess CNS depression.
- ECG monitoring for cardiac effects.

### Antidotes

- Flunitrazepam – flumazenil, a benzodiazepine antagonist.
- MDMA, GHB, and Bath Salts – none available.

### Drug(s) of Choice

#### MDMA/Bath Salts

- CNS excitation and tachycardia.
  - Acepromazine 0.05–0.1 mg/kg IV, IM, or SQ, repeat as needed.
  - Chlorpromazine 0.5–1 mg/kg IV or IM, repeat as needed.
- Serotonin syndrome – cyproheptadine 1.1 mg/kg PO or rectally (as slurry) every 4–6 hours as needed.
- Muscle tremors – methocarbamol 55–220 mg/kg, repeat as needed.
- Seizures.
  - Phenobarbital – 12–20 mg/kg IV once OR 2 mg/kg IV every 20–30 minutes to effect with maximum 24-hour dose of 24 mg/kg.
  - Levetiracetam – 30–60 mg/kg IV (dog) or 20 mg/kg IV (cat) slow bolus over 5–15 minutes.
  - Propofol – 6 mg/kg IV bolus followed by 0.1–0.6 mg/kg/min CRI.

#### GHB

- Seizures.
  - Diazepam – 0.5–2 mg/kg IV or midazolam 0.5–1 mg/kg IV.
  - Phenobarbital – 12–20 mg/kg IV once OR 2 mg/kg IV every 20–30 minutes to effect with maximum 24-hour dose of 24 mg/kg.
  - Levetiracetam – 30–60 mg/kg IV (dog) or 20 mg/kg IV (cat) slow bolus over 5–15 minutes.

#### Flunitrazepam

- Flumazenil – 0.01 mg/kg IV, repeat as needed (half-life approximately one hour).

### Precautions/Interactions

- Benzodiazepines (diazepam/midazolam) should be avoided with MDMA and Bath Salts exposure as paradoxical exacerbation of CNS stimulation may occur.
- Additional benzodiazepines (diazepam/midazolam) should not be administered with flunitrazepam as can worse clinical signs.

  **COMMENTS**

### Prevention/Avoidance

- Prevent exposure to illegal drugs in the home.
  - Safe storage of drugs.
  - Removal of pet (crate/room) during parties.
- Proper training and muzzling of drug-sniffing dogs.

## Possible Complications

- Contaminants or deliberate adulterants in the drug mixture.
- Unknown additional drugs ingested in addition to known drug.

## Expected Course and Prognosis

- Depends on quantity and mixture of drugs as well as time of presentation.
- At lower doses, chance of complete recovery is good.

## Synonyms

- MDMA – ecstasy, adam, bibs, blue kisses, blue niles, eve, scooby snacks, X, XTC, others.
- Bath Salts – blue silk, cloud 9, ivory wave, legal high, moon dust, white lightening, others.
- GHB – liquid ecstasy, G, liquid X, salty water, scoop, soap, others.
- Flunitrazepam – circles, forget me pills, R2, roofies, rophies, rope, wolfies, others.

## See Also

Chapter 37 Cocaine
Chapter 40 Methamphetamine
Chapter 42 Opiates and Opioids (Illicit)
Chapter 43 Phencyclidine (PCP)

## Abbreviations

See Appendix 1 for a complete list.
- GHB = gamma-hydroxybutyric acid
- MDMA = methylenedioxymethamphetamine
- MDPV = methylenedioxypyrovalerone

## Suggested Reading

Bischoff K. Toxicity of drugs of abuse. In: Gupta RC (ed.) *Veterinary Toxicology: Basic and Clinical Principles*, 3rd edn. New York: Elsevier, 2018; pp. 385–406.

Felmlee MA, Morse BL, Morris MA. Gamma-hydroxybutyric acid: pharmacokinetics pharmacodynamics, and toxicology. *J Am Assoc Pharm Sci* 2020;23(1):22.

Karch SB. A historical review of MDMA. *Open Forensic Sci J* 2011;4:20–24.

Prosser JM, Nelson LS. The toxicology of bath salts: a review of synthetic cathinones. *J Med Toxicol* 2012;8:33–42.

Ross EA, Watson M, Goldberger B. "Bath salts" intoxication. *N Engl J Med* 2011;365:967–968.

**Acknowledgment**: The authors and editors acknowledge the prior contributions of Christy A. Klatt, who authored this topic in the previous edition.

**Author**: Dijana Katan, DVM, MPH, DABT
**Consulting Editor**: Lynn R. Hovda, RPh, DVM, MS, DACVIM

# Chapter 37

# Cocaine

## DEFINITION/OVERVIEW

- Cocaine is the natural alkaloid obtained from leaves of the coca plant (shrub), *Erythroxylum coca* and *Erythroxylum monogynum*.
- Cocaine is a Schedule II drug used for topical anesthesia and vasoconstriction of mucous membranes.
- Although it has a medical use, it is one of the most commonly abused drugs in the world.
- Reported by an animal poison control center to be in the top five illicit substance exposures.
- Often sold as a solid white powdered salt, cocaine hydrochloride, varying in purity from 12% to >60% (Figure 37.1).
- Cocaine hydrochloride can be converted to the free alkaloid of cocaine and precipitated into "rocks" of crack to be smoked (Figure 37.2).
- Most street cocaine is diluted or "cut" with inert ingredients such as lactose, inositol, mannitol, corn starch, or sucrose, but can be cut with other active compounds such as other local anesthetics, caffeine, amphetamine, fentanyl, levamisole, strychnine, and xylazine.

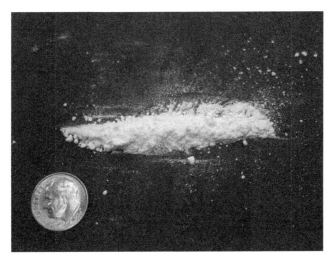

■ Figure 37.1 Cocaine powder. Source: Courtesy of Ahna G. Brutlag.

*Blackwell's Five-Minute Veterinary Consult Clinical Companion: Small Animal Toxicology*, Third Edition. Edited by Lynn R. Hovda, Ahna G. Brutlag, Robert H. Poppenga, and Steven E. Epstein. © 2024 John Wiley & Sons, Inc. Published 2024 by John Wiley & Sons, Inc.

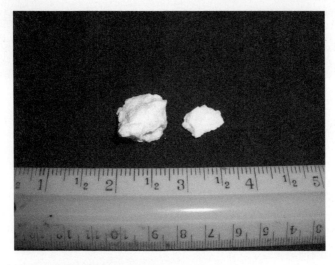

■ **Figure 37.2** Crack cocaine. Source: Courtesy of Ahna G. Brutlag.

 # ETIOLOGY/PATHOPHYSIOLOGY

- *E. coca* and *E. monogynum* originate from the Andes Mountains and grow naturally in Mexico, South and Central America, as well as the West Indies.
- 90% of cocaine in the US is brought in illegally from Colombia, the majority coming through Mexico.

## Mechanism of Action

- Strong sympathomimetic effect.
  - Increases release of catecholamines.
  - Blocks reuptake of norepinephrine, serotonin, and dopamine.
  - CNS stimulation, tachycardia, hypertension, and vasoconstriction result.
- Given IV, can have direct effect on myocardium.
  - Blocks sodium ion channels.
  - Increases calcium concentration within cardiac myocytes.
  - Can lead to thrombogenic effects.
- Norepinephrine-mediated hypothalamic effect – regulates appetite, sleep and body temperature.

## Pharmacokinetics

- Highly lipophilic and readily absorbed from all mucosal surfaces.
- Peak plasma concentrations 15 minutes to two hours after exposure.
- Readily crosses the blood–brain barrier.
- Hydrolyzed by plasma and hepatic esterases to water-soluble metabolites.
- Urinary excretion.
  - 10-20% excreted unchanged.
  - Remainder of excretion is of metabolites.

## Toxicity

- Dog.
  - IV $LD_{50}$ – 3 mg/kg.
  - Estimated PO $LD_{50}$ – 6–12 mg/kg.
  - Lowest LD – 3.5 mg/kg SQ.

■ Cat.
  • Lowest LD – 7.5 mg/kg IV.
  • Lowest LD – 16 mg/kg SQ.

## Systems Affected

■ Nervous.
■ Cardiovascular.
■ Ophthalmic.

 # SIGNALMENT/HISTORY

### Risk Factors

■ No species/ breed/sex predilections exist.
■ Environmental risk factors include:
  • animals in household with access to cocaine or crack.
  • police dogs or other drug-sniffing dogs may be predisposed.
  • performance competitions – ex. racing track.

### Historical Findings

■ Clients often reluctant to give illegal drug exposure history.
■ Access to drugs.
  • Personal use.
  • Guest or party in home.
  • Drug-sniffing working dog.

### Location and Circumstances of Poisoning

■ Cases occur anywhere cocaine and crack are available.

 # CLINICAL FEATURES

■ Central nervous system.
  • Stimulation most common – hyperactivity, hyperesthesia, tremors, seizures.
  • Can also see – obtunded/altered mentation, vocalization, weakness, ataxia.
■ Cardiovascular.
  • Tachycardia, hypertension.
■ Ophthalmic.
  • Mydriasis, anisocoria, nystagmus, blindness.
■ Gastrointestinal.
  • Vomiting, hypersalivation.
■ Other.
  • Hyperthermia.

 # DIFFERENTIAL DIAGNOSIS

■ Other stimulant drugs.
  • Amphetamines and methamphetamines.
  • Antidepressants (SSRIs, TCAs, etc.).
  • Diet pills and muscle/body building supplements.
  • Decongestants (ephedrine, pseudoephedrine, etc.).
  • Other illicit drugs – MDMA, synthetic cathinones (Bath Salts), etc.

- Other toxic causes of neurologic and cardiovascular stimulation (including tremors/seizures).
  - Methylxanthines including caffeine and theobromine.
  - Tremorgenic mycotoxins (Penitrem A).
  - Rodenticides (strychnine, bromethalin, zinc phosphate).
  - Insecticides (metaldehyde, pyrethroids).
- Other disease process that can result in tremors/seizures.
  - Thrombogenic event.
  - Neoplasia.
  - Meningitis or meningoencephalitis.
  - Hepatoencephalopathy.

 **DIAGNOSTICS**

### Clinical Pathological Findings

- Chemistry and venous blood gas.
  - Hyperglycemia, increased serum lactate or lactic acidosis, hypernatremia.
  - Less commonly: respiratory alkalosis, hyponatremia, hypochloremia.

### Other Diagnostic Findings

- ECG.
  - Sinus tachycardia.
  - Rarely increased duration of QRS complexes and P-wave abnormalities.
- Diagnostic for cocaine.
  - Over-the-counter urine multidrug test kits can be used; however, interpretation should be combined with clinical suspicion because:
    - tests are not designed for veterinary species.
    - suspected to be accurate for cocaine, but no studies available to confirm.
    - cocaine is often adulterated by other compounds.
  - Urine, plasma, or stomach contents for laboratory confirmation.
    - Thin-layer chromatography.
    - Gas chromatography/mass spectrometry.

### Pathological Findings

- Subendocardial and epicardial hemorrhage.
- Myocardial degeneration.
- Pericardial effusion.
- Pulmonary hemorrhage.

 **THERAPEUTICS**

### Detoxification

- Often not recommended/contraindicated due to delay in presentation and presence of clinical signs.
- None for inhalation/insufflation.
- Asymptomatic patient with recent and large ingestion.
  - Induce emesis.
  - Administer single dose of activated charcoal with cathartic.

- Sedated and intubated patient (cuffed endotracheal tube) with recent and large ingestion.
  - Gastric lavage.
  - Administer single dose of activated charcoal with cathartic.
- In rare case where bagged cocaine is ingested – careful endoscopic or surgical retrieval.

## Appropriate Health Care

- IV crystalloids to maintain blood volume, pH, and electrolyte balance.
- Maintain good temperature – prevent and control hyperthermia.
- Maintain adequate airway – monitor respirations and $SpO_2$.
- Avoid additional CNS stimulation – keep patient in dark, quiet area.
- ECG monitoring for cardiac effects.

## Antidote

- No specific antidote available.

## Drug(s) of Choice

- Antiemetic to prevent aspiration.
  - Maropitant 1 mg/kg SQ, IV q 24 hours.
  - Ondansetron 0.5–1 mg/kg IV q 12 hours for dogs; 0.1–1 mg/kg IV, SC, IM q 6–12 hours for cats.
- Phenothiazine sedatives to control CNS excitation and tachycardia.
  - Acepromazine 0.05–0.1 mg/kg IV, IM, or SQ, repeat as needed.
  - Chlorpromazine 0.5–1 mg/kg IV or IM, repeat as needed.
- Treatment of muscle tremors.
  - Methocarbamol 55–220 mg/kg, repeat as needed.
- Treatment of seizures.
  - Diazepam 0.5–2 mg/kg IV or midazolam 0.5–1 mg/kg IV.
  - Phenobarbital 12–20 mg/kg IV once OR 2 mg/kg IV every 20–30 minutes to effect with maximum 24-hour dose of 24 mg/kg.
  - Levetiracetam 30–60 mg/kg IV (dog) or 20 mg/kg IV (cat) slow bolus over 5–15 minutes.
  - Propofol 6 mg/kg IV bolus followed by 0.1–0.6 mg/kg/min CRI.
- Control life-threatening cardiac tachycardia.
  - Propranolol 0.02 mg/kg IV slowly, repeat as needed with a maximum dose of 1 mg/kg q 8 hours.
  - Esmolol CRI 25–100 mcg/kg/minute.
- Intralipid emulsion can be considered.
  - Initial 1.5 mL/kg IV bolus of 20% lipid solution over 5–15 minutes, followed by a 0.25 mL/kg/min for 30–60 minutes.
  - Can repeat 1.5 mL/kg bolus every 4–6 hours for a maximum of 3–5 doses.

## Surgical Considerations

- Cautious surgical or endoscopic removal if whole bag(s) of cocaine are ingested.
- Avoid rupture of bag(s).

## Patient Monitoring

- Treatment is considered effective when:
  - heart rate is maintained within normal range for the species.
  - respiratory rate is maintained within normal range for the species.
  - temperature is maintained within normal range for the species.

- Patient can be discharged once normal mentation is achieved and the above physical parameters remain normal without treatment.

 **COMMENTS**

### Prevention/Avoidance

- Prevent exposure to illegal drugs in the home.
  - Safe storage of drugs.
  - Removal of pet (crate/room) during parties.
- Proper training and muzzling of drug-sniffing dogs.

### Possible Complications

- Cardiac arrest due to cardiac vasospasm.
- Hyperthermia due to muscle activity (tremors/seizures) and vasoconstriction.

### Expected Course and Prognosis

- Hospitalization 10–30 hours.
- Good prognosis with treatment.
- Ongoing neurological or cardiovascular signs have been reported.

### Synonyms

- Cocaine – coke, bernies, snow, dust, blow, nose candy, toot, white lady, star dust, others.
- Crack cocaine – beamers, rock, crank, flake, ice.

### See Also

Chapter 15 Amphetamines
Chapter 40 Methamphetamine
Chapter 36 Club Drugs (MDMA, GHB, Flunitrazepam, Bath Salts)

### Abbreviations

See Appendix 1 for complete list.

### Suggested Reading

Bischoff K. Toxicity of drugs of abuse. In: Gupta RC (ed.) *Veterinary Toxicology: Basic and Clinical Principles*, 3rd edn. New York: Elsevier, 2018; pp. 385–408.

Llera RM, Volmer PA. Toxicologic hazards for police dogs involved in drug detection. *J Am Vet Med Assoc* 2006;228:1028–1031.

Royle K, Bandt C. Intravenous lipid emulsion to treat suspected cocaine toxicosis in a dog. *Can Vet J* 2020;61:49–52.

Swirski AL, Pearl DL, Berke O et al. Companion animal exposures to potentially poisonous substances reported to a national poison control center in the United States in 2005 through 2014. *J Am Vet Med Assoc* 2020;257:517–530.

Thomas EK, Drobatz KJ, Mandell CK. Presumptive cocaine toxicosis in 19 dogs: 2004–2012. *J Vet Emerg Crit Care* 2014;24:201–207.

### Acknowledgment

The authors and editors acknowledge the prior contributions of Karyn Bischoff and Hwan Goo Kang, who authored this topic in the previous edition.

**Author**: Dijana Katan, DVM, MPH, DABT
**Consulting Editor**: Lynn R. Hovda, RPh, DVM, MS, DACVIM

# Chapter 38

# Lysergic Acid Diethylamide (LSD)

## DEFINITION/OVERVIEW

- Lysergic acid diethylamide (LSD) was first synthesized from ergot in 1938.
- Similar compounds are present in other plants.
  - Morning glory seeds (*Ipomea violacia*).
  - Pink morning glory (*Ipomea carnea*).
  - Sleepygrass (*Stipa robusta*).
  - Hawaiian baby wood rose (*Agyreia nervosa*).

## ETIOLOGY/PATHOPHYSIOLOGY

- LSD is used as a recreational drug.
  - Banned by FDA in 1966; currently DEA Schedule I drug.
  - Decline in illegal use over last 20 years.
- LSD is dissolved in water and applied to paper, sugar cubes, gelatin cubes, or other substances for ingestion.
  - Final product in circulation today contains 0.04–0.06 mg per dose.
  - Older products (1960s) contained up to 0.25 mg LSD per sugar cube or dose.
- Difficult to predict effects on individuals.
  - Altered sensory perceptions (visual, auditory) in humans.
  - May cause euphoria or panic.

### Mechanism of Action

- Structurally similar to serotonin (5-HT).
- Agonist at $5\text{-HT}_{1A}$, $5\text{-HT}_{2A}$, and $5\text{HT}_{2C}$ serotonin receptors, D2 dopamine receptors, and alpha-2-adrenergic receptors.
- Mild agonist to alpha-1, D1, and D3 receptors.
- Increases glutamate release in the cerebral cortex.

### Pharmacokinetics

- Data from human subjects are available.
- Rapid gastrointestinal absorption.
- Peak plasma concentrations within six hours.
- Highly protein bound.
- Hepatic hydroxylation and glucuronide conjugation.
- Predominantly fecal elimination, biliary elimination in cats.

*Blackwell's Five-Minute Veterinary Consult Clinical Companion: Small Animal Toxicology*, Third Edition.
Edited by Lynn R. Hovda, Ahna G. Brutlag, Robert H. Poppenga, and Steven E. Epstein.
© 2024 John Wiley & Sons, Inc. Published 2024 by John Wiley & Sons, Inc.

- Elimination half-life 2–5 hours.
- Clinical signs often last a few hours but may persist for up to 12 hours.

## Toxicity

- Effective dose in humans – 0.05–0.20 mg.
- Toxic dose in humans – 0.70–2.80 mg/kg BW.
- Clinical signs seen in cats dosed with IP LSD.
  - 0.0025 mg/kg BW – mild signs
  - 0.0500 mg/kg BW – marked signs.
- Rat IV $LD_{50}$ – 16 mg/kg BW.

## Systems Affected

- Nervous – ranges from excitation to complete disorientation.
- Cardiovascular – tachycardia from stimulation of autonomic nervous system.
- Endocrine/metabolic – malignant hyperthermia reported in humans.
- Ophthalmic – mydriasis.

 **SIGNALMENT/HISTORY**

- Young animals, particularly puppies, predisposed to ingesting foreign material.

## Risk Factors

- Police dogs used to detect drugs may be more susceptible.

## Historical Findings

- Access to drugs.
  - Teenagers in the home.
  - Guests or party in the home.
- Owner may be reluctant to provide a complete history.
- May be combined with other drugs.

## Location and Circumstances of Poisoning

- Animals residing in neighborhoods with known drug use.

 **CLINICAL FEATURES**

- Disorientation.
- Mydriasis.
- Vocalization.
- Excitation or sedation.
- Tachycardia.
- Signs reported in cats.
  - Hallucinatory behavior – tracking and pouncing on unseen objects.
  - Compulsive scratching in litter.
  - Bizarre sitting and standing postures.
  - Increased grooming, which may be incomplete.
  - Increased play behavior (chasing tails, pawing, biting, sniffing).
  - Vomiting.

# DIFFERENTIAL DIAGNOSIS

- Other hallucinogenic or dissociative drugs.
  - Ketamine.
  - MDMA.
  - Mescaline.
  - PCP.
  - *Psilocybe* spp. mushrooms.
  - Salvia (*S. divinorum*).
  - Ayahuasca.

# DIAGNOSTICS

## Clinical Pathological Findings

- No specific serum chemistry abnormalities.

## Other Diagnostics

- Laboratory analysis to confirm exposure. Results will take several days to be returned and cannot be used to guide therapy.
  - Immunoassays.
  - HPLC.
  - LC/MC.
  - TLC.
- Over-the-counter urine test kits may not be effective due to fecal elimination.
- Causes of false positives include amitriptyline, chlorpromazine, diltiazem, doxepin, fentanyl, fluoxetine, metoclopramide, trazodone, bupropion, buspirone, risperidone, sertraline, verapamil, methylphenidate.

## Pathological Findings

- No specific lesion. LSD is not reported as a direct cause of death.

# THERAPEUTICS

- Treatment is generally limited to symptomatic and supportive care with close observation until clinical signs have resolved. Up to 12 hours may be required after a large ingestion.

## Detoxification

- Gastrointestinal detoxification is not useful due to rapid absorption and onset of clinical signs.

## Appropriate Health Care

- Minimize sensory stimulation.
  - Keep in a darkened, quiet area.
  - Avoid excessive restraint.
- Monitor and symptomatic care for tachycardia and hyperthermia.
- Most animals will recover within 12 hours if kept in a dark, quiet room.

## Antidote

- No specific antidote available.

## Drug(s) of Choice

- IV fluids as needed to stabilize cardiovascular system.
- Diazepam 0.25–0.5 mg/kg IV for anxiety, seizures in cats and dogs.
- Midazolam 0.1 to 0.3 mg/kg in dogs.
- Haloperidol has been used successfully in humans.

## Precautions/Interactions

- Selective serotonin reuptake inhibitors can aggravate CNS effects and should be avoided.

## Patient Monitoring

- Monitor heart rate and body temperature regularly over 12 hours post exposure.
- Minimize sensory stimulation for 12 hours.

 **COMMENTS**

## Prevention/Avoidance

- Avoid access to illegal drugs.
- Keep animals away from parties and other possible sources.
- Police dogs wear a muzzle to prevent ingestion of contraband.
- Monitor teenagers who might intentionally expose companion animals to drugs.

## Possible Complications

- Tachycardia reported in humans.
- Hyperthermia reported in humans. Associated with restraint.
- Injury of animal or caretaker possible because of behavioral changes.

## Expected Course and Prognosis

- Deaths have not been directly attributed directly to LSD abuse.
- Fatal accidents are possible due to behavioral changes.

## Synonyms

Acid, blotter, dots, purple haze, sugar cubes, window pane.

## See Also

Chapter 36 Club Drugs (MDMA, GHB, Flunitrazepam, Bath Salts)
Chapter 41 Miscellaneous Hallucinogens and Dissociative Agents

## Abbreviations

See Appendix 1 for a complete list.

## Suggested Reading

ASPCApro. Urine Drug Screens for Pets: What You Need to Know. www.aspcapro.org/resource/urine-drug-screens-pets-what-you-need-know

Fantegrossi WE, Murnane KS, Reissig CJ. The behavioral pharmacology of hallucinogens. *Biochem Pharmacol* 2008;75:17–33.

Jacobs BL, Trulson ME, Stern WC. Behavioral effects of LSD in the cat: proposal of an animal behavior model for studying the actions of hallucinogenic drugs. *Brain Res* 1977;132:301–314.

Oster E, Čudina N, Pavasović H et al. Intoxication of dogs and cats with common stimulating, hallucinogenic, and dissociative recreational drugs. *Vet Anim Sci* 2023;19:100288.

Volmer PA. Recreational drugs. In: Peterson ME, Talcott PA (eds) *Small Animal Toxicology*, 3rd edn. St Louis: Elsevier, 2013; pp. 309–334.

**Author:** Karyn Bischoff, DVM, MS, DABVT, MPH
**Consulting Editor:** Lynn R. Hovda, RPh, DVM, MS, DACVIM

# Chapter 39

# Marijuana (THC)

## DEFINITION/OVERVIEW

- THC – the use of phytocannabinoids has increased greatly worldwide. The recent evolution in the legal status, decriminalization, and medicinal use of psychoactive cannabinoids, notably Δ9-tetrahydrocannabinol (THC) and its isomers Δ10-THC and Δ8-THC, has strongly influenced an increase in animal exposures.
  - Other forms of THC include tetrahydrocannabinolic acid (THCA) and tetrahydrocannabivarin (THCV), which are nonintoxicating.
  - Conversely, recently discovered Δ-9-tetrahydrocannabutol (THCB) and tetrahydrocannabiphorol (THCP) are of significantly increased potency. These are not yet available through legal or illegal sources, but they may be of future importance.
- Definitions.
  - Marijuana – dried flower buds, leaves, and stems of the female *Cannabis sativa* and *C. indica* plant. THC concentrations may vary from 0.4% to 20%. The average 1 g joint contains 150 mg of THC.
  - Cannabis – the plant genus, historically used synonymously with marijuana. Shifts in legal status and federal scheduling have driven the updated and preferred terminology to hemp-derived Cannabis and marijuana-derived Cannabis.
  - Cannabinoids/phytocannabinoids – chemical compounds in *Cannabis* that may hold pharmacological benefit.
  - Hashish – resin collected from the surfaces of hair-like leaf structures. THC concentration is approximately 10%.
  - Sinsemilla – seedless female *Cannabis* plant tended to prevent pollination, imparting a higher THC concentration.
  - Hemp – *Cannabis* plant used for either industrial or medicinal purposes. THC concentration is 0.3% or less.
  - Concentrates.
    - Hash or hash oil: nonsolvent or water-based extracts containing 20–50% THC.
    - Dabs: solvent-based extracts containing up to 80–90% THC. These may include shatters, waxes, oils, budders, etc.
- Therapeutic benefits of *Cannabis* have been used since 2700–2600 BCE. Current FDA-approved THC-based medications or analogs, dronabinol and nabilone respectively, aid in managing inappetence and nausea in chemotherapy and AIDS patients. Sativex®, a 1:1 ratio of THC:CBD, is approved in many countries to manage spasticity due to multiple sclerosis, but it remains unapproved in the United States.
- Formulations include plant material (Figures 39.1, 39.2), edibles (baked goods, gummies, candy, butter, etc.), oils, tinctures, topicals, capsules, vaping liquids, hashish, and concentrates (Figures 39.3, 39.4).

*Blackwell's Five-Minute Veterinary Consult Clinical Companion: Small Animal Toxicology*, Third Edition.
Edited by Lynn R. Hovda, Ahna G. Brutlag, Robert H. Poppenga, and Steven E. Epstein.
© 2024 John Wiley & Sons, Inc. Published 2024 by John Wiley & Sons, Inc.

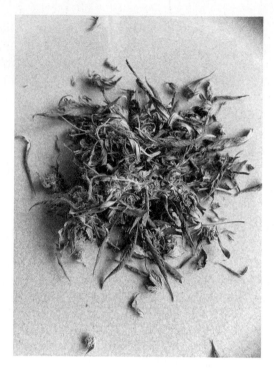

■ **Figure 39.1** Dried *Cannabis sativa* material used for recreational and fiber-dying purposes. Source: Courtesy of J. Berlin.

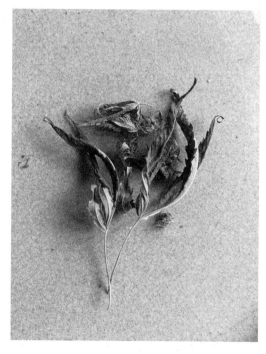

■ **Figure 39.2** *Cannabis sativa* plant material. Source: Courtesy of J. Berlin.

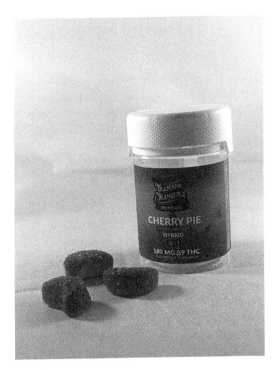

■ **Figure 39.3** Example of edible THC product. Source: Courtesy of Holly Hommerding (chapter contributor).

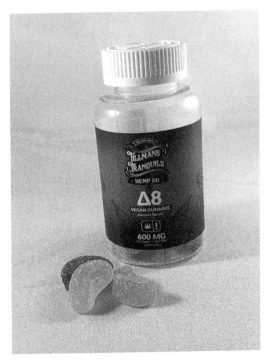

■ **Figure 39.4** Example of edible THC product. Source: Courtesy of Holly Hommerding (chapter contributor).

# ETIOLOGY/PATHOPHYSIOLOGY

## Mechanism of Action

- The endocannabinoid system (ECS) is integral to both embryonic development and physiologic maintenance in mature animals. Naturally occurring endocannabinoids interact with cannabinoid receptors (CB1 and CB2) in cell membranes to inhibit neurotransmitter release.
  - The ECS displays extensive cross-reactivity with other receptor systems, including opiate, NMDA, GABA, muscarinic acetylcholine, 5HT serotonin, dopamine, and MDR1 receptors.
- THC is an exogenous cannabinoid that is 4–20× more potent than endocannabinoids and has a longer duration of action.
  - CB1 receptors are responsible for intoxicating and psychotropic effect. Interactions in the CNS affect cognitive function, emotion, movement, hunger, and neuroprotection. Interactions in the peripheral sensory and autonomic nervous system affect the cardiovascular, gastrointestinal, respiratory, and pain perception status of the patient.
    - THC actions/agonism on CB1 receptors can inhibit the release of neurotransmitters including acetylcholine, dopamine, GABA, serotonin, histamine, glutamate, and noradrenaline.
  - CB2 receptors impart a non-intoxicating effect. Interactions in the peripheral nervous system, and to a lesser degree in the CNS, help to manage pain and inflammation.
- Interspecies differences in endocannabinoid receptor distribution and quantity may account for variability in sensitivity to THC and associated signs.
  - Dogs have a higher population of CB1 receptors in the cerebellum and medulla oblongata, which likely contributes to ataxia, cardiovascular, and respiratory effects.

## Pharmacokinetics/Toxicokinetics

- The lipophilic nature of THC results in biphasic absorption, rapid tissue distribution, and a short plasma but long biological half-life.
- Absorption.
  - Inhalation – rapid; onset of signs within minutes.
  - Ingestion – $T_{max}$ and onset of signs: 1–2 hours, up to four hours in fasted dogs.
  - Bioavailability – 6–20%.
- Distribution.
  - Rapid tissue distribution.
  - Protein bound – 90–95%.
- Metabolism.
  - Primary – hepatic by hydroxylation and oxidation via CYP450.
    - Extensive first-pass metabolism limits bioavailability.
  - Secondary – brain, intestines, lungs via alternate cytochrome pathways.
- Excretion.
  - 85% feces, 15% renal.
  - Half-life (biological) – 30 hours.
  - 80% is excreted within five days.
  - Undergoes enterohepatic recirculation.
  - Elimination time is nonlinear, highly variable, fastest from the liver and slowest from adipose tissue.

## Toxicity

- Toxic dose – mild signs at 0.3–0.5 mg/kg, moderate signs at 2 mg/kg. Variability in product consistency and lack of regulatory oversight make assessment difficult.

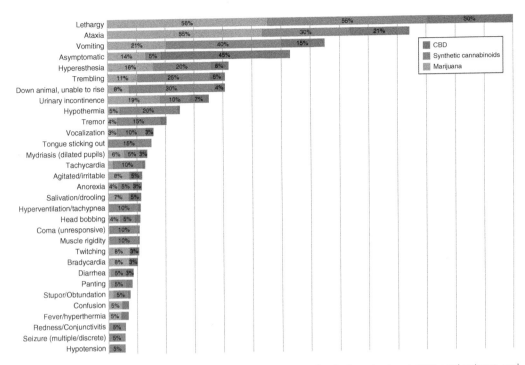

■ **Figure 39.5** A comparison of the incidence rate of clinical signs for THC-predominant, CBD-predominant, and synthetic cannabinoid products as reported to Pet Poison Helpline, January 2018–January 2023. Source: Courtesy of Holly Hommerding (chapter contributor).

- Lethal dose – >3–9 g/kg of THC-dominant plant material, >3 g/kg THC.
- $LD_{50}$ – not established in dogs or cats.

## Systems Affected (Figure 39.5)

- Nervous – CNS depression/lethargy, ataxia, hyperesthesia, agitation, trembling/twitching/tremor, vocalization, stupor/obtundation, confusion, rare seizures.
- Gastrointestinal – vomiting, hypersalivation, anorexia.
- Renal/urological – urinary incontinence.
- Ophthalmic – mydriasis.
- Cardiovascular – bradycardia, tachycardia, hypotension.
- Endocrine/metabolic – hypothermia, hyperthermia.
- Respiratory – rare respiratory depression.
- Musculoskeletal – muscle weakness.

## SIGNALMENT/HISTORY

### Risk Factors

- Indiscriminate eaters.
- Police or active-duty dogs.
- MDR1 mutation – ECS interacts with the MDR1 receptors and may impart some degree of sensitivity to phytocannabinoids in these patients. This interaction is taken into consideration with therapeutic use of CBD, but the clinical consequences of phytocannabinoid overdose in these patients have not yet been evaluated.

## Historical Findings

- Owners may be reluctant to admit exposure. Careful and compassionate questioning may aid in diagnosis.
- Due to the rapid onset, animal owners often report their pet to have neurological and gastro-intestinal signs.

## Location and Circumstances of Poisoning

- Use of recreational and medicinal marijuana and edible products is widespread, and cases occur throughout the country.

 **CLINICAL FEATURES**

- Gastrointestinal and neurological signs are common and include vomiting, salivation, lethargy, ataxia, and hyperesthesia.
- Other signs may include agitation, bradycardia, abnormal body temperature, urinary incontinence, mydriasis, tremors, and vocalization.
- Seizures and respiratory depression are rare.

 **DIFFERENTIAL DIAGNOSIS**

- Pharmaceuticals – depressants: opiates, benzodiazepines, tricyclic antidepressants, atypical antipsychotics, macrocyclic lactones.
- Pharmaceuticals – stimulants: amphetamines, methylphenidate, methylxanthines.
- Other drugs – LSD, PCP, opiates, psilocybin, synthetic cannabinoids.
- Alcohols.
- Xylitol.
- Bromethalin.

 **DIAGNOSTICS**

- Diagnosis relies on accurate history paired with clinical signs.

### Clinical Pathological Findings

- Exposure – specific changes are not expected.

### Other Diagnostics

- Point-of-care urine drug screens are indicated for use in humans but are rarely helpful in the diagnosis of THC exposure in animals. Interspecies metabolite variation often results in a false-negative test.
- Gas chromatography/mass spectrometry is effective in diagnosis, but its clinical application is limited at this time.

### Pathological Findings

- Exposure-specific changes are not expected.

 **THERAPEUTICS**

### Detoxification

- Inhalation – remove from the source.
- Emesis – asymptomatic patients only, best performed within one hour of ingestion.

- Activated charcoal – asymptomatic patients only: initial dose with sorbitol 1 g/kg. Consider follow-up doses without sorbitol q 8 hours for 1–2 doses.
- Gastric lavage – rarely indicated unless massive quantities consumed.
- Endoscopic removal – rarely indicated unless a bag of product is ingested, emesis is either contraindicated or unsuccessful, and/or patient is unlikely to pass the product.

### Appropriate Health Care

- Intravenous fluids – perfusion and hydration.
- Nursing care – vitals and blood pressure monitoring, eye lubricant, and rotating patients q 4 hours, thermoregulation.
- Low-stimulus environment.

### Alternative Therapy Plan (Inpatient Therapy Declined)

- Antiemetic.
- Subcutaneous fluids as needed for hydration in vomiting patients.
- Sedation with butorphanol or acepromazine if agitated.
- Animal owner to monitor patient mobility, body temperature, and heart rate q 4 hours if able, returning to clinic if signs progress.

### Drug(s) of Choice

- Antiemetics.
  - Maropitant 1 mg/kg SQ, IV q 24 hours.
  - Ondansetron 0.5–1 mg/kg IV q 12 hours for dogs; 0.1–1 mg/kg IV, SC, IM q 6–12 hours for cats.
- Sedation.
  - Butorphanol 0.2–0.4 mg/kg IV.
  - Diazepam 0.25–0.5 mg/kg IV.
  - Acepromazine 0.02–0.2 mg/kg IV (normotensive patients only).
- Tremor/seizure management.
  - Methocarbamol 55–220 mg/kg IV to effect.
  - Diazepam 0.25–0.5 mg/kg IV, levetiracetam 30 mg/kg q 8 hours IV, phenobarbital 4–8 mg/kg IV.
- Intravenous lipid emulsion (intralipids): may be considered in severely affected cases.
  - 1.5 mL/kg bolus followed by 0.25 mL/kg/min CRI × 30–60 minutes. Either repeat the 1.5 mL/kg bolus q 4–6 hours or start CRI of 0.5 mL/kg/h for up to one day. Monitor for lipemia, withholding intralipids if noted.

### Precautions/Interactions

- CBD – may be antagonistic or synergistic. Outcome may depend on the THC:CBD ratio and administration of the cannabinoids in temporal relation to one another.
- Opiates – synergistic, may require dose reduction.
- Benzodiazepines – concomitant interaction at GABA receptors may potentiate effects, may require dose reduction.
- Antiepileptic drugs – though cannabinoids and phenobarbital both metabolically utilize CYP450, recent CBD studies have indicated concomitant use does not affect the pharmacokinetic profile. Dose adjustments may not be necessary.
- Gabapentin – synergism can be therapeutically beneficial, but dose reduction may be required.
- Serotonin reuptake inhibitors (SSRIs) – concomitant interaction at 5-HT receptors may increase risk for serotonin syndrome.

- Coingestions.
  - A fatty meal will increase absorption of THC.
  - Baked goods or edibles may contain chocolate, raisins, macadamia nuts, or xylitol.
  - Marijuana butter may contain higher concentrations of THC; edibles made with marijuana butter can pose higher risk.
  - THC concentrates: may be contaminated with solvents, pesticides, and other chemicals.
  - Uncommonly, ingestion of human feces from individuals who use *Cannabis* recreationally or medicinally can lead to clinical signs.

## Extracorporeal Therapy

- Generally not indicated, but successful use of charcoal hemoperfusion and hemodialysis in series is reported.

## Surgical Considerations

- Monitoring of heart rate, blood pressure, and body temperature is indicated with concomitant anesthetic use.

## Patient Monitoring

- Vitals – bradycardia, less commonly tachycardia, hypothermia or hypothermia.
- Blood pressures – hypotension.

## Diet

- Gastrointestinal diet as needed.

 ## COMMENTS

### Prevention/Avoidance

- Prevent patient access to THC products.
- Police-duty dogs may benefit from a muzzle in high-risk environments.

### Possible Complications

- Rare aspiration pneumonia.

### Expected Course and Prognosis

- Prognosis – generally good.
- High morbidity, low mortality.
- Recovery time may be prolonged in large ingestions, concentrate exposures, or in dogs with excess adipose tissue.
- Full recovery – 1–3 days.

### Synonyms

Weed, pot, grass, ganja, Mary Jane, reefers, hemp, devil weed, hashish, dabs, shatter, budder, butter, wax, resin, hash oil, hash, edibles, delta8, delta10, delta9, and many others.

### See Also

Chapter 35 Cannabidiol
Chapter 44 Synthetic Cannabinoids

## Abbreviations

See Appendix 1 for a complete list.

- CYP = cytochrome
- ECS = endocannabinoid system
- NMDA = N-methyl-D-aspartate
- THC = tetrahydrocannabinol
- THCA = tetrahydrocannabinolic acid

## Suggested Reading

Brutlag A, Hommerding H. Toxicology of marijuana, synthetic cannabinoids, and cannabidiol in dogs and cats. *Vet Clin North Am Small Anim Pract* 2018;48(6):1087–1102.

Chicoine A, Illing K, Vuong S et al. Pharmacokinetic and safety evaluation of various oral doses of a novel 1: 20 THC: CBD cannabis herbal extract in dogs. *Front Vet Sci* 2020;7:583404.

Cital S, Kramer K, Hughston L et al. *Cannabis Therapy in Veterinary Medicine: A Complete Guide.* Cham: Springer International Publishing, 2021.

Culler CA, Vigani A. Successful treatment of a severe cannabinoid toxicity using extracorporeal therapy in a dog. *J Vet Emerg Crit Care* 2019;29(6):674–679.

Fitzgerald KT, Bronstein AC, Newquist KL. Marijuana poisoning. *Top Comp Anim Med* 2013;28(1):8–12.

**Acknowledgment:** The author and editors acknowledge the prior contributions of Christy A. Klatt, DVM, and Kelly Sioris, PharmD, CSPI, who authored this topic in the previous editions.

**Author:** Holly Hommerding, DVM, DABT, DABVT
**Consulting Editor:** Lynn R. Hovda, RPh, DVM, MS, DACVIM

# Chapter 40

# Methamphetamine

## DEFINITION/OVERVIEW

- Methamphetamine is a crystalline-like substance that was first synthesized around 1920.
- Routinely used medically in the 1930s and continues to be prescribed for a range of indications.
- Increasing popularity as an illicit substance and for recreational use.
- Methamphetamine is a DEA Schedule II stimulant under the Controlled Substances Act.
- Crystal methamphetamine (Figure 40.1) is the most potent form and is smoked (primarily) or injected for human use.
- Base can vary in appearance and is a damp or oily substance that is white, yellow, or brown in color. Base is injected or (less frequently) ingested by humans.
- Powdered methamphetamine is the least potent form and is adulterated with other substances. This is generally snorted, injected, or ingested by humans. Powdered methamphetamine may be pressed into pills.
- Severity of toxicity is related to the amount and type of exposure.
- Clinical signs are commonly related to cardiovascular and neurological involvement with secondary sequelae.

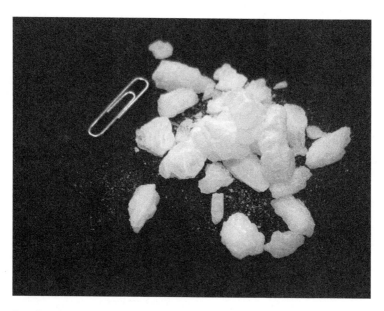

■ **Figure 40.1** Crystal methamphetamine. Source: Courtesy of Ahna G. Brutlag.

*Blackwell's Five-Minute Veterinary Consult Clinical Companion: Small Animal Toxicology*, Third Edition.
Edited by Lynn R. Hovda, Ahna G. Brutlag, Robert H. Poppenga, and Steven E. Epstein.
© 2024 John Wiley & Sons, Inc. Published 2024 by John Wiley & Sons, Inc.

# ETIOLOGY/PATHOPHYSIOLOGY

- Exposure may occur with ingestion (most frequently) or inhalation (less frequently).
- Methamphetamine use is widespread.
  - Cases may be underreported due to stigma and fear of legal repercussions.

## Mechanism of Action

- Results in neurotransmitter (catecholamine) release via binding to dopaminergic, noradrenergic, adrenergic, glutamatergic, and serotonergic receptors.
  - Membrane transporters may be altered.
  - Release of neurotransmitters may occur following interaction with the vesicle transporters or altered pH in the cytoplasm and vesicles.
  - Potential blocking of catecholamine reuptake.
- Monoamine oxidase inhibition.

## Pharmacokinetics

- Rapid absorption via the GI tract with an onset of signs within approximately 15–30 minutes following oral ingestion.
- Metabolism occurs in the liver and includes hydroxylation, N-dealkylation, and deamination.
  - Metabolites include amphetamine, which also is of clinical significance.
- Excretion of methamphetamine and amphetamine is primarily renal.

## Toxicity

- The $LD_{50}$ following ingestion of methamphetamine is 9–11 mg/kg.
- Adulterants are typically unknown and may pose additional toxicity concerns.

## Systems Affected

- Cardiovascular – hypertension, tachycardia, dysrhythmia, cardiac failure.
- Nervous – agitation, hyperthermia, lethargy, serotonin syndrome, coma.
- Neuromuscular – weakened, recumbency, seizures, tremors, uncontrollable movements, head bobbing, circling.
- Ophthalmic – mydriasis.
- Skin/exocrine – hyperthermia, erythema, petechiae.
- Gastrointestinal – diarrhea (+/- blood), vomiting, hypersalivation, abdominal discomfort, ileus.
- Respiratory – panting, tachypnea, respiratory failure.
- Hepatobiliary – hepatocellular trauma secondary to persistent hyperthermia or seizure activity.
- Hemic/lymphatic/immune – rhabdomyolysis, thrombocytopenia, disseminated intravascular coagulation (DIC).
- Renal/urological – myoglobinuria leading to acute kidney injury.

# SIGNALMENT/HISTORY

## Risk Factors

- Dogs are the most affected small animal due to their propensity for dietary indiscretion.
- Working dogs engaged in drug-sniffing training or work are at higher potential risk of exposure.
- Living in or visiting households or areas where methamphetamine production or use occurs.

### Historical Findings

- History of known or suspected exposure.
- Clinical signs noted by owners can include agitation, pacing, tremors, seizures, mydriasis; typically with a rapid onset of clinical signs.

### Location and Circumstances of Poisoning

- Cases may occur throughout the United States and worldwide following accidental (or, less commonly, intentional) exposure of pets to methamphetamine.

# CLINICAL FEATURES

- Signs may be noted within 30 minutes of exposure.
- Route, type, and amount of exposure as well as individual variation can impact progression of toxicity.
- Early signs may include agitation, tremors, seizures, mydriasis, tachycardia, hyperthermia.
- Depending on severity and persistence of signs such as seizures and hyperthermia, patients are at risk for secondary complications including DIC.
- Other clinical signs, as listed previously under Systems Affected, have been reported.
- Clinical signs may persist for days.

# DIFFERENTIAL DIAGNOSIS

- Toxicants.
  - Stimulants including amphetamine, methylphenidate, cocaine, ephedrine, pseudoephedrine, phenylephrine, methylxanthines, herbal stimulants (ephedra, ma huang), and other prescription or illicit drugs.
  - Pesticides – strychnine, metaldehyde.
  - Tremorgenic mycotoxins.
  - Cane toad (*Rhinella marinus*) intoxication.
  - Cyanobacteria.
- Nontoxicological causes including trauma and underlying neurological disease that can cause neurological signs.

# DIAGNOSTICS

### Clinical Pathological Findings

- CBC – hemoconcentration.
- Chemistry.
  - Elevated ALT, ALP.
  - Hypoglycemia.
- Prothrombin time (PT) elevated; activated partial thromboplastin time (aPTT) elevated.
- Blood gas –metabolic acidosis.

### Other Diagnostics

- Radiology/ultrasound: evidence of ileus such as distended small and large intestines.
- Urine drug immunoassay test based on history and clinical presentation.
- Analysis of urine, stomach contents, blood, liver, vitreous humor via LC/MS or GC/MS.

### Pathological Findings

- There are no pathognomonic changes identified.

- Changes may occur following significant clinical signs.
  - Congestion and hemorrhage present following persistent seizures, hyperthermia, and DIC.
  - Further signs depending on clinical progression.

 # THERAPEUTICS

- Treatment is focused on monitoring and providing supportive and symptomatic care.

## Detoxification

- Home induction of emesis is not recommended due to the rapid onset of neurological signs.
- Emesis or gastric lavage may be considered, as deemed safe, by the treating clinician, within 15 minutes of ingestion. Logistical time constraints typically do not allow this.
- Activated charcoal with a cathartic × 1 dose, as deemed safe by the treating clinician.
- Urine acidification to aid in methamphetamine elimination has been described in human methamphetamine intoxication but is not routinely performed in veterinary medicine.

## Appropriate Health Care

- Hospitalization for monitoring and supportive/symptomatic care.
- Monitor vitals, electrocardiogram, blood pressure, and neurological status.
  - Frequency of monitoring depends on clinical status.
- Minimize stimulation.
- Cooling measures for hyperthermia.

## Antidote

- No antidote is available.

## Drug(s) of Choice

- Note: Dosages are for dogs, unless otherwise specified.
- Fluid therapy.
  - Intravenous balanced crystalloid fluids as needed to maintain hydration, perfusion, and temperature. Adjust rate as needed. If myoglobinuria or other signs of rhabdomyolysis are present, aggressive intravenous fluid therapy is indicated.
- Agitation.
  - Phenothiazines (acepromazine 0.05–0.1 mg/kg IV, IM, or SQ).
  - Opioids (butorphanol 0.1–0.3 mg/kg IV or IM; can combine with acepromazine).
- Anticonvulsant agents.
  - Barbiturates (phenobarbital 4–8 mg/kg IV PRN).
  - Levetiracetam (30–60 mg/kg IV slow bolus over 5–15 minutes).
  - Benzodiazepines (diazepam 0.5–1 mg/kg IV or per rectum; midazolam 0.25–0.5 mg/kg IV). Continue with either further IV boluses or CRI depending on clinician preference and response to treatment. Adjust doses as needed. See note in Precautions/Interactions.
- Antitremorgenic agent.
  - Methocarbamol 55–220 mg/kg IV. Recommend not to exceed a maximum total dose of 330 mg/kg/day.
- Serotonin syndrome.
  - Cyproheptadine 1.1 mg/kg PO or per rectum (dogs) or 2–4 mg/cat PO or per rectum (cats).
- Tachycardia and hypertension.
  - Beta-blocker (propranolol 0.02 mg/kg IV slowly, titrate dose up to a maximum of 0.1 mg/kg and repeat as needed).

- Ventral premature contractions, ventricular tachycardia, and other ventricular dysrhythmias as needed.
  - Lidocaine.
    - Dogs – 2–4 mg/kg IV slowly, repeat q 15 minutes or CRI 25–75 mcg/kg/min.
    - Cats – 0.25–0.75 mg/kg IV slowly; cats are sensitive to lidocaine, use cautiously.
- If severe acidosis (pH <7.15 and $HCO_3^-$ <12 mEq/L) develops.
  - Sodium bicarbonate at 0.3 × base deficit (mEq) × kg body weight. Administer 1/2 slowly IV over six hours, then reevaluate acid–base status and adjust therapy as needed.

## Precautions/Interactions

- Adjust treatment as needed based on progression of clinical signs and response to treatment.
- Use of benzodiazepines may lead to paradoxical excitation or dysphoria; use judiciously and discontinue if worsening of clinical signs develops.

## Alternative Drugs

- In cases with severe signs, intravenous lipid emulsion (ILE) (1.5 mL/kg initial bolus of 20% ILE followed by 0.25 mL/kg/min for 30–60 minutes. Repeat boluses every 4–6 hours once serum is no longer lipemic.

## Extracorporeal Therapy

- Plasmapheresis has been described in human medical literature and may be beneficial in cases with rhabdomyolysis and myoglobinuria.

## Surgical Considerations

- Cardiovascular, respiratory, and neurological status should be evaluated and treated accordingly if anesthesia is considered.

## Patient Monitoring

- Monitor vitals, electrocardiogram, blood pressure, and neurological status.
- Frequency of monitoring depends on clinical status.

## Diet

- If the patient is unable to swallow, temporarily discontinue oral feeding and oral water intake. Otherwise, no dietary changes are required.

 **COMMENTS**

- Given the illicit nature of many sources of methamphetamine, contamination with other cointoxicants should also be considered.
- Use appropriate personal protection equipment, as residues on fur and presence in emesis may present human medical concerns.

## Prevention/Avoidance

- Removal of methamphetamine sources from the animal's environment to reduce risk of further or ongoing exposure.

## Possible Complications

- Chronic exposure may result in permanent cardiovascular and/or neurological damage.

## Expected Course and Prognosis

- Good with mild signs and/or aggressive early intervention.
- Poor to guarded in cases with persistent seizures, seizures refractory to care, persistent severe hyperthermia, DIC, rhabdomyolysis with secondary acute kidney injury, cardiovascular failure, and respiratory failure.

## Synonyms

- Prescription product – Desoxyn®.
- Illicit product – crystal meth, speed, crank, ice, glass, crystal, tina, others.

## See Also

Chapter 15 Amphetamines
Chapter 37 Cocaine
Chapter 36 Club Drugs (MDMA, GHB, Flunitrazepan, Bath Salts)

## Abbreviations

See Appendix 1 for a complete list.

## Suggested Reading

Buchweitz JP, Johnson M, Wixson M et al. Quantitation of methamphetamine and amphetamine in postmortem canine tissues and fluids. *J Anal Toxicol* 2022;46(2):92–96.

Chłopaś-Konowałek A, Tusiewicz K, Wachełko O et al. A case of amphetamine and methamphetamine intoxication in cat. *Toxics* 2022;10(12):749.

Ghadiri A, Etemad L, Moshiri M et al. Exploring the effect of intravenous lipid emulsion in acute methamphetamine toxicity. *Iran J Basic Med Sci* 2017;20(2):138.

Llera RM, Volmer PA. Toxicologic hazards for police dogs involved in drug detection. *J Am Vet Med Assoc* 2006;228(7):1028–1032.

Smith MR, Wurlod VA. Severe rhabdomyolysis associated with acute amphetamine toxicosis in a dog. *Case Rep Vet Med* 2020;2020:2816373.

**Author**: Sarah R. Alpert, DVM, DABT
**Consulting Editor**: Lynn R. Hovda, RPh, DVM, MS, DACVIM

# Chapter 41

# Miscellaneous Hallucinogens and Dissociative Agents

 ## DEFINITION/OVERVIEW

- Several hallucinogens and dissociative agents are of concern due to their widespread abuse. They are inexpensive, relatively easy to obtain, and frequently found at parties and in homes where pets live. Exposure can be due to voluntary ingestion or malicious poisoning.
- Hallucinogens.
  - LSD (see Chapter 38).
  - Lysergic acid amide substances (LSAs) are closely related to LSD and provide a similar experience.
    - Seeds from morning glory plant – *Ipomoea* spp.
    - Seeds from Hawaiian baby woodrose plant – *Argyreia nervosa*.
    - Endophyte infected sleepy grass – *Stipa robusta*.
  - *Amanita* mushrooms – *A. muscaria* and *A. pantherine*.
- Dissociative agents.
  - Ketamine (DEA Schedule III) is often obtained by theft from veterinary clinics. Many consider it the ideal substance of abuse as it provides the effects of LSD, opiates, and cocaine in one drug.
  - Phencyclidine (PCP) (5–90% pure), also known as angel dust, is mainly used recreationally for its significant mind-altering effects (see Chapter 43).
- Others worthy of mention but not addressed further in this chapter.
  - Dextromethorphan (CCC, Dex, DMX, triple C, rojo, skittles [gelatin capsules]) (see Chapter 46).
    - Dissociative agent readily available in nonprescription cough syrups and cold remedies. The mechanism of action is very similar to ketamine and phencyclidine. In human beings, approximately 360 mg causes a mild stimulant effect and >1500 mg a completely dissociative state. Toxicosis is rare and treatment is supportive and activated charcoal can be given if caught early.
  - Plants containing tropane alkaloids – atropine, hyoscyamine, and scopolamine.
    - Deadly nightshade (*Atropa belladonna*), Jimson weed (*Datura stramonium*).
    - Seeds are chewed, powdered, or smoked for hallucinogenic properties. Clinical signs include diaphoresis, decreased salivation, mydriasis, hyperthermia, and psychoactive effects.
  - Nutmeg.
    - Seeds from the fruit of an evergreen tree (*Myristica fragrans*) are chewed or powdered and smoked for hallucinogenic properties. The hallucinogenic properties are attributed to myristicin and elemicin. The tree is native to the South Pacific, Trinidad, and Grenada. In human beings, the toxic dose is estimated to be three

*Blackwell's Five-Minute Veterinary Consult Clinical Companion: Small Animal Toxicology*, Third Edition.
Edited by Lynn R. Hovda, Ahna G. Brutlag, Robert H. Poppenga, and Steven E. Epstein.
© 2024 John Wiley & Sons, Inc. Published 2024 by John Wiley & Sons, Inc.

whole nutmegs or 10–15 g (about one tablespoonful) of the dried spice. Clinical signs include decreased salivation, hypothermia, and vomiting.
- Peyote (mescaline).
  - The peyote cactus (*Lophophora williamsii*) contains the hallucinogen mescaline. The cactus is found in northern Mexico and the southwestern United States. Crowns or tops of the cactus are harvested and dried; ingestion is generally by chewing on the dried pieces or brewing them and drinking the liquid. In some countries, peyote oil and cream compounded for topical use are heated and concentrated into dry peyote. Clinical signs include early vomiting, diaphoresis, and mydriasis followed by a 12-hour period of psychoactivity resembling that of LSD. Dogs are reported to recover in about 10 hours.
- Psilocybin (magic mushrooms or shrooms).
  - Psilocybin and psilocin are psychoactive agents found in many species of hallucinogenic mushrooms. The mechanism of action is unknown but may be serotonergic in nature. Peak plasma concentration is reached 80–100 minutes after ingestion and lasts approximately 4–6 hours. Psilocybin is rapidly dephosphorylated into psilocin and approximately 50% of ingested psilocin is absorbed after oral administration. Roughly 65% is eliminated by the kidneys in the urine and about 15–20% is eliminated through the bile. Mushrooms can be ingested directly, brewed into tea, or dried and chewed.
- Salvia (*Salvia divinorum*).
  - Leafy green plant native to the Sierra Mazateca region of Mexico but can be grown outside in warm, subtropical climates (California and Hawaii) and can be grown inside anywhere. The seeds are generally purchased on the internet from specific *Salvia divinorum* sites. Most common forms are the dried leaves, which are chewed or smoked, and the fluid extract, which can be ingested or added to drinks. Salvorin-A is the active toxin and is a kappa (κ) receptor agonist; may act on CB1 receptor and has no effect on serotonin receptors. It has a very rapid onset of signs, is well absorbed through oral mucosa and recovery is expected in 1–2 hours. Clinical signs include abnormal mentation and vocalization.
- N,N-dimethyltryptamine (DMT).
  - Several plants including *Psychotria viridis* produce DMT which is used to make Ayahuasca tea; historically used by indigenous people in the Amazon as a form of medicine and source of knowledge. DMT acts as an agonist of several serotonin receptors. DMT can also be administered via inhalation or injection. The inhalation dose is 20–40 mg and lasts 5–15 minutes.
  - Ayahuasca tea blends DMT, beta-carbolines and harmala alkaloids which are reversible MAO inhibitors. Peak effects of Ayahuasca are felt around 1.5 hours after consumption and sessions last 4–6 hours. Clinical signs include hallucinations, vomiting, diarrhea and dizziness.

 **ETIOLOGY/PATHOPHYSIOLOGY**

- LSAs.
  - Plants are grown throughout the USA and seed packages can be purchased online and in most nurseries.
  - Seeds must be germinated, soaked in water, and crushed before ingestion or they are not effective.

- Ketamine.
  - DEA Schedule III drug and has one-tenth the potency of phencyclidine.
  - Liquid form is odorless, flavorless, and colorless and often added to party punches or individual drinks.
  - It can also be dried and powdered for smoking and inhalation.
- *Amanita* mushrooms – *A. muscaria* and *A. pantherine* (see Chapter 115).
  - Two species most frequently implicated in the pantherine-muscaria poisoning syndrome in humans.
    - Characterized by signs of CNS dysfunction including hallucinations, tremors, convulsions, and somnolence.
  - *A. muscaria*, commonly known as the fly agaric, has been recognized for its psychoactive properties and is voluntarily ingested for both recreational and ritualistic purposes.

## Mechanism of Action

- LSAs.
  - Incompletely understood.
  - Structurally like serotonin and acts as serotonin receptor antagonist.
  - Action at 5-HT$_{2A}$ receptor may be responsible for hallucinogenic effects.
  - LSD increases the release of glutamate and has a high affinity for dopamine (D$_1$ and D$_2$) and adrenergic (alpha-1 and alpha-2 receptors).
- Ketamine.
  - Incompletely understood.
  - Acts on the cerebral cortex, thalamus, and limbic system.
  - Dissociative anesthetics as they produce feelings of detachment from the environment and self.
  - Antagonizes the action of glutamate at the NMDA receptor by binding at the phencyclidine-binding site, which reduces receptor activity of glutamate (an excitatory neurotransmitter).
  - Inhibits the biogenic amine reuptake complex (NE, dopamine, serotonin).
  - Sympathomimetic effects can cause increases in cardiac output, heart rate and blood pressure.
- *Amanita* mushrooms.
  - Ibotenic acid and mucimol interfere with normal glutamate and gamma-aminobutyric acid (GABA)-mediated neurotransmission and are responsible for the CNS derangements and clinical manifestations of pantherine-muscaria syndrome in humans.
  - Muscarine has been isolated from *A. muscaria* and functions as a competitive muscarinic receptor agonist in the peripheral nervous system and is not subject to acetylcholinesterase receptor degradation. Receptors capable of binding muscarine are found in the highest concentrations in the cardiac muscle and nodes, smooth muscle, and glands, eliciting cholinergic signs such as vomiting, diarrhea, heart blocks, miosis, and ptyalism.

## Pharmacokinetics

- LSAs.
  - Little is reported; presumed to follow LSD.
  - Clinical signs in 60–90 minutes with a duration of action of several hours.
- Ketamine.
  - Well absorbed IM and IV.
  - Poorly absorbed orally, high first-pass effect.

- Distributed to brain, liver, lung, and other tissues.
- Undergoes hepatic metabolism by demethylation or hydroxylation.
- Renal excretion.
- $T_{1/2}$ cat = 67 minutes after IM dose.

## Toxicity

- LSAs.
  - 1/10 as potent as LSD.
  - 150–300 seeds associated with clinical effects in human beings.
- Ketamine.
  - Species dependent.
  - Cats – labeled dose (FDA approved) is 11 mg/kg IM for restraint and up to 22–33 mg/kg IM for diagnostic or minor surgical procedures; an accidental overdose of 100 mg/kg led to cardiopulmonary arrest.
  - Dogs – 5–10 mg/kg IM has resulted in seizures.

## Systems Affected

- LSAs.
  - CNS – primarily hallucinations with bizarre behaviors and vocalization.
  - Ophthalmic – mydriasis.
  - Musculoskeletal – rhabdomyolysis.
- Ketamine.
  - CNS – wide variety of signs from ataxia to hallucinations to bizarre or violent behaviors.
  - Musculoskeletal – increased muscle tone, spasms, rigidity, tonic-clonic convulsions, and hyperthermia.
  - Cardiovascular – tachycardia, hypertension, and arrhythmias.
  - Ophthalmic – vertical, horizontal, or rotary nystagmus, fixed stares.
  - Respiratory – can cause apneustic breathing and can cause respiratory suppression at high doses.
- *Amanita* mushrooms.
  - Seizures and muscle tremors typically develop within 4–12 hours due to ibotenic acid acting on glutamate receptors and lasts for 12–24 hours. CNS depression occurs in the final phase of intoxication and is due to the GABA synergistic effects of muscimol. Full recoveries typically occur within 24–48 hours.
  - If *A. muscaria* is ingested, the clinical signs are described as above, but acute muscarinic signs precede CNS dysfunction.

# SIGNALMENT/HISTORY

## Historical Findings

- The owners are often very reluctant to provide any information regarding these substances.

## Location and Circumstances of Poisoning

- Dogs and cats may be exposed by inhaling smoke, drinking leftover "party" punch, chewing on seed packages, digging up and mouthing plants, or finding a stash of "chews."

# CLINICAL FEATURES

- LSAs.
  - Primarily CNS signs including disorientation, vocalization, depression, or excitation. Behavioral changes reported in cats given IP injections of LSD included head and body shaking, bizarre sitting and standing positions, compulsive scratching at the litter, tracking, staring at and batting or pouncing at objects that were not apparent to the observer.
  - Onset of signs in 1–2 hours with recovery in 6–12 hours.
- Ketamine.
  - Cats – forelimb extensor rigidity, opisthotonos, mydriasis with a dazed staring expression. Hypersalivation with ingestion. Recovery in 10–12 hours.
  - Dogs – CNS excitation with tonic-clonic seizures. May develop rhabdomyolysis secondary to seizures.

# DIFFERENTIAL DIAGNOSIS

- Other intoxications.
  - Club drugs such as GHB (gamma-hydroxybutyrate) and MDMA (ecstasy/molly) and synthetic cathinones (Bath Salts).
  - Opiates or opioids (illicit or otherwise).
- CNS diseases with dissociative effects.
- Hepatic encephalopathy.

# DIAGNOSTICS

## Clinical Pathological Findings

- Acidemia, hypoglycemia, increased AST and CPK.

## Other Diagnostics

- Seeds or plant pieces found in emesis material.
- In humans, ibotenic acid and muscimol appear in urine in quantities detectable by ion-interaction HPLC within one hour of mushroom ingestion.
- LC/MS and GC/MS are useful tools but have a long turnaround time.

## Pathological Findings

- No specific lesions.

# THERAPEUTICS

## Detoxification

- LSAs.
  - Absorption is rapid and effects are self-limiting, therefore gastrointestinal decontamination is unlikely to be beneficial and emesis is not advised.
- Ketamine.
  - Liquid product so emesis only if witnessed and early.

- Activated charcoal binds phencyclidine and prevents enterohepatic recycling. Repeated dosing is recommended only in animals with normal mentation and swallowing reflexes.
- *Amanita* mushrooms.
  - Treatment includes GI decontamination and emesis can be induced only in animals with normal mentation and swallowing reflexes. Activated charcoal is advised to facilitate adsorption of the remaining toxin.

## Appropriate Health Care

- LSAs.
  - Minimize sensory stimulation by keeping the pet in a quiet, dark room.
- Ketamine.
  - Correct acid–base disturbances, and hypoglycemia if present.
  - Forced diuresis with mannitol or furosemide will increase the rate of drug clearance.
  - Muscle rigidity and seizure activity can be treated with benzodiazepines.
  - In cats, yohimbine may act as a partial antagonist to ketamine.
- *Amanita* mushrooms.
  - Seizure control using a benzodiazepine or phenobarbital but because both work as GABA agonists and may work synergistically with muscimol, the pet must be monitored carefully for worsening CNS depression.
  - Muscle tremors are largely controlled with methocarbamol.

## Antidote

- No specific antidote is available.

## Drug(s) of Choice

- IV fluids as needed to replace losses and protect kidneys if rhabdomyolysis occurs.
- Seizures, excitation, muscle rigidity.
  - Diazepam 0.25–0.5 mg/kg IV.
  - Midazolam 0.1–0.5 mg/kg IM or IV, 0.2 mg/kg intranasal.
    - CRI 0.05–0.5 mg/kg/h; start low and titrate upward until seizures are controlled.
  - Phenobarbital 3–5 mg/kg IV every 20–30 minutes; maximum total dose is 20–24 mg/kg IV.
  - Methocarbamol 44 mg/kg IV for moderate conditions, 55–220 mg/kg IV for controlling severe conditions.
    - Total cumulative dose should not exceed 330 mg/kg IV.
    - Administer IV no faster than a rate of 2 mL/minute.
- Yohimbine for a partial ketamine antagonism in cats 0.1 mg/kg IV.
- Atropine for SLUDGE signs secondary to muscarinic mushroom toxicity; 0.02–0.2 mg/kg; administer ¼ dose IV and the remainder IM or SC.

## Precautions/Interactions

- SSRIs and clomipramine should not be used as they can aggravate the mental changes that occur with intoxication.

## Patient Monitoring

- Keep in a dark, quiet area and minimize excess stimulation. Monitor closely for early signs of self-mutilation or psychosis and treat accordingly.
- Monitor body temperature for hyperthermia and treat with cooling vest, a fan, etc. Do not overcool. Stop when temperature reaches 103–103.5 °F. Rarely, hypothermia may develop.
- Minimize activity and limit restraint until clinically normal.

# COMMENTS

## Possible Complications

- None expected with a single exposure.
- Repeated exposures in human beings have resulted in "flashbacks" and permanent psychosis.

## Expected Course and Prognosis

- Prognosis is excellent with supportive care. The onset of seizures or rhabdomyolysis or the development of aspiration pneumonia complicates treatment and lowers the prognosis for a complete recovery.

## Synonyms

- LSAs – heavenly blues, flying saucers, pearly gates.
- Ketamine – special K, cat Valium, green K.
- Salvia – diviner's sage, shepherdess' herb, Mexican mint, Sally D.

## See Also

Chapter 38 Lysergic Acid Diethylamide (LSD)
Chapter 43 Phencyclidine (PCP)
Chapter 50 Dextromethorphan
Chapter 115 Mushrooms

## Abbreviations

See Appendix 1 for a complete list.

## Suggested Reading

Bischoff K. Toxicity of drugs of abuse. In: Gupta RC (ed.) *Veterinary Toxicology: Basic and Clinical Principles*, 3rd ed. New York: Elsevier, 2018; pp. 385–408.

Calina D, Carvalho F, Docea AO. Toxicity of psychedelic drugs. In: Tsatsakis A (ed.) *Toxicological Risk Assessment and Multi-System Health Impacts from Exposure*. New York: Elsevier, 2021; pp. 545–556.

Cortes YE, Holme JL. Successful cardiopulmonary resuscitation and use of short-term mechanical ventilation following inadvertent ketamine overdose in a cat. *J Vet Emerg Crit Care* 2008;(18)2:165–169.

Halpern JH. Hallucinogens and dissociative agents naturally growing in the USA. *Pharmacol Ther* 2004;102:131–138.

Rossmeisl JH, Higgins MA, Ellis ME, Jones DE. Amanita muscaria toxicosis in two dogs. *J Vet Emerg Crit Care* 2006;16(3):208–214.

**Author:** Deanna Lombardo, DVM, DACVECC
**Consulting Editor:** Lynn R. Hovda, RPh, DVM, MS, DACVIM

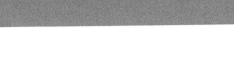
# Opiates and Opioids (Illicit)

## DEFINITION/OVERVIEW

- The opiate and opioid group includes more than 25 different drugs; most are legal prescription drugs.
- Several of these drugs are abused for their psychoactive effects. Among the most frequently abused are opium, morphine, codeine, heroin, oxycodone, hydromorphone, meperidine, fentanyl and its analogs.
- Heroin, a morphine derivative, is perhaps the most widely abused because it is inexpensive and more available than other opiates or opioids.
  - Often sold as "black tar heroin," a sticky black substance, or "Mexican brown powder," a white to dark brown powder (Figure 42.1).
  - Generally contains fillers or additives such as sugar, starch, talcum powder, quinine, strychnine, levamisole, or others.
  - Increasingly may contain illicitly manufactured fentanyl and its analogs.
  - Most recently, xylazine, an alpha-2 receptor agonist, has been used to cut heroin, fentanyl and other illicit drugs. The combination is often deadly.

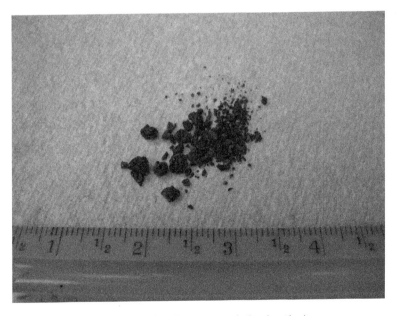

■ **Figure 42.1** Black tar heroin. Source: Courtesy of Lynn R. Hovda (book author).

*Blackwell's Five-Minute Veterinary Consult Clinical Companion: Small Animal Toxicology*, Third Edition.
Edited by Lynn R. Hovda, Ahna G. Brutlag, Robert H. Poppenga, and Steven E. Epstein.
© 2024 John Wiley & Sons, Inc. Published 2024 by John Wiley & Sons, Inc.

- Animals can be exposed in a variety of different manners.
  - Drug-detecting dogs in active service are at the highest risk for accidental intoxication either by inhalation or ingestion.
  - Puppies have been used as "pack dogs" to transport heroin and cocaine; bags are surgically placed in their abdomens prior to shipping the dogs into the United States.
  - Sporadic cases of malicious heroin injections exist. Staffordshire terriers received at Scottish rescue centers were deliberately injected with heroin by drug dealers to make them more aggressive and attack police officers.
  - Rarely, animal owners want to "share" their experiences with pets.
  - Accidental exposure to owner's supply.
- Clinical signs vary depending on the species, but death, when it occurs, is generally from respiratory depression and arrest.

 ## ETIOLOGY/PATHOPHYSIOLOGY

- Opiates – natural opium, morphine, codeine, and other alkaloids are derived from the seeds and sap of the poppy plant (*Papaver somniferum*) (Figure 42.2).
- Opioids – broad term covering all compounds with morphine-like activity.
  - Heroin, oxycodone, and hydromorphone are semisynthetic derivatives.
  - Meperidine and fentanyl are strictly synthetic drugs.
- Exposure in animals generally occurs from ingestion, inhalation, or rupture of implanted abdominal packets.

### Mechanism of Action

- Varies depending on the particular drug.
  - Full agonist – morphine, codeine, heroin, fentanyl, meperidine.
  - Full antagonist – naloxone.

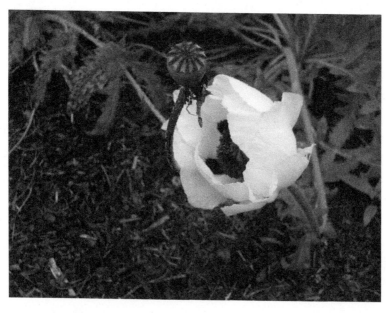

■ **Figure 42.2** White opium flower (*Papaver somniferum*). Source: Courtesy of Lynn R. Hovda (book author).

- Agonist/antagonist – butorphanol, nalorphine.
- Partial agonist – tramadol, buprenorphine.
- Both opiates and opioids bind to opioid receptors.
- Opioid receptors are G protein-coupled receptors (GPCR) that respond to endogenous peptides (e.g., endorphins, enkephalins) as well as exogenous substances (e.g., heroin, morphine, fentanyl).
  - At this time, the major identified opioid receptors (in humans) are designated as mu (MOR), kappa (KOR), delta (DOR), nociceptin (NOR, also called opioid receptor-like receptor 1, ORL1), epsilon, lambda, iota, and zeta (ZOR).
  - Sigma receptor is no longer classified as an opioid receptor because it is not a GPCR.
  - Opioid receptors are found throughout the body and their functions are complex, interrelated, and incompletely understood.
  - They are most recognized for their role in analgesia and addiction. Opioid receptors are also involved in signal transduction and mediate a wide variety of pathways including hormones, neurotransmitters, development and the senses.

## Pharmacokinetics

- Absorption.
  - Oral absorption is generally rapid and occurs in the small intestine.
  - Subcutaneous absorption is rapid.
- Distribution.
  - Well distributed to most organ systems (CNS, intestine, kidney, liver, lungs, placenta, spleen, and skeletal muscle).
  - Lipophilic drugs, including heroin and fentanyl, cross the blood–brain barrier (BBB) more efficiently.
- Metabolism.
  - Readily metabolized in liver by hydrolysis, oxidation, and N-dealkylation.
  - Morphine undergoes glucuronidation to morphine-6-glucuronide, an active metabolite.
  - Enterohepatic recirculation of morphine and its metabolite occurs.
- Excretion.
  - Renal, primarily as metabolites.
  - Some biliary excretion via feces.

## Toxicity

- Very limited animal data available.
- Codeine – IV $LD_{50}$ in dogs is 69 mg/kg.
- Heroin – minimum lethal dose.
  - Dog – 25 mg/kg SQ.
  - Cat – 20 mg/kg PO.
- Morphine – minimum lethal dose parenterally.
  - Dog – 110–210 mg/kg SQ.
  - Dog – 133 mg/kg IV $LD_{50}$.
  - Cat – 40 mg/kg BW given SQ.
- Meperidine.
  - >20 mg/kg BW causes excitation in cats.
  - 30 mg/kg BW causes seizures in cats.

## Systems Affected

- Varies depending on drug and species involved.
  - Respiratory – respiratory depression leading to death.
  - CNS – depression or excitation.

- Cardiovascular – instability with hypotension; heart block and other arrhythmias with propoxyphene overdose.
- Gastrointestinal – decreased GI motility with constipation.
- Ophthalmic – miosis or mydriasis (species variation).
- Endocrine/metabolic – meperidine and tramadol have some serotonergic activity.

 **SIGNALMENT/HISTORY**

- All breeds and ages are susceptible.
- Cats and dogs present with different clinical signs when exposed to the same opiate or opioid, primarily due to the location of opioid receptors in the CNS.

### Risk Factors

- Age.
  - Pediatric animals may have an incomplete BBB and show more severe signs, especially with highly lipophilic substances such as fentanyl and heroin.
  - Neonatal animals may have underdeveloped liver systems and be unable to adequately metabolize opiates or opioids.
  - Geriatric animals may have impaired liver and renal systems, causing inadequate metabolism and excretion of drugs.
- Cats, due to their lack of glucuronyl transferase, may inefficiently metabolize morphine.
- Police dogs, airport dogs, and other narcotic dogs in active service are at greater risk of exposure.

### Historical Findings

- These drugs are illicit, and the owners may not provide an accurate history.

### Location and Circumstances of Poisoning

- Intoxication can occur anywhere these drugs are found.
- Some dogs have been used as "drug mules" to illegally smuggle heroin or codeine across national borders.

 **CLINICAL FEATURES**

- Dogs.
  - CNS – early excitation followed by lethargy, ataxia, frank stupor, seizures, coma, death.
  - Respiratory – tachypnea followed by bradypnea.
  - Gastrointestinal – hypersalivation, vomiting, defecation, urination.
  - Cardiovascular – hypotension, arrhythmias related to propoxyphene metabolite.
  - Ophthalmic – miosis.
  - Endocrine/metabolic – hypothermia, decreased pain response, possible serotonin syndrome.
- Cats.
  - CNS – aggression, excitation, seizures, or depression.
  - Respiratory – variable early on, but eventually bradypnea.
  - Gastrointestinal – stasis with lack of emesis, constipation.
  - Cardiovascular – hypotension and arrhythmias.

- Ophthalmic – mydriasis (more common), miosis.
- Endocrine/metabolic – hypothermia, decreased pain response, possible serotonin syndrome.

# DIFFERENTIAL DIAGNOSIS

- Various encephalopathies.
- CNS depressants.
  - Alcohols.
  - Amitraz.
  - Barbiturates.
  - Benzodiazepines.
  - Ethylene glycol.
  - Marijuana.
  - Synthetic cannabinoids.
- CNS stimulants.
  - Amphetamines/methylphenidate/methamphetamine/MDMA.
  - Cocaine.
  - Metaldehyde.
  - Strychnine.

# DIAGNOSTICS

### Clinical Pathological Findings

- No specific findings.

### Other Diagnostics

- The Quick Screen Pro Multi Drug Screening Test is a human testing kit that has been successfully used in animals. It may provide a rapid and accurate diagnosis if the drug is present in high enough concentrations and the time frame is appropriate.
- Urine and serum can be submitted to human hospitals for analysis or to a laboratory for GC/MS or LC/MS/MS. Both take several days for results to be returned and will not provide information rapidly enough to guide therapy.

### Pathological Findings

- No specific findings.

# THERAPEUTICS

- The goal of therapy is to provide early decontamination, careful use of an opioid antagonist, and supportive care.

### Detoxification

- Induce emesis either at home or in veterinarian's clinic if no clinical signs have developed. Emesis may be successful for 1–2 hours after ingestion due to decreased GI motility.
- Activated charcoal with cathartic × 1 dose. Repeat doses of activated charcoal may be necessary for drugs such as morphine that undergo enterohepatic recirculation.
- Gastric lavage if large doses ingested or clinical signs preclude emesis.
- Drug-detecting dogs may have ingested bags full of narcotics; be careful that these are not ruptured. Surgical removal may be necessary.

## Appropriate Health Care

- Hospitalize and monitor closely for CNS and respiratory depression. Be prepared to intubate and ventilate if needed.
- Heart monitor with ECG as needed.
- Monitor body temperature and treat accordingly. Warm but do not overheat.
- Monitor urine output and fluid status.

## Antidote

- Naloxone, a pure opioid antagonist, may be used to reverse CNS and respiratory depression. It has no effects on the GI signs seen in dogs.
  - Injectable product – 0.01–0.04 mg/kg BW IV or IM.
    - The high end of the dosage range may be needed in massive overdoses.
    - Duration of action is generally 45–90 minutes.
    - If effective, dose may need to be repeated.
  - Human intranasal spray – 4 mg commercial spray product has been used successfully in dogs.
    - Rapid onset.
    - Few noted side-effects.
- If naloxone is not available, butorphanol 0.05–0.1 mg/kg IV may be used to partially reverse pure mu agonists.
- If incomplete or unsatisfactory response to naloxone, consider atipamezole trial to reverse potential xylazine as contaminant. Dose: 25–50 mcg/kg IM or IV (slowly) for cats; 50 mcg/kg IM for dogs.

## Drug(s) of Choice

- IV fluids as needed to replace losses and correct hypotension.
- Seizures.
  - Diazepam 0.25–0.5 mg/kg IV, midazolam 0.1–0.3 mg/kg IM, IV, other benzodiazepine drugs.
  - Levetiracetam 30–60mg/kg IV q 8 hours.
  - Phenobarbital 4–8 mg/kg IV.
- Arrhythmias.
  - Lidocaine.
    - Dogs: 2–4 mg/kg IV to effect while monitoring ECG.
    - Cats: 0.25–0.5 mg/kg slow IV while monitoring ECG. Use judiciously in cats.
  - Other drugs at discretion and ability of DVM.

## Precautions/Interactions

- Naloxone is ineffective for seizures caused by normeperidine, tramadol, or propoxyphene toxicity and may exacerbate signs.
- Naloxone will not reverse propoxyphene-induced cardiotoxicity or the effects of drugs cut or diluted with xylazine or other alpha-2-adrenergic agonists.
- Many of the drugs, especially heroin, are "cut" with or contain additives such as sugar, starch, dry or powdered milk, chalk, talcum powder, quinine, strychnine, xylazine, or levamisole.
- Veterinarians should consider opioid exposures in patients exposed to street drugs with unexpected clinical signs consistent with opioid overdose
  - Heroin and other illicit nonopioid drugs may be contaminated with illicitly manufactured fentanyl, intensifying or adding to the toxic profile of the animal's exposure.

- • Fentanyl, heroin, and other illicit drugs may be contaminated cut or diluted with xylazine, an alpha-2-adrenergic agonist. Naloxone is ineffective against xylazine.
- ■ Coingestion/administration with tramadol, tricyclic antidepressants, selective serotonin reuptake inhibitors, or monoamine oxidase inhibitors may lead to serotonin syndrome.

### Surgical Considerations

- ■ Cautious surgical removal of packets in GIT or abdomen of drug-packing dogs.

### Patient Monitoring

- ■ Baseline labs with attention to BUN, creatinine, and CK, especially if seizures occur.
- ■ Blood gases as needed.
- ■ ECG in the event of arrhythmias.

# COMMENTS

### Prevention/Avoidance

- ■ Animals should be kept away from parties where these drugs are used. Personal stashes should be locked up and kept out of reach.
- ■ Party drinks and other goodies should be cleared away before animals have access to the area.
- ■ Police and active drug-detecting dogs that are voracious eaters should wear a muzzle.
- ■ Naloxone should be available for police and drug-detecting dogs in active service.

### Expected Course and Prognosis

- ■ The onset of signs is rapid, occurring within 30–120 minutes. The duration of signs depends on the particular opiate or opioid ingested or inhaled.
- ■ The prognosis is generally excellent, especially when naloxone has been used to reverse the signs.
- ■ Death rarely occurs.

### Synonyms

- ■ Heroin – dope, heaven, Lady Jane, skag, smack, speedball.
- ■ Fentanyl – China white, tango and cash.

### See Also

Chapter 31 Opiates and Opioids

### Abbreviations

See Appendix 1 for a complete list.

### Suggested Reading

Bischoff K. Toxicity of drugs of abuse. In: Gupta RC (ed.) *Veterinary Toxicology: Basic and Clinical Principles*, 3rd edn. New York: Elsevier, 2018; pp. 385–406.

Daily Record. Revealed: Drug dealers injecting dogs with heroin to make them more aggressive. www.dailyrecord.co.uk/news/scottish-news/revealed-drug-dealers-injecting-pet-1366869

Fairbairn N, Coffin PO, Walley AY. Naloxone for heroin, prescription opioid, and illicitly made fentanyl overdoses: challenges and innovations responding to a dynamic epidemic. *Int J Drug Policy* 2017;46:172–179.

French D. The challenges of LC-MS/MS analysis of opiates and opioids in urine. *Bioanalysis* 2013;5(22):2803–2820.

Independent News (UK). Colombian vet arrested for implanting heroin inside puppies to smuggle to U.S. www.independent.co.uk/news/world/americas/puppies-heroin-injected-vet-colombia-us-smuggle-drug-cartel-mules-a8769981.html

Volmer PA. Recreational drugs. In: Peterson ME, Talcott (eds) *Small Animal Toxicology*, 3rd edn. St Louis: Elsevier, 2013; pp. 309–333.

Wahler BM, Lerche P, Pereira CH et al. Pharmacokinetics and pharmacodynamics of intranasal and intravenous naloxone hydrochloride administration in healthy dogs. *Am J Vet Res* 2019;80(7):696–701.

**Authors:** Shannon Jarchow, DVM and Colleen Almgren, DVM, DABT, DABVT
**Consulting Editor:** Lynn R. Hovda, RPh, DVM, MS, DACVIM

# Chapter 43

# Phencyclidine (PCP)

## DEFINITION/OVERVIEW

- PCP (1-[phenylcyclohexyl] piperidine), or phencyclidine, was introduced in the 1950s as a human surgical anesthetic but was discontinued a few years later because of disagreeable and often violent side-effects such as hallucination, mania, delirium, and disorientation.
- It was marketed in 1967 as a veterinary anesthetic (Sernylan®) but withdrawn in 1978 because of similar side-effects, long half-life, and potential as a drug of abuse.
- Currently a DEA Schedule II synthetic drug.
- Easily synthesized in clandestine laboratories in both the powder and liquid form.
- More than 80 known analogs. Ketamine, one of the analogs, is widely used in veterinary medicine, but it has a shorter half-life and 1/10 to 1/20 potency of PCP.

## ETIOLOGY/PATHOPHYSIOLOGY

### Mechanism of Action

- Dissociative agent, but the precise mechanism is not fully understood.
- Inhibits glutamate at NMDA receptors in the cerebral cortex, thalamus, and limbic system.
- Inhibits dopamine and norepinephrine reuptake.
- Binds acetylcholine and GABA receptors.

### Pharmacokinetics

- PCP is a weak base with poor gastric absorption and significant intestinal absorption.
- Inhaled PCP is well absorbed via the respiratory system.
- Slower GI absorption.
- Highly lipophilic.
  - Crosses the blood–brain barrier.
  - Partitions to the CNS, which may increase half-life.
- Metabolism varies with species.
  - In dogs, 68% of a single dose is metabolized in the liver and 32% is excreted unchanged by the kidney.
  - In cats, 88% is excreted unchanged by the kidney and has a short elimination half-life.

### Toxicity

- Oral administration.
  - Severe signs of toxicosis.
    - Dogs 2.5–10.0 mg/kg BW PO.
    - Cats 1.1–12.0 mg/kg BW PO.
  - Lethal PO dose in dogs is 25 mg/kg BW.

*Blackwell's Five-Minute Veterinary Consult Clinical Companion: Small Animal Toxicology*, Third Edition.
Edited by Lynn R. Hovda, Ahna G. Brutlag, Robert H. Poppenga, and Steven E. Epstein.
© 2024 John Wiley & Sons, Inc. Published 2024 by John Wiley & Sons, Inc.

- IV administration – clinical signs in dogs at 1 mg/kg BW IV.
- IM administration in dogs.
    - 2 mg/kg BW – muscle incoordination.
    - 5 mg/kg BW – immobilization and seizures.

## Systems Affected

- Nervous – variable, from depression to stimulation; may last several days.
- Neuromuscular – tremors, tetany, loss of motor function.
- Cardiovascular – tachycardia, hypo- or hypertension, arrhythmias.
- Endocrine/metabolic – hyperthermia.
- Musculoskeletal – rhabdomyolysis.
- Renal/urological – acute renal failure secondary to myoglobinuria.

 # SIGNALMENT/HISTORY

### Risk Factors

- Ingestion of illegal PCP.
- Police dogs may be predisposed.

### Historical Findings

- Access to drugs.
    - Teenagers in the home.
    - Guests or party in the home. Owners may be reluctant to give a complete history.
    - Contaminant in other drugs.
        - Owner/user may be unaware of what is in illicit drugs.

### LOCATION AND CIRCUMSTANCES OF POISONING

- Animals residing in neighborhoods with known drug use.
- May be combined with other drugs.

 # CLINICAL FEATURES

### ACUTE

- Behavioral effects vary depending on dosage.
    - Depression at low dose.
    - Stimulation at high dose with the potential for tetany and seizures.
- General signs include hypertension, tachycardia, nausea, vomiting, hypersalivation, fever, sweating, and convulsion.
- Dogs dosed with PCP showed muscular rigidity, facial grimacing, increased motor activity, head weaving, stereotyped sniffing behaviors, jaw snapping, salivation, blank staring, incoordination, nystagmus, coma, tonic-clonic convulsions, and hyperthermia.
- Cardiovascular effects include tachycardia, hypertension, and cardiac arrhythmias.

### Chronic

- Not reported.

# DIFFERENTIAL DIAGNOSIS

- Hallucinogenic mushrooms.
- Ketamine.
- LSD.
- Marijuana and synthetic cannabinoids.
- Amphetamines, cocaine, cathinone derivatives, methylxanthines, other stimulants.
- Serotonin syndrome.

 # DIAGNOSTICS

## Clinical Pathological Findings

- Serum chemistry may show acidosis, hypoglycemia, electrolyte imbalances, and increases in CPK and AST.

## Other Diagnostics

- Over-the-counter urine test kits.
  - High urinary elimination of parent compound.
  - False positives have been associated with tramadol, diphenhydramine, ketamine, lamotrigine, venlafaxine, dextromethorphan, doxylamine, and ibuprofen.
- Urine, blood, plasma, or gastric contents for laboratory analysis.
  - Urine is the most analyzed sample. PCP may be detected for more than two weeks after exposure.
  - Blood concentrations do not correlate with clinical findings.

## Pathological Findings

- Nonspecific.
- Subendocardial and epicardial hemorrhage.

 # THERAPEUTICS

- Treatment of poisoning is generally symptomatic and supportive.

## Detoxification

- Emesis only if very recent ingestion of large doses. Use with caution, as animals may develop seizures at any time.
- Activated charcoal with a cathartic × 1 dose.

## Appropriate Health Care

- Monitor for urine output and adjust IV fluids as needed.
- Monitor for hyperthermia and treat accordingly.
- Monitor blood pressure and treat accordingly.
- Obtain baseline BUN, creatinine, and blood glucose. Repeat as needed.
- Keep animal in a darkened, quiet, low-stress environment and minimize sensory stimulation.

## Antidote

- No specific antidote is available.

## Drug(s) of Choice

- IV fluids to correct hypoglycemia and electrolyte abnormalities. IV rate, at a minimum, should be two times maintenance for renal and cardiovascular support.
- After rehydration, forced diuresis with mannitol or furosemide can be used to increase the rate of clearance.
  - Furosemide CRI at 1 mg/kg/hour in cats or dogs.
  - Mannitol bolus at 1–2 g/kg slow IV in cats or dogs.
- Tremors and seizures.
  - Midazolam 0.1–0.3 mg/kg IV in dogs.
  - Diazepam 0.25–2.0 mg/kg IV in dogs, lower in cats.
  - Phenobarbital 2–5 mg/kg IV, can be repeated up to twice at 20-minute intervals.

## Precautions/Interactions

- Phenothiazine tranquilizers exacerbate anticholinergic effects and produce hypotension.

## Patient Monitoring

- Monitor body temperature regularly over 12 hours post exposure.
- Monitor BUN, creatinine, CK, and blood glucose.
- Monitor urine for evidence of myoglobinuria.

    **COMMENTS**

## Prevention/Avoidance

- Police dogs can wear a muzzle to prevent ingestion of illegal drugs.
- Prevent exposure to illegal drugs.
  - Keep animals away from illegal drug stash.
  - Keep animals confined during parties where drugs may be used.

## Possible Complications

- Self-induced trauma or rhabdomyolysis may complicate treatment.

## Expected Course and Prognosis

- Depends on the clinical condition of the animal at the time of presentation.
- Prognosis is generally good with early decontamination, monitoring, and supportive care.
- Dogs injected IM with low dose of PCP.
  - 1 mg/kg – recovered in a little over one hour.
  - 5 mg/kg – recovered within two hours.
- Poor prognosis if self-induced trauma or rhabdomyolysis is evident.

## Synonyms

Angel dust, angel hair, boat, dummy dust, jet fuel.

## See Also

Chapter 39 Marijuana (THC)
Chapter 41 Miscellaneous Hallucinogens and Dissociative Agents

## Abbreviations

See Appendix 1 for a complete list.

## Suggested Reading

ASPCApro. Urine Drug Screens for Pets: What You Need to Know. www.aspcapro.org/resource/urine-drug-screens-pets-what-you-need-know

Ortega J. Phencyclidine for capture of stray dogs. *J Am Vet Med Assoc* 1967;150:772–776.

Oster E, Čudina N, Pavasović H et al. Intoxication of dogs and cats with common stimulating, hallucinogenic, and dissociative recreational drugs. *Vet Anim Sci* 2023;19:100288.

Volmer PA. Recreational drugs. In: Peterson ME, Talcott PA (eds) *Small Animal Toxicology*, 3rd edn. St Louis: Elsevier, 2013; pp 309–334.

**Author**: Karyn Bischoff, DVM, MS, DABVT, MPH
**Consulting Editor**: Lynn R. Hovda, RPh, DVM, MS, DACVIM

# Chapter 44

# Synthetic Cannabinoids

## DEFINITION/OVERVIEW

- Synthetic cannabinoid receptor agonists were originally developed in the 1960s for pioneering the research of cannabinoid receptors and the endocannabinoid system. This evolved into studies that then investigated their pharmaceutical potential.
- Synthetic cannabinoids (SCBs) are now manufactured as recreational drugs that have grown significantly in popularity and prevalence since the 2000s, escalating in popularity in 2009. These were initially legal and made available in gas stations, tattoo parlors, specialty shops, and the internet. The Synthetic Drug Control Act of 2011 banned SCBs, and they are now classified as a Schedule I drug.
- SCBs are powders that are dissolved in solvents and applied to dried herbaceous plant material to make them appear more natural. This material is usually smoked in a pipe, water pipe, or rolled cigarette, but may be formulated into edible baked goods, vaped, or inhaled.
- SCBs are structurally unrelated to THC but are cannabimimetic in that they act on cannabinoid receptors and cause similar but more profound clinical signs. They are designed to impart a much more potent effect.
- Both inhalation and oral exposures may result in clinical signs in pets.
- Common names include K2, Spice, Kronic, Skunk, Wild Greens, Purple Haze, Crazy Monkey, Happy Tiger, and Black Mamba, among many others.
- Scientific names are often derived from acronyms of the chemical name or the initial developer or research institution. Examples include:
  - the JWH series (John William Huffman).
  - the CP series (Charles Pfizer).
  - the HU series (Hebrew University).
  - APINACA, AB-CHMINACA, among many others.
- Often labeled with "warning" indicating "not for human consumption" and marketed as "incense" or "potpourri" to reduce risk of detection.
- May be laced with other stimulant substances such as caffeine.

## ETIOLOGY/PATHOPHYSIOLOGY

### Mechanism of Action

- The endocannabinoid system (ECS) is integral to both embryonic development and physiologic maintenance in mature animals. Naturally occurring endocannabinoids interact with cannabinoid receptors (CB1 and CB2) in cell membranes to inhibit neurotransmitter release.
- The ECS displays extensive cross-reactivity with other receptor systems, including opiate, NMDA, GABA, muscarinic acetylcholine, 5-HT serotonin, dopamine, and MDR1 receptors.

*Blackwell's Five-Minute Veterinary Consult Clinical Companion: Small Animal Toxicology*, Third Edition. Edited by Lynn R. Hovda, Ahna G. Brutlag, Robert H. Poppenga, and Steven E. Epstein. © 2024 John Wiley & Sons, Inc. Published 2024 by John Wiley & Sons, Inc.

- SCBs are potent and complete CB1 receptor agonists, in contrast to marijuana's psychotropic phytocannabinoid, THC, a partial CB1 agonist. SCBs impart profound psychotropic effects with more significant stimulatory consequences. On average, many SCBs carry greater than a 100× higher affinity (ranging from 2 to 800×) for CB1 receptors compared to THC.
- When compared to THC, SCBs are 2–3× more likely to cause stimulatory affects, 5× more likely to lead to hallucinations, and much more likely to cause seizures. Though these signs are influenced by the potency of SCBs and their higher affinity for CB1 receptor agonism, the absence of antiepileptic phytocannabinoids and phytochemicals found in the marijuana plant may also play a role in the more severe clinical outcome.
- THC has some degree of antiepileptic effect. Given SCBs cause a much higher incidence of seizures, there may be notable differences in the functional groups between the two.

## Pharmacokinetics

- Pharmacokinetics (PK) are not well established for SCBs and may vary significantly by chemical/drug and product.
- PK are likely similar to those of phytocannabinoids THC and CBD.
- Absorption and distribution: suspected to be rapid due to onset of signs, and likely similar to that of phytocannabinoids.
  - Oral bioavailability is likely lower, as human ingestion of baked goods caused milder signs of shorter duration.
- Metabolism.
  - Poorly established; may vary by SCB/chemical.
  - JWH-018 and AM-2201: hydroxylated to metabolites in the liver, conjugated by glucuronosyltransferases in humans.
  - APINACA: oxidative metabolism via CYP3A4 in humans.
- Excretion.
  - Half-life 72–96 hours.
  - Recovery typically within 24 hours, may be shorter with ingestion (4–10 hours).

## Systems Affected

- PPH data: less than 4% of cases remained asymptomatic from January 2010 to January 2023 (see Chapter 39, Figure 39.5).
- Both inhalation and oral exposures may result in signs.
- Nervous/neuromuscular: ataxia, lethargy, recumbency, tremor, twitching, hyperesthesia, agitation, vocalization, seizure, confusion, stupor/obtundation, coma.
- Gastrointestinal: vomiting, anorexia.
- Ophthalmic: mydriasis.
- Renal/urological: urinary incontinence.
- Cardiovascular: bradycardia, tachycardia, hypertension.
- Endocrine/metabolic: hypothermia or hyperthermia.
- Respiratory: tachypnea, respiratory depression.
- Musculoskeletal: weakness.
- Of note: acute kidney injury, liver damage, liver failure, and death have been reported in humans.

 # SIGNALMENT/HISTORY

## Risk Factors

- Indiscriminate eaters.
- Police or active-duty dogs.

- Underlying liver or renal disease.
- MDR1 mutation: the ECS interacts with the MDR1 receptors and may impart some degree of sensitivity to phytocannabinoids in these patients. This interaction is taken into consideration with therapeutic use of CBD, but the clinical consequences of phytocannabinoid or synthetic cannabinoid overdose in these patients have not yet been evaluated.

### Historical Findings

- Owners may also be clinically affected in inhalation exposures and require emergency medical care.
- Pets often present symptomatic due to rapid absorption and onset of signs, but they may present as asymptomatic following the very recent ingestion of herb-like plant material.
- Owners may be reluctant to admit exposure. Careful and compassionate questioning may aid in diagnosis.

### Location and Circumstances of Poisoning

- Because many SCBs are manufactured internationally and distributed widely through many sources including but not limited to the tnternet, exposures may be prevalent world-wide.

 CLINICAL FEATURES

- Initial gastrointestinal signs and lethargy may be reported, but animals may quickly progress to display stimulatory signs including agitation, aggression, vocalization, disorientation, ataxia, twitching or tremors, and seizures. Cardiovascular changes may be noted.

 DIFFERENTIAL DIAGNOSIS

- Consumer over-the-counter stimulants: caffeine, nicotine, 5-HTP (*Griffonia* seed extract), methylxanthines, decongestants (pseudoephedrine, phenylephrine).
- Prescription drugs: THC, amphetamines, methylphenidate, methylxanthines, 5-fluorouracil, baclofen, SSRIs, TCAs.
- Nonprescription or illicit drugs: THC, amphetamines, cocaine, MDMA (ecstasy/molly), LSD (acid).

 DIAGNOSTICS

- Renal and hepatic profile monitoring given reports of acute kidney injury and liver failure in humans.
- Urinalysis if severe tremors or seizure are noted.
- Blood glucose and electrolyte monitoring intermittently in severely symptomatic patients.
- Venous blood gas and lactate analysis in severely symptomatic patients.
- Point-of-care urine drug screens are ineffective in the detection of synthetic cannabinoids.
- Gas chromatography/mass spectrometry is effective in confirmation/diagnosis, but its clinical application is limited at this time.

### Clinical Pathological Findings

- CBC – no exposure-specific findings expected.
- Chemistry – renal and hepatic enzyme elevations reported in humans.
- Venous blood gas – mild respiratory acidosis.
- Lactate – may be elevated in severely affected patients.

## Pathological Findings

- Exposure-specific changes are not expected.

# THERAPEUTICS

- **Detoxification**
  - Inhalation – remove from the source.
  - Emesis – asymptomatic patients only, best performed within one hour of ingestion.
  - Activated charcoal – asymptomatic patients only: initial dose with sorbitol: 1 g/kg. Consider follow-up doses without sorbitol q 8 hours for 1–2 doses.
  - Gastric lavage – symptomatic patients if large quantities consumed.
  - Endoscopic removal – rarely indicated unless a bag of product is ingested, emesis is either contraindicated or unsuccessful, and/or patient is unlikely to pass the product.

## Appropriate Health Care

- Most SCB exposures require inpatient hospitalization.
- Intravenous fluids: perfusion and hydration.
- Thermoregulation.
- Low-stimulus environment.
- Nursing care – vitals and blood pressure monitoring, eye lubricant, and rotating patients q 4 hours if needed.
- Ventilation as needed.

## Drug(s) of Choice

- Antiemetics.
  - Maropitant 1 mg/kg SQ, IV q 24 hours.
  - Ondansetron 0.5–1 mg/kg IV q 12 hours for dogs; 0.1–1 mg/kg IV, SC, IM q 6–12 hours for cats.
- Sedation as needed.
  - Butorphanol 0.2–0.4 mg/kg IV.
  - Diazepam 0.25–0.5 mg/kg IV.
  - Acepromazine 0.02–0.2 mg/kg IV (normotensive patients only).
- Tremor/seizure management.
  - Methocarbamol 44–220 mg/kg IV to effect.
  - Diazepam 0.25–0.5 mg/kg IV; diazepam was ineffective in controlling seizures in one canine case report. Multimodal therapy or other anticonvulsants may be a more effective choice.
  - Levetiracetam 60 mg/kg loading dose, 30 mg/kg q 8 hours.
  - Phenobarbital 4–8 mg/kg IV.

## Alternative Drugs

- Intravenous lipid emulsion (intralipids): the lipophilicity of SCBs has not been established. As of February 2023, there is one canine case report indicating successful use of intralipid therapy. Clinical signs improved within 15 hours, allowing for extubation of the intubated patient. Intralipids may be considered in severely affected cases, but efficacy is not established, and its use may hinder the effectiveness of other therapeutic drugs.
- 1.5 mL/kg bolus followed by 0.25 mL/kg/min CRI × 30–60 minutes. Either repeat the 1.5 mL/kg bolus q 4–6 hours or start CRI of 0.5 mL/kg/h for up to one day. Monitor for lipemia, withholding intralipids if noted.

## Precautions/Interactions

- A drug or medication interaction profile is not available for SCBs. Interactions are unlikely on an acute basis. Chronic drug interactions are not likely applicable, but may reflect those noted with THC.

## Extracorporeal Therapy

- Use of extracorporeal therapy has not been reported or evaluated in animals exposed to SCBs.

## Surgical Considerations

- Monitoring of heart rate, blood pressure, and body temperature is indicated with concomitant anesthetic use.

## Patient Monitoring

- Vitals – tachycardia, bradycardia, hyperthermia, hypothermia.
- Blood pressures – hypertension.

## Diet

- Gastrointestinal diet as needed.

    **COMMENTS**

- Coingestions – baked goods or edibles may contain chocolate, raisins, macadamia nuts, or xylitol.
- SCBs be laced with other stimulant drugs such as caffeine.

## Prevention/Avoidance

- Prevent patient access to SCB edibles, smoke, and vapor.
- Police-duty dogs may benefit from a muzzle in high-risk environments.

## Possible Complications

- Aspiration pneumonia.
- Rare myoglobinuria.
- Liver or renal damage.

## Expected Course and Prognosis

- As based on case reports, recovery is expected within 24 hours for most patients.
- The duration of signs may be shorter with ingestion of edible products.
- Severe signs of liver failure, acute kidney injury, and death have been reported in humans.

## See Also

Chapter 35 Cannabidiol (CBD)
Chapter 36 Club Drugs (MDMA, GHB, Flunitrazepam, Bath Salts)
Chapter 39 Marijuana (THC)

## Abbreviations

- SCB = synthetic cannabinoid
- THC = tetrahydrocannabinol
- ECS = endocannabinoid system
- LSD = lysergic acid diethylamide
- MDMA = 3,4-methyl enedioxy methamphetamine

## Suggested Reading

Cital S, Kramer K, Hughston L et al. *Cannabis Therapy in Veterinary Medicine: A Complete Guide.* Cham: Springer International Publishing, 2021.

Kelmer E, Shimshoni JA, Merbl Y et al. Use of gas chromatography–mass spectrometry for definitive diagnosis of synthetic cannabinoid toxicity in a dog. *J Vet Emerg Crit Care* 2019;29(5):573–577.

Obafemi AI, Kleinschmidt K, Goto C et al. Cluster of acute toxicity from ingestion of synthetic cannabinoid-laced brownies. *J Med Tox* 2015;11:426–429.

Solimini R, Busardò FP, Rotolo M et al. Hepatotoxicity associated to synthetic cannabinoids use. *Eur Rev Med Pharmacol Sci* 2017;21(1 Suppl):1–6.

Williams K, Wells RJ, McLean MK. Suspected synthetic cannabinoid toxicosis in a dog. *J Vet Emerg Crit Care* 2015;25(6):739–744.

## Acknowledgment

The author and editors acknowledge the prior contributions of Kelly Sioris, PharmD, CSPI, who authored this topic in the previous edition.

**Author**: Holly Hommerding, DVM, DABT, DABVT
**Consulting Editor**: Lynn R. Hovda, RPh, DVM, MS, DACVIM

# Drugs: Over the Counter

# Chapter 45

# Acetaminophen

## DEFINITION/OVERVIEW

- Acetaminophen is the active ingredient in many over-the-counter and human prescription analgesics and fever reducers.
- It is also known as paracetamol.
- It is primarily used to treat pain and fever in humans and is available in various concentrations for children and adults.
- It can also be used in dogs to manage fever and mild pain at dosages of 10–15 mg/kg every 8–12 hours. However, there is no safe use in cats.
- It is available in liquid, tablet, capsule, caplet, gel caps/gel tabs, chewable, and extended-release forms.
- It can be found in hundreds of products, and is often combined with other active ingredients in medicines used to treat allergy, cough, colds, flu, pain, and insomnia.
- Toxicosis can occur when it is administered to dogs and cats and by accidental ingestions. Some formulations are flavored and can entice dogs and cats if found in the household.
- Cats are particularly susceptible to toxicosis.

## ETIOLOGY/PATHOPHYSIOLOGY

### Mechanism of Action

- Acetaminophen is a centrally acting analgesic and antipyretic with minimal antiinflammatory properties.
- The mechanism of action for reducing pain is unknown but may be related to inhibition of prostaglandin synthesis.
- It reduces fever by inhibiting the formulation and release of prostaglandins in the CNS and by the inhibiting endogenous pyrogens at the hypothalamic thermoregulator center.
- Intoxication after ingestion of supratherapeutic doses is related to the biotransformation of the parent compound to reactive metabolites.

### Pharmacokinetics or Toxicokinetics – Absorption, Distribution, Metabolism, Excretion

- In dogs, oral bioavailability is variable, ranging from 45% to 98% after oral administration.
- Absorption is not different between fasted and fed dogs.
- Protein binding is low with only 10–25% bound to plasma proteins.
- Distribution is wide throughout the body except fat and similar in dogs and cats.

---

*Blackwell's Five-Minute Veterinary Consult Clinical Companion: Small Animal Toxicology*, Third Edition.
Edited by Lynn R. Hovda, Ahna G. Brutlag, Robert H. Poppenga, and Steven E. Epstein.
© 2024 John Wiley & Sons, Inc. Published 2024 by John Wiley & Sons, Inc.

- Metabolism in the liver is extensive, and biotransformation to toxic metabolites is responsible for the toxicity seen.
- Biotransformation to nontoxic metabolites is primarily through phase 2 conjugation with sulfate and glucuronide. Because cats have relatively poor capacity for glucuronide conjugation, a majority of ingested doses undergoes oxidation via phase 1 cytochrome P450 isoenzyme metabolism.
- Toxic reactive metabolites can undergo further detoxification through glutathione conjugation, but this pathway can saturate quickly after toxic doses.
- Methemoglobinemia is thought to occur due to *p*-aminophenol, a reactive toxic metabolite formed in red blood cells that oxidizes hemoglobin to methemoglobin. Dogs and cats lack the enzyme N-acetyltransferase (NAT) isoform 2 which would convert *p*-aminophenol back to acetaminophen.
- The half-life (oral) in dogs is ~1–4 hours and five hours in cats.
- Excretion is primarily through renal clearance, with a small amount undergoing biliary excretion.

## Toxicity

- Dogs.
  - Keratoconjunctivitis sicca (KCS) has been reported at 30–40 mg/kg.
  - Hepatotoxicity has been reported at 100–150 mg/kg although, in some dogs, this many not occur until 600 mg/kg.
  - Methemoglobinemia may occur starting at 100–200 mg/kg, with 200 mg/kg being a more common dose of concern.
- Cats.
- Methemoglobinemia and death reported in one feline at 10 mg/kg although 40–50 mg/kg is a more commonly considered toxic dose.

## Systems Affected

- Hepatobiliary.
  - Once sulfation and glucuronide detoxification pathways have been saturated, biotransformation to highly reactive metabolites occurs, which also quickly exhausts cellular glutathione.
  - The result is the rapid increase in the highly reactive N-acetyl-p-benzoquinone imine (NAPQI), which covalently binds with protein macromolecules in hepatocytes, causing cell death and centrilobular degeneration of the liver.
  - Liver cell death also occurs from free radical injury produced by acetaminophen.
  - Microcirculatory changes induced through neutrophil activation and microvascular plugging exacerbate hepatic injury and extend necrosis through ischemic infarction of the periacinar region.
- Hemic/lymphatic/immune.
  - Heinz body and methemoglobin formation occurs with subsequent hemolytic anemia due to oxidative injury to red blood cells and hemoglobin molecules.
  - Methemoglobin is commonly seen in cats, but seldom in dogs.
- Renal/urological.
  - Experimental studies in mice have resulted in proximal tubular necrosis through covalent binding of reactive metabolites.
- Ophthalmic.
  - KCS may occur with overdose.

## SIGNALMENT/HISTORY

### Risk Factors

- Toxic doses are significantly lower in cats, and any exposure in cats should be considered potentially life-threatening.
- Because acetaminophen is commonly available as an over-the-counter analgesic, it may be administered by well-meaning pet owners who are unaware of its potential for toxicity, especially in cats.
- Accidental exposures can occur when medications containing acetaminophen are left out with easy access by pets. Many formulations for children are flavored and may entice pets to ingest them when easily accessible.
- It is critically important to ask owners about possible exposures especially since many may not be aware of its potential toxicity.

### Historical Findings

- Owners may initially observe a change in appetite with or without vomiting.
- Lethargy may occur during the acute phase of toxicity before hepatotoxic findings are observed.
- In cats, distal forelimb and facial swelling may be observed.

## CLINICAL FEATURES

- In cats, facial and distal forelimb swelling may be noted. This rarely occurs in dogs.
- Abdominal tensing and tenderness on palpation.
- Liver tenderness or swelling on palpation.
- Icterus/jaundice from hepatotoxicity.
- Cyanotic or grey mucous membranes may be observed in the presence of methemoglobinemia.
- Pale mucous membranes may be observed in the presence of anemia.
- Ocular discharge and other signs associated with KCS may occur.

## DIFFERENTIAL DIAGNOSIS

- Any toxin that can result in acute hepatonecrosis, including:
  - aflatoxins
  - amatoxin mushroom ingestions (i.e., *Amanita phalloides*)
  - certain drug exposures (carprofen, ketoconazole, lomustine, methimazole, mitotane, sulfonamides, and others)
  - cyanobacteria (i.e., blue-green algae)
  - sago palm
  - xylitol.
- Other causes of anemia and methemoglobinemia.
  - Oxidative damage to red blood cells (onions, garlic, zinc).

## DIAGNOSTICS

### Clinical Pathological Findings

- Serum ALT and AST concentrations may rise within 24 hours after ingestion and peak within 48–72 hours.
- Serum bilirubin concentrations may begin to rise within 24 hours of exposure.

- Serum albumin concentrations may decrease 2–3 days after exposure as liver function declines.
- Hypoglycemia and prolongation of clotting parameters such as PT/PTT may be associated with severe liver failure.
- Excessive Heinz bodies or Heinz body anemia and/or methemoglobinemia may occur.

## Other Diagnostics

- Serum acetaminophen analysis is not commonly available, but if possible to measure, a four-hour postexposure concentration can confirm toxic exposures.
- Schirmer tear test (STT) if KCS is suspected.

## Pathological Findings

- Zone 3 (centrilobular or distal acinar) degeneration with hepatocellular necrosis.
- Acute proximal tubular necrosis in some cases.

# THERAPEUTICS

## Detoxification

- Induce vomiting within two hours of ingestion so long as the patient is able to protect their airway with an intact gag reflex.
- Administer one dose of activated charcoal (1–2 g/kg) with a cathartic (e.g., sorbitol) within a few hours of presentation. Multiple doses of activated charcoal are not indicated.

## Appropriate Health Care

- Supportive care to include administration of IV fluids and correction of electrolyte imbalances, especially in cases with acute vomiting.
- Provide supplemental oxygen as indicated.
- Administer packed red blood cells as indicated.

## Antidote

- The antidote is N-acetylcysteine (NAC) which is used for prevention of acute liver injury by limiting the formation of toxic metabolites, providing a substrate for sulfation, replenishing glutathione substrates, and binding directly to toxic metabolites.
  - NAC is available as a human pharmaceutical as an injectable solution (20%) and as an inhalation/oral solution (10% or 20%) which can be administered IV or orally. If charcoal has recently been administered, IV dosing is recommended. Oral capsules are also available but not recommended for first-line use in a poisoning scenario.
    - IV dosing: dilute using D5W to a 3–4% solution. If using the oral/inhalation solution, filter with a 0.22 micron filter prior to diluting.
    - Oral dosing using oral/inhalation solution: dilute to at least a 5% solution using enticing liquid or soft food to reduce the risk of tissue irritation/spontaneous emesis. Because of an offensive, sulfurous odor and taste, a feeding tube may be required.
  - Loading/initial dosage of 140–180 mg/kg (slowly IV), followed by 70 mg/kg q 4–6 hours for 7–17 doses total.

## Drug(s) of Choice

- Antioxidant therapy.
  - S-adenosyl-methionine (SAMe) 18 mg/kg/day orally to help reduce oxidative damage.

- • Ascorbic acid (vitamin C) 30 mg/kg orally, SQ, or IV q 6 hours as an antioxidant to reduce methemoglobin to oxyhemoglobin.
- ■ Antiemetic therapy.
  - • Maropitant (1 mg/kg SC or IV over 1–2 minutes), ondansetron, and dolasetron at standard doses as needed for vomiting.

### Precautions/Interactions

- ■ Use caution when administering activated charcoal with other oral therapeutic agents such as N-acetylcysteine and antiemetics as it may reduce their effects. It is best to administer therapeutic drugs at least two hours before or after activated charcoal administration.

### Alternative Drugs

- ■ Fresh frozen plasma 10–20 mL/kg IV over 3–4 hours as indicated for coagulopathy due to severe hepatic dysfunction, based on PT/PTT results.
- ■ Vitamin $K_1$ 2.5–5 mg/kg, SQ or orally with fatty meal, given once per day, or in divided doses every 12 hours, as adjunctive therapy for coagulopathy due to severe hepatic dysfunction.
- ■ Methylene blue, 1% solution, 1–1.5 mg/kg slow IV over several minutes for 1–2 doses to treat severe methemoglobinemia. Must be used with caution in cats because it can cause Heinz body anemia.

### Patient Monitoring

- ■ CBC and serum biochemistry panel on presentation and every 4–6 hours to monitor for serial changes in ALT, AST, and bilirubin concentrations, and possible development of anemia and methemoglobinemia.
  - • Methemoglobin may be recognized as dark brown blood.
  - • Blood smears can be used to identify Heinz bodies on the surfaces of red blood cells.
- ■ Hypoglycemia and hypoalbuminemia may be present with worsening hepatic function.
- ■ Coagulopathy as evidenced by prolonged PT/PTT may also be present in cases of severe hepatic dysfunction.

### Diet

- ■ Standard maintenance diet as tolerated, but may need to premedicate with antiemetics during acute phase of toxicity, and while administering N-acetylcysteine.

 **COMMENTS**

### Prevention/Avoidance

- ■ Acetaminophen should never be administered to cats.
- ■ Acetaminophen should only be used in dogs with direct veterinary supervision and guidance.
- ■ Pet proofing and client education are critically important to avoid accidental and intentional exposures.

### Possible Complications

- ■ Methemoglobinemia may present as a life-threatening emergency. However, it is important to remember that even if the cat or dog is treated and recovers from methemoglobinemia, severe hepatic dysfunction may ensue if appropriate therapies to prevent it are not implemented soon after exposure. Therefore, administration of NAC is recommended while undergoing therapy for methemoglobinemia in the initial hours after exposure.

## Expected Course and Prognosis

- Evidence of improvement includes resolving respiratory distress associated with resolution of methemoglobinemia along with normalization of mucous membrane color, improvement of laboratory values, resolving facial and distal forelimb edema, normal appetite and tolerance of food and water, and normal affect and energy levels.
- A good prognosis is associated with serum concentrations of AST, ALT, and bilirubin trending back to reference range values.
- Ongoing severe hepatic dysfunction with changes in mentation, coagulopathy, and worsening hemodynamic stability are associated with a poor prognosis.

## Synonyms

- Tylenol toxicosis.
- Paracetamol toxicosis.

## Abbreviations

- KCS = keratoconjunctivitis sicca
- NAC = N-acetylcysteine
- NAPQI = N-acetyl-p-benzoquinone imine
- NAT = N-acetyltransferase
- STT = Schirmer tear test

## Suggested Reading

Bischoff K. Toxicity of over-the-counter drugs. In: Gupta RC (ed.) *Veterinary Toxicology*, 3rd edn. San Diego: Academic Press Elsevier, 2018.

McConkey SE, Grant DM, Cribb AE. The role of para-aminophenol in acetaminophen-induced methemoglobinemia in dogs and cats. *J Vet Pharmacol Ther* 2009;32(6):585–590.

Nelson K. Paracetamol toxicity in dogs. *Vet Rec* 2019;184(19):594.

Sartini I, Lebkowska-Wieruszewska B, Lisowski A, Poapolathep A, Cuniberti B, Giorgi M. Pharmacokinetics of acetaminophen after intravenous and oral administration in fasted and fed Labrador Retriever dogs. *J Vet Pharmacol Ther* 2021;44:28–35.

**Author:** John H. Tegzes, MA, VMD, Dipl. ABVT
**Consulting Editor:** Ahna G. Brutlag, DVM, MS, DABT, DABVT

# Aspirin

## DEFINITION/OVERVIEW

- Aspirin (acetylsalicylic acid, ASA), is a common NSAID and antipyretic medication.
- Indications in veterinary medicine are antithrombotic therapy (dogs/cats), osteoarthritis pain (dogs), and fever reduction (dogs/cats).
- Toxic effects are dose dependent, ranging from GI side-effects to multiple organ failure and death.

## ETIOLOGY/PATHOPHYSIOLOGY

### Mechanism of Action

- Nonselective prostaglandin inhibitor.
- Causes irreversible inhibition of COX needed to produce thromboxane, prostacyclin, and other prostaglandins.
- Inhibition of thromboxane and prostacyclin disrupts platelet aggregation, altering hemostasis.
- Inhibition of $PGE_2$ production disrupts normal GI and renal blood flow.
- Salicylates alter the Krebs cycle, leading to organ dysfunction from uncoupling of oxidative phosphorylation.

### Pharmacokinetics or Toxicokinetics – Absorption, Distribution, Metabolism, Excretion

- Easily and rapidly absorbed in the stomach and proximal small intestine.
- Metabolized by the liver, intestines, and RBCs to salicylic acid.
- Salicyclic acid is highly protein bound (70–90%) and conjugated with glucuronate and glycine.
- Conjugated forms of salicyclic acid are excreted in urine.
- Half-life of aspirin at 25 mg/kg dose: dog 4–6 hours, cat 38–45 hours. Half-life increases with repeated exposure up to 18–28 hours.
- Cats have a prolonged half-life due to decreased amounts of glucuronyl transferase.
- When large quantities of aspirin are ingested, glucuronide conjugation is saturated, decreasing the excretion rate.
- Excreted metabolites of aspirin lower the urinary pH, enabling renal tubular reabsorption and therefore prolonging the half-life

*Blackwell's Five-Minute Veterinary Consult Clinical Companion: Small Animal Toxicology*, Third Edition.
Edited by Lynn R. Hovda, Ahna G. Brutlag, Robert H. Poppenga, and Steven E. Epstein.
© 2024 John Wiley & Sons, Inc. Published 2024 by John Wiley & Sons, Inc.

## Toxicity

- Intoxication is dose dependent.
- Single dose of 25 mg/kg in dogs has provoked gastric bleeding which started within 24 hours.
- Mild toxicity (≤50 mg/kg) limited to GI side-effects (vomiting, inappetence, and/or diarrhea).
- Significant toxicity reported with 100–500 mg/kg in dogs and multiple doses of 80 mg/kg in cats.
- Exposures to ≥100 mg/kg has fatal potential.
- Chronic administration of 23 mg/kg PO q 8 hours for ≥6 days produced gastric lesions in an experimental dog model.
- Enteric-coated aspirin tablets are less likely to lead to GI ulceration/intoxication.

## Systems Affected

- Gastrointestinal – vomiting, hematemesis, diarrhea, melena, GI ulceration/erosions.
- Hematological – anemia from GI hemorrhage, primary bone marrow suppression, or Heinz body formation (cats).
- Renal/urological – azotemia, ARF, anuria, sodium retention, fluid overload.
- Hepatobiliary – hepatopathy documented with high doses in cats.
- Respiratory – respiratory depression secondary to muscle weakness from hypokalemia and CNS depression, pulmonary edema.
- Nervous – CNS depression, seizures, cerebral edema (rare), coma, and death.
- Endocrine/metabolic – respiratory alkalosis progressing to metabolic acidosis

 # SIGNALMENT/HISTORY

- Intoxication occurs by accidental ingestion of OTC medication, complications from prescribed chronic administration, or well-meaning attempts of the pet owner that exceed therapeutic dosages.

## Risk Factors

- Patients with coagulopathy, underlying renal disease, and/or hypoalbuminemia are more susceptible to toxicity.
- Cats are at greater risk given their prolonged half-life due to decreased amounts of glucuronyl transferase.
- Concurrent steroid or prescription NSAIDs administration will increase risk of GI ulceration.
- Concurrent furosemide increases aspirin activity, especially at higher aspirin doses.
- Old and/or expired aspirin may have more toxic effect as already degraded into salicylic and acetic acid active forms.

## Historical Findings

- Chewed bottle or aspirin containers found by owner at home.
- Owners report they medicated their pet with OTC medications containing aspirin-related products (including Pepto-Bismol® which contains bismuth subsalicylate).
- Owners report current aspirin administration or NSAID prescriptions.

 # CLINICAL FEATURES

- Signs usually apparent within several hours after ingestion, but some clinical signs may be delayed for several days (e.g., melena from GI ulceration, septic peritonitis from GI perforation).

- GI signs (vomiting/diarrhea with or without melena) which may lead to dehydration.
- Abdominal pain may be noted secondary to GI cramping, GI ulceration, or septic peritonitis.
- Pale mucous membranes, prolonged CRT, and poor femoral pulse quality may be present secondary to anemia or hypovolemia from gastrointestinal blood loss.
- Altered mentation from obtundation to severe coma.
- Seizures possible at high doses.
- Tachypnea, increased respiratory effort, or dyspnea due to pain or metabolic acidosis.
- Pulmonary crackles on auscultation if pulmonary edema is present.
- Hyperthermia may be present due to uncoupling of oxidative phosphorylation.
- If pregnant, possible stillbirth or abortion complications.

 # DIFFERENTIAL DIAGNOSIS

- Intoxication from other substances containing salicylates such as Pepto-Bismol (bismuth subsalicylate), headache remedies, topical analgesics such as Bengay® (methyl salicylate), oxycodone with aspirin combinations, and oil of wintergreen (methyl salicylate).
- NSAID toxicosis (e.g., carprofen, grapiprant, meloxicam).
- Steroid-induced GI signs.
- Primary or secondary coagulopathy (e.g., thrombocytopenia, etc.).
- Primary gastrointestinal disease (usually more chronic signs).
- Metabolic disease (e.g., renal, hepatic, hypoadrenocorticism).

 # DIAGNOSTICS

## Clinical Pathological Findings

- PCV/TS to evaluate for anemia from GI ulceration.
- If anemia is present without blood loss, perform a blood smear to screen for the presence of Heinz bodies, particularly in cats.
- Electrolytes checked for hypokalemia and hypernatremia due to dehydration and GI losses.
- Liver function parameters as increased liver enzymes (e.g., ALP, AST, ALT, and GGT) can be seen with hepatotoxicity. These signs may be delayed.
- Kidney values and USG should be monitored to evaluate renal status. Signs may be delayed. Recommended to repeat values 24–48 hours after presentation to help monitor for development of ARF/AKI.
- Blood gas analysis may show an early respiratory alkalosis with progressive metabolic acidosis as poisoning progresses.
- Increased anion gap may be seen due to increased lactate, ketone production, and the presence of salicylates themselves.
- Blood glucose should be initially evaluated and monitored.
- Patients exhibiting bleeding tendencies and/or hepatic insufficiency warrant evaluation of the hemostatic system, which may include platelet count, PT, PTT, ACT, BMBT, or rarely TEG.

## Other Diagnostics

- Thoracic radiographs are indicated to evaluate for pulmonary edema if dyspnea, tachypnea, or hypoxemia is observed and/or pulmonary crackles are auscultated.
- Focused ultrasound of the abdomen (AFAST) should be performed to evaluate for the presence of free abdominal fluid.

# THERAPEUTICS

## Detoxification

- Induce emesis if ingestion occurred up to several hours before presentation, provided the patient is asymptomatic and able to protect their airway.
- If emesis unsuccessful and high-dose exposure, then consider gastric lavage only if ingestion was within 1–2 hours and an abdominal radiograph confirms the presence of gastric contents. If performed, should be done under anesthesia with patient intubated to protect airway.
- Activated charcoal with a cathartic in massive overdose cases of sustained-release or enteric-coated tablets.
- Repeated doses of activated charcoal (without cathartic) should be given orally every 6–8 hours for 24 hours to prevent enterohepatic circulation.

## Appropriate Health Care

- IV fluids to prevent dehydration, treat hypovolemia, and promote renal and GI perfusion, and vasodilate renal vessels.
- Urine alkalinization therapy, with target urine pH within 7.5–8.0 and systemic pH within 7.35–7.5. This is usually attained by adding 1–2 mEq/kg of sodium bicarbonate, diluted with sterile water in a 1:1 ratio and administered IV over 1–2 hours. Once target range is reached, repeat urine and blood pH q 2–4 hours.
- In severely hypoproteinemic patients, consider enteral nutrition using liquid feedings via a nasoesophageal or nasogastric tube if patient is not eating.
- If severe blood loss (typically from the GIT), consider whole blood or packed red blood cell transfusions.
- If hepatopathy with concurrent coagulopathy is present, initiate vitamin $K_1$ supplementation and/or S-adenosyl-methionine (SAMe) supplementation.
- If pulmonary edema present leading to hypoxemia/dyspnea, then oxygen supplementation via oxygen cage, nasal cannula, or other means of low flow oxygen is indicated.
- Consider desmopressin SQ therapy in patient if active blood loss with prolonged BMBT.

## Antidotes

- No antidote.

## Drug(s) of Choice

- Misoprostol (2–5 mcg/kg, PO q 8 hours) has been demonstrated to help prevent aspirin-induced GI ulceration.
- GI protectant (e.g., sucralfate 250–1000 mg, PO q 6–8 hours). Make sure separated from other medications or feedings by 1–2 hours.
- Proton pump inhibitors (e.g., pantoprazole 1 mg/kg, IV q 12 hours or omeprazole 1 mg/kg, PO q 12 hours).
- $H_2$-blockers (e.g., famotidine 1 mg/kg, IV, SC, or PO q 12 hours).
- Consider antiemetics (e.g., ondansetron 0.5–1 mg/kg IV/PO q 8 hours or maropitant 1 mg/kg, SQ/IV q 24 hours) for persistent vomiting if contraindications such as a GI perforation/septic abdomen have been ruled out.
- If high-dose toxicosis, then cholestyramine (0.3–0.5 g/kg, dissolved in liquid and administered orally every 6–8 hours for 3–5 days) can be added to therapy.

## Precautions/Interactions

- Concurrent NSAIDs or steroid should be avoided.
- Other protein-bound drugs may alter metabolism of aspirin.
- Aspirin may increase active amount of digoxin in blood and prolong its half-life.
- Aspirin may be more active in patients on concurrent furosemide therapy.

## Extracorporeal Therapy

- CRRT/hemodialysis should only be considered for patients who develop ARF, fluid overload, or persistent acidosis, or have deterioration of their neurological status.

## Surgical Considerations

- Abdominal surgery is reserved for those patients who develop a septic abdomen from a perforated GI ulcer or those with GI ulcers causing excessive hemorrhage.

## Patient Monitoring

- Electrolytes at least daily with IV fluid therapy, or more if indicated.
- Blood glucose should be monitored at baseline and then if clinically indicated thereafter.
- Acid–base status to help guide alkanization therapy and help offset progressive metabolic acidosis.
- Monitor respiratory effort/rate closely. Consider $SPO_2$, arterial blood gas monitoring, thoracic radiographs, and/or TFAST exam if concerns for hypoxia arise.
- For high-dose toxicity exposure, urinary catheter placement can be considered to monitor UOP due to potential for AKI to develop.
- UA may show evidence of renal damage (e.g., casts prior to the development of azotemia).
- Monitor neurological status; if cerebral edema suspected, mannitol should be administered (0.5–1.0 g/kg, IV over 20 minutes using an in-line IV filter).

## Diet

- A bland diet is recommended for those showing GI signs (vomiting, diarrhea).

 **COMMENTS**

### Prevention/Avoidance

- Prevention includes educating owners to store all OTC medication out of reach and refrain from using aspirin for treatment as analgesic/antiinflammatory/antipyrexic in pets.

### Possible Complications

- Chronic renal damage may be a problem for those dogs and/or cats that develop azotemia after toxic exposures.

### Expected Course and Prognosis

- Prognosis varies depending on amount ingested.
- For lower doses (≤50 mg/kg), prognosis is likely good with supportive care for GI side-effects.
- For higher exposures (≥50 mg/kg), prognosis can be poor to guarded if multiple organ dysfunction develops, to fair if patient is treated aggressively and early.

## Synonyms

- Salicylate toxicity, acetylsalicylic acid toxicity, ASA toxicity, NSAID toxicity, nonsteroidal antiinflammatories.

## See Also

Chapter 51 Human NSAIDs (Ibuprofen, Naproxen)
Chapter 61 Veterinary NSAIDs

## Abbreviations

- OTC = over the counter
- ARF = acute renal failure
- AKI = acute kidney injury

## Suggested Reading

Alwood AJ. Salicylates. In: Silverstein DC, Hopper K (eds) *Small Animal Critical Care Medicine*. St Louis: WB Saunders, 2009.

Curry SL, Cogar SM, Cook JL, Nonsteroidal anti-inflammatory drugs: a review. *J Am Anim Hosp Assoc* 2005;41:298–309.

Khan SA, McLean M. Toxicology of frequently encountered nonsteroidal anti-inflammatory drugs in dogs and cats. *Vet Clin North Am Small Anim Pract* 2012;42(2):289–306.

Lee J. *Decontamination of the Poisoned Patient: What's the Evidence and Does it Work?* Western Veterinary Conference, Las Vegas, 2020.

Steele C, Stefanovski D. Clinical outcomes and prognostic factors associated with nonsteroidal anti-inflammatory drug overdose in dogs presented to an emergency room. *J Vet Emerg Crit Care* 2021;31(5):638–646.

**Author**: Megan Kaplan, DVM, DACVECC
**Consulting Editor**: Ahna G. Brutlag, DVM, MS, DABT, DABVT

# Chapter 47

# Calcium Supplements

## DEFINITION/OVERVIEW

- Calcium supplements come in a variety of formulations and concentrations, available both over the counter and by prescription.
- Commonly available calcium salts include calcium carbonate, calcium gluconate, calcium chloride, calcium acetate, and calcium citrate.
- Vomiting and diarrhea are the most common clinical signs associated with calcium supplement intoxication and are typically mild and self-limiting.
- If a very large quantity of calcium supplements is ingested, transient hypercalcemia may occur.
- Calcium alone is generally poorly absorbed by the GI tract, therefore many calcium supplements also contain vitamin $D_3$ which enhances calcium absorption and can increase risk of intoxication.

## ETIOLOGY/PATHOPHYSIOLOGY

### Mechanism of Action

- Ingestion of calcium salts (without vitamin $D_3$) typically only causes irritation to the GI tract.
- Ingestion of large quantities of calcium can result in transiently elevated blood calcium concentrations.
- Hypercalcemia can lead to:
  - increased excitation threshold of nerve and muscle cells, causing cardiac arrhythmias, weakness, and lethargy.
  - decreased contractility of smooth muscle in GI tract potentially causing constipation.
  - increased gastrin secretion leading to increased hydrochloric acid secretion, which in turn causes GI irritation.
  - inhibited ADH receptors in the renal tubules, leading to polyuria with compensatory polydypsia (secondary nephrogenic diabetes insipidus).
- Persistent hypercalcemia can lead to development of calcium deposits in the kidneys, cardiac vessels, and GI tract.
- Deposition of calcium in the renal tubules causes mineralization and kidney failure.
- Hypercalcemia, metabolic alkalosis, and kidney damage due to chronic use of oral calcium carbonate supplements have been described in humans. This is known as calcium-alkali syndrome and is characterized by the following:

*Blackwell's Five-Minute Veterinary Consult Clinical Companion: Small Animal Toxicology*, Third Edition.
Edited by Lynn R. Hovda, Ahna G. Brutlag, Robert H. Poppenga, and Steven E. Epstein.
© 2024 John Wiley & Sons, Inc. Published 2024 by John Wiley & Sons, Inc.

- Hypercalcemia caused by increased oral intake of calcium exceeding renal excretion of calcium.
- Decreased GFR caused by increased sodium excretion and fluid loss secondary to hypercalcemia.
- Development of metabolic alkalosis due to hypovolemia-induced reabsorption of calcium and bicarbonate in the kidney.

## Pharmacokinetics or Toxicokinetics – Adsorption, Distribution, Metabolism, Excretion

- Calcium salts are poorly absorbed from the GI tract.
- Activated vitamin $D_3$ is necessary for calcium absorption.
- A small portion of calcium is distributed to the intracellular and extracellular fluid. The majority of calcium is taken up by bone.
- Approximately 80% of calcium is eliminated in the feces, and 20% is eliminated by the kidneys.

## Toxicity

- Acute ingestions of calcium supplements do not typically result in clinical signs of hypercalcemia and toxicosis in healthy animals.
- Vitamin $D_3$ in the supplement significantly increases risk of clinically relevant hypercalcemia.

## Systems Affected

- Gastrointestinal – vomiting, diarrhea, anorexia, constipation.
- Endocrine/metabolic – transient hypercalcemia.
- Musculoskeletal – weakness.
- Nervous – depression.
- Renal/urological – PU/PD, rarely azotemia, oliguria, decreased GFR, renal mineralization, nephroliths, cystic calculi.
- Cardiovascular – arrhythmias.

 # SIGNALMENT/HISTORY

- All breeds and species are susceptible to GI irritation.

## Risk Factors

- Patients with renal impairment are at increased risk of complications associated with hypercalcemia.

## Historical Findings

- Owners most commonly report lethargy, vomiting, and diarrhea. PU/PD may occur if sustained hypercalcemia develops.

## Location and Circumstances of Poisoning

- Most ingestions will occur at home but calcium overdose may occur within the hospital setting.

 # CLINICAL FEATURES

- Mild and self-limiting GI distress (vomiting, diarrhea) are the most likely clinical signs following an acute ingestion of calcium supplements.
- Though transient hypercalcemia may occur following ingestion, it is rarely clinically significant.

- If enough vitamin D$_3$ has been ingested in conjunction with the calcium ingestion, clinical signs of hypercalcemia could be expected (PU/PD, weakness, lethargy, nausea, vomiting, diarrhea, constipation).

# DIFFERENTIAL DIAGNOSIS

- Other causes of gastrointestinal upset:
  - Pancreatitis.
  - Dietary indiscretion.
  - GI obstruction.
  - Infectious or inflammatory GI diseases.
- Other causes of hypercalcemia:
  - Vitamin D intoxication.
  - Hypercalcemia of malignancy.
  - Hyperparathyroidism.
  - Fungal disease.
  - Feline idiopathic hypercalcemia.
  - Hypoadrenocorticism.
  - Renal disease.

# DIAGNOSTICS

### Clinical Pathological Findings

- Acute ingestion of calcium supplements without vitamin D$_3$ is unlikely to result in biochemical abnormalities.
- Chemistry panel should be performed in sick patients and may identify the presence of hypercalcemia, hyperphosphatemia, and azotemia.

### Pathological Findings

- With acute ingestion of calcium supplements, GI irritation may be seen.
- With hypercalcemia, calcification in the kidneys, GI tract walls, and cardiac vessels may be found.

# THERAPEUTICS

### Detoxification

- Induction of emesis can be performed if a large quantity of calcium supplements has been ingested.
- In most cases of calcium supplement ingestion without vitamin D$_3$, no further intervention will be required.
- Unless toxic amounts of vitamin D$_3$ have been consumed along with the calcium supplement, no activated charcoal is required.

### Appropriate Health Care

- If prolonged GI distress develops, symptomatic and supportive care can be provided with fluids (IV or SQ crystalloids depending on severity), antiemetics, and antidiarrheals.

### Drug(s) of Choice

- Antiemetic such as maropitant (1 mg/kg SQ or IV q 24 hours).

## Precautions/Interactions

- The concomitant ingestion of vitamin $D_3$ along with calcium significantly increases the risk of clinically significant hypercalcemia.
- Oral calcium administration has the potential to decrease the GI absorption of several medications including fluoroquinolones, levothyroxine, mycophenolate, oral phosphates, sotalol, and tetracyclines.
- Concurrent use of thiazide diuretics or vitamin A increases the risk of hypercalcemia.

 **COMMENTS**

### Expected Course and Prognosis

- Clinical signs are typically mild and self-limiting in healthy patients and prognosis is good.
- If there is previous renal compromise, the prognosis will depend on the amount of the ingestion, the timing of intervention, and the degree of previous compromise.
- Concomitant vitamin D ingestion will require more aggressive treatment and may change prognosis.

### See Also

Chapter 55 Vitamins and Minerals
Chapter 124 Cholecalciferol

### Suggested Reading

Green T, Chew DJ. Calcium disorders. In: Silverstein DC, Hopper K (eds) *Small Animal Critical Care Medicine*, 2nd edn. St Louis: Saunders Elsevier, 2015; pp. 274–280.
Hiromichi Y, Yoshiyuki M, Kusano E. Renal injury in calcium-alkali syndrome. *J Nephrol Ther* 2012;S3:006.
Messinger JS, Windham WR, Ward CR. Ionized hypercalcemia in dogs: a retrospective study of 109 cases (1998–2003). *J Vet Intern Med* 2009;23(3):514–519.
Plumb DC. Calcium salts. In: *Plumb's Veterinary Drug Handbook*, 9th edn. Ames: Wiley-Blackwell, 2018.

### Acknowledgment

The authors and editors acknowledge the prior contributions of Catherine M. Adams, DVM, who authored this topic in a previous edition.

**Author:** Tracy Julius, DVM, DACVECC
**Consulting Editor:** Ahna G. Brutlag, DVM, MS, DABT, DABVT

# Decongestants (Imidazolines)

## DEFINITION/OVERVIEW

- Imidazolines are a class of drugs commonly found in OTC nasal decongestants and ophthalmic preparations for the relief of redness and inflammation due to their topical vasoconstrictive activity. Examples include oxymetazoline, tetrahydrozoline, naphazoline, and tolazoline.
  - There are several FDA-approved products: Upneeq® (0.1% oxymetazoline ophthalmic solution) used to treat ptosis, Rhofade® (1% oxymetazoline topical cream) used to treat facial erythema associated with rosacea, and Kovanaze® (tetracaine and oxymetazoline nasal spray) used for regional anesthesia for dental procedures.
- They are from a broader class of drugs known as sympathomimetics.
- While generally safe and well tolerated in adult humans, oral overdoses in children have resulted in significant toxicosis. This is because overdosed amounts of the drug tend to have a central effect.
- The central action of the drug leads to significant CNS depression.

## ETIOLOGY/PATHOPHYSIOLOGY

### Mechanism of Action

- Imidazolines are sympathomimetic compounds specific to alpha-2-adrenergic and imidazoline receptors.
- Oxymetazoline and naphazoline have no effect on histamine $H_1$ and $H_2$ receptors.
- Tetrahydrozoline and tolazoline may influence $H_2$ receptors but not $H_1$.
- Imidazolines do not influence beta-adrenergic receptors.
- While imidazolines may bind to both central and peripheral receptors, central binding tends to predominate in overdose situations.
  - Central receptor binding will result in the inhibition of norepinephrine, leading to a decreased sympathetic response. Common side-effects of this binding are hypotension, bradycardia, and lethargy.
  - Peripheral receptor binding will result in vasoconstriction (topical application) and hypertension.

### Pharmacokinetics or Toxicokinetics – Adsorption, Distribution, Metabolism, Excretion

- Information on companion animal pharmacokinetics is limited.
- Systemic absorption may follow topical administration.
- Imidazolines are readily absorbed from the GIT.

*Blackwell's Five-Minute Veterinary Consult Clinical Companion: Small Animal Toxicology*, Third Edition. Edited by Lynn R. Hovda, Ahna G. Brutlag, Robert H. Poppenga, and Steven E. Epstein.
© 2024 John Wiley & Sons, Inc. Published 2024 by John Wiley & Sons, Inc.

- The half-life of most imidazolines is 2–4 hours (humans).
- Widely distributed throughout the body. Though imidazoline receptors have been found in the brain, human studies have shown that their concentrations there were relatively low.
- Human *in vitro* studies show minimal liver metabolism.
- Imidazolines are eliminated, mostly unchanged, in the urine.

## Toxicity

- Imidazolines have a narrow safety margin.
- Oxymetazoline oral $LD_{50}$ (mice): 4700 **mcg/kg**.
- No therapeutic dose known in veterinary literature.

## Systems Affected

- Gastrointestinal – vomiting/GI irritation.
- Nervous – may present as lethargic (most common) or agitated. Lethargy can progress to the point of coma.
- Cardiovascular – initial hypertension progressing to severe hypotension, bradycardia, weakness/lethargy, prolonged CRT, and hypoperfusion.
- Neuromuscular – animals may develop tremors or seizures.
- Respiratory – depression.
- Ophthalmic – miotic pupils.

 # SIGNALMENT/HISTORY

## Risk Factors

- Animals with renal insufficiency may have reduced drug clearance, resulting in more severe or prolonged clinical signs.
- Neonates and geriatric animals may be more severely affected.
- Drugs of this class have a narrow safety margin and unknown therapeutic range.

## Historical Findings

- Witnessed ingestion or administration.
- Discovery of chewed nasal decongestant or "eye-drop" containers.
- The owner may find the animal vomiting, lethargic or in a state of collapse.

## Location and Circumstances of Poisoning

- Exposures generally occur in the home due to unsecured medications.

 # CLINICAL FEATURES

- Onset of symptoms is generally rapid (within 15 minutes).
- Animals may present with initial hypertension and agitation but will likely progress to depression and bradycardia.
- Cardiovascular collapse may be noted.

 # DIFFERENTIAL DIAGNOSIS

- Dependent on the stage of toxicosis.
    - Toxicities – amphetamines, cocaine, other CNS stimulants (early stages).
    - Toxicities – sedatives, opioids, tranquilizers (later stages).

- Primary cardiac disease resulting in bradycardia, hypotension, syncope, etc.
- Trauma or blood loss leading to collapse.

# DIAGNOSTICS

## Clinical Pathological Findings

- Chemistry panel – in severe cases, blood glucose and electrolytes (especially potassium) should be monitored.

## Other Diagnostics

- ECG – may show tachycardia or bradycardia depending on stage of presentation.
- Blood pressure monitoring – may vary between hypertension and hypotension, trending toward hypotension.
- As these cases may be critically ill, 24/7 intensive care (along with the ability to perform blood pressure monitoring) is essential.

## Pathological Findings

- No specific gross or histopathological findings.

# THERAPEUTICS

## Detoxification

- It is NOT recommended to induce vomiting due to the rapid absorption and onset of clinical signs.
- Often, patients present already symptomatic due to rapid onset of signs rendering a risk instead of a benefit. If a patient presents asymptomatic and in the early stages of ingestion, activated charcoal with a cathartic may be administered once.
- Eyes should be flushed with tepid water if ocular exposure occurs.
- Patient should be bathed with liquid dishwashing detergent if dermal exposure occurs to limit oral exposure secondary to grooming.

## Appropriate Health Care

- Hypotension – aggressive IV fluids (e.g., a balanced electrolyte crystalloid at 20–30 mL/kg IV over 20–30 minutes, repeat 2–3× as needed) should be used to correct hypotension, as needed to effect. Diuresis does not enhance drug elimination.
- If patient is persistently hypotensive, vasopressors may be necessary (e.g., dopamine, 5–20 mcg/kg/min IV CRI).
- Frequent monitoring of TPR, HR, blood pressure, mentation, and UOP.

## Antidote

- No specific antidotes are available; however, alpha-2-adrenergic antagonists may be helpful. They may need to be administered multiple times during the course of treatment as their half-life may not be as long as the imidazoline agent.
  - Atipamezole, 50 mcg/kg, to reverse severe sedation and bradycardia. Give one quarter of the dose IV and the remaining three-quarters of the dose IM to avoid worsening hypotension. Another one quarter to one half dose may be considered IV if patient has not responded in 30–60 minutes.
  - Yohimbine, 0.1 mg/kg IV, to reverse severe sedation and bradycardia.

### Drug(s) of Choice

- Diazepam, 0.1–0.5 mg/kg IV or midazolam 0.1–0.3 mg/kg SC, IM, or IV as needed for tremors and hyperactivity.
- Antiemetics if vomiting is protracted (e.g., maropitant, 1 mg/kg SQ q 24 hours).
- Atropine, 0.01–0.02 mg/kg IV, IM, SQ, as needed for bradycardia – see Precautions/ Interactions. While atropine may be considered, there is potential for it to cause a significant increase in mean arterial pressure. Fluids and alpha antagonists are typically the mainstay of treatment.

### Precautions/Interactions

- Do not induce vomiting in symptomatic animals.
- Do not attempt to induce vomiting in a cat exposed to imidazolines with xylazine or medetomidine. This may exacerbate toxicosis.
- Any drug that may decrease blood pressure (e.g., beta-blockers, acepromazine, ACE inhibitors) should be used cautiously.
- Atropine: the concurrent use of atropine with dexmedetomidine, an alpha-2-adrenergic agonist, can increase arterial blood pressure, heart rate, and cardiac work, and may increase the risk for arrhythmias in dogs and is not recommended. There is no evidence to suggest this occurs with imidazoline decongestants but appropriate monitoring is recommended.

### Alternative Drugs

- While most imidazolines are lipophilic, intravenous lipid emulsion therapy is not generally used due to the availability and successful use of alpha-adrenergic antagonists.

### Extracorporeal Therapy

- Hemodialysis is unlikely to be effective due to large volume of distribution.

### Surgical Considerations

- No surgical considerations unless the animal has ingested large amounts of the container, and radiographic evidence or clinical signs of foreign body obstruction are present.

### Patient Monitoring

- Observation may be required for as long as 24–36 hours.
- Patients should be monitored for 4–6 hours after alpha-adrenergic antagonist administration. Alpha-adrenergic antagonists may need to be administered multiple times during the course of treatment as their half-life may not be as long as the imidazoline agent.

### Diet

- Animal may return to normal diet at discharge or may be given several days of bland diet if GI irritation is persistent.

 ## COMMENTS

### Prevention/Avoidance

- Imidazolines are not intended for use in companion animals.
- Imidazolines are readily available in multiple topical preparations and their toxicity is widely underestimated for this reason. Pet owners and clinicians may not make the connection between exposure and signs.
- Store human and veterinary medications separately to avoid mix-ups.

## Possible Complications

- In severe cases, or if treatment is delayed, end-organ damage may be possible due to lack of perfusion.

## Expected Course and Prognosis

- Generally good if treated promptly.
- Patients generally recover in 24–36 hours.
- Follow-up is generally minimal in uncomplicated cases or cases in which clinical signs are easily controlled.

## Synonyms

Oxymetazoline, naphazoline, tetrahydrozoline, tetrazolina, tetryzoline, xylometazoline.

## See Also

Chapter 56 Alpha-2-adrenergic Agonists

## Abbreviations

See Appendix 1 for a complete list.
- ACE = angiotensin-converting enzyme
- UOP = urine output

## Suggested Reading

Khan S. Decongestants (Toxicity) – Toxicology. Merck Veterinary Manual online. 2022. www.msdvetmanual.com/toxicology/toxicities-from-human-drugs/decongestants-toxicity

Means C. Decongestants: imidazolines. In: Plumlee KH (ed.) *Clinical Veterinary Toxicology*. St Louis: Mosby, 2004; pp. 310–311.

**Author**: Kirsten Waratuke, DVM, DABT, DABVT
**Consulting Editor**: Ahna G. Brutlag, DVM, MS, DABT, DABVT

# 49

# Decongestants (Pseudoephedrine, Phenylephrine)

## DEFINITION/OVERVIEW

- Pseudoephedrine (PSE) and phenylephrine (PE) are sympathomimetic drugs with alpha- and beta-adrenergic properties.
- PSE and PE are primarily used by humans for their vasoconstrictive effects; PSE is a stereoisomer of ephedrine (from *Ephedra* spp.; see Chapter 86, Ephedra [Ma Huang]).
- PSE and PE are most commonly found in cough/cold preparations, allergy and asthma medications (PSE), diet pills (PSE), nasal sprays (PE), and hemorrhoid preparations (PE). When present in cough/cold or allergy medications, the presence of PE or PSE is often indicated by a "-D" (for decongestant) suffix in the name (e.g. Claritin-D®).
- In veterinary medicine, PE has been used IV to treat hypotension and shock, intranasally to treat sinusitis, and intraocularly for treatment of ocular disorders and as a diagnostic aid (e.g. Horner syndrome). Oral PSE has been used as an aid in increasing urethral sphincter tone in dogs and as a decongestant in dogs and cats.
- Clinical signs of toxicosis include CNS stimulation, tachycardia, hypertension, decreased appetite, vomiting, mydriasis, and seizures.

## ETIOLOGY/PATHOPHYSIOLOGY

### Mechanism of Action

- PE and PSE stimulate both alpha- and beta-adrenergic receptors by increasing norepinephrine levels.
  - PE stimulates beta-adrenergic receptors only at high doses.
- Pharmacological effects include increased vasoconstriction, heart rate, blood pressure, and coronary blood flow; mild CNS stimulation; increased urethral tone (PSE); and decreased nasal congestion and appetite.

### Pharmacokinetics or Toxicokinetics – Adsorption, Distribution, Metabolism, Excretion

- In humans, PE is extensively metabolized in the GI tract and liver, resulting in a relatively low oral bioavailability. Peak plasma levels are achieved within 30 minutes and the half-life is 2–3 hours. PE crosses the BBB and placenta and passes into the milk. It is excreted primarily unchanged via the urine, with higher excretion rates in acidic urine. Similar data for cats/dogs is not available.
- PSE is well absorbed orally in dogs with bioavailability of 58% and peak plasma levels achieved within 24 minutes. Onset of action is generally less than 30–60 minutes and the

*Blackwell's Five-Minute Veterinary Consult Clinical Companion: Small Animal Toxicology*, Third Edition. Edited by Lynn R. Hovda, Ahna G. Brutlag, Robert H. Poppenga, and Steven E. Epstein. © 2024 John Wiley & Sons, Inc. Published 2024 by John Wiley & Sons, Inc.

half-life is approximately 1.5 hours. PSE is poorly bound to plasma proteins (~20%), crosses the BBB and placenta, and passes into the milk. It is partially metabolized to norpseudoephedrine, an active metabolite. PSE is excreted via the urine, primarily as parent drug, in a pH-dependent fashion.

## Toxicity

- The low bioavailability of PE makes it less toxic orally than other sympathomimetics.
- PE-based hemorrhoid medications may have higher toxicity as their ointment bases may enhance oral transmucosal absorption, bypassing GI first-pass metabolism.
- Hypertension was noted in dogs that ingested 7 mg/kg and 11.9 mg/kg of PE from hemorrhoidal preparations. Hypertension was not reported in dogs ingesting unknown amounts of PE in nasal spray or ocular drops nor in dogs ingesting tablet or capsule forms in dosages ranging from 0.23 to 30 mg/kg.
- PSE has a very narrow window of safety in veterinary medicine, with therapeutic dosages in dogs of 1–2 mg/kg (some dogs show mild signs at therapeutic doses), and moderate-to-severe clinical signs possible at 5–6 mg/kg. Dosages of 10–12 mg/kg have caused fatalities in dogs.

## Systems Affected

- Cardiovascular – peripheral vasoconstriction leads to increased systemic vascular resistance and hypertension with tachycardia or reflex bradycardia. Beta-adrenergic stimulation results in tachycardia, increased contractility/output, and tachyarrhythmias.
- Nervous – stimulation results from endogenous catecholamine release and adrenergic stimulation.
- Metabolic/endocrine – hyperthermia secondary to adrenergic effects (severe).
- Ophthalmic – alpha-adrenergic stimulation causes mydriasis.
- Hemic – DIC (sequela to prolonged seizure activity and hyperthermia).
- Renal – myoglobinuria (sequela to prolonged seizure activity and hyperthermia).

 # SIGNALMENT/HISTORY

## Risk Factors

- All species and breeds are susceptible. Dogs may be at increased risk of accidental exposure due to their inquisitive nature and indiscriminate eating habits.
- Patients with underlying conditions such as cardiovascular disease, seizure disorders, renal insufficiency, narrow-angle glaucoma, or concurrent disease predisposing to hypertension (e.g., immune-mediated hemolytic anemia, hyperthyroidism) are at risk for more severe intoxications.

## Historical Findings

- Intentional exposures due to owners medicating patients with OTC products containing decongestants (e.g., Claritin-D versus regular Claritin).
- Accidental ingestion of owner's medication by pets.
- Acute onset of restlessness, pacing, agitation in previously normal dog or cat.

## Location and Circumstances of Poisoning

- Most patients are exposed to decongestants in the home.

# CLINICAL FEATURES

- Signs generally occur within 30–60 minutes of exposure but can be delayed if extended/sustained/controlled-release products are ingested.
- Clinical signs of PE toxicosis in dogs have included vomiting, lethargy, diarrhea, bradycardia, tachycardia, trembling, and hypertension.
  - Signs reported to an animal poison control center in dogs exposed to PE include vomiting (83%), lethargy (8%), hyperactivity (5%), trembling (5%), panting (3%), diarrhea (3%), bradycardia (2%), tachycardia (2%), and hypertension (1%).
- Clinical signs of PSE toxicosis can include hyperactivity, agitation, mydriasis, vomiting, tachycardia, hypertension (+/− reflex bradycardia), ventricular arrhythmias, hyperthermia, cyanosis, hypersalivation, tremors, and possible seizures. Rarely, cerebral hemorrhage may occur.
  - Patients that exhibit severe or sustained CNS signs and hyperthermia typically have a poorer prognosis.

 # DIFFERENTIAL DIAGNOSIS

- Intoxications: amphetamines, baclofen, ethylene glycol, *Humulus lupulus* (hops), isoniazid, methylxanthines, nicotine, phenylpropanolamine, strychnine.
- Malignant hyperthermia, hypernatremia, encephalitis.

 # DIAGNOSTICS

## Clinical Pathological Findings

- Minimum baseline blood work, including blood glucose, potassium, and venous blood gas, should be performed; no specific changes expected, although hypoglycemia, acidosis or electrolyte abnormalities may occur.
- Geriatric patients or those with underlying metabolic disease should have more extensive blood work done, including CBC, serum chemistry panel, and creatine kinase.

## Other Diagnostics

- PSE will frequently cause a positive reaction for amphetamines in many OTC urine drug test kits for humans.

## Pathological Findings

- No specific pathological lesions are expected.

 # THERAPEUTICS

- The goals of treatment are to prevent absorption, support the cardiovascular and neurological systems, and provide supportive care.

## Detoxification

- If emesis was not induced at home, and the patient is asymptomatic, prompt emesis should be performed by the veterinarian.
- Activated charcoal with a cathartic may be given for one dose in asymptomatic patients.

■ Multidose activated charcoal may be given to patients ingesting sustained-release formulations.
■ Acidifying the urine may enhance excretion of PSE and phenylephrine. Note: severely symptomatic patients may already be acidotic, so evaluation of acid–base status is recommended.

## Appropriate Health Care

■ IV fluid therapy should be administered to aid in perfusion and excretion of the drug, maintain hydration, and help cool the patient (if hyperthermic).
■ Cooling measures for hyperthermia; cooling measures should be discontinued at 103.5 °F.

## Antidote

■ There is no antidote for PE or PSE intoxication.

## Drug(s) of Choice

■ In patients demonstrating agitation or anxiety, sedation should be used; phenothiazines are preferred as they block dopaminergic and alpha-adrenergic activity (see Precautions/Interactions).
  • Acepromazine 0.02–1.0 mg/kg, IV slowly, IM, or SC PRN to effect; select dose based on severity of signs and titrate to effect.
  • Chlorpromazine 0.5–1 mg/kg, IV or IM PRN to effect; select dose based on severity of signs and titrate to effect. Cumulative dosages up to 10–15 mg/kg have been necessary.
■ In patients with tachycardia (dog >180 bpm; cat >220 bpm), a fast-acting beta-blocker should be used.
  • Propranolol 0.02 mg/kg IV slowly, up to a maximum of 0.1 mg/kg.
  • Esmolol 0.25–0.5 mg/kg, IV slow load, then 10–200 **mcg**/kg/min CRI.
  • Carvedilol 0.5 mg/kg PO q 12 hours was used to successfully manage tachycardia and hypertension in a dog that ingested 50 mg/kg PSE and whose CNS signs persisted for two days.
■ With severe toxicosis, seizures may be seen and should be treated with anticonvulsant therapy (see Precautions/Interactions).
  • Phenobarbital 4 mg/kg, IV × 4–5 doses to effect PRN.
  • Propofol 3–6 mg/kg IV slowly or 0.1 mg/kg/min IV as continuous rate infusion.
  • Levetiracetam 20–60 mg/kg IV q 8 hours or as needed.

## Precautions/Interactions

■ Benzodiazepines are **not** recommended as they may exacerbate signs.
■ PE and PSE can enhance the CNS and/or cardiovascular toxicity of other sympathomimetics (e.g., phenylpropanolamine), methylxanthines (e.g., caffeine, theobromine), and MAO inhibitors (e.g., selegiline).

## Alternative Drugs

■ Urinary acidification in dogs can be used to aid in excretion but must be done with caution.
  • Ammonium chloride 50 mg/kg, PO q 6 hours.
  • Ascorbic acid 20–30 mg/kg, SC, IM or IV q 8 hours.

### Extracorporeal Therapy

■ No information on use of extracorporeal therapy for PE or PSE toxicosis was found in the veterinary literature; currently, the human literature considers sympathomimetic agents to be poor candidates for extracorporeal therapy.

### Patient Monitoring

■ Patients should be monitored under veterinary care for 18–24 hours after detoxification if asymptomatic, or until clinical signs resolve.
■ If the product was sustained release, the patient should be monitored for 24–72 hours, or until clinical signs resolve.
■ Monitor body temperature, heart rate, and respiratory rate frequently.
■ Monitor blood pressure and heart rhythm (with continuous ECG monitoring).
■ Ensure appropriate urine output (1–2 mL/kg/hour) and treat accordingly.
■ Minimize stimulation or excitement.

 **COMMENTS**

### Prevention/Avoidance

■ Advise owners to keep medications out of the reach of pets, preferably stored in locked cabinets or cabinets located high off the ground.
■ Keep purses, gym bags, full shopping bags, etc. out of reach of pets.
■ When recommending OTC allergy medications for use in pets, instruct owners to avoid products with a "-D" (indicating decongestant) suffix in the name (e.g., Benadryl®-D).

### Possible Complications

■ DIC, rhabdomyolysis, and myoglobinuria (with subsequent ARF) may occur with prolonged, untreated tremors/seizures or hyperthermia.

### Expected Course and Prognosis

■ The earlier the patient is treated, the better the prognosis.
■ Signs generally resolve within 1–24 hours for regular formulations, and within 24–72 hours for sustained-release formulations.
■ Patients that exhibit severe or sustained CNS signs and hyperthermia typically have a poorer prognosis.
■ Patients with DIC or myoglobinuria have a poorer prognosis and will need aggressive therapy, including 24-hour care, aggressive IV fluid therapy, FFP transfusions, and aggressive monitoring.

### Synonyms

■ Ephedrine, ephedra; methamphetamine; weight loss supplements, Sudafed®.

### See Also

Chapter 15 Amphetamines
Chapter 40 Methamphetamine
Chapter 59 Phenylpropanolamine
Chapter 86 Ephedra (Ma Huang)

## Abbreviations

See Appendix 1 for a complete list.

- PE = phenylephrine
- PSE = pseudoephedrine

## Suggested Reading

Bischoff K, Mukai M. Toxicity of over-the-counter drugs. In: Gupta RC (ed.) *Veterinary Toxicology: Basic and Clinical Principles*, 2nd edn. New York: Elsevier, 2012; pp. 443–468.

Kang MH, Park HM. Application of carvedilol in a dog with pseudoephedrine toxicosis-induced tachycardia. *Can Vet J* 2012;53:783–786.

Wegenast C. Toxicology Brief: Phenylephrine ingestion in dogs: what's the harm? http://dvm360.com/toxicology-brief-phenylephrine-ingestion-dogs-whats-harm

**Author**: Sharon Gwaltney-Brant DVM, PhD, DABVT, DABT
**Consulting Editor**: Ahna G. Brutlag, DVM, PhD, DABVT, DABT

# Dextromethorphan

## DEFINITION/OVERVIEW

- Dextromethorphan is the most common OTC antitussive or cough suppressant used in people.
- It is available as a single active ingredient or in combination with other OTC cough and cold medications such as acetaminophen, NSAIDs, decongestants, expectorants, and/or antihistamines.
- Drug formulations include tablets, capsules, liquid forms including sprays, lozenges, chewable tablets, or dissolvable oral strips. Some preparations may contain xylitol which is toxic to dogs.
- Dextromethorphan has been used extra-label in veterinary medicine as an antitussive, although it is not generally considered effective. It is recommended as a treatment for reduction of compulsive behaviors in dogs. There are anecdotal reports of its use for adjunctive pain management in cats.

## ETIOLOGY/PATHOPHYSIOLOGY

### Mechanism of Action

- Dextromethorphan is structurally similar to the opioids and ketamine. It is the d-isomer of the opioid levorphanol.
- It works as an antitussive in the CNS by stimulation of sigma receptors, reducing cough receptor sensitivity in the medullary cough center.
- It does not appear to bind to kappa, mu, or delta opioid receptors, even in toxic doses.
- It is also an N-methyl-D-aspartate (NMDA) receptor antagonist, which in toxic doses is thought to cause many of the CNS effects.
- In toxic doses, it also may inhibit serotonin reuptake.

### Pharmacokinetics – Absorption, Distribution, Metabolism, Excretion

- It is rapidly orally absorbed with poor oral bioavailability in dogs (11%).
- Peak plasma levels in humans vary from 1.6 to 3 hours.
- Extensive (>90%) metabolism. Significant first-pass metabolism via CYP-450s to the active metabolite dextrorphan (3–4 times less potent than dextromethorphan *in vitro*).
- In a pharmacokinetics study in dogs, only glucuronide conjugates of dextrorphan were detected in plasma, indicating it is likely rapidly converted.
- Half-life in dogs is from 1.3 hours (oral) to two hours (IV). May be prolonged with supratherapeutic dosages.
- Metabolites are excreted in urine; <1% of the parent compound recovered in the urine.

*Blackwell's Five-Minute Veterinary Consult Clinical Companion: Small Animal Toxicology*, Third Edition.
Edited by Lynn R. Hovda, Ahna G. Brutlag, Robert H. Poppenga, and Steven E. Epstein.
© 2024 John Wiley & Sons, Inc. Published 2024 by John Wiley & Sons, Inc.

## Toxicity

- Therapeutic dose in dogs: 2 mg/kg PO twice daily.
- 5 mg/kg PO resulted in vomiting in one of six dogs.
- There is no reported oral $LD_{50}$ in dogs or cats.
- $LD_{50}$ SQ dog: 157 mg/kg; IV dog: 30 mg/kg.
- $LD_{50}$ IV cat: 19.8 mg/kg.
- $LD_{50}$ oral mice: 201mg/kg.
- Toxicity is dose dependent.

## Systems Affected

- Nervous – variable agitation or sedation, aggression, disorientation, nystagmus, ataxia, tremors, seizures.
- Cardiovascular – hypertension and tachycardia, or bradycardia, depending on CNS status.
- Respiratory – tachypnea or hypoventilation, depending on CNS status. Respiratory arrest is rare.
- Musculoskeletal – a distinctive, stiff, ataxic gait has been described in humans.
- Endocrine/metabolic – hyperthermia, typically secondary to excess muscle activity, which may also lead to metabolic acidosis, hypoglycemia, or DIC.
- Renal – with excessive tremors/seizures/hyperthermia, there is a risk for myoglobinuria-induced renal impairment.
- Gastrointestinal – vomiting, diarrhea.

 # SIGNALMENT/HISTORY

### Risk Factors

- Due to the extensive hepatic metabolism of dextromethorphan, there is potential increased risk for toxicosis in animals with underlying hepatic insufficiency or with concurrent hepatotoxicities, although there is no published data to support this.
- Cats may be more sensitive due to their reduced capacity for glucuronidation, although this has not been specifically studied.
- In humans, dextromethorphan is metabolized by CYP-450 2D6 (CYP2D6). Polymorphism results in poor metabolizers which can greatly contribute to toxicity. Polymorphism is also recognized in the canine ortholog CYP2D15, but the clinical relevance is unclear.

### Historical Findings

- Discovery of chewed or spilled bottles of tablets or liquids.
- The animal owner may notice behavioral changes such as sedation or agitation, aggression, and ataxia.

### Location and Circumstances of Poisoning

- Exposures likely to occur at home.

 # CLINICAL FEATURES

- Clinical signs will vary with dose ingested.
- Effects will vary from sedation to extreme agitation. Ataxia is common while tremors and seizures are possible. Nystagmus has been noted. Hallucinations or a dissociative state are described in people.
- Tachycardia, hypertension, or bradycardia, depending on overall state.

- Hyperthermia with extreme agitation, tremors or seizures.
- GI upset (vomiting, diarrhea).
- With coingestion of an anticholinergic (antihistamines), flushed skin, dry mucous membranes, mydriasis, urinary retention, and ileus may be noted.
- With coingestion of a stimulant (decongestants), agitation, tachycardia, hyperthermia, and hypertension may be amplified.
- Serotonin syndrome is possible, which includes clinical signs such as muscle tremors, agitation, disorientation, excessive salivation, and seizure activity.
- Respiratory arrest is rare with dextromethorphan toxicity.

 # DIFFERENTIAL DIAGNOSIS

- Illicit/recreational drugs (ketamine, PCP, other stimulants, sedatives or hallucinogens).
- Other medications – amphetamines, sedatives, antihistamines, decongestants, SSRIs.
- Other toxins – chocolate, caffeine, nicotine.
- Primary CNS disease causing ataxia and other behavioral changes.
- Other metabolic disorders – hypoglycemia, hepatic encephalopathy.

 # DIAGNOSTICS

## Clinical Pathological Findings

- No specific findings unless secondary to clinical effects.
- Baseline CBC, chemistry, electrolytes and venous blood gas should be assessed and monitored in severely affected patients.
- With excessive hyperthermia/tremors/seizures, development of hypoglycemia, metabolic acidosis, DIC, and myoglobinuria-induced renal impairment may occur.

## Other Diagnostics

- Dextromethorphan serum levels are not widely available and unlikely to be helpful in making a diagnosis.
- Dextromethorphan is not routinely detected in urine drug screen tests although may yield a false positive for PCP and opioids.

 # THERAPEUTICS

## Detoxification

- Emesis is recommended in recent ingestions with asymptomatic patients.
- If >1 hour since ingestion, there is a risk of triggering seizure activity with emesis, so this should only be done with caution.
- Emesis is not recommended in symptomatic patients, as the drug has already been absorbed and there is a greater risk for aspiration.
- A single dose of activated charcoal with a cathartic is recommended within one hour of ingestion if the patient is asymptomatic.

## Appropriate Health Care

- Treatment is symptomatic and supportive.
- Symptomatic patients should be hospitalized until clinical signs resolve.
- Monitor vitals closely (temperature, pulse, respirations, blood pressure, CNS status).

- If body temperature exceeds 103.5 °F, cooling measures should be instituted, such as fans or cooling blankets. Discontinue cooling measures once body temperature reaches 103.5 °F.
- IV fluids are recommended to maintain hydration and adequate urine output. Because dextromethorphan is renally excreted, IV fluids may help to increase elimination, although there is no data to support this.
- If serotonin syndrome is suspected, then cyproheptadine is recommended.
- Seizure activity should be treated with standard anticonvulsant dosing.
- Tremors can be treated with methocarbamol at standard dosing.
- Metabolic acidosis, hypoglycemia, or other abnormalities should be treated supportively.

## Antidote

- There is no antidote.

## Drug(s) of Choice

- Acepromazine (0.05–0.1 mg/kg IV, IM, SQ) for sedation.
- Cyproheptadine (1.1 mg/kg – dogs, and 2–4 mg *total* per cat q 4–6 hours until signs resolve) for serotonergic signs. Can be administered orally or rectally.
- Naloxone (0.001–0.04 mg/kg IV, IM, SQ, with doses up to 0.1–0.2 mg/kg suggested based on severity of clinical signs) may help to reverse some of the toxic effects such as sedation or respiratory depression (rare). IV doses may be repeated every 2–3 minutes as necessary. If given IM or SQ, effects may be delayed up to five minutes.

## Precautions/Interactions

- Benzodiazepines can exacerbate serotonin syndrome in dogs, so should be avoided if serotonin syndrome is suspected.
- There is a theoretical increased risk for increased toxicity with concurrent administration of CYP2D15 inhibitors (clomipramine, fluoxetine, ketoconazole, loperamide, quinidine, etc.) and potentially also amantadine, given its similar mechanism (NMDA receptor antagonism).
- There is an increased risk for serotonin syndrome with concurrent administration of monoamine oxidate inhibitors (MAOIs; amitraz, selegiline), serotonergic agents (fluoxetine, tramadol, trazodone, etc.), and opioids.

## Patient Monitoring

- Monitor vital signs closely, including temperature, pulse, respirations, blood pressure, and CNS status.
- With severely agitated or aggressive patients, care should be taken to prioritize staff safety.
- Agitated patients will benefit from minimal stimulation and should be kept in a darkened, quiet area.
- Monitor hydration status and urine output.

 **COMMENTS**

- Dextromethorphan often comes in combination with other active ingredients that can also pose a toxicity risk, such as acetaminophen, NSAIDs, decongestants, etc. Some preparations contain xylitol. It is important to verify active and inactive ingredients from packaging provided by the animal owner.

## Prevention/Avoidance

- Medication should be stored out of reach by pets.

## Possible Complications

- If excessive hyperthermia/tremors/seizures are not controlled, there is a risk for myoglobinuria-induced renal impairment.

## Expected Course and Prognosis

- In otherwise healthy animals receiving adequate treatment, prognosis is expected to be good.

## See Also

Chapter 45 Acetaminophen
Chapter 46 Aspirin
Chapter 48 Decongestants (Imidazolines)
Chapter 49 Decongestants (Pseudoephedrine, Phenylephrine)
Chapter 51 Human NSAIDs (Ibuprofen, Naproxen)

## Abbreviations

- NMDA = N-methyl-D-aspartate
- PCP = phencyclidine

## Suggested Reading

Barnhart JW. Urinary excretion of dextromethorphan and three metabolites in dogs and humans. *Toxic App Pharm* 1980;55:43–48.

Kukanich B, Papich MG. Plasma profile and pharmacokinetics of dextromethorphan after intravenous and oral administration in healthy dogs. *J Vet Pharmacol Ther* 2004;27(5):337–341.

Liang IE, Boyer EW. Dissociative agents: phencyclidine, ketamine and dextromethorphan. In: Shannon MW, Borron SW, Burns M (eds) *Haddad and Winchester's Clinical Management of Poisoning and Drug Overdose*, 4th edn. New York: Saunders, 2007.

Martinez MN, Antonovic L, Court M et al. Challenges in exploring the cytochrome P450 system as a source of variation in canine drug pharmacokinetics. *Drug Metab Rev* 2013;45(2):218–230.

Neerman MF, Uzoegwu L. Is dextromethorphan a concern for causing a false positive during urine drug screening? *Lab Med* 2010;41(8):457–460.

**Author:** Tiffany Romelhardt, DVM
**Consulting Editor:** Ahna G. Brutlag, DVM, MS, DABT, DABVT

# Chapter 51

# Human NSAIDs (Ibuprofen, Naproxen)

## DEFINITION/OVERVIEW

- NSAIDs are a group of compounds that suppress inflammation and that are not steroidal in structure.
- They include a variety of prescription and over-the-counter agents that are often supplied alone, but also in combination with other agents such as analgesics.
- Over-the-counter formulations are available in tablet, chewable tablet, capsule, and liquid suspension forms for oral administration.
- Ibuprofen is a propionic acid and is perhaps the most widely available form.
- Naproxen is also a propionic acid derivative NSAID.
- These drugs are used for their analgesic, antiinflammatory, and antipyretic actions in people.

## ETIOLOGY/PATHOPHYSIOLOGY

### Mechanism of Action

- The mechanism of action of the NSAIDs generally involves inhibition of cyclooxygenase (COX-1 and COX-2), thereby reducing the production of prostaglandins.
  - Prostaglandins mediate pain and inflammation.
  - Prostaglandins also mediate physiological functions such as maintenance of renal blood flow, protection of the stomach by regulating gastric acid secretion, and platelet aggregation.
- Other mechanisms of action have been proposed and include a reduction in some proinflammatory cytokines and peptides.

### Pharmacokinetics or Toxicokinetics – Absorption, Distribution, Metabolism, Excretion, Toxicity

- Ibuprofen.
  - Rapid and complete absorption in dogs with peak plasma concentrations occurring within 15 minutes once ingested doses reach the duodenum.
  - Lipid soluble and 95% of circulating drug is plasma protein bound.
  - Undergoes metabolism primarily in the liver via glucuronidation.
  - More than 50% excreted in urine and about 25% via the bile with some enterohepatic recirculation.
  - Elimination half-life of 2.5–5.3 hours in dogs.
- Naproxen.
  - Rapid absorption that is not impacted by food. Oral bioavailability of 68–100% in cats and dogs.

---

*Blackwell's Five-Minute Veterinary Consult Clinical Companion: Small Animal Toxicology*, Third Edition.
Edited by Lynn R. Hovda, Ahna G. Brutlag, Robert H. Poppenga, and Steven E. Epstein.
© 2024 John Wiley & Sons, Inc. Published 2024 by John Wiley & Sons, Inc.

- Peak plasma concentrations in 0.5–3 hours.
- Highly bound to plasma proteins.
- Metabolism in the dog is thought to be primarily hepatic with metabolites excreted in the bile. Feline metabolism is not well described.
- In dogs, elimination is primarily biliary with significant enterohepatic recirculation. The half-life is very long—up to 74 hours (35–74). Feline elimination is primarily renal/urinary.

## Toxicity

- Ibuprofen.
  - Before the availability of veterinary approved NSAIDs, ibuprofen had been recommended in dogs at 5 mg/kg. This is no longer recommended as significant adverse effects can be seen.
  - >8 and <50 mg/kg: chronic use (and occasionally acute dosing) in dogs may cause mild gastritis, and gastric erosions/ulcers.
  - 50–60 mg/kg: acute ingestion in dogs can lead to mild to severe GI upset and GI ulceration. Potential for renal compromise in sensitive breeds/populations (e.g. German shepherds, pediatric/geriatric, etc.).
  - 100–300 mg/kg: reported to produce acute kidney injury in dogs.
  - >400 mg/kg: can lead to CNS effects such as seizures, ataxia, CNS depression, or coma in dogs.
  - Cats are susceptible to adverse effects at approximately half the doses required to cause issues in dogs.
- Naproxen.
  - Toxic doses >5 mg/kg are associated with gastrointestinal signs; >25 mg/kg with renal injury; and >50 mg/kg with CNS effects.
  - Limited data is available for cats but they are more sensitive than dogs. Assume adverse effects occur at approximately half the doses required to cause issues in dogs.

## Systems Affected

- Gastrointestinal.
  - Abdominal pain.
  - Anorexia, vomiting (+/– hematemesis), diarrhea (+/– melena, hematochezia).
  - GI irritation, GI ulceration and sloughing, gastric and duodenal perforation.
  - Septic peritonitis.
- Renal/urological.
  - Acute kidney injury (oliguric or anuric).
  - Renal papillary necrosis.
  - Transient tubular damage.
  - Polyuria, polydipsia.
- Nervous.
  - CNS depression, ataxia.
  - Seizures or coma rarely occur.
- Endocrine/metabolic.
  - Metabolic acidosis leading to tachypnea and shock.
- Hemic/lymphatic/immune.
  - Anemia (with concurrent panhypoproteinemia) secondary to severe GIT ulceration; thrombocytopathia may occur as a result of altered platelet aggregation.

# SIGNALMENT/HISTORY

## Risk Factors

- Cats are more susceptible to NSAID intoxication than dogs.
- Underlying intestinal or renal pathology.
- Dehydration.
- Concurrent use of other NSAIDs or corticosteroids.
- Animals with liver disease (delays metabolism).
- Geriatric and neonatal animals at higher risk for toxicity.
- Hypoalbuminemia increases the risk for toxicity due to degree of protein binding.
- German shepherd dogs appear to be more susceptible and may need to be managed aggressively.

## Historical Findings

- Witnessed NSAID ingestion, owner administration of NSAID to pet, chewed medication container found in household.
- Clinical signs secondary to NSAID administration may be detected by the owner, including anorexia, vomiting (± hematemesis), diarrhea (± melena), weakness, abdominal pain, and sudden onset of CNS signs (e.g., altered mentation, seizures).

## Location and Circumstances of Poisoning

- Pet owners may unknowingly administer OTC human NSAIDs to dogs in pain, not understanding the potential risks. This can be especially problematic when administered to pets that are not adequately hydrated.

# CLINICAL FEATURES

- GI signs often develop within 2–6 hours of ingestion.
- Abdominal pain with signs of GI hemorrhage, ulceration, or perforation may be delayed 12 hours to 4–5 days following ingestion.
- Lower doses of ibuprofen (<50 mg/kg in dogs) are usually associated with milder signs (inappetence, vomiting, diarrhea), while higher doses (>50–100 mg/kg) are more likely to cause bleeding, ulceration, and/or perforation.
- Clinical signs related to acute kidney injury may develop as early as 12 hours following ingestion or be delayed several days, and can include polydipsia, polyuria or oliguria/anuria, pain on renal palpation, vomiting, and anorexia.
- High-dose exposures can result in decreased mentation, respiratory depression, seizures, and delayed or absent PLRs.

# DIFFERENTIAL DIAGNOSIS

- Toxin exposures that cause GI signs and/or acute kidney injury.
  - Ethylene glycol toxicosis.
  - Grapes/raisins in dogs.
  - Lilies (*Lilium* sp. and *Hemerocallis* sp.) in cats.
  - Other NSAIDs (human or veterinary).
  - Selected mushroom ingestions.

## DIAGNOSTICS

### Clinical Pathological Findings

- Serum BUN and creatinine concentrations may become elevated. Renal values should be monitored every 24 hours for 72 hours (minimum), especially for naproxen exposures.
- Check urinalysis with urine specific gravity prior to starting fluid therapy, especially if a nephrotoxic dose has been ingested. As toxicosis progresses, look for evidence of isosthenuria, hematuria, casts, etc.
- PCV/TS may decrease due to GI hemorrhage or increase due to dehydration.

### Other Diagnostics

- Abdominal radiographs and/or abdominal ultrasound may be helpful when abdominal pain or significant GI signs are present to rule out GI perforation and septic peritonitis.
- Abdominal ultrasound may be used to evaluate kidneys.

### Pathological Findings

- Gastrointestinal erosion and/or ulcerations.
- Degeneration and/or necrosis in the renal papilla in severe cases.

## THERAPEUTICS

### Detoxification

- Typically, for emesis to be effective, it should be induced within 30 minutes of ingestion (due to rapid GI absorption).
- If large amounts of tablets were ingested, emesis within 3–6 hours of ingestion may be effective as ibuprofen has been shown to form gastric concretions that may result in delayed breakdown and/or gastric emptying.
- If the animal has CNS signs, emesis should be avoided to prevent aspiration. Instead, secure the airway and perform gastric lavage.
- Administer one dose of activated charcoal (1–2 g/kg) with a cathartic (e.g., sorbitol) followed by cholestyramine (0.3–1 g/kg q 8 hours) for three days. Cholestyramine can be mixed into canned food or into water and then applied to the food. Ensure the formulation does not contain xylitol and the patient is well hydrated prior to use.
- If cholestyramine is not available, multiple doses of activated charcoal (0.5 g/kg) without a cathartic should be repeated q 8 hours for 24–48 hours (due to extensive enterohepatic recirculation).

### Appropriate Health Care

- Supportive care.
  - Urine output should be monitored in animals exposed to a nephrotoxic dose of NSAIDs.
  - An indwelling urinary catheter and closed collection system should be used if oliguric (<1 mL/kg/h).
  - If volume depleted and oliguric, IV fluid boluses (10 mL/kg over 30 minutes) can be used to expand the intravascular volume.
  - If volume expanded and oliguric, furosemide (1–2 mg/kg IV) and/or mannitol (1 g/kg, IV, over 15 minutes) can be administered to encourage urine production.

## Antidote

- While not truly an antidote, misoprostol (2–5 **mcg**/kg, PO q 8 hours) is a synthetic prostaglandin that can help to prevent GI ulceration by replacing the prostaglandins inhibited by NSAIDs.

## Drug(s) of Choice

- Gastroprotection (5–7 days ibuprofen, two weeks for naproxen).
  - Misoprostol (2–5 mcg/kg, PO q 8 hours).
  - H$_2$-blockers (e.g., famotidine 0.5 mg/kg, PO, IV, SQ q 12 hours).
  - Proton pump inhibitors (e.g., omeprazole 0.7–1.4 mg/kg, PO q 12–24 hours or esomeprazole 0.7 mg/kg, IV q 12–24 hours).
  - Sucralfate (0.25–1 **g/patient**, not mg/kg, PO q 6–8 hours).
- Antiemetics for protracted vomiting (e.g., maropitant 1 mg/kg SQ or IV slowly once daily for up to five days).
- IV fluid therapy should be used to maintain euvolemia, hydration, and renal perfusion.
  - Fluid diuresis (at least 6 mL/kg/hour of an isotonic crystalloid) should be performed for 48 hours with ibuprofen ingestions approaching nephrotoxic doses.
  - Following toxic doses of naproxen, fluid diuresis should ensue for 72 hours.
- If hypoproteinemia results, artificial colloid therapy (e.g., Hetastarch at 1–2 mL/kg/hour) should be considered to maintain colloid osmotic pressure.
- Blood transfusion with pRBC as needed to maintain PCV ≥15–20% if gastric hemorrhage noted.
- Seizures should be treated with anticonvulsants such as diazepam, phenobarbital, or levetiracetam. Diazepam should be used to stop ongoing seizures (0.25–0.5 mg/kg, IV, to effect PRN) while phenobarbital loading (4 mg/kg, IV q 2–12 hours × 4–5 doses) should be used when cluster seizures occur.

## Precautions/Interactions

- Activated charcoal and sucralfate should be dosed at least two hours prior to other oral medications.
- Other NSAIDs, aspirin, or corticosteroids should be withheld from any animal with signs of toxicosis for 7–14 days, depending on the severity of toxicity.

## Extracorporeal Therapy

- Therapeutic plasma exchange (TPE) is helpful for NSAID intoxications because NSAIDs have small molecular weights, are extensively protein bound, and have a low volume of distribution.
- The basic principle of TPE relies on the removal of plasma that contains the protein-bound toxicant from the patient and subsequent administration of replacement solutions including donor plasma, colloidal solutions, and crystalloid solutions.
- Outcomes can be excellent using TPE even with very high-dose NSAID exposures.

## Patient Monitoring

- Appetite, vomiting, diarrhea, melena.
- Water intake and urine output.
- Renal parameters (BUN, creatinine, phosphorus).
- Monitor PCV/TS daily to evaluate for severity of blood loss, hemodilution, and hydration status.

## Diet

- Renal diet is indicated in presence of azotemia.

**COMMENTS**

### Prevention/Avoidance

- Pet owners should be instructed never to administer OTC NSAIDs to their pets unless under direct instruction of their veterinarian.
- There are several NSAIDs that have been specifically formulated and undergone extensive FDA testing and approval for veterinary patients. Veterinary-approved COX-selective NSAIDs may reduce the toxic side-effects from NSAIDs. Whenever possible, veterinarians should recommend these medications instead of human OTC NSAIDs.

### Possible Complications

- Severe gastrointestinal hemorrhage.
- Gastrointestinal ulcerations and/or perforations.
- Acute kidney injury.

### Expected Course and Prognosis

- Prognosis is variable depending on the dose ingested and the duration of time elapsed from ingestion to admission to a veterinary clinic. Dehydration following large-dose exposures can precipitate renal injury.
- Outcomes have been excellent even with high-dose exposures when TPE instituted.

### Synonyms

- OTC NSAIDs (Advil®, Aleve®, Motrin®, etc.).

### See Also

Chapter 46 Aspirin
Chapter 61 Veterinary NSAIDs
Chapter 45 Acetaminophen

### Abbreviations

- COX = cyclooxygenase
- NSAIDs = nonsteroidal antiinflammatory drugs
- OTC = over the counter
- TPE = therapeutic plasma exchange

### Suggested Reading

Butty EM, Suter SE, Chalifoux NV et al. Outcomes of nonsteroidal anti-inflammatory drug toxicosis treated with therapeutic plasma exchange in 62 dogs. *J Vet Intern Med* 2022;36:1641–7.
Khan SA, McLean MK. Toxicology of frequently encountered nonsteroidal anti-inflammatory drugs in dogs and cats. *Vet Clin North Am Small Anim Pract* 2012;42:289–306.
Wolff EDS, Bandt C, Bolfer L. Treatment of ibuprofen intoxication with charcoal haemoperfusion in two dogs. *N Z Vet J* 2020;68:255–260.

**Author:** John H. Tegzes
**Consulting Editor:** Ahna G. Brutlag, DVM, MS, DABT, DABVT

# Loperamide

# DEFINITION/OVERVIEW

- Loperamide is an over-the-counter peripheral opioid receptor agonist used for the treatment of diarrhea.
- Loperamide can cause vomiting, lethargy, sedation, ataxia, bradycardia, hypothermia, and rarely tremors or excitation.
- Patients with the ABCB1-1Δ mutation genotype are more susceptible to clinical signs of loperamide toxicosis.
- Treatment generally consists of supportive care, naloxone, and potentially intravenous lipid emulsion therapy.

# ETIOLOGY/PATHOPHYSIOLOGY

## Mechanism of Action

- Loperamide is a peripheral mu-opioid agonist that acts on opioid receptors in the intestinal wall. It has a direct depressant effect on the circular and longitudinal smooth muscle to inhibit peristalsis. Loperamide has additional effects that aid in the control of diarrhea, such as antisecretory activity and inhibition of calmodulin.
- Loperamide toxicosis is thought to be due to its opioid effects.
- Loperamide is transported out of the brain via P-glycoprotein (P-gp), an efflux pump. In normal animals, therapeutic doses of loperamide do not result in opioid effects due to the P-gp pump. In patients with decreased P-gp or if P-gp is saturated due to large exposures to loperamide, signs of toxicosis can be seen due to increased loperamide levels in the central nervous system.
  - Dogs with the ABCB1-1Δ are not able to synthesize functional P-gp, and are deficient, increasing their susceptibility to loperamide toxicosis.

## Pharmacokinetics or Toxicokinetics – Absorption, Distribution, Metabolism, Excretion

- Absorption.
  - In dogs, 20% of an oral dose is absorbed and is 46–67% bioavailable.
  - Peak concentrations are reached in 1–3.6 hours in dogs.
  - Since loperamide alters GI motility, it may alter its own absorption.
- Distribution.
  - 97% albumin bound in humans. Not determined in dogs or cats.
  - Loperamide is a substrate for P-gp, which is a transmembrane protein efflux pump found in the blood–brain barrier and other tissues. Dogs that have the ABCB1-1Δ mutation have dysfunctional P-gp, resulting in increased loperamide levels in the central nervous system.

*Blackwell's Five-Minute Veterinary Consult Clinical Companion: Small Animal Toxicology*, Third Edition.
Edited by Lynn R. Hovda, Ahna G. Brutlag, Robert H. Poppenga, and Steven E. Epstein.
© 2024 John Wiley & Sons, Inc. Published 2024 by John Wiley & Sons, Inc.

- Metabolism.
  - Extensive first-pass metabolism.
  - Metabolized via oxidated n-demethylation and glucuronidation.
  - The ABCB1-1Δ mutation does not affect metabolism.
- Elimination: undergoes enterohepatic recirculation. In dogs the plasma half-life is 6–14 hours.

## Toxicity

- In patients with the ABCB1-1Δ mutation, signs of loperamide toxicosis can be seen at therapeutic dosages.
- In patients without the mutation, signs of toxicosis have been reported at 1.25–5 mg/kg.
- Signs are typically seen within six hours of ingestion.

## Systems Affected

- Gastrointestinal – vomiting, hypersalivation, anorexia, diarrhea, ileus.
- Nervous – lethargy, depression, sedation, hyperexcitability, vocalization.
- Neuromuscular – ataxia, weakness, hindlimb paresis, tremors.
- Ophthalmic – mydriasis.
- Cardiovascular – bradycardia, arrhythmias (widening of the QRS complex, prolonged QT interval), hypotension.
- Respiratory – respiratory depression.

 # SIGNALMENT/HISTORY

## Risk Factors

- Patients that are heterozygous or homozygous for the ABCB1-1Δ mutation are at higher risk for toxicosis even at therapeutic dosages.
  - Breeds that more commonly have this mutation include collies, Australian shepherds, North American shepherds, Old English sheepdogs, longhaired whippets, Shetland sheepdogs, Skye terriers, and silken windhounds.
- Patients taking medications that inhibit P-gp (e.g., carvedilol, erythromycin, ketoconazole, itraconazole, and verapamil) can increase loperamide plasma concentrations.
- Cats are more susceptible due to their limited ability to glucuronidate.

## Historical Findings

- Known dosing error.
- Ingestion of the owner's medications by the pet.
- Acute onset of vomiting, lethargy, or sedation.

 # CLINICAL FEATURES

- Vomiting.
- Hypersalivation.
- Diarrhea.
- Lethargy.
- Sedation.
- Ataxia.
- Bradycardia.
- Hypothermia.
- Mydriasis.

- Excitation.
- Tremors.
- Respiratory depression.
- Hypotension.

 # DIFFERENTIAL DIAGNOSIS

- Toxicosis with the following: other opioid medications, marijuana, ivermectin, antidepressants, or centrally acting muscle relaxants.

 # DIAGNOSTICS

## Clinical Pathological Findings

- No specific clinical pathological abnormalities are expected.

## Other Diagnostics

- ECG: widened QRS complex, prolonged QT interval.
- Blood pressure: hypotension.
- Loperamide concentrations can be determined in the plasma and urine, although are not clinically useful.

 # THERAPEUTICS

## Detoxification

- Emesis within one hour of exposure if the pet is asymptomatic.
  - Avoid the use of apomorphine or opioids such as hydromorphone as they can increase sedation or respiratory depression.
- Activated charcoal is not recommended due to loperamide-induced alterations in GI motility, such as ileus.

## Appropriate Health Care

- Intravenous fluid therapy: balanced electrolyte solution should be used as needed to maintain hydration and support cardiovascular function and perfusion.
- Monitor blood pressure for hypotension.
- Monitor ECG.
- Monitor body temperature and provide warming support as needed.
- Oxygen therapy may be needed if severe respiratory depression is seen. Ventilatory support is unlikely to be needed.

## Antidote

- Naloxone, an opioid antagonist, may be used to reverse the CNS and respiratory depressant effects of loperamide. 0.001–0.04 mg/kg IV. Repeat doses may be necessary since the duration of naloxone action is shorter than the duration of loperamide effect.

## Drug(s) of Choice

- Antiemetic for vomiting.
  - Maropitant 1 mg/kg IV or SQ.
  - Metoclopramide 0.25–0.5 mg/kg IV or SQ.
  - Ondansetron 0.1–1 mg/kg IV (slow).

- If IV fluid therapy is not effective at improving the blood pressure, consider vasopressors.
  - Norepinephrine: 0.05–0.1 mcg/kg/minute CRI. titrated to effect. Maximum rate 1–2 mcg/kg/minute.
  - Dopamine: 2.5–5 mcg/kg/min IV CRI titrated to effect. Maximum rate of 5–20 mcg/kg/minute.
- Intravenous lipid emulsion: may be used for cases where severe CNS or respiratory depression are seen, although may not be effective in patients with the ABCB1-1Δ mutation (see Chapter 1).
  - 20% solution: 0.25 mL/kg/min IV CRI for 30–60 minutes.
  - May be repeated in four hours if poor response and serum is not lipemic.
- Diphenhydramine may be used for extrapyramidal or dystonic signs, such as vocalizing or excitation – 2 mg/kg IM.

## Precautions/Interactions

- Loperamide can increase the concentrations of the following drugs by interfering with their metabolism or elimination.
  - Ketamine.
  - Midazolam.
  - Propofol.
  - Metoprolol.
  - Propranolol.
  - Cyclosporine.
  - Tacrolimus.
  - Desmopressin.
  - Moxidectin.
- The following medications inhibit P-gp and increase concentrations of loperamide since it is a P-gp substrate.
  - Amiodarone.
  - Carvedilol.
  - Erythromycin.
  - Ketoconazole.
  - Itraconazole.
  - Quinidine.
  - Verapamil.
- Sulfamethoxazole/trimethoprim can also increase loperamide concentrations because it inhibits first-pass metabolism of loperamide.

## Extracorporeal Therapy

- No evidence that extracorporeal therapy is effective for loperamide toxicosis.

## Patient Monitoring

- Continuous or intermittent blood pressure monitoring.
- Continuous or intermittent ECG monitoring.
- Intermittent temperature monitoring.

 **COMMENTS**

### Prevention/Avoidance

Store medications out of reach of patients and keep animal medications separate from human ones.

## Expected Course and Prognosis

- Signs are expected within six hours of ingestion.
- Signs in most patients may last 24 hours. In patients with the ABCB1-1Δ mutation, signs may be prolonged up to several days.
- Prognosis is usually good.

## Synonyms

- Imodium®.

## See Also

Chapter 31 Opiates and Opioids

## Abbreviations

- P-gp = P-glycoprotein
- ABCB1-1Δ was formerly known as MDR-1 or multidrug resistance 1 mutation

## Suggested Reading

Cortinovis C, Pizzo F, Caloni F. Poisoning of dogs and cats by drugs intended for human use. *Vet J* 2015;203:52–58.

Hugnet C, Cadore JI, Buronfosse F et al. Loperamide poisoning in the dog. *Vet Human Toxicol* 1996;38:31–33.

Long WM, Sinnott VB, Bracker K, Thomas D. Use of 20% intravenous lipid emulsion for the treatment of loperamide toxicosis in a Collie homozygous for the ABCB1-1Δ mutation. *J Vet Emerg Crit Care* 2017;27:357–361.

Sartor LL, Bentjen SA, Trepanier L, Mealey KL. Loperamide toxicity in a collie with the MDR1 mutation associated with ivermectin sensitivity. *J Vet Intern Med* 2007;18:117–118.

El Bahri L. Loperamide – investigating a human medication toxic to pets. www.vettimes.co.uk/app/uploads/wp-post-to-pdf-enhanced-cache/1/loperamide-investigating-a-human-medication-toxic-to-pets.pdf

**Author:** Cristine L. Hayes, DVM, DABT, DABVT
**Consulting Editor:** Ahna G. Brutlag, DVM, MS, DABT, DABVT

# Chapter 53

# Minoxidil

## DEFINITION/OVERVIEW

- Minoxidil is a potent, direct-acting arteriolar dilator. It is used as a prescribed oral medication for the treatment of severe and malignant hypertension in humans.
- Minoxidil also stimulates hair follicles and produces hypertrichosis in humans and animals. Available as an OTC topical formulation for people, it is applied to the scalp to slow hair loss/increase hair growth. It has also been used off-label for various alopecic conditions in dogs, cats, and horses.
- Cats are particularly susceptible to toxicosis.
- Cats and dogs can be exposed through topical and oral routes. The most common poisoning scenarios involve unintentional ingestion of topical product from application sites or accidental ingestion of topical or minoxidil tablets.

## ETIOLOGY/PATHOPHYSIOLOGY

### Mechanism of Action

- Minoxidil is a prodrug. It selectively dilates arterioles without affecting venous capacitance after its conversion in the liver to an active, sulfated metabolite which interacts directly and irreversibly with ATP-sensitive potassium channels to lengthen their open time and increase potassium permeability in arteriolar smooth muscle cells. This action limits the availability of calcium required for smooth muscle contraction.
- Hypotension caused by systemic vasodilation induces baroreflex activation of the sympathetic nervous system, leading to an increase in heart rate and myocardial oxygen consumption.
- The exact pathogenesis of cardiac lesions in dogs is unknown, but is thought to result from vasodilation-induced ischemic injury and cardiac stimulation-induced myocardial hyperperfusion and hypoxia.
- After topical application, minoxidil affects the hair cycle by stimulating anagen in resting hair follicles and shortening the telogen phase.

### Pharmacokinetics – Absorption, Distribution, Metabolism, Excretion

- Minoxidil is administered as an oral formulation (2.5 or 10 mg tablets) for hypertension or as topical formulations (2% or 5% in liquid or foam) to stimulate hair growth.
- Minoxidil has high oral bioavailability (>90%), is rapidly absorbed, reaching peak plasma concentration within 2.5 hours, and has a plasma half-life of approximately two hours in beagle dogs. It has lower systemic bioavailability ($\approx$40%) when applied to healthy, intact skin in dogs. Limited pharmacokinetic data are available for cats.

*Blackwell's Five-Minute Veterinary Consult Clinical Companion: Small Animal Toxicology*, Third Edition. Edited by Lynn R. Hovda, Ahna G. Brutlag, Robert H. Poppenga, and Steven E. Epstein. © 2024 John Wiley & Sons, Inc. Published 2024 by John Wiley & Sons, Inc.

- Peak hypotensive and reflex tachycardic effects of minoxidil occur within 4–8 hours after oral administration to beagle dogs.
- Minoxidil is rapidly and widely distributed throughout the body; it is not extensively bound to plasma proteins. Studies in rats indicate that it does not cross the blood–brain barrier.
- After oral administration, minoxidil undergoes phase 1 and phase 2 metabolism in the liver and other body tissues, including skin and hair follicles. Its phase 1 metabolite, 4′-hydroxy-minoxidil, is the principal metabolite excreted by dogs, and its phase 2 glucuronide conjugate is the major metabolite produced in primates, including humans. Biotransformation of minoxidil is limited after its topical administration, and the parent drug is the main compound present at the site of application.
- A minor sulfonated metabolite, minoxidil N-O-sulfate, represents the biologically active form of the drug. This chemically reactive metabolite is hydrophobic and can accumulate in arteriolar smooth muscle cells, where it produces prolonged (>24 hours) vasorelaxant activity due to its irreversible action on ATP-sensitive potassium channels.
- It has been hypothesized that cats are more susceptible than dogs to minoxidil toxicity because of their poorer ability to conjugate the drug to glucuronic acid, thereby exposing more of it to sulfate conjugation. However, there is no evidence to support this idea.
- Minoxidil and its metabolites are cleared by glomerular filtration and excreted in the urine.

## Toxicity

- The toxic signs produced by minoxidil represent extensions of its potent hypotensive action.
- Acute $LD_{50}$ values for dogs and cats have not been published.
- Oral $LD_{50}$ (mice and rats): 1.4–2.5 mg/kg.
- Dogs: in canine studies, short-term administration of 2.5–5 mg/kg of oral minoxidil causes a variety of cardiac lesions. However, dermal application of topical minoxidil does not produce these lesions. In a large retrospective case series, the amount ingested was so low that exposure could not be quantified through traditional units of measurement, and a few licks were sufficient to cause clinical signs. When a toxic dose could be quantified, the lowest dose at which signs developed was 0.79 mg/kg.
- Cats: case literature suggests that as little as one drop ingested leads to clinical signs. However, 5% minoxidil applied topically for 30 days to a cat did not result in any adverse effects.

## Systems Affected

- Cardiovascular – severe and prolonged hypotension with reflex tachycardia, shift in coronary blood flow from endocardium to epicardium, pericardial effusion, and reduced cardiac function.
- Respiratory – dyspnea, cyanosis, pleural effusion and pulmonary edema.
- Renal – salt and water retention.
- Nervous – lethargy, hypothermia.
- Gastrointestinal – potential vomiting with ingestion of large numbers of tablets or hypersalivation with ingestion of topical formulation.

 # SIGNALMENT/HISTORY

### Risk Factors

- Species: cats are more susceptible to minoxidil toxicity than dogs.
- No breed, sex, or age predilection.
- Animals with preexisting cardiovascular, respiratory, or renal disease or those receiving antihypertensive or antiadrenergic medications may manifest a more severe toxicosis.

### Historical Findings

- Intentional topical application of human hair products containing minoxidil to alopecic areas on pets.
- Ingestion secondary to grooming of fur or hair on other animals or humans to which minoxidil has been applied.
- Spillage of hair loss products resulting in animal contact with minoxidil.
- Ingestion of or contact with sites where product has been applied (pillowcase, cotton swab) or applicator/bottle.
- Ingestion of minoxidil tablets.

### Location and Circumstances of Poisoning

- Exposures to minoxidil in dogs are most commonly due to exploratory behavior, i.e., licking or chewing on application materials or medication bottle.
- Exposures in cats are most commonly through unintentional delivery, i.e., licking product off owner's skin or product spilled on cat.
- Exposure can also occur after intentional application of hair loss products to pets.

 ## CLINICAL FEATURES

- In dogs and cats, vomiting and/or hypersalivation may occur immediately to within a few hours after exposure.
- The onset of minoxidil's cardiovascular action (hypotension with tachycardia) may be delayed 1–3 hours after exposure.
- Animals may not present until severe respiratory signs have developed, which may be days after exposure.
- Once severe signs have developed, death usually occurs within 24 hours.
- For those animals that survive aggressive supportive care, treatment may be prolonged (3–5 days).
- Clinical signs and physical examination findings most commonly noted include the following.
  - Cardiovascular – tachycardia (dogs) or bradycardia (cats), pale mucous membranes, cyanosis, poor pulse quality, muffled heart sounds due to pleural/pericardial effusion.
  - Respiratory – dyspnea, tachypnea, crackles and wheezes, decreased lung sounds secondary to pleural effusion.
  - Nervous – lethargy, recumbency, trembling, tcollapse, hypothermia.
  - Skin – areas of alopecia where topical product may have been applied.
- Death occurs secondary to cardiopulmonary congestion and cardiovascular collapse due to prolonged and severe hypotension.

 ## DIFFERENTIAL DIAGNOSIS

- Toxicants.
  - Baclofen, opiates (hypotension with *bradycardia*).
  - Cardiotoxic antineoplastic drugs, such as doxorubicin, cyclophosphamide, 5-fluorouracil.
  - Other antihypertensive drugs, including calcium channel blockers and beta-adrenergic antagonists (hypotension with *bradycardia*).
- Primary respiratory disease.
  - Bronchitis, asthma.
  - Noncardiogenic pulmonary edema (near drowning, acute upper airway obstruction, electrocution, post seizure).

- Pneumonia, hemorrhage, neoplasia.
- Pleural effusion (pyothorax, hemothorax, chylothorax, FIP, neoplasia, hypoproteinemia).
■ Primary cardiac disease.
■ Acute anaphylaxis causing collapse, dyspnea, and hypotension.

 # DIAGNOSTICS

### Clinical Pathological Findings

■ Chemistry panel may be normal or liver enzymes (ALT, AST) and renal values (BUN, creatinine) may be above normal due to hypotension and decreased perfusion.
■ Blood gas analysis – metabolic acidosis and elevated lactate due to decreased perfusion.

### Other Diagnostics

■ Echocardiography to determine if cardiac lesions are present and rule out other causes of cardiac disease. Findings with minoxidil toxicosis include septal thickening, thickening of the left ventricular posterior wall, increased ejection fraction, decreased end-diastolic and systolic volumes and pericardial effusion.
■ Thoracic radiography to rule out other causes of respiratory signs. Possible findings include pleural effusion and pulmonary edema.
■ Thoracocentesis to characterize fluid and rule out other causes of pleural effusion. Fluid from affected animals is expected to be a transudate.

### Pathological Findings

■ Dogs: changes reported in the heart and vasculature of dogs with multiple oral doses of minoxidil include lesions involving the right atrium, left ventricular papillary muscle, and myocardial arteritis. Other lesions include subendocardial and papillary muscle necrosis, coronary arterial medial hemorrhage and necrosis, and multifocal to diffusely extensive areas of hemorrhage over the right atrial epicardium.
■ Cats: postmortem examination of myocardial tissues from poisoned cats revealed evidence of interstitial edema and acute ischemia, lesions that were different from those seen in dogs.
■ Other lesions include pleural effusion, failure of lung collapse due to extensive pulmonary congestion and edema, pericardial effusion, pale streaks interspersed with hemorrhage in the heart chambers extending from epicardial to endocardial surface. Cardiac weights and valvular measurements may be normal. Histologically, marked myocardial interstitial edema in all heart chambers, unevenly distributed areas of myodegeneration, and pleocellular myocarditis.

 # THERAPEUTICS

■ The objectives of treatment are decontamination to prevent further toxicant exposure in those animals presenting acutely in stable condition.
■ In those animals already exhibiting clinical signs, treatment is aimed at stabilization and aggressive supportive care.
■ In animals that survive, chronic management may be necessary if significant and permanent cardiac injury has occurred.

### Detoxification

■ Topical exposure – once stabilized, bathe areas where minoxidil was applied with liquid dishwashing detergent, even up to 48–72 hours after initial exposure.
■ Oral exposure – if stable and asymptomatic, induce emesis if ingestion occurred within one hour. Activated charcoal and cathartic can reduce further intestinal absorption.

## Appropriate Health Care

- Hospitalization for aggressive cardiovascular and respiratory monitoring.
- Dyspneic animals should receive immediate oxygen supplementation via facemask or oxygen cage; those severely affected may require intubation and mechanical ventilation.
- If pulmonary edema is present, diuretics can be given PRN until signs have improved.
- Intravenous crystalloids may be indicated to support blood pressure and facilitate removal of the drug and metabolites in the urine. However, cardiac function must be considered prior to fluid administration.
- Vasopressor agents may be indicated if hypotensive.
- Thermoregulation may be necessary if hypothermic.

## Antidote

- None.

## Drug(s) of Choice

- Antiemetics.
  - Maropitant 1 mg/kg IV or SQ q 24 hours.
  - Ondansetron 0.1–0.3 mg/kg IV q 8–12 hours.
- Pulmonary edema.
  - Furosemide (2 mg/kg IM or IV PRN) or other loop diuretic to reduce fluid and salt retention.
- Hypotension.
  - An alpha-1-adrenergic pressor agent such as dopamine (5–20 mcg/kg/min IV CRI titrated to effect) or norepinephrine (0.1–0.2 mcg/kg/min IV CRI titrated to effect) to maintain blood pressure.
- Persistent tachycardia despite normalization of blood pressure.
  - Beta-1-adrenergic receptor antagonists, such as esmolol (0.25–0.5 mg/kg IV over 1–2 minutes, followed by CRI of 10–200 **mcg**/kg/min) or atenolol (0.2–1 mg/kg PO or IV q 12 hours, titrated to effect), to reduce reflex sympathetic activity.
- Intralipid emulsion therapy (ILE) 20% solution.
  - ILE may improve cardiac function or act as a lipid sink/shuttle, whereby fat-soluble toxic agents are sequestered into a newly formed lipid compartment within the intravascular space and then eliminated.
  - With a logP of 1.33, minoxidil is considered lipophilic (>1).
  - 1.5 mL/kg IV bolus over 1–15 minutes. Follow immediately with a CRI 0.25 mL/kg/min over 30–60 minutes.

## Precautions/Interactions

- Electrolytes, acid–base, and renal values should be monitored in patients receiving diuretic therapy.
- When using diuretics, other potentially nephrotoxic drugs should not be used or used with extreme caution (NSAIDs, ACE inhibitors, aminoglycosides).
- If beta-1-adrenergic receptor antagonists are used, blood pressure should be closely monitored and the agents discontinued if hypotension occurs.
- If administering ILE, the potential impact of its action on concurrently administered lipid-soluble medications must be considered.

## Surgical Considerations

- Sedation/general anesthesia should be avoided in these patients due to potential cardiovascular instability.

## Patient Monitoring

- The extent and type of patient monitoring will depend on the stability of the patient. Certain diagnostics such as thoracic radiographs and echocardiography may not be possible until the patient is stable.
- Patients should be hospitalized for frequent monitoring of respiratory rate/effort, thoracic auscultation, pulse oximetry, blood pressure, and ECG to assess for response to therapy and determine duration of treatment.

## Diet

- A nasoesophageal feeding tube or other means of parenteral nutrition may be necessary in animals with prolonged clinical signs that are unable or unwilling to eat or drink.

 **COMMENTS**

### Prevention/Avoidance

- Clients should be educated about the toxicity of minoxidil tablets and topical preparations.
- Stress the importance of keeping medications secure.
- Explain that clients should never apply minoxidil or any medication topically to their pet unless directed to do so by a veterinarian.
- If topical minoxidil is used in the household, take measures to prevent access to the medication (prevent pets from licking human skin, keep pets away from bedding, tissues used during application, etc.).

### Possible Complications

- In dogs, hypotension and reflex tachycardia lead to significant, irreversible cardiac lesions.
- In cats, death occurs secondary to cardiopulmonary congestion and cardiovascular collapse due to prolonged and severe hypotension.
- For severely affected patients, referral to a 24-hour facility with mechanical ventilation capabilities may be necessary.

### Expected Course and Prognosis

- Previous case reports suggested a poor to grave prognosis in cats. However, newer publications report a more favorable prognosis after minoxidil exposure.
- In patients that develop clinical signs, most developed moderate or major illness.
- Death occurred in 13% of cats that developed clinical signs after the pet owner's minoxidil use.
- In those animals responsive to therapy, prolonged hospitalization may be necessary.
- For those animals that survive, permanent cardiac damage may be present.

### Abbreviations

See Appendix 1 for a complete list.
- FIP = feline infectious peritonitis

### Suggested Reading

DeClementi C, Bailey KL, Goldstein SC, Orser MS. Suspected toxicosis after topical administration of minoxidil in 2 cats. *J Vet Emerg Crit Care* 2004;14:287–292.

Hanton G, Gautier M, Bonnet P. Use of M-mode and Doppler echocardiography to investigate the cardiotoxicity of minoxidil in beagle dogs. *Arch Toxicol* 2004;78:40–48.

Jordan TJ, Yaxley PE, Culler CA, Balakrishnan A. Successful management of minoxidil toxicosis in a dog. *J Am Vet Med Assoc* 2018;252:222–226.

Mesfin GM, Robinson FG, Higgins MJ et al. The pharmacologic basis of the cardiovascular toxicity of minoxidil in the dog. *Toxicol Pathol* 1995;23:498–506.

Tater KC, Gwaltney-Brant S, Wismer T. Topical minoxidil exposures and toxicoses in dogs and cats: 211 cases (2001–2019). *J Am Anim Hosp Assoc* 2021;57:225–231.

Thomas RC, Hsi RS, Harpootlian H et al. Metabolism of minoxidil, a new hypotensive agent I: absorption, distribution, and excretion following administration to rats, dogs, and monkeys. *J Pharm Sci* 1975;64:1360–1366.

**Authors:** Julie Schildt, DVM, DACVECC and David R. Brown, PhD
**Consulting Editor:** Ahna G. Brutlag, DVM, MS, DABT, DABVT

# Chapter 54

# Nicotine and Tobacco

## DEFINITION/OVERVIEW

- Most tobacco products contain the plant *Nicotiana tabacum*.
- Nicotine is a natural insecticide in tobacco leaves and, historically, was used in commercial pesticide products.
- Nicotine is a rapid-onset, dose-dependent nicotinic ganglion depolarizer causing neurological and cardiovascular stimulation followed by depression.
- Products that contain nicotine include cigarettes, cigarette butts, cigars, chewing tobacco, snuff, nicotine gum, patches, inhalers (smoking cessation aids), vape pens and electronic cigarettes, "E-juice" or "E-liquid" that fill electronic cigarettes or vape pens, nasal sprays, lozenges, and sublingual tablets.

## ETIOLOGY/PATHOPHYSIOLOGY

### Mechanism of Action

- Low-dose and early high-dose intoxications cause neurological stimulation due to depolarization and excitation of the nicotinic receptors in the sympathetic and parasympathetic ganglia, adrenal medulla, CNS, spinal cord, neuromuscular junctions, and chemoreceptors. Subsequent nervous system depression may occur due to persistent depolarization causing a blockade of the nicotinic receptors.
- Vagal nerve stimulation can cause cardiovascular depression.
- Blockade of the autonomic ganglia can cause skeletal muscle paralysis.
- Vomiting is caused by stimulation of the chemoreceptor trigger zone.

### Pharmacokinetics or Toxicokinetic – Adsorption, Distribution, Metabolism, Excretion

- Nicotine is water soluble and rapidly absorbed through the respiratory tract, skin, and oral mucous membranes; however, absorption is pH dependent. It is slowly absorbed from the stomach due to low pH of the environment and increases in the intestines due to the alkaline environment.
- Oral products are buffered to increase absorption through oral mucous membranes. Clinical signs have been seen from buccal exposure alone in dogs.
- Oral bioavailability is 20–45% with oral peak plasma concentration in about one hour.
- Widely distributed throughout body tissues with the highest affinity for the liver, kidney, spleen, lungs, and brain.
- Can be present in milk and crosses the placenta.

*Blackwell's Five-Minute Veterinary Consult Clinical Companion: Small Animal Toxicology*, Third Edition.
Edited by Lynn R. Hovda, Ahna G. Brutlag, Robert H. Poppenga, and Steven E. Epstein.
© 2024 John Wiley & Sons, Inc. Published 2024 by John Wiley & Sons, Inc.

**TABLE 54.1 Nicotine contents of common products.**

| Product | Nicotine content | Notes |
|---|---|---|
| Bidi cigarette | 3.3–12.4 mg/bidi | |
| Cigarette | 9–30 mg/cigarette | Dose inhaled during smoking is only 0.3–2 mg |
| Cigarette butt | 5–7 mg/butt | |
| Low yield or "light" cigarette | 3–8 mg/cigarette | |
| Cigar | 15–40 mg/cigar | Wrapped in nicotine-containing paper |
| Chewing tobacco | 6–8 mg/g | May be flavored which could increase palatability |
| Vape pens or electronic cigarette | 6–24 mg/cartridge | May be flavored which could increase palatability |
| E-liquid or E-juice refill | 0 to >100 mg/mL | May be flavored which could increase palatability |
| Nicotine gum | 2–4 mg/piece | May contain xylitol |
| Nicotine transdermal patch | 8.3–114 mg/patch | Used patches still contain nicotine |
| Snuff | 12–16 mg/g | |

- Metabolized primarily in the liver and excreted mainly by the kidneys. Mostly the metabolites are excreted but about 2–35% is excreted unchanged.
- In dogs 4–5% is excreted in the bile and feces.
- Half-life in humans is two hours and is completely excreted by 16 hours in humans.
- Rate of excretion may increase with low urine pH.
- Renal failure decreases renal clearance.

## Toxicity

- Minimum lethal dose in dogs and cats is 20–100 mg (total) which may require only a small amount to be ingested (see Table 54.1).
- The minimum lethal dosage is 9.2 mg/kg with a canine (oral) $LD_{50}$ of 9–12 mg/kg.
- Signs can be seen at 1 mg/kg.
- In spite of low toxic dosages, toxicosis is rare. This could be due to the bitter taste of some products, the acidic environment of the stomach which slows absorption, and/or because nicotine stimulates the chemoreceptor trigger zone, often causing spontaneous emesis.

## Systems Affected

- Gastrointestinal – emesis/retching, nausea, hypersalivation, increased peristalsis, diarrhea.
- Nervous – stimulation then depression, excitement, agitation, twitching, tremors, seizures/convulsions, depression/lethargy, ataxia, weakness, disorientation.
- Cardiovascular – tachycardia, hypertension, vasoconstriction, bradycardia, hypotension, vasodilation. Increases myocardial work and oxygen demand which can cause arrhythmias, cardiac standstill, and sudden death.
- Ophthalmic – mydriasis, miosis.
- Respiratory – panting, tachypnea, respiratory depression, and arrest.
- Neuromuscular – paralysis of respiratory muscles, skeletal muscle paralysis.

 # SIGNALMENT/HISTORY

- No breed or sex predilection.

## Risk Factors

- Indiscriminate eating behavior. Puppies and birds seem to be most at risk.
- Chewing tobacco, "E-liquid," and gum can have added sugars and flavors that may increase palatability.
- Access to places nicotine products are stored such as a purse or backpack.
- Access to cigarette butts such as litter in public places or from an ashtray in the car or home.
- Some products such as gum and liquids can contain xylitol.
- Preexisting renal or cardiovascular disease.
- Neonatal and geriatric pets may be more susceptible to intoxication.

## Historical Findings

- Witnessed ingestion.
- Discovery of disturbed ashtrays or chewed products/packaging containing nicotine.
- Discovery of products containing nicotine in emesis or feces.
- Signs of intoxication including agitation, emesis, lethargy, ataxia, or depression.

# CLINICAL FEATURES

- Rapid onset of signs, sometimes within minutes, but usually less than four hours. Duration of signs in mild cases is 1–2 hours; in severe cases 18–24 hours.
- Initially, neurological signs are due to stimulation of nicotinic receptors in the CNS and include excitement, ataxia, tremors, and seizures. Continued stimulation leads to blockade of the neuromuscular junctions resulting in weakness and paralysis.
- Common cardiovascular signs are tachycardia and hypertension due to stimulation of the sympathetic ganglia, adrenal medulla, and the chemoreceptors of the carotid and aortic bodies.
- Respiratory signs such as tachypnea are due to stimulation of the medulla oblongata and chemoreceptors of the carotid and aortic bodies.
- Parasympathetic stimulation and stimulation of the chemoreceptor trigger zone cause gastrointestinal signs such as salivation, emesis, and diarrhea.
- Vagal nerve stimulation can cause bradycardia and cardiac standstill. Blockade of the autonomic ganglia can cause skeletal and respiratory muscle paralysis, potentially leading to death.

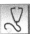

# DIFFERENTIAL DIAGNOSIS

- Intoxications: strychnine, theobromine and chocolate, caffeine, tremorigenic mycotoxins, organophosphates and carbamates, depressants, amphetamines, cocaine, phenylpropanolamine, pyrethrins, xylitol (weakness/seizures due to hypoglycemia).
- Primary cardiac disease that may cause tachycardia, bradycardia, arrhythmias, or hypertension.
- Other causes of hypotension such as fluid or blood loss.
- Primary neurological disease or other causes of CNS signs such as hypoglycemia or liver failure.
- Neuromuscular disease such as tick paralysis.

# DIAGNOSTICS

## Clinical Pathological Findings

- CBC and chemistry: no significant changes expected unless secondary to nicotine-induced clinical signs (e.g., dehydration/GI losses from vomiting/diarrhea, acid–base abnormalities secondary to tachypnea or hypoventilation).
- Monitor serum sodium and electrolytes if giving activated charcoal.

## Other Diagnostics

- Serum nicotine assay can be done but is rarely clinically useful due to rapid onset of signs and need for rapid treatment.
- Nicotine can be detected in blood, stomach contents, urine, liver, and kidney tissue either pre or postmortem.

## Pathological Findings

- Gross and histopathological findings are typically nonspecific although internal organ congestion has been reported.

 # THERAPEUTICS

- Treatment is mainly decontamination followed by symptomatic and supportive care.

## Detoxification

- Gastrointestinal decontamination: induce emesis for solid products (liquid products are absorbed rapidly) only if patient is asymptomatic. Many patients spontaneously vomit soon after ingestion.
- Can consider gastric lavage if large amount ingested.
- Give one dose activated charcoal with a cathartic (e.g., sorbitol) once if there is no risk of aspiration. For sustained-release products, such as transdermal patches, consider redosing charcoal *without* a cathartic for two mores doses q 8 hours while hospitalized.

## Appropriate Health Care

- Treatment in hospital is recommended until asymptomatic with frequent monitoring of heart rate, blood pressure, and neurological status.
- Antiemetics as needed.
- Sedation for agitation, tachycardia, or hypertension.
- IV fluids may increase renal elimination and are used for hypotension.
- Urine acidification may increase elimination but is not routinely recommended as it may cause other complications. It should only be done if the patient's electrolytes and acid–base status can be closely monitored.
- Oxygen and mechanical ventilation for respiratory depression or distress.
- Anticonvulsants for seizures.
- Further neurological or cardiovascular support as needed, see below.

## Antidote

- None.

## Drug(s) of Choice

- Antiemetic: maropitant 1 mg/kg SQ or IV (over 1–2 minutes) q 24 hours.
- Sedation for agitation.
    - Diazepam (0.5–1 mg/kg IV) or midazolam.
    - Acepromazine 0.05–0.1 mg/kg IM, SQ, IV PRN. Use cautiously as may exacerbate impending hypotension. Do **not** use if hypotensive.
    - Butorphanol 0.1–0.5 mg/kg IM, SQ, IV.
- Cardiovascular support.
    - Tachycardic (dog >180–190 bpm, cat >220–230 bpm) *with* hypertension: start with sedation. If persistent and nonresponsive to sedation, consider beta-blockers (i.e., propranolol 0.02–0.06 mg/kg, IV slowly to effect).

- Bradycardia (dog <50 bpm, cat <120 bpm): atropine 0.02–0.04 mg/kg IM, IV.
  - Hypotension: a balanced electrolyte crystalloid can be administered in small aliquots (i.e., 20–30 mL/kg IV over 20–30 minutes, repeat 2–3× to effect) until blood pressure improves.
- Neurological support and anticonvulsant therapy.
  - Diazepam 0.5–1 mg/kg IV to effect.
  - Phenobarbital 4–8 mg/kg slow IV.
  - Levetiracetam (extra-label) 30 mg/kg IV.
  - Tremors: methocarbamol 55–220 mg/kg slow IV to effect.

### Precautions/Interactions

- Avoid antacids (e.g., $H_2$-blockers, proton pump inhibitors) as alkalization of stomach contents hastens absorption.

### Surgical Considerations

- Surgical or endoscopic removal of transdermal patches or cartridges from vaping pens may be needed from the stomach or intestines to stop nicotine absorption and reduce the chance of a foreign body obstruction.

### Patient Monitoring

- Frequent monitoring of heart rate, respiratory rate, ECG, blood pressure, and neurological status.

## COMMENTS

### Prevention/Avoidance

- Keep ashtrays/cigarette butts, packs of cigarette, gum, patches, E-liquid, or any other nicotine-containing products out of reach of pets.
- Monitor closely when on walks outside for ingestion of cigarette butts or other discarded products.
- Warn owners that some products have sugars and flavors added to them that could increase palatability.
- Some products such as gum contain xylitol.
- Warn owners that some products are wrapped in tobacco-containing paper (e.g., cigars) and ingestion of these alone can be toxic.

### Possible Complications

- Usually if treated appropriately and signs resolve, no long-term changes are expected.
- There has been one report of pericardial effusion after nicotine ingestion in a dog.

### Expected Course and Prognosis

- Small ingestions and patients displaying only mild signs generally have a good prognosis.
- Large ingestions can have a poor to grave prognosis.
- If the patient survives the first four hours, then prognosis is usually good.

### See Also

Chapter 15 Amphetamines
Chapter 71 Chocolate and Caffeine
Chapter 37 Cocaine
Chapters 48 and 49 Decongestants

## Suggested Reading

Hackendahl NC, Sereda CW. Toxicology brief: the dangers of nicotine ingestion in dogs. *Vet Med* 2004;March:218–222.

Herman EH, Vick JA, Strong JM et al. Cardiovascular effects of buccal exposure to dermal nicotine patches in the dog: a comparative evalution. *J Toxicol Clin Toxicol* 2001;39(2):135–142.

Kim JH, Lim JH. Acute fatal pericardial effusion induced by accidental ingestion of cigarette butts in a dog. *Can Vet J* 2016;57(2):151–156.

Novotny TE, Hardin SN, Hovda LR, Novotny DJ, Mclean MK, Khan S. Research Paper: tobacco and cigarette butt consumption in humans and animals. *Tobacco Control* 2011;20: i17–i20.

Plumlee KH. Nicotine. In: Peterson ME, Talcott PA (eds) *Small Animal Toxicology*, 3rd edn. St Louis: Elsevier Saunders, 2013; pp. 683–686.

**Author:** Crystal Davis, BVM&S
**Consulting Editor:** Ahna G. Brutlag, DVM, MS, DABT, DABVT

# Chapter 55

# Vitamins and Minerals

## DEFINITION/OVERVIEW

- Vitamins, in the form of single nutrient formulations, multivitamins, and prenatal vitamins, are readily available in many homes. However, there is a paucity of veterinary literature describing toxicosis resulting from vitamin and mineral ingestion in small animals.
- In the United States, a multivitamin/mineral supplement is defined as a supplement containing three or more vitamins and minerals but does not include herbs, hormones, or drugs. Each nutrient is at a dose below the tolerable upper level determined for humans by the FDA to not cause a risk for adverse health effects.
- Among the common vitamins and minerals found within readily available multivitamin, prenatal, and single nutrient formulations, the most dangerous ingredients resulting in toxicosis following acute ingestion are **vitamin A**, **vitamin D$_3$**, and **iron**.
- Management of patients who have ingested any medication containing vitamins or minerals entails calculation of amount consumed, emesis if appropriate, specific antidote therapy if indicated, monitoring, and supportive care.
- Prognosis following vitamin and/or mineral toxicosis depends on ingested ingredient(s), health status of the pet, prompt and appropriate care, and response to treatment.
  - Vitamin and mineral supplements labeled "high potency" are required to have 100% of the recommended daily value for at least two-thirds of the ingredients contained within the supplement, as dictated by the FDA.
  - Prenatal vitamins may contain many of the same ingredients found in multivitamins but tend to have higher compositions of folic acid, calcium, and iron.
  - Many formulations are available in order to appeal to the vast array of consumer demands health needs, desired dosing regimen, and preferred formulation type (Figure 55.1). Formulations such as gummies, sublingual tablets, chewables, and liquids may contain xylitol or other sweeteners. Besides looking at the active ingredients, be certain to review the inert/other ingredients.

## ETIOLOGY/PATHOPHYSIOLOGY

### Pharmacokinetics – Absorption, Distribution, Metabolism, Excretion

- Vitamin absorption depends mostly on the solubility of the vitamin: fat-soluble vitamins require bile salts and fat in order to be passively absorbed in the duodenum and ileum, whereas water-soluble vitamins require active transport for uptake from the GIT.
- Mineral absorption depends on solubility, density, and mineral–mineral interactions in both the GIT and tissue storage level.

*Blackwell's Five-Minute Veterinary Consult Clinical Companion: Small Animal Toxicology*, Third Edition.
Edited by Lynn R. Hovda, Ahna G. Brutlag, Robert H. Poppenga, and Steven E. Epstein.
© 2024 John Wiley & Sons, Inc. Published 2024 by John Wiley & Sons, Inc.

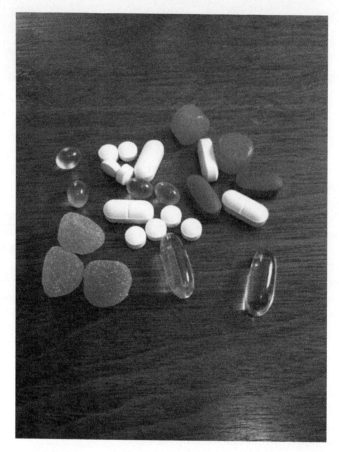

■ **Figure 55.1** An assortment of vitamin and mineral supplements in different shapes, sizes, and formulations. Source: Courtesy of Ahna G. Brutlag.

- **Vitamin A** is stored in the liver and can undergo enterohepatic circulation. Cats require preformed vitamin A, since they lack an enzyme necessary for beta-carotene cleavage.
- **Vitamin B$_1$ (thiamine)** is absorbed primarily in the jejunum after intestinal phosphatases hydrolyze thiamine to free thiamine. Active, carrier-mediated transport is the primary mechanism of absorption; however, passive diffusion is also utilized during periods of increased thiamine intake. It is transported in red blood cells and plasma to the tissues.
- **Vitamin B$_2$ (riboflavin)** requires hydrolysis prior to absorption in the GIT. Absorbed riboflavin is bound in approximately equal percentages to albumin and globulin. Excess riboflavin is renally excreted.
- **Vitamin B$_3$ (niacin)** is readily absorbed by the mucosa of the stomach and small intestine and is taken up by tissues, where it is often required for cofactor synthesis. Excessive amounts are excreted by the kidneys following methylation.
- **Vitamin B$_6$ (pyridoxine)** is absorbed via passive diffusion in the small intestine, but only small quantities are stored. Products of vitamin B$_6$ metabolism are renally excreted.
- **Vitamin B$_{12}$ (cobalamin)** absorption depends on both intake and GIT function, as it undergoes several transformations (hydrolysis, intrinsic factor binding, ileal absorption, protein-bound transport, and cell surface receptor-mediated uptake) in order to be utilized.

- **Vitamin C (ascorbic acid)**, though not technically a vitamin, can be synthesized from glucose by cats and dogs. Additional vitamin C is absorbed by passive diffusion. It is transported by albumin, distributed throughout the body, and excreted via urine, feces, and sweat.
- **Vitamin D ($D_3$, cholecalciferol)** can be synthesized by the skin after exposure to UV light. It is also absorbed in the small intestine, using bile salts, and subsequently transported with vitamin D-binding protein to tissues where it is contained within lipid deposits.
- **Vitamin E** is absorbed in the small intestine by passive diffusion; however, it is absorbed with poor efficacy. Absorption can be increased by consuming fats at the same time. Transport to circulation is facilitated by the lymphatics. There is minimal metabolism of vitamin E, and the majority of it is fecally excreted.
- **Biotin** is released via protein hydrolysis in order to permit intestinal absorption and subsequent transfer from the blood to the tissues. In addition, intestinal microbes synthesize approximately half of the biotin requirements. Excessive biotin is excreted by the kidneys.
- **Calcium** absorption is variable in the GIT and can be achieved using three possible mechanisms. In the duodenum and jejunum, there is an active, transcellular method using a vitamin D-dependent, calcium-binding protein. The other two methods are passive and facilitated absorption, which are primarily localized to the distal GIT. Most calcium in dietary supplements is in the form of calcium salts, which are poorly absorbed by the GIT.
- **Copper** can be absorbed along the entire length of the GIT, though most is absorbed within the small intestine, by both active and passive mechanisms. The liver is the main site of copper metabolism, and excretion is via feces and bile.
- **Folic acid (folate)** is hydrolyzed in the intestine before enterocyte absorption. There are no folate reserves in the body; therefore, it must be ingested daily in the diet.
- **Iodine** within the plasma is trapped by the thyroid glands to ensure adequate supplies of thyroid hormone.
- **Iron** must be ionized in order to be absorbed. It is absorbed into mucosal cells lining the intestinal lumen, particularly in the duodenum and jejunum. The absorbed iron is then transferred to ferritin or transferrin. No distinct mechanism for iron excretion exists, which contributes to toxicosis with iron ingestion.
- **Magnesium** is absorbed is either actively or passively from the intestines, depending on the intraluminal concentration. The kidney is essential for magnesium homeostasis and is responsible for filtration, excretion, and reabsorption of this mineral.
- **Pantothenic acid** is released via protein hydrolysis within the intestinal lumen. Most of the vitamin is contained within erythrocytes.
- **Phosphorus** is well absorbed in the intestines, particularly when found in animal-based ingredients. Calcium and phosphorus absorption, metabolism, and hemostasis are under the delicate and intricate control of hormonal and renal influences.
- **Zinc** absorption is not completely understood, though the majority of absorption occurs in the duodenum, jejunum, and ileum. The liver is responsible for zinc metabolism, and excretion of excess zinc occurs via the feces.

## Toxicity

- Of the common vitamins and minerals nutrient supplements, **vitamins A, $D_3$,** and **iron** are the most likely to cause toxicosis.
- The remaining vitamins and minerals are likely to cause mild GIT signs, such as vomiting, diarrhea, and anorexia, when ingested in large quantities. Specific vitamin or mineral toxicity is otherwise uncommon.
- **Vitamins E, K, $B_2$, $B_3$,** and **$B_6$** are considered to be minimally toxic. No toxicosis has been associated with supplements containing **pantothenic acid, folic acid, biotin,** and **zinc.**

- **Calcium, phosphorus, iodine**, and **magnesium** may be associated with specific clinical signs or end-organ damage (see Systems Affected).
- **Vitamin A** – for acute vitamin A toxicosis, clinical signs are usually associated with ingested amounts that exceed 10–1000× the daily requirement.
- **Vitamin C** (ascorbic acid) – large doses greater than 1 g/kg can cause urine calcium oxalate crystals.
- **Vitamin D$_3$** – ingested doses <0.1 mg/kg can cause mild GIT signs, whereas doses >0.1 mg/kg can lead to hypercalcemia and AKI. To calculate the amount of vitamin D$_3$ ingested, it is important to note that 1 IU of vitamin D$_3$ equals 0.025 mcg or 0.000025 mg of vitamin D$_3$. See Chapters 23 (Calcipotriene/Calcipotriol) and 124 (Cholecalciferol).
- **Iron** – in dogs ingesting less than 20 mg/kg of elemental iron, no clinical signs have been reported. When amounts between 20 and 60 mg/kg of elemental iron are consumed, mild clinical signs may be seen. Doses above 60 mg/kg may cause severe clinical signs, and death may result from doses between 100–200 mg/kg. See Chapter 103 (Iron).
- Massive ingestion of capsules or tablets can result in bezoar formation and may require gastric lavage for removal.

## Systems Affected

- Gastrointestinal.
  - Vomiting, diarrhea, anorexia – may be seen with ingestion of any vitamin or mineral.
  - Gastrointestinal bleeding – seen with **iron** toxicosis.
  - Gastrointestinal strictures – late complication seen with **iron** toxicosis.
  - Hematochezia – associated with **vitamin B$_3$ (niacin)** toxicosis.
- Nervous.
  - Flaccid paralysis – associated with **magnesium** toxicosis.
  - Tremors/convulsions – associated with **vitamin A** and B$_3$ toxicosis.
  - Paralysis – seen with **vitamin A** toxicosis.
  - Ataxia – seen with vitamin B$_6$ **(pyridoxine)** toxicosis.
  - Abnormal reflexes – associated with vitamin B$_{12}$ **(cobalamin)** toxicosis.
- Musculoskeletal.
  - Lameness – associated with calcium and **vitamin D$_3$** toxicosis.
  - Soft tissue calcifications – associated with **phosphorus** and **vitamin D$_3$** toxicosis.
  - Cervical spondylosis – seen with **vitamin A** toxicosis.
  - Long bone fractures – seen with **vitamin A** toxicosis.
- Renal/urological.
  - AKI – seen with **vitamin D$_3$** toxicosis.
  - Uroliths – seen with **vitamin C, calcium, phosphorus**, and **magnesium** toxicosis.
- Endocrine/metabolic.
  - Hypercalcemia – seen with **calcium** and **vitamin D$_3$** toxicosis.
  - Secondary hyperparathyroidism – seen with **phosphorus** toxicosis.
- Hemic/lymphatic/immune.
  - Coagulopathy – associated with **vitamin A and E** toxicosis.
  - Anemia – seen with **vitamin A** toxicosis.
- Hepatobiliary.
  - Hepatitis/increased liver enzymes/decreased hepatic function – seen with **vitamin A** and **copper** toxicosis.
- Cardiovascular.
  - Hypotension and bradycardia – associated with **vitamin B$_1$ (thiamine)** toxicosis.
- Skin/exocrine.
  - Rough haircoat – associated with chronic **iodine** toxicosis.

# SIGNALMENT/HISTORY

- There are no breed, sex, or age predilections for nutritional supplement toxicosis.
- While no mean age has been reported, it is likely that younger animals are more frequently affected given their increased incidence of ingesting foreign objects.
- Some pet owners may give high doses of vitamins based on internet searches, or the theory that "more is better."

## Risk Factors

- Animals living in homes or areas where vitamin or mineral supplements are stored.
- Animals with renal disease could be at increased risk of more severe consequences after **vitamin D₃** or **calcium** ingestion.
- Although by definition, vitamins should not contain additional herbs or drugs, many do. Labels should be read carefully. For example, words like "active metabolism" may indicate that the product contains significant amounts of caffeine. The following is a list of common added ingredients that could potentially cause clinical signs.
  - 5-HTP (5-hydroxytryptophan).
  - Caffeine (guarana, green tea).
  - Citrus aurantium (synephrine).
  - Fluoride.
  - Methionine.
  - Thioctic acid (alpha-lipoic acid).
  - Tryptophan.
  - Xylitol (as a sweetener).

## Historical Findings

- The owner may suspect or witness ingestion of vitamin or mineral supplements based on damaged packaging or spilled supplements.
- Owners may witness vomiting (which may or may not contain supplements), diarrhea, and neurological changes.

## Location and Circumstances of Poisoning

Ingestion often occurs when plastic baggies or plastic weekly pill holders are used to store medications temporarily, or when dogs learn to open suitcases, backpacks, and purses.

# CLINICAL FEATURES

- Gastrointestinal – vomiting, diarrhea, anorexia, GIT bleeding, hematochezia.
- Nervous – abnormal reflexes, ataxia, tremors, convulsions, flaccid paralysis, paralysis.
- Musculoskeletal – lameness, soft tissue calcification, cervical spondylosis, long bone fractures.
- Renal/urological – pain on abdominal (specifically, kidney or bladder) palpation.
- Cardiovascular – bradycardia, poor pulse quality.
- Skin/exocrine – rough haircoat.

# DIFFERENTIAL DIAGNOSIS

- Vomiting, diarrhea, anorexia, and GIT bleeding due to other primary or secondary GIT disease.
- ARF.

- Liver dysfunction or failure.
- Ataxia, tremors, and paralysis due to other primary or secondary neurological disease.

## DIAGNOSTICS

### Clinical Pathological Findings

- A baseline CBC and serum chemistry should be considered in most animals where multivitamin/multimineral/prenatal supplement ingestion is suspected, especially when the ingested amount is unknown.
- In animals known to have ingested near-toxic or toxic amounts of **vitamin D$_3$** and calcium, total calcium, ionized calcium, BUN, creatinine, and urinalysis (including urine specific gravity) should be measured. Monitor calcium and phosphorus (especially in puppies) daily for four days. Monitor BUN and creatinine on day 1 and 4. If at 96 hours post exposure the pet is asymptomatic, further treatment is not needed.
- For patients ingesting near-toxic or toxic amounts of **vitamin A** and **copper**, special attention should be directed toward liver enzymes and measures of liver function (e.g., BUN, glucose, albumin, and cholesterol).
- For animals ingesting toxic or near-toxic doses of **vitamin A**, a complete coagulation panel (e.g., PT, PTT, platelets, and d-dimers) should be measured.
- For patients with severe tremors from **multivitamin** ingestion, serum AST and CK, as well as blood lactate, should be monitored.
- For patients ingesting 1 g/kg of **vitamin C**, baseline chemistry and urinalysis should be obtained.
- For any patient ingesting elemental **iron** at toxic or near-toxic doses, serum iron concentration and total iron-binding capacity should be measured.

### Pathological Findings

- Gross necropsy findings in pets that have ingested toxic amounts of vitamin or mineral supplements may include whole or partial tablets or capsules within the GIT, GIT bleeding (**iron**), GIT stricture formation (**iron**), soft tissue mineralization (**calcium, phosphorus**), long bone fracture (**vitamin A**), cervical spondylosis (**vitamin A**), nephroliths/uroliths (**calcium, phosphorus, vitamin C**), renomegaly due to ARF (**vitamin D$_3$**), and hepatomegaly associated with hepatitis (**copper**).
- Histopathological lesions seen in pets ingesting toxic amounts of vitamin or mineral supplements include GIT ulceration (**iron**), fibrous tissue deposition within the GIT (iron), acute tubular necrosis (**vitamin D$_3$**), hepatitis (**copper**), and soft tissue calcification (**phosphorus, calcium**).

## THERAPEUTICS

If an animal is healthy and did not ingest a toxic or near-toxic amount of any vitamin or mineral, no further action is needed aside from monitoring by the owner.

### Detoxification

- In general, animals ingesting a toxic or near-toxic dose of any vitamin or mineral, or those with preexisting hepatic or renal dysfunction, should have emesis induced and activated charcoal with a cathartic should be administered.
  - For the most dangerous vitamin and mineral toxicoses (**vitamin A**), repeat doses of activated charcoal (without a cathartic) may be considered.

- Toxic **vitamin D₃** ingestions should receive one dose of activated charcoal, followed by cholestyramine (300 mg/kg q 8 hours × 4 days). This is a bitter powder, so mix with tasty food. Verify the cholestyramine was not presweetened with xylitol.
- Activated charcoal does not bind to **iron** well and is not indicated.

■ For neurologically inappropriate patients who have ingested multivitamins, initial treatment should be aimed at managing neurological signs, such as paralysis, tremors, or convulsions. Appropriate sedation, intubation (to protect the airway), and gastric lavage should be considered to facilitate decontamination if the supplements are still suspected to be within the stomach.

■ As massive ingestion may result in a gastric bezoar, gastric lavage may be indicated for decontamination.

## Appropriate Health Care

■ In general, fluid therapy (either IV or SQ, depending on the severity of the toxicosis and clinical symptoms) should be used to manage hydration and prevent hypovolemia. 24 hours of fluid diuresis should be considered in large **vitamin C** overdoses.

■ Aggressive IV saline diuresis and medications to increase calciuresis may be necessary for patients with **vitamin D₃** toxicosis.

■ For patients with tremors or convulsions, body temperature, patient comfort, hydration, and blood lactate should be closely monitored.

## Antidotes

■ Iron – chelation with deferoxamine (see Chapter 103).

■ Vitamin D₃ – pamidronate (a bisphosphonate) for hypercalcemia (see Chapter 124).

## Drug(s) of Choice

■ Gastroprotectants and antiemetics may be necessary with multivitamin toxicity, including the following.
- Famotidine 0.5–1.0 mg/kg IV q 12–24 hours.
- Pantoprazole 0.7–1 mg/kg IV over 15 minutes q 24 hours.
- Sucralfate suspension 0.5–1 g PO q 8 hours, administered 30–60 minutes after any medication aimed at decreasing gastric acid production.
- Ondansetron 0.1–0.2 mg/kg IV q 8–12 hours.
- Maropitant 1 mg/kg SQ q 24 hours.

■ In patients at risk of **iron** toxicosis or those that are showing clinical signs, chelation therapy and gastroprotectants are indicated.

■ Patients with severe tremors or convulsions secondary to vitamin or mineral supplement toxicosis should be controlled with diazepam (0.5–1 mg/kg IV) or midazolam (0.2–0.5 mg/kg IV). For patients with ongoing tremors or convulsions, a diazepam (0.25–1 mg/kg/hour) or midazolam (0.1–0.5 mg/kg/hour) CRI may be needed.

## Patient Monitoring

■ With hypercalcemia from **vitamin D₃** toxicosis, serum total and ionized calcium should be monitored every 12–24 hours, and more frequently if therapy to treat hypercalcemia is being used. Electrolytes (e.g., sodium, potassium, and chloride) should be monitored every 12–24 hours if furosemide therapy is used. For patients at risk for or those with AKI, renal values, PCV/TS, and assessment for hydration (e.g., skin turgor, chemosis, peripheral edema, PCV/TS, weight) should also be measured at least every 12–24 hours. Urine output should be measured every 2–4 hours. Patients should be weighed every 6–8 hours to help assess fluid balance.

- If **iron** toxicosis, serum iron concentration and total iron-binding capacity should be measured at presentation and during chelation therapy.
- If there are elevations in liver enzymes, reassessment should be performed every 3–7 days depending on clinical course.
- In hepatic failure, blood glucose should be monitored every 2–4 hours and supplemented as needed.
- If coagulopathic, clotting times should be measured at least every 24 hours and more frequently if being treated with FFP to assess success of therapy.
- Neurological status should be monitored every 2–4 hours, as well as body temperature, gag reflex, and blood lactate in any patient with tremors, paralysis, or other neurological impairment.

## Diet

For patients with any neurological compromise, vomiting, or regurgitation, oral food and water should be withheld until the patient is neurologically appropriate and GIT signs have resolved.

 ## COMMENTS

### Prevention/Avoidance

- Education about proper storage and handling of vitamin and mineral supplements will help prevent reexposure.
- Clients should be advised that pets being fed an AAFCO-approved, balanced commercial diets do not require additional vitamin or mineral supplementation; therefore, they should not administer any nutritional supplements unless specifically instructed by a veterinarian.

### Possible Complications

- Chronic renal failure after resolution of AKI.
- Liver failure/hepatitis.
- GIT hemorrhage.
- GIT stricture.
- Paralysis, tremors.

### Expected Course and Prognosis

- For patients that did not consume a toxic amount of any vitamin or mineral, owners can expect self-limiting GIT signs that should resolve on their own within 12–48 hours.
- There are four stages associated with **iron** toxicosis: the first stage starts within six hours of iron ingestion, and the fourth stage may not be seen for 2–6 weeks after ingestion. Without aggressive supportive care, monitoring, and chelation therapy, acute iron poisoning is potentially lethal in animals. For more see Chapter 103.
- For patients with hypercalcemia secondary to **vitamin D$_3$** toxicosis, prognosis and clinical course will depend on how soon treatment for hypercalcemia is initiated and response to therapy. For patients that develop AKI secondary to hypercalcemia, even though aggressive care is absolutely warranted, a guarded prognosis must be given.
- The prognosis for **vitamin A** toxicosis is likely favorable with appropriate treatment and supportive care.

### Synonyms

Multivitamin toxicosis, multimineral toxicosis, prenatal vitamin/mineral toxicosis, vitamin or mineral supplement toxicosis

## See Also

Chapter 47 Calcium Supplements
Chapter 124 Cholecalciferol
Chapter 103 Iron
Chapter 105 Zinc

## Abbreviations

See Appendix 1 for a complete list.
- AAFCO = Association of American Feed Control Officials
- FDA = Food and Drug Administration
- FFP = fresh frozen plasma
- UV light = ultraviolet light

## Suggested Reading

Albretsen A. The toxicity of iron, an essential element. *Vet Med* 2006;February:82–90.

Gross KL, Wedekind KJ, Cowell CS et al. Nutrients. In: Hand MS, Thatcher CD, Remillard RL et al. (eds) *Small Animal Clinical Nutrition*, 4th edn. Marceline: Walsworth, 2000.

Khan SA. Vitamin A toxicosis. In: Cote E (ed.) *Clinical Veterinary Advisor*, 3rd edn. St Louis: Mosby, 2015; pp. 1071–1072.

McKnight KL. Ingestion of over-the-counter calcium supplements. www.vetfolio.com/learn/article/toxicology-brief-ingestion-of-over-the-counter-calcium-supplements

Murphy LA. Toxicities from over the counter drugs. In: Kahn CM (ed.) *Merck Veterinary Manual*, 9th edn. Whitehouse Station: Merck, 2005.

**Author:** Charlotte Means, DVM, MLIS, DABVT, DABT
**Consulting Editor:** Ahna G. Brutlag, DVM, MS, DABT, DABVT

# Drugs: Veterinary Prescription

# Chapter 56

# Alpha-2-adrenergic Agonists

## DEFINITION/OVERVIEW

- Detomidine, dexmedetomidine, xylazine, romifidine, clonidine, brimonidine, guanfacine, and tizanidine are all examples of alpha-2-adrenergic agonists used in veterinary or human medicine.
  - These medications can be found in a variety of forms, such as injectables, tablets, transdermal patches, topical and oromucosal gels, sublingual films, and ophthalmic solutions.
- Alpha-2-adrenergic agonists are widely used in veterinary medicine to reduce anesthetic requirements by providing dose-dependent sedation, analgesia, and muscle relaxation.
  - Currently available FDA-approved veterinary options include xylazine, detomidine, romifidine, clonidine, dexmedetomidine, and medetomidine (including a combination product with vatinoxan).
- Alpha-2-adrenergic agonists are also used in human medicine for common medical conditions such as hypertension, glaucoma, attention-deficit/hyperactivity disorder, agitation associated with schizophrenia or bipolar I or II disorder in adults, stimulant intoxication, withdrawal symptoms from sedatives and narcotics, and as an aid in smoking cessation.
- All drugs in this class can be rapidly and completely reversed with use of an alpha-2 antagonist.

## ETIOLOGY/PATHOPHYSIOLOGY

### Mechanism of Action

- These agents have agonist actions on the alpha-adrenergic receptors.
  - Alpha-1 receptors produce arousal, excitement, and increased locomotor activity.
  - Alpha-2a receptors mediate sedation, supraspinal analgesia, bradycardia, and hypotension. Found mainly in the central nervous system.
  - Alpha-2b receptors mediate the initial increase in vascular resistance and reflex bradycardia. Found on vascular smooth muscle and mediate vasopressor effects.
  - Alpha-2c receptors mediate hypothermia. Found mainly in the central nervous system.
- Receptor selectivity ratios, alpha-2/alpha-1, are as follows.
  - Xylazine 160:1
  - Clonidine 220:1
  - Detomidine 260:1
  - Romifidine 340:1
  - Brimonidine 1000:1
  - Dexmedetomidine/Medetomidine 1620:1
- Inhibition of norepinephrine and dopamine storage and release.

*Blackwell's Five-Minute Veterinary Consult Clinical Companion: Small Animal Toxicology*, Third Edition.
Edited by Lynn R. Hovda, Ahna G. Brutlag, Robert H. Poppenga, and Steven E. Epstein.
© 2024 John Wiley & Sons, Inc. Published 2024 by John Wiley & Sons, Inc.

## Pharmacokinetics – Absorption, Distribution, Metabolism, Excretion

- Alpha agonists are well absorbed from all routes, including across the oral mucosa.
- Rapid absorption can lead to rapid onset of clinical signs.
- Widely distributed to virtually all organs of the body, particularly throughout the CNS.
- Metabolized via biotransformation in the liver to inactive metabolites.
- Excreted primarily in the urine.
- Half-life can vary depending on the drug and the formulation.
  - The half-life of xylazine is 30 minutes in dogs and cats; however, clonidine has a half-life over 12 hours (up to 19 hours with transdermal products).
  - The half-life of dexmedetomidine IV is 40–60 minutes in dogs and cats; however, dexmedetomidine oromucosal gel has a half-life of 0.5–3.0 hours.

## Toxicity

- Dogs exposed to just small amounts of brimonidine ophthalmic solution from puncturing the bottle have showed clinical effects including hypotension and bradycardia.
- Clonidine doses as low as 0.01 mg/kg have caused lethargy, ataxia, and bradycardia in dog cases reported to the ASPCA Animal Poison Control Center.
- Toxicosis from the injectable veterinary alpha-2-adrenergic agonists has been seen with up to five times the normal IV dose and up to 10 times the normal IM dose.
- Intensity and duration of effect are dose dependent.

## Systems Affected

- Cardiovascular – **hypotension** common. Initially, marked peripheral vasoconstriction is caused by activation of peripheral postsynaptic alpha-2 receptors, which leads to a dramatic increase in arterial blood pressure and rise in systemic vascular resistance. Vascular smooth muscle contraction and vasoconstriction results, which causes both a decrease in cardiac output by 30–50% and heart rate (reflex **bradycardia**). AV block can also be seen following administration of alpha-2 agonists.
- Nervous – **CNS depression** (as evidenced by sedation), analgesia (somatic and visceral), and muscle relaxation occur. **Hypothermia** may occur from inhibition of the noradrenergic mechanism of body temperature regulation and reduced muscle activity.
- Gastrointestinal – **vomiting** is common immediately following administration. There may be decreased GI secretions, motility, and varying effects on intestinal muscle tone.
- Endocrine – receptor-mediated inhibition of insulin release from the pancreatic beta cells leading to hyperglycemia. Inhibition of ACTH and cortisol secretion.
- Respiratory – depression, decreased respiratory rate, and possible apnea can occur. These drugs may potentiate the respiratory depressant effects of other drugs, such as opioids.
- Urinary – promotion of diuresis through inhibiting ADH release, promoting ANP secretion, and increasing GFR.
- Reproductive – some drugs, such as clonidine, can cross the placenta and be excreted into the milk, but other drugs have insufficient safety data available. Generally, use of these drugs is not recommended for pregnant or lactating animals.

 # SIGNALMENT/HISTORY

### Risk Factors

- Geriatric or pediatric animals, those with renal, hepatic, or cardiovascular disease, and those with a seizure disorder or respiratory compromise may be at a higher risk of developing clinical signs.

### Historical Findings

- Owner may report an ingestion of an alpha-2-adrenergic agonist if one is witnessed or if packaging for the product at home is found.

### Location and Circumstances of Poisoning

- Iatrogenic administration of an improper dose of injectable veterinary alpha-2-adrenergic agonists in a veterinary setting.
- Inadvertent overdose of oromucosal gels at home.
- Accidental exposure (pet chewing on the owner's pills, patch, or bottle of ophthalmic solution) of human alpha-2-adrenergic agonists at home.

 # CLINICAL FEATURES

- The onset of clinical signs is generally rapid.
- The duration of signs depends on the drug. However, as all are easily reversible, signs typically only last until the reversal agent is administered.
- Nervous – CNS depression, ataxia, sedation, and hypothermia. Paradoxical excitation (aggression), muscle twitching, and seizures are possible but rare.
- Cardiovascular – bradycardia, AV block, decreased myocardial contractility and cardiac output, initial hypertension followed by hypotension. Pale (or cyanotic) oral mucous membranes may also be seen.
- Respiratory – respiratory depression with decreased respiratory rate, hypoventilation, and possible apnea.
- Gastrointestinal – vomiting and drooling.
- Urinary – increased urination.
- Clinical signs may exhibit dose-related amplification. Death may occur from circulatory failure and severe pulmonary congestion.

 # DIFFERENTIAL DIAGNOSIS

- Intoxication with beta-blockers, calcium channel blockers, ivermectin, marijuana, or opioids.

 # DIAGNOSTICS

### Clinical Pathological Findings

- Serum chemistry: with the exception of possible hyperglycemia due to decreased insulin, no significant changes expected.

### Other Diagnostics

- ECG – sinus bradycardia and second-degree AV block.
- Blood pressure – hypertension followed by hypotension.

### Pathological Findings

- Dose-related hepatic intracytoplasmic eosinophilic inclusions have been noted in dogs receiving 2.5× and 12.5× the recommended clinical dose of dexmedetomidine for four weeks. No specific gross or histopathological findings noted for other products.

# THERAPEUTICS

- All drugs can be rapidly and completely reversed with alpha-2 antagonists.
- Treatment consists of administration of a reversal agent, supportive care, protection of the airway, and intensive monitoring.
- Monitor heart rate and rhythm, blood pressure, ventilation, body temperature, and glucose levels.

## Detoxification

- If the product was a pill or patch and was ingested, induction of emesis is recommended within 15 minutes if the patient is asymptomatic. Otherwise, gastric lavage can be performed within one hour of ingestion.
- Activated charcoal, if given early for a pill or patch ingestion, may reduce the amount of systemically absorbed drug, though absorption is typically rapid.
- Clinical signs following oral exposure to brimonidine ophthalmic solutions or dexmedetomidine gels are usually due to absorption across the oral mucosa, so emetics and activated charcoal are not warranted.

## Appropriate Health Care

- Prompt administration of a reversal agent (see Antidotes).
- IV crystalloid fluids to treat hypotension and increase urine output.
- Antiemetic as needed for nausea and vomiting.
- Thermoregulation to prevent or correct hypothermia.
- Mechanical ventilation if too sedate or respiratory depression.

## Antidotes

- There are three available antagonists: atipamezole (Antisedan®), yohimbine, and tolazoline.
- Atipamezole is highly selective for the alpha-2 receptors and does not create significant hypotension.
    - Atipamezole is marketed as the reversal agent for dexmedetomidine but will also reverse all other alpha-2 agonist drugs. Reversal should occur within 5–10 minutes.
    - It is recommended to give atipamezole IM due to the potential to create excitement and tachycardia. It can be given IV in emergency situations.
    - Take into consideration the amount of agonist given and the time duration since the agonist was administered.
    - Dose for dexmedetomidine – give the same volume of atipamezole as was given of dexmedetomidine.
    - Dose for other alpha-2 agonist drugs – 50 mcg/kg IM.
- Yohimbine (0.1 mg/kg IV slowly) and tolazoline (4 mg/kg IV slowly) produce variable effects as they also antagonize alpha-1 receptors. This can lead to hypotension.
- It is better to underdose the antagonist, as side-effects from an overdose include excitement, muscle tremors, hypotension, tachycardia, salivation, and diarrhea. Large doses of antagonists will also reverse analgesia.
- An additional dose of the antagonist may be needed if the clinical signs reoccur. The half-life of atipamezole is longer than yohimbine so may need less frequent dosing.

## Precautions/Interactions

- Atropine: generally, treatment with a reversal agent is enough to correct any bradycardia and hypotension. If the animal remains severely bradycardic and hypotensive, IV atropine or glycopyrrolate can be given to effect but use with caution due to the possibility of heart block, VPCs, tachycardia, or hypertension.

## Patient Monitoring

- Continuous ECG is preferable, otherwise frequent monitoring of heart rate and rhythm.
- Blood pressure.
- Blood glucose should be checked at least daily.
- Respiratory rate and effort should be closely monitored until the animal is fully recovered.
- Body temperature needs to be checked frequently until the animal has completely recovered.
- Monitor fluid balance due to increased urination.

## Diet

- For animals with any vomiting, sedation, or neurological compromise, food and water should not be provided orally until the clinical signs have resolved.

 # COMMENTS

### Prevention/Avoidance

- Be aware of proper dosing and drug concentration.
- Inform owners of the risk their alpha-2 agonist drugs present to their pets if ingested.

### Possible Complications

- Mechanical ventilation may be required for respiratory support if the pet develops hypoventilation from respiratory depression or becoming too sedated.
- Potential for apprehensive or aggressive behavior in animal emerging from sedation.

### Expected Course and Prognosis

- The prognosis for alpha-2 agonist overdose is excellent with proper supportive care and prompt use of a reversal agent.

### Synonyms

- Alpha-2-adrenergic agonist intoxication, alpha-2-adrenergic agonist poisoning.

### See Also

Chapter 97 Amitraz
Chapter 48 Decongestants (Imidazolines)

### Abbreviations

See Appendix 1 for a complete list.
- ACTH = adrenocorticotrophic hormone
- ADH = antidiuretic hormone
- ANP = Atrial natriuretic peptide
- AV = atrioventricular
- GFR = glomerular filtration rate

### Suggested Reading

Baumgartner K, Doering M, Mullins ME, for the Toxicology Investigators Consortium. Dexmedetomidine in the treatment of toxicologic conditions: a systematic review and review of the toxicology investigators consortium database. *Clin Toxicol* 2022;60:1356–1375.

Giovannitti JA, Thoms SM, Crawford JJ. Alpha-2 adrenergic receptor agonists: a review of current clinical applications. *Anesth Progress* 2015;62(1):31–38.

Lemke KA. Anticholinergics and sedatives. In: Tranquilli WJ, Thurmon JC, Grimm KA (eds) *Lumb & Jones Veterinary Anesthesia and Analgesia*, 4th edn. Ames: Blackwell, 2007; pp. 203–239.

Plumb DC. *Plumb's Veterinary Drug Handbook: Pocket*, 8th edn. Ames: John Wiley & Sons, 2015.

Rolfe NG, Kerr CL, McDonell WN. Cardiopulmonary and sedative effects of the peripheral α2-adrenoceptor antagonist MK 0467 administered intravenously or intramuscularly concurrently with medetomidine in dogs. *Am J Vet Res* 2012;73:587–594.

**Author**: Amanda Gross, DVM

**Consulting Editor**: Ahna G. Brutlag, DVM, MS, DABT, DABVT

# Chapter 57

# Isoxazolines

## DEFINITION/OVERVIEW

- Novel class of insecticide and acaracide.
- Common isoxazoline insecticides include afoxolaner, fluralaner, lotilaner, and sarolaner.
- Afoxolaner, lotilaner, and sarolaner are labeled for oral administration for prevention and treatment of flea and certain species of tick infestations in the dog. They are additionally used off-label for the treatment of demodectic mange, sarcoptic mange, and ear mite infestations.
- Fluralaner is used topically in dogs and dermally in dogs and cats for the same indications.
- Isoxazoline insecticides can come in combination with milbemycin oxime, moxidectin, pyrantel, and/or selamectin, which can represent additional toxicologic concerns, especially in overdose situations.
- Isoxazoline insecticides can cause clinical signs at therapeutic dosages, but signs are more commonly seen in overdose situation. Common clinical signs observed are vomiting, ataxia, fasciculations, tremors, seizures, hyperesthesia, vocalization, and disorientation.
- Hypothermia can additionally be seen with symptomatic cats.
- Dogs with an underlying seizure disorder are more prone to developing seizures, especially at therapeutic dosages.
- Onset of clinical signs can be rapid or can be delayed to about 20 hours post exposure.
- Clinical signs generally resolve within 24 hours. Occasionally, some cases can show clinical signs for longer than 24 hours, though hospitalization is generally not needed over 24 hours.

## ETIOLOGY/PATHOPHYSIOLOGY

### Mechanism of Action

The mechanism of action for adverse effects in mammals is not completely understood. In insects, isoxazoline insecticides inhibit glutamate and gamma-aminobutyric (GABA) gated chloride channels. Vertebrates do not possess glutamate-gated chloride channels. Studies have shown that isoxazoline insecticides preferentially inhibit invertebrate versus vertebrate GABA-gated chloride channels, but this may be a potential mechanism of action for adverse effects in mammals.

*Blackwell's Five-Minute Veterinary Consult Clinical Companion: Small Animal Toxicology*, Third Edition.
Edited by Lynn R. Hovda, Ahna G. Brutlag, Robert H. Poppenga, and Steven E. Epstein.
© 2024 John Wiley & Sons, Inc. Published 2024 by John Wiley & Sons, Inc.

## Pharmacokinetics or Toxicokinetics – Adsorption, Distribution, Metabolism, Excretion

### Absorption

- Peak plasma.
  - Afoxolaner: 2–6 hours.
  - Fluralaner.
    - Oral, dog: 24 hours.
    - Topical, dog: 25 days.
    - Topical, cat: 6–9 days.
  - Lotilaner: 2–4 hours.
  - Sarolaner: less than 24 hours.
- Bioavailability.
  - Afoxolaner: oral, dog: 26%.
  - Fluralaner.
    - Oral, dog: 26%.
    - Dermal, dog: 25%.
    - Dermal, cat: 25%.
- Lotilaner.
  - Oral, dog, fasted: 24%.
  - Oral, dog, fed: 82%.
  - Oral, feline, fasted: 8%.
  - Oral, feline, fed: 100%.
- Sarolaner.
  - Oral, canine, fasted: 86%.
  - Oral, canine, fed: 107%.

### Distribution

- Afoxolaner.
  - Dog, oral: 2.7 L/kg.
- Fluralaner.
  - Dog, oral: 3.1 L/kg.
  - Cat, oral: 3.5 L/kg.
- Lotilaner
  - Dog, oral: 6.5 L/kg.
  - Cat, oral: 5.4 L/kg.
- Sarolaner.
  - Dog, oral: 2.8 L/kg.

### Metabolism

- Minimal.

### Excretion

- Biliary/feces.
- Half-life.
  - Afoxolaner.
    - Dog, oral: 16 days.
  - Fluralaner.
    - Dog, oral: 12–15 days.
    - Dog, dermal: 19 days.
    - Feline, dermal: 12 days.

- Lotilaner.
    - Dog, oral: 30 days.
    - Cat, oral: 30 days.
- Sarolaner.
    - Dog, oral: 11–12 days.

## Toxicity

Adverse effects, including seizures, can be seen at therapeutic dosages with isoxazoline insecticides, especially in animals with a history of seizure disorders. However, significant neurologic signs are more commonly seen at dosages at least 2–3 times therapeutic.

## Systems Affected

- Gastrointestinal – vomiting, hypersalivation, diarrhea.
- Skin/exocrine – (dermally applied products only) erythema, pruritus, hyperesthesia, alopecia, dermatitis.
- Nervous – ataxia, vocalization, hyperesthesia, disorientation, vocalization, hypothermia (cats).
- Neuromuscular – muscle fasciculations, tremors, seizures.
- Ophthalmic – (ocular exposures only) ocular irritation and conjunctivitis.
- Reproductive – fluralaner administration during pregnancy has been associated with the development of limb deformity, enlarged heart and spleen, and cleft palate in puppies.

 # SIGNALMENT/HISTORY

### Risk Factors

- Pets with a history of idiopathic epilepsy are predisposed to developing seizures at a therapeutic dosage.

### Historical Findings

- Pet owners often report the pet accidentally ingesting supratherapeutic amounts of these agents or a recent therapeutic exposure to the agent.

 # CLINICAL FEATURES

- Pets with isoxazole insecticide toxicosis can present with vomiting, ataxia, fasciculations, tremors, seizures, hyperesthesia, vocalization, and disorientation.
- Cats may also present with hypothermia, despite a history of stimulatory neurologic signs.
- Seizures are often short and may not recur after a single seizure. Rarely, intermittent seizures have been reported lasting several weeks.
- Clinical signs can occur less than pme hour post exposure or may be delayed out to 20 hours post exposure.
- The most severe clinical signs are expected to resolve within 24 hours post exposure.

 # DIFFERENTIAL DIAGNOSIS

### Intoxications

- Permethrin (cats) – permethrin exposure is accompanied by a history of the application of a dog spot-on flea and tick product. It is important to obtain a thorough history and the packaging material of the product applied dermally to the cat. Tremors for permethrin tend to be more refractory to treatment and last longer than those associated with isoxazoline insecticides.

- Bromethalin – may also cause acute-onset seizures. However, seizures are generally refractory to treatment and signs do not tend to resolve. Pet may have a history of ingesting rodenticide and abnormally colored stool may be present on rectal exam.
- Bifenthrin – may also cause similar acute neurologic and gastrointestinal signs. Cases may present similarly and are treated similarly, though clinical signs often are more refractory to treatment and may be more severe and last longer. Bifenthrin toxicosis often has a history of recent application of bifenthrin insecticide to the lawn or exposure to stored granules.
- Xylitol – may also cause acute-onset seizures. Hypoglycemia and potentially increased liver enzymes as well as a history of ingesting human food containing xylitol or powdered xylitol.
- Tremorgenic mycotoxins – may present with a history of GI upset and tremors. Patients will typically have a history of getting into the garbage, compost pile, or other mold foodstuff. Tremors will usually be more severe and require higher doses of methocarbamol to stop.

 # DIAGNOSTICS

## Clinical Pathological Findings

- None expected. May see some mild changes secondary to the CNS signs.

 # THERAPEUTICS

## Detoxification

- Oral – consider emesis if recent ingestion of pills and patient is asymptomatic. Emesis is unlikely to be of benefit with topical solutions that are ingested but can consider administering a small amount of milk or canned food to help with a taste reaction to the bitter taste of the agent. Activated charcoal is not generally indicated due to the rapid absorption and inconsistent development of clinical signs.
- Aural – clean and flush ears thoroughly if accidentally applied into the ear canals.
- Dermal – when pet is stable, consider bathing whole patient with hand dish soap, if they were recently treated with the dermal formulation.
- Ophthalmic – flush eyes with sterile eye irrigation solution, tepid water, or normal saline for 20–30 minutes following accidental ocular exposure.

## Appropriate Health Care

- Asymptomatic patients with lower dosages can be monitored at home but should seek emergency medical care if neurologic signs occur. Patients with very high dosages or those showing neurologic signs should be hospitalized and monitored closely.
- Thermoregulation – body temperature in cats should be monitored closely and warming measures should be instituted if hypothermic.

## Antidote

- None.

## Drug(s) of Choice

- Antiepileptics for seizures.
    - Midazolam 0.1–0.3 mg/kg IV (preferred) or IM.
    - Diazepam 0.5–1.0 mg/kg IV.
    - Levetiracetam 30–60 mg/kg IV. Note: in rare cases where patients continue to have intermittent seizures, oral levetiracetam is recommended for at-home therapy at 20 mg/kg PO TID or 30 mg/kg PO BID.

- Antiemetics for cases of refractory vomiting.
  - Ondansetron 0.1–0.2 mg/kg PO or slow IV.
  - Maropitant 1.0 mg/kg SQ or slow IV.
- Tremors.
  - Methocarbamol 55–220 mg/kg slow IV to effect until tremors have stopped.
  - Diazepam 0.5–1.0 mg/kg IV.
- IV crystalloid fluids as needed to maintain normal hydration.

### Precautions/Interactions

- None known.

### Alternative Drugs

- Phenobarbital, propofol, or gas anesthesia could be used for refractory seizures, but are unlikely to be needed as seizures are typically readily controlled.

### Extracorporeal Therapy

- Due to the short-lived nature of the most severe signs of the toxicosis, extracorporeal therapy is not likely to be of benefit.

### Surgical Considerations

- Clinical signs should fully resolve before elective surgery is considered.

### Patient Monitoring

- Patient should be monitored for the resolution of neurologic signs until the duration of action of therapeutic medication used for treatment has passed. This is typically 6–8 hours after the last medical intervention is needed.

### Diet

- Patient can and should be continued per normal, as long as the patient is mentally appropriate and can safely ingest food. A bland diet for a couple of days can be considered in patients experiencing gastrointestinal distress.

 **COMMENTS**

### Prevention/Avoidance

- Use of isoxazoline insecticides should be avoided in patients who have had a previous adverse reaction.
- Caution should be used when considering therapeutic use in patients with a history of seizures.
- Chewable medication should be kept out of reach of pets to prevent accidental suprathera-peutic ingestion.
- Products labeled for use in dogs should not be used on cats.

### Possible Complications

- No long-term effects are expected.

### Expected Course and Prognosis

- Onset of clinical signs can be rapid or can be delayed to about 20 hours post exposure.
- Clinical signs generally resolve within 24 hours. Although some may last longer, hospitalization is generally not needed beyond 24 hours.
- Prognosis is generally good with prompt treatment.

## Synonyms

- Bravecto®, Bravecto Plus®
- Credelio®
- NexGard®
- Revolution Plus®
- Simparica®, Simparica Trio®

## Suggested Reading

Bravecto New Animal Drug Application. 2016. https://animaldrugsatfda.fda.gov/adafda/app/search/public/document/downloadFoi/945

Zhou X, Hohman AE, Hsu WH. Current review of isoxazoline ectoparaciticides used in veterinary medicine. *J Vet Pharmacol Ther* 2022;45:1–15.

**Author**: Laura Stern, DVM, DABVT

**Consulting Editor**: Ahna G. Brutlag, DVM, MS, DABT, DABVT

# Chapter 58

# Macrocyclic Lactones

## DEFINITION/OVERVIEW

- Ivermectin, milbemycin, selamectin, doramectin, eprinomectin, moxidectin, and abamectin are macrocyclic lactone derivatives indicated for use either as anthelmintics and heartworm preventives in veterinary medicine (Figure 58.1) or as environmental pesticides (e.g., abamectin, an insecticide).
- Toxicosis can occur when small animals ingest formulations intended for use as pesticides, for use in large animals, or when excessive amounts of products for small animals are

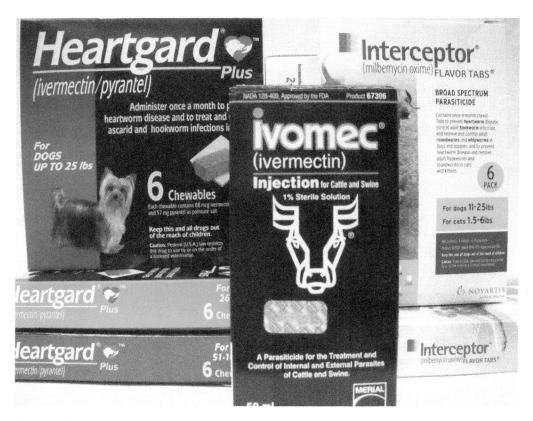

■ **Figure 58.1** Selected large animal products containing macrocyclic lactones. Because of the high concentration of macrocyclic lactones in large animal formulations, very small volumes can be toxic to dogs and cats, especially those with defective P-glycoprotein function.

*Blackwell's Five-Minute Veterinary Consult Clinical Companion: Small Animal Toxicology*, Third Edition. Edited by Lynn R. Hovda, Ahna G. Brutlag, Robert H. Poppenga, and Steven E. Epstein.
© 2024 John Wiley & Sons, Inc. Published 2024 by John Wiley & Sons, Inc.

consumed. Animals with P-glycoprotein deficiency due to MDR1 (multidrug resistance) gene mutations (MDR1 or ABCB1-1Δ mutation in dogs; ABCB11930_1931del TC in cats) or dysfunction (due to drug interactions) can experience toxicosis even at therapeutic doses.

- Clinical signs of toxicosis include lethargy, ataxia, hypersalivation, mydriasis, blindness, tremors, or seizures. Toxicosis can be fatal, especially in animals with P-glycoprotein deficiency or dysfunction.
- Treatment entails decontamination, activated charcoal administration, intensive monitoring, and supportive care. The use of intravenous lipid emulsion (ILE) therapy has been explored.
- With appropriate supportive care, prognosis for complete recovery is often good. However, intensive monitoring, mechanical ventilation, and prolonged hospitalization may be necessary.

 # ETIOLOGY/PATHOPHYSIOLOGY

## Mechanism of Action

- Macrocyclic lactones are fermentation products from *Streptomyces* species with excellent activity against nematodes and arthropods.
- Selective mammalian-sparing toxicity depends on an intact BBB. Specifically, P-glycoprotein must be present and functional. Toxicosis in veterinary species results when the drug gains access to the CNS, allowing it to bind postsynaptic GABA-gated chloride channels and thereby inhibiting neuronal impulse transmission.

## Pharmacokinetics – Absorption, Distribution, Metabolism, Excretion

- Absorption after oral administration is rapid. Peak plasma concentrations at two hours (moxidectin) and four hours (ivermectin).
- While absorption after SQ drug administration is slower than after oral administration, bioavailability is greater.
- Macrocyclic lactones are highly lipophilic and extensively distributed including fat. The lipophilic nature of these drugs, combined with low plasma clearance, contributes to their long persistence in the body. Moxidectin has an approximately eight-fold longer elimination half-life than ivermectin in dogs.
- Canine ivermectin half-life: 3.3 days; moxidectin: 25.9 days.
- Ivermectin and moxidectin are primarily eliminated unchanged in the feces via P-glycoprotein-mediated biliary and enterocyte excretion.
- Eprinomectin has a 23-hour elimination half-life in cats after IV dosing and a 114-hour elimination half-life after topical application likely due to delayed absorption.
- Pharmacokinetic behavior of other macrocyclic lactones would be expected to be similar.

## Toxicity

- Toxic doses vary greatly depending on whether or not the animal expresses P-glycoprotein (harbors an MDR1 mutation) and whether P-glycoprotein is functional or inhibited.
- It is important to note that all original, brand name FDA-approved canine heartworm prevention products have been tested for safety in dogs with the MDR1 mutation and are considered safe in these dogs if used at the manufacturer's recommended dose. The same is not true for cats.
- The FDA-approved heartworm preventive product containing eprinomectin (NexGard Combo™) has caused severe neurological toxicity in cats with ABCB11930_1931del TC when used at the label dose.

### Ivermectin

- For dogs with normal P-glycoprotein function, dosages up to 2.5 mg/kg can be tolerated without clinical signs. Doses ≥2.5 mg/kg may cause mydriasis.
- Tremors can be seen at ≥5 mg/kg; severe tremors and ataxia at ≥10 mg/kg.
- Reported fatalities at 40 mg/kg.
- The reported $LD_{50}$ in experimental beagle models is 80 mg/kg.
- Dogs affected by the P-glycoprotein deletion can tolerate doses up to 0.1 mg/kg.
- Severe and potentially fatal neurological toxicity occurs in dogs with the MDR1 mutation at oral or subcutaneous doses as low as 0.15–0.2 mg/kg.
- Cats have tolerated oral doses of 0.75 mg/kg, though some reports indicate they are tolerant of higher doses.
- Clinical signs of ivermectin toxicosis in cats and kittens older than eight weeks (that do not have the MDR1 mutation) have been reported at oral or subcutaneous doses of 0.3–0.4 mg/kg.

### Moxidectin

- No clinical signs at 0.9 mg/kg (oral), which is 300 times higher than the oral pharmacological dose.
- Clinical signs were observed in a collie, presumably with the MDR1 mutation, after 0.09 mg/kg (oral).

### Milbemycin

- Beagles ingesting 100 mg/kg of milbemycin, which is 200 times the monthly oral pharmacological dose, had no adverse clinical signs.
- Hypersalivation, ataxia, mydriasis, and depression were observed in some collies at 5 mg/kg and all collies at 10 mg/kg in one study.
- Information about toxicosis of milbemycin in cats is not available.

## Systems Affected

- Nervous – affects the CNS causing cell membrane hyperpolarization and subsequent inhibition of neuronal depolarization. Severity of CNS signs increases with dose.
- Ophthalmic – mydriasis, central blindness, multifocal retinal edema, retinal folds, and ERG changes, which are usually reversible.
- Gastrointestinal – hypersalivation, vomiting, anorexia, diarrhea.
- Respiratory – severe neurological impairment secondary to macrocyclic lactone exposure can progress to respiratory failure. Aspiration pneumonia is a possible complication of this toxicosis.
- Cardiovascular – in patients with a significant microfilaria burden, anaphylactic shock after sudden microfilaria death can cause severe hypotension and shock.

## SIGNALMENT/HISTORY

- Dogs and cats of any age, breed, or sex can be affected by this toxicosis.
- Toxicosis is more commonly reported in dogs.
- In most veterinary patients over six weeks old, P-glycoprotein at the BBB prevents toxicosis when macrocyclic lactones are used at therapeutic doses.
- Many breeds of dogs, in particular collies, Australian shepherds, longhaired whippets, silken windhounds, Shetland sheepdogs, German shepherds and similar breeds, harbor a four-base pair deletion of the MDR1 gene (current nomenclature ATP-binding cassette 1 or ABCB1) known as the MDR1 mutation or ABCB1-1Δ mutation. Dogs with this mutation have either no (MDR1 mutant/mutant) or decreased (MDR1 mutant/normal) P-glycoprotein in the BBB, resulting in increased CNS penetration and neurotoxic effects of macrocyclic lactones.

■ Approximately 4% of cats have a two-base pair deletion mutation of the MDR1 (ABCB1) gene. Affected cats display the same sensitivity to macrocyclic lactones as dogs with the MDR1 mutation.

## Risk Factors

■ Use of macrocyclic lactone antiparasitic therapies.
■ Access to or treatment with large animal macrocyclic lactone formulations.
■ Ingestion of feces from large animals recently treated with macrocyclic lactones.
■ Mutations in the MDR1 (ABCB1) gene (dogs or cats).
■ Concurrent administration of drugs that inhibit P-glycoprotein function, such as spinosad, cyclosporine or ketoconazole.

## Historical Findings

■ If ingestion is witnessed by the owner or packaging material is found, the owner may report that their pet ingested a macrocyclic lactone medication or pesticide. Cats may have had topical eprinomectin applied.

## Location and Circumstances of Poisoning

■ Any area where the pet has access to either the medications (e.g., home, garage, barn, farm, etc.) or pesticides.
■ Access to areas where large animals recently treated with these medications defecate (e.g., fields, paddocks, barn, etc.).

# CLINICAL FEATURES

■ Nervous – ataxia, weakness, disorientation, paddling, head pressing (seen in cats), tremors, seizures, coma.
■ Ophthalmic – mydriasis, central blindness, retinal edema (may be multifocal), retinal folds, attenuated or extinguished ERG wave amplitude (measure of retinal function).
■ Gastrointestinal – hypersalivation, vomiting.
■ Respiratory – hypoventilation, poor chest excursions (e.g., intercostal breathing).
■ Cardiovascular – hyperthermia, hypothermia, bradycardia, hypotension.

# DIFFERENTIAL DIAGNOSIS

■ Intoxications: anticholinesterase insecticide (expect muscarinic/SLUDGE signs), tremorgenic mycotoxin (more severe tremors), cannabis/THC (typically lacks blindness and seizures are rare), ethylene glycol (elevated anion gap with metabolic acidosis and renal involvement), benzodiazepines (lacks ophthalmic signs, reversible with flumazenil), barbiturate ingestion, opioid intoxication (miosis and severe respiratory depression, reversible with naloxone), lead toxicosis (GI signs, measurable blood lead concentrations, basophilic stippling on RBCs).
■ Metabolic disease – hepatic encephalopathy, portosystemic shunt, etc.
■ Primary ophthalmic disease.

# DIAGNOSTICS

## Clinical Pathological Findings

■ Depending on the patient's clinical status, diagnostics to assess the stability of the patient should take priority over confirmatory testing. Such emergency diagnostics may include:
  • serum chemistry: electrolytes, PCV/TS, blood glucose, BUN, creatinine.

- arterial blood gas (to assess oxygenation and ventilation) or venous blood gas (to assess ventilation) and pulse oximetry.

## Other Diagnostics

- Cardiovascular status: blood pressure, ECG.
- Liquid chromatography mass spectroscopy to determine drug levels.
  - Can be performed on serum, adipose tissue, and liver samples.
  - If animal does not have an MDR1 mutation, serum levels correlate with clinical signs, as clinical signs are dependent on the concentration of the drug in the brain. The concentration of macrocyclic lactones in the brain of animals with dysfunctional P-glycoprotein will be much higher for any given serum concentration than in "normal" animals.
- MDR1 genotyping.
  - Should be considered in all dogs whose clinical signs do not correlate with the amount of macrocyclic lactone ingested.
  - Requires either a cheek swab or EDTA blood sample sent to the Program in Individualized Medicine, Washington State University, Pullman, WA 99164-6610 (https://prime.vetmed.wsu.edu).
- Fundoscopy: can be performed via direct or indirect ophthalmoscopy.
- ERG: allows for assessment of the neurosensory activity of the retina.

## Pathological Findings

There are no characteristic gross or histopathological lesions.

# THERAPEUTICS

## Detoxification

- In neurologically appropriate patients, emesis should be induced as quickly and safely as possible. Ropinirole is preferred to apomorphine as an emetic in dogs with the MDR1 mutation.
- For neurologically inappropriate sedation, intubation, and gastric lavage may be considered.
- Due to enterohepatic recirculation, repeated doses of activated charcoal are indicated. Only the first dose should contain a cathartic. Administration of activated charcoal via a stomach tube for intubated patients may be necessary, with an inflated ETT to prevent secondary aspiration pneumonia.

## Appropriate Health Care

- Seizures must be aggressively controlled to prevent cerebral edema, noncardiogenic pulmonary edema, and aspiration of GIT contents. Intubation may be necessary.
- Ventilation should be closely monitored in patients with severe neurological impairment using venous or arterial (preferred) $pCO_2$ or end-tidal capnography. Mechanical ventilation is indicated for patients with hypoventilation.
- Perform frequent lung auscultation as well as serial measurement of blood oxygenation (e.g., pulse oximetry, arterial blood gas) in patients where aspiration pneumonia is a concern. Mechanical ventilation is indicated for patients with severe hypoxemia unresponsive to supplemental oxygen therapy.
- Continuous ECG in patients with concerning bradycardia.

## Antidotes

There is no antidote.

## Drug(s) of Choice

- For control seizures, patients can be loaded with phenobarbital (2–4 mg/kg IV as needed to control seizures, up to 16 mg/kg) or levetiracetam (20 mg/kg IV q 8 hours). The lowest effect dose should be used, due to the risks of severe sedation.
- ILE: the author has experience with using ILE to help treat dogs with ivermectin toxicosis. ILE is thought to create a lipid partition or "sink" within the intravascular space, which helps to contain the lipophilic macrocyclic lactone in the vasculature, and therefore decrease brain exposure. There is also a published case report describing the use of ILE to treat a puppy with suspected moxidectin toxicosis. Unfortunately, ILE has not been helpful in treating macrocyclic lactone toxicosis in dogs with the MDR1 mutation (three cases described in the literature). The reader is encouraged to contact an established veterinary toxicology helpline or toxicologist for the most current guidance.

## Precautions/Interactions

- Concurrent administration of drugs that competitively inhibit P-glycoprotein function.
  - Spinosad.
  - Ketoconazole.
  - Verapamil.
  - Tamoxifen.
  - Cyclosporine.
- Benzodiazepines (e.g., midazolam, diazepam) should be avoided for tremor or seizure management, as these drugs may potentiate the CNS toxicosis due to GABA binding leading to prolonged recovery.
- The use of physostigmine, picrotoxin, or flumazenil is not recommended.

## Alternative Drugs

- If tremors or seizures do not respond to phenobarbital or levetiracetam, propofol (1–2 mg/kg IV bolus, 0.1–0.2 mg/kg/min CRI) or etomidate (0.5–4 mg/kg IV) may be used. Etomidate should not be used as a sole agent.

## Extracorporeal Therapy

- Not routinely recommended.
- Single-pass lipid dialysis has been described in one case report involving two Australian shepherd dogs homozygous for the ABCB1-1Δ mutation. The clinical response was minimal and both dogs remained ventilated for several days following dialysis. Ultimately, both dogs made a full recovery.

## Patient Monitoring

- Intensive neurological monitoring (e.g., mentation, menace, visual ability, pupil size, PLR, ambulation, etc.) should be carried out every 2–4 hours, especially if neurological impairment is evident at presentation.
- Care should be provided for recumbent patients, including frequent turning, passive range of motion, bladder and colon care, and eye and oral care.
- Special attention should be given to patients with central blindness to protect their corneas with frequent lubrication and prevent trauma to the eyes since patients may not blink as a protective mechanism.
- For patients with seizures and concerns for cerebral edema, a board under the head and neck, positioned at a 15–30° angle, should be used to help decrease ICP. Compression of the jugular veins (especially for venipuncture) and hyperthermia should be avoided. Supplemental oxygen via a mask should be considered for all recumbent, neurological patients.

- Body temperature should be measured frequently. Heat support should be used for patients with hypothermia but should be discontinued when the body temperature has reached 99 °F. In addition, gentle cooling measures, such as wetting of the fur and a fan, can be used for patients with hyperthermia. Cooling measures should be stopped once the patient's temperature has reached 103.5 °F to prevent rebound hypothermia.
- Serum electrolytes (e.g., sodium, potassium, glucose) should be monitored and treated if needed for patients receiving multiple doses of activated charcoal, large amounts of IV fluids, and those with seizures.

### Diet

- In patients with prolonged neurological compromise, recumbency, or those that require mechanical ventilation, a feeding tube or parenteral nutrition may be necessary.

 # COMMENTS

### Prevention/Avoidance

- Proper storage of antiparasitic medications (Figure 58.2).
- Ensuring correct dosage, particularly when large animal formulations are used.
- Preventing access to feces from large animals recently treated with these medications.
- Restricting animal's access to areas treated with macrocyclic lactone pesticides.
- MDR1 genotyping in all animals with toxicosis to rule out ABCB1 mutations.
  - MDR1 genotyping in cats prior to treatment with eprinomectin (NexGard COMBO).
  - For patients confirmed to be affected with the ABCB1 mutations, recommendations on other medications that must be avoided should be made (e.g., loperamide – see "Problem Medications" list at https://prime.vetmed.wsu.edu).

### Possible Complications

- Aspiration pneumonia.
- Hypoventilation or hypoxemia requiring mechanical ventilation.

### Expected Course and Prognosis

- The prognosis for recovery is largely dependent on dose and MDR1 genotype. Animals ingesting a larger dose, or those that lack functional P-glycoprotein at the BBB, are expected to require more intensive care and will likely have a more prolonged recovery.
- Duration to recovery can vary from days to weeks.

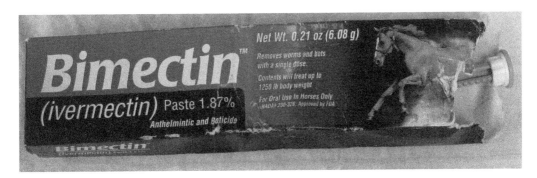

■ Figure 58.2 A tube of equine ivermectin anthelmintic chewed by a dog. Ingestion of equine macrocyclic lactone anthelmintics is the most common cause of this toxicosis reported to the Pet Poison Helpline. Source: Courtesy of Dana L. Clarke.

- Patients requiring more intensive care, especially mechanical ventilation, will also have increased costs associated with hospitalization, which may affect prognosis due to the owner's financial capabilities.
- Animals that recover usually have no long-term complications secondary to this toxicosis.

## Abbreviations

See Appendix 1 for a complete list.
- ABCB1 = ATP-binding cassette protein 1
- BBB = blood–brain barrier
- ERG = electroretinogram
- ETT = endotracheal tube
- GABA = gamma-aminobutyric acid
- ICP = intracranial pressure
- ILE = intravenous lipid emulsion
- MDR1 = multidrug resistance gene 1

## Suggested Reading

Al-Azzam SI, Fleckstein L, Cheng K et al. Comparison of the pharmacokinetics of moxidectin and ivermectin after oral administration to beagle dogs. *Biopharm Drug Disposition* 2007;28:431–438.

Beal MW, Poppenga RH, Birdsall WJ et al. Respiratory failure attributable to moxidectin intoxication in a dog. *J Am Vet Med Assoc* 1999;215(12):1813–1817.

Crandell DE, Weinberg GL. Moxidectin toxicosis in a puppy successfully treated with intravenous lipids. *J Vet Emerg Crit Care* 2009;19(2):181–186.

Hopper K, Aldrich J, Haskins SC. Ivermectin toxicity in 17 collies. *J Vet Intern Med* 2002;16:89–94.

Kenny PJ, Vernau KM, Puschner B et al. Retinopathy associated with ivermectin toxicosis in two dogs. *J Am Vet Med Assoc* 2008;233(2):279–284.

Mealey KL. Ivermectin: macrolide antiparasitic agents. In: Peterson ME, Talcott PA (eds) *Small Animal Toxicology*, 2nd edn. St Louis: Elsevier, 2006; pp. 601–608.

Mealey KL, Owens JG, Freeman E. Canine and feline P-gp deficiency: what we know and where we need to go. *J Vet Pharmacol Ther* 2023;46(1):1–16.

Wright HM, Chen AV, Talcott PA, Poppenga RH, Mealey KL. Intravenous fat emulsion as treatment for ivermectin toxicosis in three dogs homozygous for the ABCB1-1D gene mutation. *J Vet Emerg Crit Care* 2011;21(6):666–672.

**Author:** Katrina L. Mealey, DVM, PhD, DACVIM, DACVCP
**Consulting Editor:** Ahna G. Brutlag, DVM, MS, DABT, DABVT

# Chapter 59

# Phenylpropanolamine

## DEFINITION/OVERVIEW

- Phenylpropanolamine (PPA) is a sympathomimetic drug commonly used for the medical treatment of female urinary incontinence (urethral sphincter hypotonus).
- Overdoses are associated with tachycardia or reflex bradycardia, hypertension, agitation, excitability, tremors, urinary retention, and seizures.
- PPA is commonly available as flavored chewable tablets (Proin® 25, 50, and 75 mg) (Proin extended-release [ER] 18, 38, 74, and 145 mg) and liquid (Proin drops 25 mg/mL), but multiple formulations are available through various manufacturers and compounding pharmacies.
- Intoxication is often due to animals ingesting large amounts of chewable medications.

## ETIOLOGY/PATHOPHYSIOLOGY

### Mechanism of Action

- PPA is a sympathomimetic agent that primarily works via alpha-adrenergic receptor stimulation, which leads to its therapeutic effect of smooth muscle contraction in the urethra.
- The drug is also believed to increase norepinephrine release and stimulate beta-$1$ receptors but has no reported stimulation of beta-2 receptors.

### Pharmacokinetics – Absorption, Distribution, Metabolism, Excretion

- Absorption – well absorbed orally with good bioavailability, approximately 98%.
- Distribution – distributed widely throughout the body, including the CNS.
- Metabolism – partially metabolized by the liver into active metabolites, no enterohepatic recirculation.
- Excretion – immediate release: 80–90% is excreted unchanged in urine within 24 hours, longer with ER products. The half-life is approximately 3–4 hours with immediate-release products and 3–10 hours with ER products.

### Toxicity

- No known $LD_{50}$ exists in veterinary medicine.
- Mild signs can be seen at the therapeutic dose (2 mg/kg PO q 12 hours) but significant signs are not anticipated at this dose.
- Overdoses of 2–3 times the therapeutic dose should be decontaminated and monitored for at least eight hours.

*Blackwell's Five-Minute Veterinary Consult Clinical Companion: Small Animal Toxicology*, Third Edition.
Edited by Lynn R. Hovda, Ahna G. Brutlag, Robert H. Poppenga, and Steven E. Epstein.
© 2024 John Wiley & Sons, Inc. Published 2024 by John Wiley & Sons, Inc.

## Systems Affected

- Cardiovascular – hypertension often with reflex bradycardia, tachycardia, tachyarrhythmias, myocardial dysfunction.
- Gastrointestinal – anorexia, salivation, and vomiting.
- Hemic – DIC (rare sequela to prolonged seizure activity and hyperthermia).
- Hepatobiliary – elevated liver enzymes.
- Musculoskeletal – tremors, rhabdomyolysis (rare sequela to prolonged seizure/tremors).
- Nervous – agitation, hyperactivity, hyperesthesia, tremors and rarely seizures or coma.
- Ophthalmic – mydriasis (sympathomimetic stimulation), hyphema, retinal detachment, increased IOP.
- Renal/urological – urinary retention, myoglobinuria, azotemia.
- Skin – piloerection, erythema.

 # SIGNALMENT/HISTORY

### Risk Factors

- Animals with preexisting cardiovascular disease (including hypertension), hyperthyroidism, or glaucoma may develop more severe clinical signs.
- Cats – PPA is rarely prescribed for cats as they may have signs of intoxication even at therapeutic doses.

### Historical Findings

- History of accidental ingestion of medication (generally via dietary indiscretion but potentially through therapeutic error).
- Owners may report hiding, restlessness, CNS stimulation, mydriasis, piloerection, excitability, vocalization, vomiting, anorexia, tremors, or seizures.

### Location and Circumstances of Poisoning

- Although primarily prescribed for older spayed female dogs, any pet may ingest this medication.
- Dogs more commonly ingest large quantities of medication, compared to cats; however, cats are more sensitive to PPA than dogs.

 # CLINICAL FEATURES

- Clinical signs may be noted as early as 30 minutes; typically noted within eight hours after exposure.
- Agitation/hyperactivity.
- Piloerection.
- Erythema.
- Tachycardia.
- Bradycardia.
- Hyperthermia.
- Mydriasis.
- Hyphema/retinopathy.
- Ataxia.
- Tremors/twitching.
- Seizures.

# DIFFERENTIAL DIAGNOSIS

- Other intoxications that may result in similar signs include 5-HTP, albuterol, amphetamines/methamphetamines, anticholinergics, antihistamines, antipsychotics, benzodiazepines (paradoxical response), cocaine, hops, imidazoline, methylxanthines (caffeine, chocolate, etc.), marijuana, metaldehyde, methionine, tremorgenic mycotoxins, nicotine, pseudoephedrine, SSRIs, TCAs, thyroid supplements (generally very large overdoses).
- Pheochromocytoma.
- Primary CNS lesion.
- Hyperthyroidism.

# DIAGNOSTICS

## Clinical Pathological Findings

- Serum chemistry.
  - Acute renal failure and elevated liver enzymes may be noted secondary to toxicosis.
  - Serum CK to monitor for rhabdomyolysis.
- UA to evaluate renal function, check for tubular casts and monitor for pigmenturia and proteinuria.
- Coagulation panel if DIC is suspected.
- Cardiac troponin levels if suspicious for myocardial damage.
- Phenylpropanolamine concentrations can be detected in urine or blood via liquid and gas chromatography, but this is rarely done.

## Other Diagnostics

- Blood pressure monitoring for hypertension.
- ECG – may see tachyarrhythmias or reflex bradycardia secondary to hypertension.

## Pathological Findings

- Myocardial infarction.
- Pigmentary nephropathy and tubular damage.
- Hemorrhagic stroke.

# THERAPEUTICS

## Detoxification

- Induce emesis within one hour of ingestion if the animal is asymptomatic.
- Activated charcoal with a cathartic at 1 g/kg PO once.

## Appropriate Health Care

- Observation for eight hours after exposure.
- Provide symptomatic and supportive care for signs noted.
- IV fluids – rate will depend on blood pressure. High rates of IV fluids may exacerbate hypertension.
- Cooling measures as needed for hyperthermia. Stop cooling at temperature $\leq$103.5 °F.

## Antidote

- None.

## Drug(s) of Choice

- Hyperactivity and hypertension – acepromazine 0.02–1.0 mg/kg IV, IM, SQ or chlorpromazine 0.5–1.0 mg/kg IV, IM as needed for sedation. Higher doses may be required. These drugs are preferred over other sedatives (see Precautions/Interactions).
- Hyperactivity – butorphanol 0.2–0.4 mg/kg IV, IM, SQ q 6–8 hours.
- Hypertension – amlodipine 0.1–0.5 mg/kg PO q 12–24 hours or hydralazine 0.5–3 mg/kg PO q 12 hours.
- Tachycardia – propranolol 0.02–0.06 mg/kg IV slowly to effect.
- Tremors – methocarbamol 55–220 mg/kg IV to effect.
- Seizures/tremors – phenobarbital 4 mg/kg IV to effect (up to 16–24 mg/kg loading dose) or levetiracetam 30–60 mg/kg IV once then 30 mg/kg IV or PO q 8 hours.

## Precautions/Interactions

- Concurrent treatment with MAOIs, SSRIs, TCAs, amitraz, NSAIDs, and other sympathomimetic agents may increase the risk of intoxication, even at therapeutic dosages.
- Benzodiazepines (diazepam/midazolam) are not often used for sedation in sympathomimetic overdoses as they may exacerbate clinical signs.
- Drugs used to treat bradycardia such as atropine may exacerbate hypertension. Bradycardia is often secondary to hypertension and will resolve once hypertension is controlled.

## Patient Monitoring

- Patient should be monitored (TPR, BP, CNS status) for eight hours after an exposure.
- ECG and blood pressure monitoring should be frequent, ideally every 2–4 hours. Continuous ECG and blood pressure monitoring in serious cases.
- Symptomatic patients should be monitored closely for seizures.
- Uncomplicated cases do not require follow-up.
- Animals developing secondary complications such as cardiac dysfunction, rhabdomyolysis, DIC, or renal damage may require prolonged treatment.

 **COMMENTS**

### Prevention/Avoidance

- Owner should be advised of the palatability of the tablets and about securing all medications, especially chewable/flavored tablets.
- Due to the potential for drug interactions with PPA, instruct clients not to administer other medications without veterinary approval.

### Possible Complications

- Cardiac arrhythmias and myocardial dysfunction have been reported. Consultation with a cardiologist may be needed in severe cases.
- Although not reported commonly in the veterinary literature, myglobinuric renal failure and DIC may develop following prolonged seizures/tremors.
- Animals with preexisting renal or hepatic insufficiency may have decreased rate of drug clearance. These animals may require a longer and more aggressive course of treatment.

### Expected Course and Prognosis

- Prognosis is generally good if treated early.
- Signs can persist for 24–72 hours depending on formulation and dose ingested.
- Animals exhibiting severe CNS signs, cardiac arrhythmias, developing DIC, or myoglobinuria have guarded to poor prognosis.

## Synonyms

PPA, Proin, Proin drops, cystolamine, Propalin®, Propalin syrup.

## See Also

Chapter 15 Amphetamines
Chapter 49 Decongestants (Pseudoephedrine, Phenylephrine)
Chapter 86 Ephedra/Ma Huang
Chapter 40 Methamphetamine

## Abbreviations

See Appendix 1 for a complete list.

## Suggested Reading

Bacon NJ, Oni O, White RAS. Treatment of the urethral sphincter mechanism incompetence in 11 bitches with a sustained-release formulation of phenylpropanolamine hydrochloride. *Vet Rec* 2002;151:373–376.
Crandell JM, Ware WA. Cardiac toxicity from phenylpropanolamine overdose in a dog. *J Am Anim Hosp Assoc* 2005;41:413–420.
Ginn JA, Bentley E, Stepien RL. Systemic hypertension and hypertensive retinopathy following PPA overdose in a dog. *J Am Anim Hosp Assoc* 2013;49:46–53.
Peterson KL, Lee JA, Hovda LR. Phenylpropanolamine toxicosis in dogs: a review of 170 cases (2004–2009). *J Am Vet Med Assoc* 2011;239:1463–1469.

## Acknowledgment

The authors and editors acknowledge Nancy M. Gruber, DVM, for her previous contribution to this chapter.

**Author**: Katherine L. Peterson, DVM, DACVECC, DABT
**Consulting Editor**: Ahna G. Brutlag, DVM, MS, DABT, DABVT

# 60

# Pimobendan

## DEFINITION/OVERVIEW

- Pimobendan is a drug commonly used in dogs with congestive heart failure, preclinical dilated cardiomyopathy, and preclinical degenerative valve disease.
- Although not FDA approved for use in cats, pimobendan is used with increasing frequency for cardiomyopathy and heart failure.
- Pimobendan has both a positive inotropic effect and a balanced vasodilatory effect, improving cardiac output without proarrhythmic effects when administered at prescribed doses.
- The drug is available as 1.25 mg, 2.5 mg, 5 mg, and 10mg tablets under the brand name Vetmedin®.
- Overdose may occur when animals ingest large quantities due to the enhanced palatability of tablets with meat flavoring.
- Clinical signs of overdose may include anorexia, vomiting, tachycardia, hypotension, or hypertension.

## ETIOLOGY/PATHOPHYSIOLOGY

### Mechanism of Action

- Pimobendan increases forward blood flow from the left ventricle.
- Pimobendan is an inodilator, with both calcium-sensitizing properties and phosphodiesterase III inhibition.
  - Inodilators have both positive inotropic (increased contractility) and vasodilating effects.
  - Pimobendan alters sensitivity of troponin C to calcium, resulting in greater actin–myosin interaction (positive inotropy).
  - Phosphodiesterase (PDE) III is expressed mainly in the heart and vascular smooth muscle. Inhibition of PDEIII causes increased contractility and vasodilation.

### Pharmacokinetics – Absorption, Distribution, Metabolism, Excretion

- Pimobendan is absorbed rapidly when given orally and has a bioavailability of 60–65%.
- The onset of action is within one hour of administration.
- It is metabolized into its active form by the liver.
- The half-life of pimobendan and its metabolite is 0.4 hours and 2 hours, respectively, in the dog.
- The half-life of pimobendan and its metabolite is longer in cats (0.7 hours and 1.3 hours, respectively), suggesting reduced metabolism in this species.

*Blackwell's Five-Minute Veterinary Consult Clinical Companion: Small Animal Toxicology*, Third Edition.
Edited by Lynn R. Hovda, Ahna G. Brutlag, Robert H. Poppenga, and Steven E. Epstein.
© 2024 John Wiley & Sons, Inc. Published 2024 by John Wiley & Sons, Inc.

- Elimination is by excretion in the bile.
- Pimobendan is 90–95% bound to plasma proteins in circulation.

## Toxicity

### Dogs

- The labeled dosage in dogs is 0.5 mg/kg PO divided twice daily.
- Oral doses as low as 1 mg/kg have caused mild hypotension and tachycardia in dog cases reported to the ASPCA Animal Poison Control Center (APCC).
  - Doses up to 8 mg/kg PO in experimental dogs have failed to produce acute clinical signs. However, a single case report of a dog ingesting 8.24 mg/kg orally developed systolic anterior motion of the mitral valve, increased T-wave amplitude, and hypertension, which resolved at 12, 24, and 36 hours after ingestion, respectively.
  - No studies have demonstrated an increased risk of sudden death in dogs. Brief, self-limiting arrhythmias (AIVR, supraventricular tachycardia, VPCs) have been reported.
  - Long-term studies have shown development of mitral valve pathology in dogs.
  - In a four-week study of dogs, dose-dependent increases in heart rate were seen after administration of pimobendan 2 and 8 mg/kg IV.
- In a six-month toxicity study of dogs, mild heart murmurs developed in one dog at three times (1.5 mg/kg) the labeled dosage and in two dogs at five times (2.5 mg/kg) the labeled dosage; the dogs were not clinically affected by these murmurs.
  - Dogs receiving supraphysiological doses orally had elevations in alkaline phosphatase (ALP) without histological evidence of hepatotoxicity.
  - One case study demonstrated a worsening of mitral valve regurgitation in two dogs with mitral valve disease after oral pimobendan administration, which subsided upon withdrawal of the drug. Development of previously undetected heart murmurs have also been reported in overdose cases, which resolved spontaneously.
  - *In vitro* evidence of platelet inhibition has failed to translate into clinical evidence of platelet inhibition or thrombocytopenia.

### Cats

- Use in cats in cats is off-label, with prescribed dosages of 1.25 **mg per cat** or 0.25 mg/kg PO divided twice daily.
- High doses (0.5mg/kg PO q 12 h) in healthy cats showed increased numbers of idioventricular and idiojunctional escape beats that were clinically irrelevant. The drug is well tolerated at doses similar to those in dogs.

## Systems Affected

- Cardiovascular – possible hypotension, reflex tachycardia. Potential for self-limiting hypertension.
- Gastrointestinal – hyporexia, vomiting.
- Hepatobiliary – increased ALP.

 # SIGNALMENT/HISTORY

### Risk Factors

- Pimobendan is FDA approved for administration only to dogs with CHF secondary to mitral valve disease or dilated cardiomyopathy (DCM), as well as to dogs with Stage B2 preclinical myxomatous mitral valve disease. Given the pathology of mitral and tricuspid valves with naturally occurring disease, administration of clinical doses of pimobendan is unlikely to cause additional valvular damage.

- The manufacturer states that pimobendan should not be administered to dogs with hypertrophic cardiomyopathy (HCM), aortic stenosis, or conditions wherein additional augmentation of cardiac output is contraindicated. Studies of arrhythmogenesis with pimobendan have failed to demonstrate a clinically significant proarrhythmic effect.
- In cats, evidence suggests that the drug is well tolerated at doses similar to those in dogs. No adverse effects were noted in cats that had hypertrophic obstructive cardiomyopathy in several studies. Hypotension was seen in a single cat with a fixed left ventricular outflow tract obstruction in one study, but this was secondary to a complex congenital cardiac defect.

### Historical Findings

- Witnessed ingestion or discovery of a spilled/chewed pill canister.
- Clinical signs such as anorexia or vomiting may be detected by the pet owner.

### Location and Circumstances of Poisoning

- Given the palatable nature of the tablets, pets may intentionally ingest large amounts of the medication if allowed access to the container.

 ## CLINICAL FEATURES

- Signs of intoxication would be expected to develop within 1–2 hours.
- Due to pimobendan's short half-life, signs would be expected to resolve in less than 6–8 hours. Hypertension seems to resolve in approximately 8–12 hours with little or no treatment.
- Vomiting can be seen at any dose.
- Hypotension and tachycardia are the most common signs following overdose. Doses as low as 1 mg/kg have caused mild hypotension and tachycardia in dog cases reported to the APCC.
- Hypertension was observed in about 3% of dog cases reported to the APCC. The lowest dose where hypertension was observed in a dog, without underlying cardiac disease, was 3.06 mg/kg.
- Massive overdoses may cause arrhythmias (atrial fibrillation with increased ventricular ectopic beats), syncope, and weak or irregular pulses. Increased amplitude T-waves have been reported on EKG.

 ## DIFFERENTIAL DIAGNOSIS

- Other causes of gastrointestinal signs.
- Primary cardiac disease.
- Primary respiratory disease.
- Intoxication with other medications that cause hypotension, including other PDEIII inhibitors (amrinone, inamrinone, milrinone), erectile dysfunction drugs (sildenafil, tadalafil, vardenafil), nitroglycerin, and other nitrites/nitrates, ACE inhibitors, alpha-adrenergic agents, beta-blockers, and angiotensin II blockers.

 ## DIAGNOSTICS

### Clinical Pathological Findings

- Baseline CBC, chemistry profile – mild increase in ALP may occur.

## Pathological Findings

- No changes expected acutely. In chronic dosing, cardiac histopathology can be performed but may be similar to changes seen in normal progression of heart failure.
- Chronic high-dose administration results in development of myxomatous changes of the mitral valve, consistent with changes seen with other potent inotropes (milrinone).

 # THERAPEUTICS

- Pimobendan has a wide margin of safety. It is important to note that observed clinical signs may be directly related to the animal's underlying cardiac disease rather than exposure to pimobendan.
- Preexisting cardiac disease must be taken into account when considering therapeutic intervention.

## Detoxification

- With acute ingestion of large quantities of pimobendan, emesis is recommended within one hour if the patient is asymptomatic.
- Activated charcoal with a cathartic (e.g., sorbitol), given early, may reduce the amount of systemically absorbed drug. Absorption of pimobendan is rapid.

## Appropriate Health Care

- Treatment is symptomatic and supportive and based on clinical signs.
- With mild ingestions and appropriate decontamination, outpatient treatment is often sufficient.
- With larger/symptomatic ingestions, hospitalization for monitoring and supportive care is recommended.

## Antidotes

- There is no antidote.

## Drug(s) of Choice

- IV fluids (crystalloids and/or colloids) to control hypotension. Fluid therapy must be used judiciously in patients with underlying cardiac disease.
- Dopamine (1–3 mcg/kg/min titrated up to 10 mcg/kg/min IV CRI) or dobutamine (5–15 mcg/kg/min IV CRI) may be needed for hypotension nonresponsive to IV fluids. Use with care in animals with preexisting heart disease.
- Tachycardia should resolve with control of blood pressure; beta-blockers if needed, but use with care in animals with CHF or DCM.

## Precautions/Interactions

- Clinical experience of combination therapy with digoxin, sildenafil, diuretics, ACE inhibitors, and antiarrhythmic agents have failed to demonstrate significant drug interactions.
- The effects of pimobendan may be attenuated by potent negative inotropes, vasoconstrictors, or calcium channel blockers.

## Patient Monitoring

- Monitor ECG, heart rate, and blood pressure for 6–8 hours.

**COMMENTS**

## Prevention/Avoidance

- Keep all medications in an inaccessible place away from animals.

## Possible Complications

- None expected from acute overdose; chronic dosing may cause cardiac changes.

## Expected Course and Prognosis

- For symptomatic cases, hospitalization is generally short (24 hours).
- Prognosis for acute pimobendan ingestion is good.

## See Also

Chapter 16 Angiotensin-Converting Enzyme Inhibitors
Chapter 22 Beta Receptor Antagonists (Beta-blockers)
Chapter 24 Calcium Channel Blockers

## Abbreviations

See Appendix 1 for a complete list.
- AIVR = accelerated idioventricular rhythm
- VPC = ventricular premature contraction

## Suggested Reading

Oldach MS, Ueda Y, Ontiveros ES et al. Cardiac effects of a single dose of pimobendan in cats with hypertrophic cardiomyopathy: a randomized, placebo-controlled, crossover study. *Front Vet Sci* 2019;6:15.
Reinker LN, Lee JA, Hovda LR, Rishniw M. Clinical signs of cardiovascular effects secondary to suspected pimobendan toxicosis in five dogs. *J Am Anim Hosp Assoc* 2012;48(4):250–255.
Schober KE, Rush JE, Luis Fuentes V et al. Effects of pimobendan in cats with hypertrophic cardiomyopathy and recent congestive heart failure: results of a prospective, double-blind, randomized, nonpivotal, exploratory field study. *J Vet Intern Med* 2021;35(2):789–800.
Tokuriki T, Miyagawa Y, Takemura N. Overdose ingestion of pimobendan in a dog. *Adv Anim Cardiol* 2015;48(1):21–28.
Ward JL, Kussin EZ, Tropf MA et al. Retrospective evaluation of the safety and tolerability of pimobendan in cats with obstructive vs nonobstructive cardiomyopathy. *J Vet Intern Med* 2020;34(6):2211–2222.

**Authors:** Julie Schildt, DVM, DACVECC and Philip Krawec, DVM, DACVECC
**Consulting Editor:** Ahna G. Brutlag, DVM, MS, DABT, DABVT

# Chapter 61

# Veterinary NSAIDs

 **DEFINITION/OVERVIEW**

- NSAIDs are FDA approved for use in cats and dogs for the relief of pain and inflammation.
- They are inhibitors of COX-1, -2, and -3 as well as LOX enzymes, which decrease inflammation but can result in adverse effects, most commonly on the GI tract and kidneys and, at higher doses, the CNS. Hepatotoxicity has been reported but is suspected to be idiosyncratic.
- Veterinary NSAID drugs, formulations, and therapeutic doses.
  - Carprofen is available in 25, 75, and 100 mg caplets and chewable tablets and a 50 mg/mL injectable formulation. It is FDA approved for dogs only at 4.4 mg/kg/day PO, IM, or SQ; can divide into q 12 dosing.
  - Deracoxib is available in chewable tablets in 12, 25, 75, and 100 mg strength and is FDA approved for dogs only at 1–4 mg/kg PO q 24 hours. The dosage and duration are indication dependent.
  - Firocoxib is available in 57 and 227 mg chewable tablets and is FDA approved for dogs (not cats) at 5 mg/kg PO q 24 hours. Additional formulations are FDA approved for horses: 0.82% (8.2 mg/g) oral paste, 57 mg tablets, 20 mg/mL injectable solution.
  - Ketoprofen is not FDA approved for cats or dogs, only horses, and is available as a 100 mg/mL injectable solution. Oral formulations may be approved for dogs or cats in other countries. The extra-label dosage in dogs and cats is 0.25–2 mg/kg PO, IM, SQ, IV q 24 hours; dosage, administrative route, and duration of use are indication dependent.
  - Meloxicam is available as an 0.5 and 1.5 mg/mL oral suspension and a 5 mg/mL injectable solution. Multiple oral and injectable formulations are available for human use as well. Other formulations may be available in other countries. Meloxicam is FDA approved for use in dogs and cats. Dog therapeutic dose: 0.2 mg/kg PO, IV, or SQ once then 0.1 mg/kg PO q 24 hours. Cat therapeutic dose: 0.3 mg/kg SQ **once** (not FDA approved for oral dosing).
  - Robenacoxib is available in 5 mg, 10 mg, 20 mg, and 40 mg tablets for dogs; 6 mg tablets for cats; and 20 mg/mL injectable solution for both cats and dogs. Therapeutic dose dog: 2 mg/kg PO, SQ q 24, for a maximum of three days. Therapeutic cat dose: 1 mg/kg PO or 2 mg/kg SQ q 24 hours, for a maximum of three days.
  - Tepoxalin is no longer commercially available in the US. The FDA-approved therapeutic dosage in dogs was 20 mg/kg PO **once**, then 10 mg/kg PO q 24 hours.

*Blackwell's Five-Minute Veterinary Consult Clinical Companion: Small Animal Toxicology*, Third Edition. Edited by Lynn R. Hovda, Ahna G. Brutlag, Robert H. Poppenga, and Steven E. Epstein. © 2024 John Wiley & Sons, Inc. Published 2024 by John Wiley & Sons, Inc.

# ETIOLOGY/PATHOPHYSIOLOGY

## Mechanism of Action

- Carprofen, deracoxib, firocoxib, meloxicam, and robenacoxib are selective COX-2 inhibitors but may inhibit COX-1 at higher doses. Ketoprofen is a nonselective inhibitor of COX enzymes, and tepoxalin inhibits COX-1 and -2 as well as LOX enzymes.
- COX-1 enzymes serve constitutive functions in the body, which leads to the toxicity of these drugs at therapeutic doses and overdoses. COX-2 enzymes are associated with inflammation which leads to the therapeutic response.

## Pharmacokinetics – Absorption, Distribution, Metabolism, Excretion

- All veterinary NSAIDs are well absorbed orally. Food will inhibit absorption of robenacoxib.
- They are highly protein bound and metabolized in the liver via glucuronidation and other hepatic pathways.
- Enterohepatic recirculation: meloxicam (significant), carprofen (limited), ketoprofen (suspected), deracoxib (none), robenacoxib (none), tepoxalin (unknown). This will affect activated charcoal dosing during decontamination.
- Carprofen, deracoxib, firocoxib, meloxicam, robenacoxib, and tepoxalin are mainly excreted in the feces. A small amount is excreted in the urine. Ketoprofen is excreted in the urine.

## Toxicity

### Dogs

- Acute exposures: generally, doses greater than five times the therapeutic dose of most veterinary NSAIDs can result in clinical signs and requires intervention. Toxicity can vary based on patient factors such as age, underlying disease, etc.
  - Carprofen – per the manufacturer, acute doses of 22 mg/kg resulted in GI signs. Commonly suggested acute toxic doses in veterinary literature: >20 mg/kg for GI ulceration, >40 mg/kg for renal failure.
  - Deracoxib – per the manufacturer, acute doses of >10 mg/kg resulted in GI ulceration. Doses up to 100 mg/kg did not show renal damage. Commonly suggested acute toxic doses in veterinary literature: >10 mg/kg for GI ulceration, >20 mg/kg for renal failure.
  - Firocoxib – per the manufacturer, acute doses of 50 mg/kg resulted in GI signs. Other studies with repeat dosing in dogs >15–25 mg/kg clinical signs including GI ulceration.
  - Meloxicam – per the manufacturer, acute doses up to five times therapeutic dose (0.1–0.5 mg/kg) resulted in GI signs. Commonly suggested acute toxic doses in veterinary literature: 4–5× therapeutic dose for GI issues and 8–10× therapeutic for renal issues
  - Tepoxalin – per the manufacturer, acute doses from 100 to 300 mg/kg may result in GI signs.
  - No manufacturer reported renal damage in their safety studies. Manufacturer safety data may differ from postmarket experience as it is not necessarily reflective of animals of differing ages or those with underlying medical conditions.
  - Chronic exposure: therapeutic doses of all veterinary NSAIDs can result in clinical signs.

### Cats

- Acute and chronic doses of NSAIDs may cause intoxication, especially off-label use.
  - Carprofen – commonly suggested toxic doses in veterinary literature: >4 mg/kg for GI signs and >8 mg/kg for renal signs.

- Deracoxib – commonly suggested toxic doses in veterinary literature: >4 mg/kg for GI signs and >8 mg/kg for renal signs.
- Meloxicam – chronic doses of 0.3 mg/kg resulted in vomiting, diarrhea, anorexia. A black box warning for the drug states that repeated use of meloxicam in cats has been associated with acute renal failure and death.
- Robenacoxib – chronic doses of 10 mg/kg resulted in vomiting, diarrhea, anorexia, and rear limb ataxia.

## Systems Affected

- Gastrointestinal – gastroenteritis, mucosal erosions, ulceration and perforation.
- Renal – tubular damage, azotemia, oliguric to anuric renal failure.
- Hemic/immune – blood loss anemia with thrombocytopenia, platelet dysfunction, prolongation of bleeding times.
- Nervous – agitation, depression, ataxia, seizures.

 # SIGNALMENT/HISTORY

### Risk Factors

- Older animals or those with underlying kidney or liver disease or dehydration may be more susceptible to adverse effects. Younger pets may be more likely to retrieve medication bottles and chew on them.
- Concurrent use of steroids or other NSAIDs may contribute to GI ulceration and kidney damage.
- Chronic or off-label use may increase the likelihood of developing clinical signs.
- Chewable and flavored tablets pose a greater risk of massive ingestion due to palatability.
- Cats are more sensitive to NSAIDs than dogs due to decreased glucuronidation and longer elimination half-lives of most drugs. Fewer products are approved for use in cats and off-label use is common.

### Historical Findings

- Owners may report anorexia, vomiting +/– hematemesis, diarrhea, melena or hematochezia, abdominal pain, polydipsia, and polyuria.

### Location and Circumstances of Poisoning

- Most ingestions occur at home.
- Iatrogenic overdoses may occur, especially with injectable forms.

 # CLINICAL FEATURES

- Onset of clinical signs may occur within an hour after ingestion, but some signs, such as renal failure or GI perforation, may take >48–72 hours before they become evident.
- The most common signs will involve the GI tract and include vomiting, abdominal pain, melena, and diarrhea, which often causes secondary dehydration.
- Kidney damage will often manifest as increased drinking and urinating, anorexia, lethargy, and vomiting. Pale mucous membranes and tachycardia may occur after blood loss, hypovolemia, and poor perfusion develop.
- In severe toxicosis, CNS signs can develop, such as weakness, ataxia, and seizures; icterus may occur if liver damage is present.

# DIFFERENTIAL DIAGNOSIS

- Human NSAIDs may cause similar clinical signs but can result in a longer and more significant disease course due to prolonged half-lives. See Chapter 51 (Human NSAIDs).
- Gastrointestinal – gastroenteritis, IBD, HGE, metabolic disease, foreign body, pancreatitis.
- Renal/urological – acute on chronic kidney disease, pyelonephritis, dehydration, grape/raisin ingestion, ethylene glycol intoxication, ureteral obstruction, urethral obstruction.
  - Cats: *Lilium* or *Hemerocallis* plant intoxication.
- Hepatic – xylitol or mushroom intoxication, hepatitis, pancreatitis, cholangiohepatitis.
- Neurological – epilepsy, other neurological toxicants (SSRIs, stimulants, tremorgenic mycotoxins, etc.), hypoglycemia.

# DIAGNOSTICS

## Clinical Pathological Findings

- CBC – blood loss anemia, thrombocytopenia noted with blood loss, high or low WBC with GI perforation and sepsis.
- Serum chemistry profile – azotemia, liver enzyme/bilirubin elevations, elevated protein with dehydration, low albumin with liver failure, blood loss, or sepsis.
- Urinalysis – isosthenuria, urinary casts, proteinuria, glucosuria with renal tubular damage.
- Clotting profile – typically unaffected; platelet function tests can be prolonged.

## Other Diagnostics

- Abdominocentesis or diagnostic peritoneal lavage – neutrophils with intracellular bacteria, glucose differential >20 mg/dL less in abdominal fluid versus peripheral glucose is consistent with a septic abdomen secondary to GI tract perforation.
- Abdominal radiograph – loss of abdominal detail, free gas in the abdomen.
- Abdominal ultrasound – complex free fluid, gastric ulceration, ileus.

## Pathological Findings

- GI tract – erosions, ulceration, and perforation of the stomach and small intestine.
- Kidney – multifocal renal tubular necrosis, renal tubular regeneration, membranoproliferative glomerulonephritis.
- Liver – hepatocellular necrosis.

# THERAPEUTICS

- Treatment is aimed at prevention and palliation of gastric erosion, ulceration, and perforation as well as prevention of renal failure.

## Detoxification

- Induce emesis within one hour after ingestion; may be difficult to identify chewable tablets and liquid formulations in the emesis.
- Activated charcoal with a cathartic 1 g/kg. Consider multidose charcoal (without a cathartic) for drugs that undergo enterohepatic recirculation.

## Appropriate Health Care

- IV fluids as needed to correct dehydration and hypovolemia. Continue IV fluids for 24–72 hours or as needed until clinical signs abate and to support kidney perfusion.
- A blood transfusion may be needed for significant blood loss associated with GI ulceration (rare).

## Antidote

■ None.

## Drug(s) of Choice

■ GI protectants – use an $H_2$-blocker, proton pump inhibitor, or misoprostol, and sucralfate for 5–10 days after ingestion or until clinical signs resolve. Use multiple drugs if clinical signs are severe. Examples:
  • $H_2$-blocker: famotidine 0.5–1 mg/kg PO, IV (slowly), SQ q 12–24 hours. Dogs may benefit from a CRI of 8 mg/kg/day IV.
  • Proton pump inhibitor: pantoprazole 0.7–1 mg/kg IV over 15 minutes q 12 hours; omeprazole 1.0 mg/kg PO q 12 hours.
  • Misoprostol 2–5 mcg/kg PO q 8–12 hours.
  • Sucralfate 0.25–1 g PO q 8 hours.
■ Antiemetic such as maropitant 1 mg/kg SQ, IV (over 1–2 min) for cats/dogs or 2 mg/kg PO q 24 hours for dogs.

## Precautions/Interactions

■ Discontinue use of other NSAIDs and steroids and use caution with drugs listed that may have interactions with NSAIDs.
■ Animals taking or concurrently ingesting the following drugs may be more susceptible to intoxication: ACE inhibitors, anticoagulants, aspirin, bisphosphonates, corticosteroids, cyclosporine, digoxin, fluconazole, furosemide, hepatic enzyme-inducing agents (e.g., phenobarbital), highly protein-bound drugs, methotrexate, nephrotoxic drugs, other NSAIDs, probenecid.

## Alternative Drugs

■ Alternative medication to replace NSAID for postoperative pain control or arthritis pain, such as tramadol 1–4 mg/kg PO q 8–12 hours or gabapentin 10 mg/kg PO q 8 hours.
■ Hepatoprotective medications and antioxidants can be used prophylactically or if liver damage is noted (e.g., silymarin/milk thistle, SAMe).
■ IV lipid emulsion use has been reported as a treatment in veterinary NSAID toxicity. Although drugs may be lipid soluble, successful treatment with lipids may be limited due to high protein binding and routine use as a first-line treatment is not recommended for all cases.

## Extracorporeal Therapy

■ Therapeutic plasma exchange can be considered in large overdoses for drug removal due to high protein binding of most veterinary NSAIDs.

## Surgical Considerations

■ Exploratory laparotomy may include repair of GI perforation as well as copious lavage of the abdomen when a septic abdomen is identified. Standard postsurgical care as needed.

## Patient Monitoring

■ Monitor hydration, kidney values, and urine output for patients with suspected kidney damage. Recheck kidney values every 24 hours until normal or at a steady state.
■ Animals can bleed into their GI tract without obvious melena or hematochezia. Monitor PCV/TP, CRT, heart rate, blood pressure, appetite, and stool quality as abnormalities can be early indicators of blood loss.
■ Keep animals clean and dry if having diarrhea.

## Diet

- Bland diet or prescription GI diet in symptomatic animals.
- Nutritional supplementation or appetite stimulants for anorectic animals.

 # COMMENTS

### Prevention/Avoidance

- Discuss appropriate dosing of these medications and provide owners with signs to check for at home so that they can be addressed early before significant morbidity develops.
- Discuss palatability of chewable medication; keep medications out of reach. Animals may take these medications out of purses or bags if left unattended.

### Possible Complications

- Oliguria or anuria may develop and these patients need aggressive therapy and monitoring, including referral for dialysis.
- Chronic renal failure may occur after ingestion and requires lifelong therapy.
- GI perforation can occur and surgery is required for these cases. A septic abdomen and surgery will complicate recovery and may carry a poor prognosis.

### Expected Course and Prognosis

- Clinical signs generally resolve in 48–72 hours.
- Prognosis is fair to good with acute and chronic ingestion with appropriate decontamination and therapy. Surgery for GI perforation may complicate recovery; multiple surgeries may be required. Owners should be informed of the prolonged hospitalization and expense associated with these cases.
- Renal tubules may be able to regenerate with time, but full recovery may not be possible. Oliguria or anuria carries a guarded to poor prognosis.

### See Also

Chapter 46 Aspirin
Chapter 51 Human NSAIDs (Ibuprofen, Naproxen)

### Abbreviations

See Appendix 1 for a complete list.

### Suggested Reading

Enberg TB, Braun LD, Kuzme AB. Gastrointestinal perforation in five dogs associated with the administration of meloxicam. *J Vet Emerg Crit Care* 2006;16:34–43.

Lascelles BD, Blikslager AT, Fox SM, Reece D. Gastrointestinal tract perforation in dogs treated with a selective cyclooxygenase-2 inhibitor: 29 cases (2002–2003). *J Am Vet Med Assoc* 2005;7:1112–1117.

McLean MK Khan SA. Toxicology of frequently encountered nonsteroidal anti-inflammatory drugs in dogs and cats: an update. *Vet Clin North Am Small Anim Pract* 2018;48:969–984.

Monteiro-Steagall BP, Steagall PVM, Lascelles BDX. Systemic review of nonsteroidal anti-inflammatory drug-induced adverse effects in dogs. *J Vet Intern Med* 2013;27:1011–1019.

Rosenthal MG, Labato MA. Use of therapeutic plasma exchange to treat nonsteroidal anti-inflammatory drug overdose in dogs. *J Vet Intern Med* 2019;33(2):596–602.

**Author:** Katherine L. Peterson, DVM, DACVECC. DABT
**Consulting Editor:** Ahna G. Brutlag, DVM, MS, DABT, DABVT

# Envenomations and Internal Toxins

# Black Widow Spiders

## DEFINITION/OVERVIEW

- The black widow spider (*Latrodectus* spp.) is a black, shiny spider about 2–2.5 cm in length with a red or orange hourglass mark on the ventral abdomen. The immature female is brown with red to orange stripes that change into the hourglass shape as she darkens with age (Figure 62.1). Males are brown, have no hourglass marks, and are generally thought to have fangs that are too small to penetrate the skin.
- Black widow spiders are found in every state except Alaska.

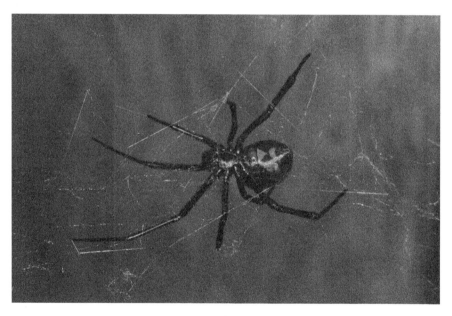

■ Figure 62.1 Black widow spider (*Latrodectus* spp.). Source: Courtesy of Richard Vetter, Department of Entomology, University of California–Riverside.

*Blackwell's Five-Minute Veterinary Consult Clinical Companion: Small Animal Toxicology*, Third Edition.
Edited by Lynn R. Hovda, Ahna G. Brutlag, Robert H. Poppenga, and Steven E. Epstein.
© 2024 John Wiley & Sons, Inc. Published 2024 by John Wiley & Sons, Inc.

# ETIOLOGY/PATHOPHYSIOLOGY

## Mechanism of Action

- The venom contains alpha-latrotoxin, a potent neurotoxin that opens cation-selective channels at the presynaptic nerve terminal. This causes massive release and then depletion of acetylcholine and norepinephrine, resulting in sustained muscular spasms.
- Some proteolytic enzymes are also present, causing minimal localized tissue inflammation and pain.

## Toxicokinetics

- After the venom is injected, it is taken up by the lymphatics, entering the bloodstream.
- In 30–120 minutes, muscle pain begins near the site of the bite.
- Within 2–3 hours, muscle pain and cramping spread to the muscles of the legs, abdomen, thorax, and back.
- Acute clinical signs generally resolve in 48–72 hours, but weakness and lethargy may continue for weeks to months.

## Toxicity

- The neurotoxin is very potent.
    - $LD_{50}$ in guinea pigs is 0.0075 mg/kg.
    - $LD_{50}$ in mice is 0.9 mg/kg.
- Cats are particularly sensitive to the venom, and many do not survive envenomation. Muscle pain and cramping can proceed to muscle, ataxia, and paralysis.

## Systems Affected

- Musculoskeletal – severe muscle pain and cramping.
- Nervous – in cats especially, ataxia, tremors, and paralysis.
- Cardiovascular – mild tachycardia and hypertension.
- Gastrointestinal – vomiting, diarrhea, hypersalivation.
- Respiratory – Cheyne–Stokes pattern prior to death.

# SIGNALMENT/HISTORY

- Diagnosis is based on history and clinical signs.

## Risk Factors

- Geriatric animals or animals with cardiac compromise may be at greater risk of complications.

## Historical Findings

- Owners have reported seeing the spider in the emesis of the animal.
- Clinical onset is usually acute but may be delayed by several days with mild envenomation.

## Location and Circumstances of Poisoning

- Spiders are often found outside in leaf litter and debris or inside houses in dark areas under cabinets and in corners. Spiders are generally shy and will bite only if threatened by curious dogs and cats.

# CLINICAL FEATURES

- Clinical signs usually develop within 30 minutes to two hours post exposure, and the duration of clinical signs is generally 48–72 hours.
- The most common signs are vomiting, diarrhea, vocalization, severe muscle spasms and cramping, pain, agitation, and restlessness.
- Examination may show abdominal rigidity without tenderness, hypertension, tachycardia, regional tenderness, and lymph node tenderness.

# DIFFERENTIAL DIAGNOSIS

- Acute abdomen.
- Acute injury (hit by car, falling downstairs, etc.).
- Back pain from intervertebral disc disease.

# DIAGNOSTICS

## Clinical Pathological Findings

- CBC – leukocytosis.
- Serum chemistry – elevated CK.

# THERAPEUTICS

- Therapeutic goals are to provide symptomatic and supportive therapy to minimize pain, muscle tremors, and agitation. If obtainable, antivenom can be used to rapidly shorten clinical signs.

## Detoxification

- None in particular.

## Appropriate Health Care

- Monitor closely for signs of allergic reaction when giving antivenom.
- Monitor for signs of tachycardia and hypertension and treat appropriately.

## Antidote

- Antivenom is the definitive antidote. It should be reserved for high-risk patients (pediatric, geriatric, metabolically compromised). In one case report, a cat was treated with antivenom 26 hours after becoming clinically compromised and quickly recovered neurological function.
  - Lycovac® Antivenin Black Widow Spider (human antivenin, equine origin); Merck, West Point, PA.
    - One vial mixed with 100 mL crystalloid solution given IV slowly with monitoring of the ventral ear pinna for evidence of hyperemia (an indicator of allergic response).
    - One dose is usually sufficient, with a response occurring within 30 minutes.
    - With proper use, reactions are rare. If an adverse reaction occurs, stop antivenin and administer diphenhydramine (2–4 mg/kg IM, lower dose in cats). Wait 5–10 minutes and restart the antivenin at a slower rate.

- A second antivenin (Aracmyn®, Instituto Bioclon, Mexico) (Also called Anawidow, Rare Disease Therapeutics, Inc., Tennessee) has completed human trials and is scheduled to be submitted to the FDA for approval in 2023. This is an equine-origin Fab2 antivenin product and may be less likely to trigger an allergic reaction.

## Drug(s) of Choice

- Judicious use of IV fluids, especially if CK is elevated.
- Muscle rigidity and anxiety.
  - Methocarbamol 55–220 mg/kg/day slow IV. Do not exceed 330 mg/kg/day.
  - Diazepam 0.25–0.5 mg/kg IV as needed.
- Opioids may be used at the lowest effective dose to control pain without compromising respiratory function.
  - Buprenorphine 0.005–0.03 mg/kg IM, IV or SQ q 6–12 hours.
  - Tramadol 4–10 mg/kg PO q 8–12 hours in dogs; 1–2 mg/kg PO q 12 hours in cats. Extra-label use for both dogs and cats.
- Antiemetics.
  - Maropitant 1 mg/kg SQ, IV q 24 hours.
  - Ondansetron 0.5–1 mg/kg IV q 12 hours for dogs; 0.1–1 mg/kg IV, SQ, IM q 6–12 hours for cats.

 **COMMENTS**

## Possible Complications

- Weakness, fatigue, and insomnia may persist for weeks to months. Pets should be monitored closely.

## Expected Course and Prognosis

- Clinical signs generally resolve within 48–72 hours.
- Prognosis is uncertain for days; envenomation in cats is usually fatal without antivenom administration.

## Abbreviations

See Appendix 1 for a complete list.

## Suggested Reading

Gwaltney-Brant SM, Dunayer EK, Youssef HY. Terrestrial zootoxins. In: Gupta RC (ed.) *Veterinary Toxicology: Basic and Clinical Principles*, 3rd edn. New York: Elsevier, 2018; pp. 781–786.
Mebs D. Black widow spider. In: Mebs D (ed.) *Venomous and Poisonous Animals*. Boca Raton: CRC Press, 2002; pp. 184–187.
Peterson ME, McNally J. Spider envenomation: black widow. In: Peterson ME, Talcott PA (eds) *Small Animal Toxicology*, 3rd ed. St Louis: Saunders, 2006; pp. 817–821.
Twedt DC, Cuddon PA, Horn TW. Black widow spider envenomation in a cat. *J Vet Intern Med* 2008;13:613–616.

**Author:** Michael E. Peterson, DVM, MS
**Consulting Editor:** Lynn R. Hovda, RPh, DVM, MS, DACVIM

# Chapter 63

# Brown Recluse Spiders

## DEFINITION/OVERVIEW

- The brown recluse spider (*Loxosceles reclusa*) is 8–13 mm in length with comparatively long legs of 20–30 mm. Its color ranges in shades of brown; there is a violin shape on the dorsal cephalothorax (Figure 63.1).
- The spider is a hunter; the web is irregular and wispy.
- Various species of the *Loxosceles* spiders range over the temperate regions of Europe, Africa, and North and South America; however, most are found in the Americas. In the United States, the range is primarily in the southern Midwest, with certain species being found in the southern western states. It is a common misconception that they are more widespread (Figure 63.2).

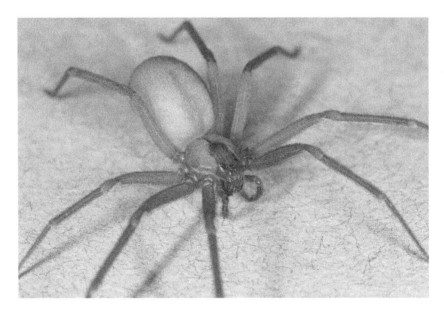

■ **Figure 63.1** Brown recluse spider (*Loxosceles reclusa*). Note the distinctive violin mark; it is often poorly demarcated in immature spiders or other species. Source: Courtesy of Richard Vetter, Department of Entomology, University of California–Riverside.

*Blackwell's Five-Minute Veterinary Consult Clinical Companion: Small Animal Toxicology*, Third Edition. Edited by Lynn R. Hovda, Ahna G. Brutlag, Robert H. Poppenga, and Steven E. Epstein. © 2024 John Wiley & Sons, Inc. Published 2024 by John Wiley & Sons, Inc.

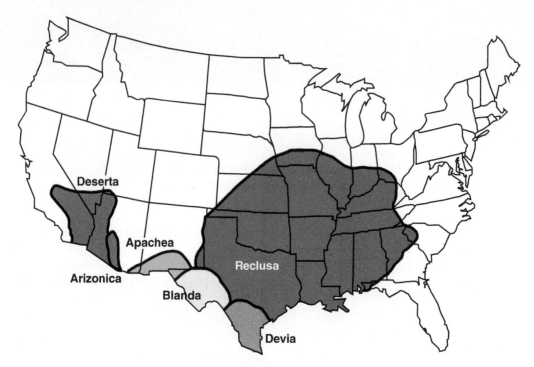

■ **Figure 63.2** North American distribution of the most widespread species of *Loxosceles* spiders. Source: Courtesy of Richard Vetter, Department of Entomology, University of California–Riverside.

 # ETIOLOGY/PATHOPHYSIOLOGY

## Mechanism of Action

■ The venom is a mixture of proteases and phospholipases, causing local and systemic clinical signs.
■ Sphingomyelinase D, present in the venom, causes platelet aggregation, complement cascade, cellular lysis, apoptosis, and an immune response that leads to dermonecrosis.
■ There appears to be tremendous variability between species regarding the extent of the response and susceptibility to the venom.
  • Rabbits and humans had similar dermonecrotic lesions, but the rabbit's lesions healed more quickly.
  • Dogs had a milder version of the dermonecrotic lesion with a similar dose of venom.

## Toxicokinetics

■ After venom injection, little or no pain may be felt initially.
■ Within 3–8 hours after envenomation, the area develops pruritus, pain, swelling, and a target lesion. The center may form a vesicle that later becomes a black scab (eschar).
■ Tissue around the lesion, along with the scab, may slough after 2–5 weeks, leaving a deep, slowly healing ulcer that usually spares muscle tissue.
■ Less commonly, hemolytic anemia with hemoglobinuria may occur within the first 24 hours.
■ Other systemic signs (tachycardia, fever, vomiting, dyspnea, renal failure, coma) may develop 6–72 hours after envenomation.

## Toxicity

- Severity of signs varies with the amount of venom injected and the victim's immune response, so even minute amounts can cause severe clinical signs. Bites to fatty tissues are more severe.
- Very little research has been done, and since the clinical signs mimic many other rule-outs, the concern is that misdiagnosis of spider venom may prevent correct diagnosis of another illness with more serious consequences, such as MRSA, Lyme disease, corrosive injury, dermal infection, and others.
- Little animal-related scientific data is available. There have been only two *in vivo* studies done in dogs to determine the effects of envenomation and no studies in cats.

## Systems Affected

- Skin/exocrine – localized pruritus, pain, swelling, classic target lesion, scabbing, ulceration.
- Hemic/lymphatic/immune – leukocytosis, hemolytic anemia, thrombocytopenia, prolonged coagulation times.
- Renal/urological – renal failure.
- Hepatobiliary – elevations in hepatic enzymes.
- Endocrine/metabolic – fever, lethargy.
- Gastrointestinal – vomiting.

 **SIGNALMENT/HISTORY**

- Diagnosis is based on history, clinical signs, and appropriate geographic environment.
  - In humans, over 60% of "recluse" bite diagnoses are made in areas with no endemic brown recluse spider populations (see Figure 63.2).
- No breed or sex predilection.

### Risk Factors

- Geriatric or pediatric patients may be at more risk of developing systemic effects.

### Location and Circumstances of Poisoning

- The brown recluse spider is a shy, nocturnal creature that hides in dark areas under leaf litter, tree bark, or rocks. Inside houses, it hides in bedding, basements, under piles of clothes, and anywhere it will have protection.
- The spider will bite only if disturbed, attacking quickly and leaving immediately, making accurate identification difficult.

 **CLINICAL FEATURES**

- Two distinct forms are seen in humans.
  - Cutaneous – after an initial mild edema or erythema, the bite area becomes necrotic. An eschar forms over the area, covering a deep ulcerating wound that heals very slowly. Secondary infection may occur.
  - Viscerocutaneous – rare systemic reactions are more likely in pediatric or geriatric patients. Severe hemolytic anemia, with hemoglobinuria, hematuria, and thrombocytopenia, may occur within 6–24 hours. Renal failure may be a sequela.

# DIFFERENTIAL DIAGNOSIS

- In humans, the primary misdiagnosis is MRSA.
- Immune-mediated disease.
- Injury.
- Primary infections, including parasitic, fungal, bacterial, viral causes.
- Neoplastic cutaneous disease.
- Secondary cutaneous disease (diabetic ulcer, septic embolism).
- Vascular disease.

# DIAGNOSTICS

## Clinical Pathological Findings

- Baseline CBC with platelet count and serum chemistry in those animals with evidence of systemic disease.

## Other Diagnostics

- There are no specific tests for the disease.
- Other tests should be used to rule out other diseases (Lyme test, autoimmune tests, coagulation tests, chemistry panel, CBC, UA) and to predict treatment in the case.

## Pathological Findings

- Dermal necrosis and ulceration with possible secondary infection.

# THERAPEUTICS

- The treatment goals are to provide symptomatic and supportive care (rest, antibiotics if needed, IV fluids, blood transfusion).
- There have been many suggested treatments, including surgical removal, dapsone, hyperbaric oxygen, anticoagulants, shock therapy, steroids, antihistamines, vitamin C, and meat tenderizer, but none has proven to be effective.

## Detoxification

- None other than good wound care.

## Appropriate Health Care

- Clean wound well with soap and water; prevent secondary infection.
- Cool compresses. Avoid application of heat as this may exacerbate the condition.
- Elevation of area.

## Antidote

- No specific antidote or antivenom is available.

## Drug(s) of Choice

- IV fluids as needed for dehydration and cardiovascular support.
- Blood products as needed.
- Broad-spectrum antibiotics if wound becomes infected.

- Analgesics for pain.
  - NSAIDs.
    - ○ Carprofen – dogs 2.2 mg/kg PO q 12–24 hours.
    - ○ Robenacoxib 2 mg/kg SQ q 24 hours (maximum three days).
  - Opioids.
    - ○ Buprenorphine 0.005–0.02 mg/kg IM, IV or SQ q 6–12 hours.
    - ○ Tramadol 4–10 mg/kg PO q 8–12 hours in dogs; 1–2 mg/kg PO q 12 hours in cats. Both are extra-label.
- Antiemetics.
  - Maropitant 1 mg/kg SQ, IV q 24 hours.
  - Ondansetron 0.5–1 mg/kg IV q 12 hours for dogs; 0.1–1 mg/kg IV, SQ, IM q 6–12 hours for cats.
- Antihistamines for pruritus.
  - Diphenhydramine 2–4 mg/kg IM or PO as needed.

## Surgical Considerations

- Wound debridement with Burrow's solution or dilute hydrogen peroxide followed by bandaging may be necessary.

# COMMENTS

## Possible Complications

- Prolonged wound care may be necessary.

## Expected Course and Prognosis

- Full recovery may take weeks to months, but prognosis is good if systemic signs are not seen.

## Abbreviations

See Appendix 1 for a complete list.

## Suggested Reading

Gwaltney-Brant SM, Dunayer EK, Youssef HY. Terrestrial zootoxins. In: Gupta RC (ed.) *Veterinary Toxicology: Basic and Clinical Principles*, 3rd edn. New York: Elsevier, 2018; pp. 78–1786.

Mebs D. Brown or fiddleback spiders. In: Mebs D (ed.) *Venomous and Poisonous Animals*. Boca Raton: CRC Press, 2002; pp. 188–189.

Pace L, Vetter R. Brown recluse spider (*Loxosceles recluse*) envenomation in small animals. *J Vet Emerg Crit Care* 2009;19(4):329–336.

Peterson ME, McNally J. Spider envenomation: brown recluse. In: Peterson ME, Talcott PA (eds) *Small Animal Toxicology*, 3rd ed. St Louis: Saunders, 2013; pp. 823–826.

**Author:** Michael E. Peterson, DVM, MS
**Consulting Editor:** Lynn R. Hovda, RPh, DVM, MS, DACVIM

# Crotalids (Pit Vipers)

## DEFINITION/OVERVIEW

- Local and systemic venom-induced toxicity may both occur following bites by snakes in the subfamily Crotalinae (pit vipers), which is composed of three genera: *Agkistrodon* (cottonmouths [water moccasins] and copperheads – Figures 64.1, 64.2), and *Crotalus* and *Sistrurus* (rattlesnakes) in North America (Figures 64.3–64.6).
- Identified by retractable fangs, a heat-sensing pit between the nostril and eye (appearance of four nostrils), vertically elliptical pupils (live snakes in light), and a triangular-shaped head (see Figures 64.3 and 64.5).
- Venomous snakebite does not necessarily mean envenomation has occurred; in human beings, 25% of bites are "dry bites" with no venom injected.
- Typically, signs are evident within 30–45 minutes of the bite. However, in some cases, the onset of clinical signs may be delayed up to six hours.
- Good emergency and supportive care coupled with antivenom therapy are key components for achieving an optimal outcome in cases of venomous snakebite.

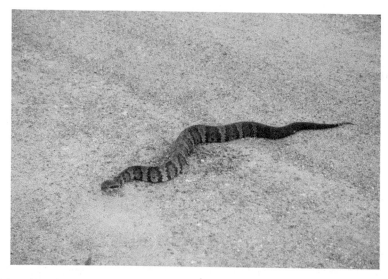

■ **Figure 64.1** *Agkistrodon conanti* (cottonmouth, also known as a water moccasin), North Carolina. Source: Courtesy of Daniel E. Keyler (chapter contributor).

*Blackwell's Five-Minute Veterinary Consult Clinical Companion: Small Animal Toxicology*, Third Edition.
Edited by Lynn R. Hovda, Ahna G. Brutlag, Robert H. Poppenga, and Steven E. Epstein.
© 2024 John Wiley & Sons, Inc. Published 2024 by John Wiley & Sons, Inc.

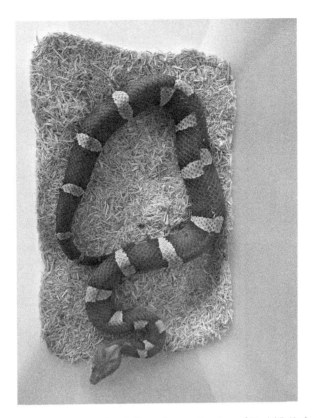

■ **Figure 64.2** *Agkistrodon laticinctus* (copperhead), Texas. Source: Courtesy of Daniel E. Keyler (chapter contributor).

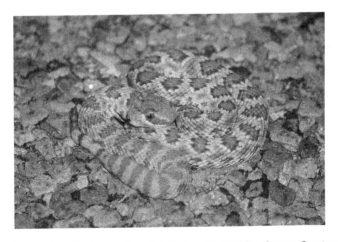

■ **Figure 64.3** *Crotalus scutulatus* (Mojave rattlesnake), Rodeo, New Mexico. Source: Courtesy of Daniel E. Keyler (chapter contributor).

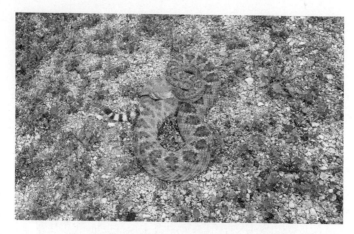

■ **Figure 64.4** *Crotalus atrox* (western diamondback rattlesnake), Texas. Source: Courtesy of Daniel E. Keyler (chapter contributor).

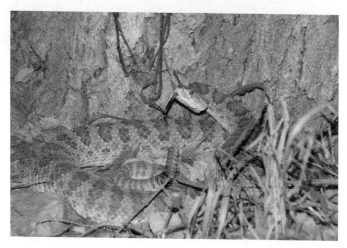

■ **Figure 64.5** *Crotalus viridis* (prairie rattlesnake), South Dakota. Source: Courtesy of Daniel E. Keyler (chapter contributor).

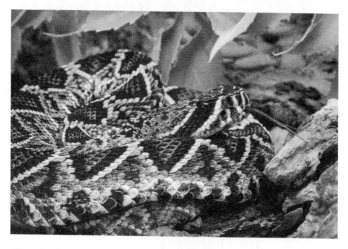

■ **Figure 64.6** *Crotalus adamanteus* (eastern diamondback rattlesnake). Source: Courtesy of Barney Oldfield.

# ETIOLOGY/PATHOPHYSIOLOGY

- Inquisitive companion animals living in regions where venomous snakes are indigenous (particularly the southeastern and southwestern regions of the US).
- Bites – frequently to face and front legs due to the curious nature of dogs and cats when they encounter a snake (Figures 64.7).
- Fang punctures may be evident but can be missed due to hair.
- Venom quantity delivered with a bite is highly variable, and a small animal may receive the same venom dose as a large animal, or none at all. Thus, careful clinical monitoring for symptoms is essential in directing treatment.
- When envenomation has occurred, swelling, pain, and skin discoloration are the usual early signs that envenomation has occurred.
  - Airway obstruction consistently occurs with bites to the tongue and occasionally with bites to the face (Figures 64.8).
  - Neurotoxic venom may exhibit minimal or no local signs other than bite wounds.
- Coagulopathy – typically occurs in cases of more severe envenomation.
- Edema, swelling, and wound necrosis should be monitored.

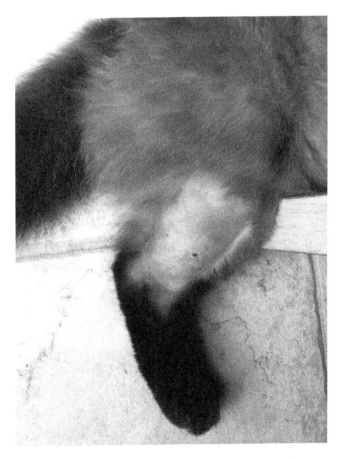

■ **Figure 64.7** Timber rattlesnake bite to cat. Source: Courtesy of Daniel E. Keyler (chapter contributor).

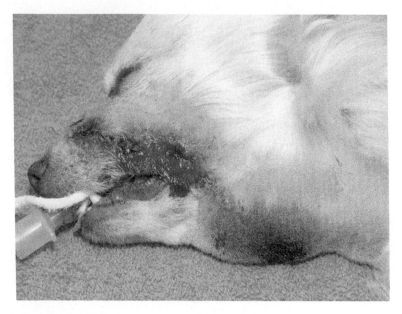

■ **Figure 64.8** Dog with airway compromise after bite from prairie rattlesnake (*Crotalus viridis*). Source: Courtesy of Barney Oldfield.

## Mechanism of Action

■ Pit viper venoms are primarily composed of numerous proteins (both enzymatic and nonenzymatic) and small peptides (neurotoxic components). These typically will work in concert to produce insults to blood clotting and tissue integrity, alter fluid (blood and serum) distribution, and in some cases (depending on the species of snake) affect central nervous system function.

■ Envenomation frequently results in hypotension, due to fluid redistribution or hemorrhage resulting in central blood volume loss and consequent shock. Pooling of blood within the splanchnic (dogs) and pulmonary (cats) vessels may further compromise respiratory efforts.

■ Blood clotting factors can be inhibited, and the function of fibrinogen and platelets may be compromised, potentially producing significant consumptive coagulopathy.

■ Red blood cell morphology can be altered (echinocyte-like or burring appearance), rendering them dysfunctional, and RBCs may distribute to the extravascular space, further reducing function.

## Toxicokinetics

■ The multiple toxins that compose snake venom all have their own individual toxicokinetics but the toxins function collectively to enhance the absorption and distribution of specific toxins to target tissues and organs. Increased vascular permeability, third-spacing of fluids, and altered clotting system functions may result.

■ The rate of distribution of venom toxins to target tissues and organs can be quite rapid in the case of intravenous bites, slower with intramuscular bites, and slowest with more superficial or subcutaneous bites (majority).

■ Bites to the face and extremities generally have slower venom uptake than bites to the torso; peritoneal and tongue envenomations have rapid absorption.

■ Metabolism and excretion kinetics are complex and, because of the multitoxin composition of venom, have not been well studied. However, some venom components or toxins may persist for weeks, and this is one reason why recurrent coagulopathy can occur.

- Toxins may remain depot at a bite site, disrupting local tissue integrity and resulting in a slower sustained-release systemic absorption. Toxins that penetrate deeper tissues may redistribute with time back into the systemic circulation, resulting in recurrent toxicity. This process of redistribution can occur days, and in some instances weeks, after the bite.

## Toxicity

- General ranking of potential systemic venom toxicity: (1) rattlesnakes, (2) water moccasins, (3) copperheads.
- Several species of rattlesnakes have subpopulations with venom containing a potent neurotoxin.
  - Mohave rattlesnake – *Crotalus scutulatus* of southern Arizona.
  - Southern Pacific rattlesnake – *Crotalus helleri* of California.
  - Timber/canebrake rattlesnake – *Crotalus horridus* of South Carolina and Georgia.
- It is possible for a snake to have both neurotoxic and coagulopathic venom actions. Strictly neurotoxic venoms produce minimal or no evidence of coagulopathy.
- Venom delivery route influences the time to venom component-induced effects, and the level of systemic venom dosage (mg venom/kg BW).
- 85% of victims have altered laboratory values and clinically important swelling.
- Systemic toxic effects are greatest in highly perfused tissues, with certain organ systems being more susceptible to thrombocytopenia, hypofibrinogenemia (hyperfibrinogenemia, which is a result of volume depletion in the vascular circulation), and resultant coagulopathy.

## Systems Affected

- Hemic/lymphatic/immune – coagulopathies and vascular hemorrhage.
- Respiratory – fluid shifts to lungs, respiratory compromise secondary to neuromuscular complications.
- Skin/exocrine – tissue destruction.
- Cardiovascular – shock.
- Renal/urological – renal failure.
- Gastrointestinal – vomiting and diarrhea.
- Neuromuscular – generalized weakness.

 # SIGNALMENT/HISTORY

- Cats and dogs of any age may encounter venomous snakes that are indigenous to their region.
- The veterinarian should be aware of the venomous snake species indigenous to the geographic area in which they practice.

## Risk Factors

- Important factors include species of snake, size of snake, size of cat/dog, site of bite, age of cat/dog, venom quantity injected, and time to treatment.
- Smaller patients, those with predisposing health problems (cardiac, diabetic, renal), and older animals are at greater risk of more severe medical complications.
  - Smaller animals – venom dose (mg/kg BW of victim) may be quite large.
  - Geriatric animals lack resilience in their physiological systems.
- Animals receiving medications for existing medical problems.
  - NSAIDs may predispose to clotting anomalies.
  - Corticosteroids may decrease natural defenses.
  - Beta-blockers may mask the onset of anaphylaxis.

- Aggressiveness and motivation of snake.
  - Defensive strike – more likely to be "dry"; no venom injected.
  - Feeding strike – more venom injected.
  - Agonal bite – most of available venom injected.

### Historical Findings

- If snake is not observed biting the animal, puncture wounds from fangs can frequently be observed; may require clipping hair in affected area.
- Owners should be questioned as to whether antivenom has ever been given in the past as prior antivenom treatment may increase the chances of allergic reaction.

### Location and Circumstances of Poisoning

- Copperheads account for most of the venomous snakebites in areas where they are endemic (eastern USA). Frequently found around human habitation. Significantly, copperhead envenomation to dogs rarely results in coagulopathic complications and rarely requires the use of antivenom.
- Owners may find their pet carrying around a snake that they have killed and chewed on. These patients should be checked carefully for multiple bite sites and are at high risk for agonal bites. If the snake has been killed (or photo available), it is useful in correct identification.

 ## CLINICAL FEATURES

- Local signs may include the following.
  - Angioedema.
  - Fang punctures – not always two, may be multiple, not always visible.
  - Edema and swelling.
  - Bleeding from the bite site.
  - Erythema, ecchymosis.
  - Lymphangitis.
  - Necrosis.
- Systemic signs may include the following.
  - Hypotension.
  - Respiratory changes (dyspnea).
  - Weakness/ataxia.
  - Bleeding – epistaxis, gingival, hematuria, melena, retinal hemorrhage.
  - Excessive salivation.
  - Myokymia/fasciculations.
  - Vomiting – hematemesis.
  - Diarrhea.
  - Oliguria – hematuria.
  - Acute kidney injury (AKI).

 ## DIFFERENTIAL DIAGNOSIS

- Animal bites – nonsnake (e.g., scorpion, spider, rodents, shrews, etc.).
- Hymenoptera venom-induced angioedema. When touched, these swollen areas are generally not significantly painful, in contrast to pit viper envenomation.
- Toxicants – brodifacoum or warfarin-based rodenticides, ethylene glycol.
- Trauma-induced puncture wounds (e.g., nails, barbed wire fence, etc.).
- Sepsis.

# DIAGNOSTICS

- If snake (or photo) available, confirm identification – venomous or nonvenomous.
- Examine animal for fang marks, clip hair in affected area, examine for local tissue damage and ecchymosis.

## Clinical Pathological Findings

- CBC, serum chemistry, UA, and coagulation profile – initial bloodwork sets a baseline reference for monitoring progression and resolution of envenomation syndrome.
  - CBC – if venom has been injected, 89% have echinocytosis (non-EDTA blood).
  - Creatine kinase (CK) elevation with intramuscular envenomation.
- Urinalysis – hemoglobinuria or myoglobinuria secondary to rhabdomyolysis.
- Coagulation parameters (INR, Plts, PT, PTT, Fib, FDP).
  - International normalized ratio (INR) – prolonged.
  - Prothrombin time (PT), partial thromboplastin time (PTT) – prolonged.
  - Platelets (Plts) – decreased.
  - Fibrinogen (Fib) – decreased.
  - Fibrinogen degradation products (FDP) – increased.

## Other Diagnostics

- ECG – ventricular arrhythmias may be detected in severely depressed patients.

## Pathological Findings

- There are no characteristic gross or histopathological lesions. Tissue necrosis is common at the bite site with hemorrhage and edema seen. Other lesions may be present depending on the severity of the envenomation.

# THERAPEUTICS

## Detoxification

- Superficially wash wound area to remove any residual venom at bite site.
- Transport to animal care facility for treatment.
- Remove collars and other restrictive devices prior to transport.
- Clip and clean bite area.

## Appropriate Health Care

- Minimize exercise/movement.
- Observe closely for airway obstruction and be prepared to intubate.
- Monitor cardiovascular system closely.
- Blood pressure (fluid replacement may be needed).

## Antivenoms

- Antivenom is the definitive antidote for venomous snakebite. In the United States, there are potentially five antivenom products available for treating crotalid envenomation.
  - Three are USDA approved and licensed for veterinary use (available from most veterinary supply distributors).
  - Two are FDA approved and licensed for human use in North America.
- In the absence of availability of the veterinary products, human antivenom products can be successfully used. Availability and economic factors (wide range of product costs to DVM) may determine whether antivenom therapy is an option.

- *The earlier antivenom is administered, the more effective it is*; one vial early is equal to several later.
- Antivenom has been used successfully in pregnant humans but specific studies in animals are lacking. Therapeutically, what is good for the mother should be good for the fetus. Consequences in the absence of antivenom therapy must be considered.
- Specifics of use (for further details refer to product package insert).
  - Lyophilized antivenom should be reconstituted with diluent and can be gently flushed and swirled to hasten solubilization and allow for more antivenin to be readily withdrawn. Dilute in 250 mL (reduce volume if small animal) of crystalloids and administer IV slowly, looking for any sign of allergic reaction – pruritus, hyperemia of pinna, piloerection. If allergic-type reaction occurs, stop antivenom infusion.
  - Reaction is usually a complement-mediated anaphylactoid-type response to foreign proteins given too rapidly. Stop infusion, give diphenhydramine (2–4 mg/kg IM or PO), wait five minutes and begin antivenom again at a slower rate. If problem persists, seek veterinary toxicology consult.
  - Anaphylactic reactions may also occur and the clinician should be prepared to respond. Epinephrine may be required for acute reactions.

## Veterinary Antivenoms

- Specific USDA-approved veterinary products are available in the USA.
- **Special notes.**
  - Antivenoms listed provide coverage for all North American pit vipers (Crotalinae: rattlesnakes, copperheads, cottonmouths). All three snake antivenoms for veterinary use have been shown to be therapeutically effective. The particular use of any one of the three products may depend on the timely availability of a given product, the patient's medical history (prior exposures/allergic reactions, age, other pathologies), cost differences, and DVM prior experience with use of a given antivenom.
  - Considerations should be given to total fluid volume and animal size when administering any antivenom, particularly important in smaller patients.
- Antivenin (Crotalidae, polyvalent, equine origin) – IgG.
  - Boehringer-Ingelheim, Ridgefield, CT.
  - Canine indication.
  - Dose varies from one to five vials IV depending on severity of symptoms.
  - 95% of cases controlled with a single vial.
  - Lyophilized product, requires reconstitution.
- Venom Vet® (antivenin, polyvalent, Crotalidae (F(ab')$_2$, equine origin) – injectable solution.
  - MT Venom, LLC, Canoga Park, CA.
  - Species indication not provided.
  - No reconstitution necessary. Does require further dilution.
  - Dose 1–2 vials.
- Rattler Antivenin (antivenin, Crotalidae, polyvalent, equine origin)
  - Mg Biologics, Ames, IA.
  - Canine and equine indication.
  - Liquid plasma preparation (50 mL IV bag).
  - One or two doses (50–100 mL) typically adequate.

## Alternative Antivenoms (Human)

- Doses not precisely determined for veterinary use.
- CroFab® (Crotalidae, polyvalent, immune Fab, ovine).
  - BTG International Inc., West Conshohocken, PA.
  - Supplied as a carton of two vials.

- Anavip® (Crotalidae, immune (Fab')$_2$, equine).
  - Instituto Bioclon, Mexico.
  - Maintained by multiple hospitals and zoos in United States.

## Drug(s) of Choice

- IV crystalloid fluids for volume resuscitation. The vast majority of cases are started on fluid therapy while antivenom is being prepared. Some envenomation syndromes can be controlled with IV fluids alone. Do not fluid overload.
- Blood products (FFP, whole blood) may be needed for animals with marked hypoproteinemia. Coagulopathies rarely corrected with blood products alone, and persistent defects require additional antivenom.
- Pain management.
  - Buprenorphine 0.005–0.03 mg/kg IM, IV or SQ q 6–12 hours.
  - Tramadol 4–10 mg/kg PO q 8–12 hours for dogs; 1–2 mg/kg PO q 12 hours for cats.
  - Fentanyl transdermal patch appropriate for weight of animal or fentanyl IV.
- Antiemetics for persistent vomiting.
  - Maropitant 1 mg/kg SQ, IV q 24 hours.
  - Ondansetron 0.5–1 mg/kg IV q 12 hours for dogs; 0.1–1 mg/kg IV, SQ, IM q 6–12 hours for cats.
- Antibiotics are not routinely needed in cases of snakebite unless localized tissue damage is severe and there is confirmed evidence of infection. Fluoroquinolone antimicrobials improved survival in one study, but wound infection was not assessed. No other antimicrobial agent had an effect on survival.

## Precautions/Interactions

- Antivenom reactions.
  - Antibodies are foreign proteins and may precipitate allergic complications. This sometimes results from too rapid administration or when antivenom solution is too concentrated; appropriate dilution or simply slowing/stopping the infusion rate may reduce risk of this complication.
- Other drugs.
  - Corticosteroids have no documented value in the treatment of venomous snakebite; evidence suggests they may worsen the condition.
  - Colloids are avoided since they can alter coagulation and may pull fluids out of the extra- or intervascular space through damaged vessel walls.
  - DMSO enhances uptake and spread of venom.
  - Heparin should not be used as the coagulopathies induced by pit viper venoms work by a different mechanism. It has no clinical value and may worsen the condition.
  - Opiates (buprenorphine, fentanyl, oxymorphone) may be used for pain. However, in cases of neurotoxic envenomation, they may confound the interpretation of signs. Morphine can cause histamine release reactions similar to early anaphylaxis and should be used with caution.
  - NSAIDS should be avoided.
- Rattlesnake vaccine for dogs (Red Rock Biologics, Woodland, CA) – intended prophylaxis for western diamondback rattlesnake envenomation. Published documentation of efficacy suggests no significantly protective effect, and anaphylaxis has been reported.
- Environmental factors such as excessive heat and humidity may be additional burdens beyond the effects of snake venom alone. Careful and selective use of medications to maintain euthermia and homeostasis is key to optimal outcome.

- Because of the complex makeup of snake venom with numerous different toxins, there is the potential for interaction with many drugs. See Risk Factors.

## Patient Monitoring

- Baseline laboratory values should be obtained and repeated as necessary, particularly coagulation panel, packed cell volume, and total protein.
- Recurrence of clinical signs or coagulation abnormalities can occur with any antivenom. If patient's initial coagulopathy resolved with antivenom use, recurrence can occur usually within the next week (most commonly the next few days), although rarely as severe as initial defect. There have been no documented veterinary cases of clinical bleeding from subsequent coagulopathy; however, the clinician should be aware of the possibility.
- Renal complications may develop consequent to coagulopathy, and maintaining adequate renal function is important. Urinalysis and monitoring renal function are useful.

 **COMMENTS**

## Prevention/Avoidance

- Clients should be aware of venomous snakes in their region and be mindful when taking pets on hikes in known areas where venomous snakes live. Stay on the trail and keep the pets on a leash.
- Client can attempt to eliminate dark areas or hiding spots in their yard or area where their pets spend most of their time at home.

## Expected Course and Prognosis

- Animals may also suffer recurrent symptoms following an apparent recovery. These may be both local and systemic, and as such warrant that animals are closely monitored for up to several weeks (as outpatients) following the snakebite and associated treatments.
- Prognosis is good with early medical intervention.

## See Also

Chapter 65 Elapids (Coral Snakes)

## Abbreviations

See Appendix 1 for a complete list.

## Suggested Reading

Gilliam LL, Brunker J. North American snake envenomation in the dog and cat. *Vet Clin North Am Small Anim Pract* 2011;41:1239–1259.

Katzenbach JE, Foy DS. Retrospective evaluation of the effect of antivenom administration on hospitalization duration and treatment cost for dogs envenomated by *Crotalus viridis*: 113 dogs (2004–2012). *J Vet Emerg Crit Care* 2015;25:655–659.

Lee BM, Zersen KM, Shissler JR et al. Antivenin-associated serum sickness in a dog. *J Vet Emerg Crit Care* 2019;29:558–563.

Martinez J, Londoner L, Schaer M. Retrospective evaluation of acute kidney injury in dogs with pit viper envenomation (2008–2017): 56 cases. *J Vet Emerg Crit Care* 2019;30:698–705.

Pashmakova MB, Bishop MA, Black DM et al. Multicenter evaluation of the administration of crotalid antivenom in cats: 115 cases (2000–2011). *J Am Vet Med Assoc* 2013;243:520–525.

Petras KE, Wells RJ, Pronko J. Suspected anaphylaxis and lack of clinical protection associated with envenomation in two dogs previously vaccinated with *Crotalus atrox* toxoid. *Toxicon* 2018;142:30–33.

Pritchard JC, Birkenheuer AJ, Hanel RM et al. Copperhead (*Agkistrodon contortrix*) envenomation of dogs: 52 cases (2004–2011). *J Am Anim Hosp Assoc* 2014;50:5.

**Authors**: Dominic Tauer, DVM, DABT, DABVT and Daniel E. Keyler, RPh, BS, Pharm D, FAACT
**Consulting Editor**: Lynn R. Hovda, RPh, DVM, MS, DACVIM

# Elapids (Coral Snakes)

## DEFINITION/OVERVIEW

- Elapidae family – frontal maxillary fixed fangs.
- Two genera in the United States (*Micrurus* and *Micruroides*).
- Three species in North America.
    - Eastern coral snake (*Micrurus fulvius*) – southeastern North Carolina and eastern South Carolina; southern Georgia, Alabama, and Mississippi; southeastern Louisiana; all of Florida (Figure 65.1).
    - Sonoran coral snake (*Micruroides euryxanthus*) – southern half of Arizona, and southwestern New Mexico (Figure 65.2).
    - Texas coral snake (*Micrurus tener*) – west of Mississippi; southern Arkansas, western Louisiana, and southeastern half of Texas (Figure 65.3).
- Identification.
    - Brilliant glossy color pattern – red, yellow, and black bands (in this order) fully encircling the body (red and yellow colors touch each other; see Figures 65.1 and 65.3).
    - Same sequence pattern is observed in the Sonoran coral except colors are red, white, and indigo blue bands (see Figure 65.2).

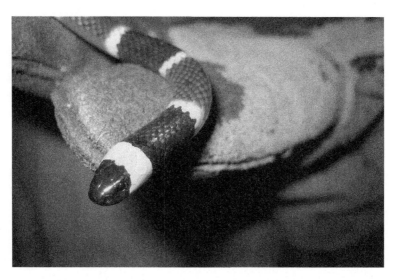

■ **Figure 65.1** Eastern coral snake (*Micrurus fulvius*); red and yellow bands touch each other; head is small with black snout. Source: Courtesy of David Seerveld, AAAnimal Control, Orlando, Florida.

---

*Blackwell's Five-Minute Veterinary Consult Clinical Companion: Small Animal Toxicology*, Third Edition. Edited by Lynn R. Hovda, Ahna G. Brutlag, Robert H. Poppenga, and Steven E. Epstein. © 2024 John Wiley & Sons, Inc. Published 2024 by John Wiley & Sons, Inc.

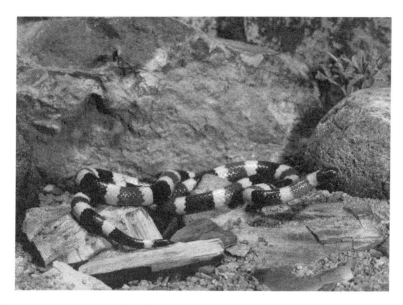

■ **Figure 65.2** Sonoran coral snake (*Micruroides euryxanthus*); red and white bands touch each other; head is small with black snout. Source: Courtesy of Barney Oldfield.

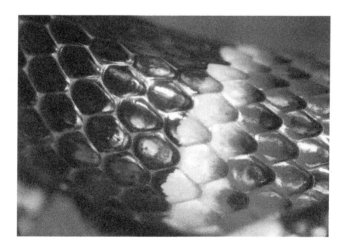

■ **Figure 65.3** Skin from Texas coral snake (*Micrurus tener*); black tips on the red scales are characteristic of the Texas coral snake. Source: Courtesy of Daniel E. Keyler.

- Relatively small head – black-sock-snout that extends to behind the eyes, round pupils, no narrow demarcation between the head and neck.
■ Nonvenomous "mimic" species (similar color/size) and geographic range of eastern coral and Texas coral snakes.
- Scarlet snake (*Cemophora coccinea*).
- Scarlet king snake (*Lampropeltis triangulam elapsoides*).
- Color pattern shows yellow bands with black bands on each side, yellow does not touch red.

# ETIOLOGY/PATHOPHYSIOLOGY

- Coral snakes – usually timid/nonaggressive; bites to animals usually occur because the animal is harassing the snake.
- Fixed small fangs – typically need to chew or hang on when biting to inject venom.
- Bites infrequent due to reclusive/fossorial behavior and nocturnal habits.
- Bites may occur in any month of the year.
- Early identification important.
    - Bite marks by nonvenomous mimic species may look like coral snake bite marks.
    - These snakes also chew when biting.

## Mechanism of Action

- Bite wounds to soft tissues – primarily to lips, tongue, mouth (gums), and webbing of paws. Fang marks may or may not be distinctly observed; may appear as scratches.
- Envenomation usually associated with a protracted bite and puncture of skin.
- Venom is neurotoxic, causing descending muscle paralysis, CNS depression, respiratory and cardiovascular failure.
    - Primary site of action – neuromuscular junction. Presynaptic and postsynaptic blockade actions may occur. More rarely, cardiotoxin-like actions are observed.
    - Acetylcholinesterase inhibition is not a major action of coral snake venom.

## Toxicokinetics

- Onset of clinical signs may be delayed several hours (up to 12–18 hours) after envenomation.
- Duration of venom effects may persist for days.

## Toxicity

- Eastern coral snake envenomations – typically more severe and neurological in effect than the Texas coral snake.
- Sonoran coral snake bites quite rare; however, neurological venom effects have been reported to occur following envenomation.

## Systems Affected

- Neuromuscular – depolarization in muscle fibers.
- Respiratory – respiratory depression.
- Cardiovascular – antagonism of acetylcholine receptors.

# SIGNALMENT/HISTORY

- Dogs and cats – equally affected.
- Cats – more difficult time surviving if prolonged respiratory support needed.

## Risk Factors

- Species of snake.
- Size of snake.
- Size of cat/dog.
- Site of bite.
- Age of cat/dog.
- Venom quantity injected.
- Time to treatment.

# CLINICAL FEATURES

- Cats – primarily neurological: CNS depression, respiratory depression (erratic breathing), ascending flaccid quadriplegia, hypotension, anisocoria, hypothermia, reduced nociception, loss of spinal cutaneous trunci reflexes, vocalization, delayed pupillary light reflex.
- Dogs – CNS depression, generalized weakness/lethargic, shallow abdominal breathing (dyspnea/tachypnea), ptosis, hyperreflexia, tremor, sialorrhea, vomiting, bulbar paralysis affecting cranial motor nerves, delayed pupillary light reflex, acute flaccid quadriplegia, dysphoria, hypotension, ventricular tachycardia, hemolysis resulting in anemia and hemoglobinuria.
- Both cats and dogs – animals may appear ataxic/staggering, salivating excessively, and disoriented.
- Signs may appear within an hour of being bitten, but lack of signs does not mean envenomation has not occurred. Onset of signs may be delayed for up to 18 hours following a coral snake bite.
- Humans – Texas coral snake envenomation in humans primarily presents as painful paresthesias, mild swelling, and erythema without significant paralytic symptoms.

# DIFFERENTIAL DIAGNOSIS

- Adverse drug reaction.
- Botulism.
- Myasthenia gravis.
- Polyradiculoneuritis.
- Spider bite (*Latrodectus* – widow spider species).
- Tick bite paralysis.
- Toxicant-induced neuropathies.
- Trauma puncture wounds, small, and not bite related.

# DIAGNOSTICS

- If snake or photo of snake is available, accurate identification is useful in confirmation of coral snake envenomation.
- Bite site – often difficult to determine if a bite has occurred. Fangs are very small. Use of magnifying glass and good lighting can aid in determination of skin penetration. Important to examine particularly facial soft tissue areas, tongue, and gums for bite/fang or scratch-like marks.
- Coagulopathy and pain are not typically observed.

## Clinical Pathological Findings

- CBC – PCV/TPP for dehydration and evidence of anemia.
- Serum chemistry – ALP, AST, and CK (elevated), electrolyte abnormalities.
- Urinalysis.
  - Hemoglobinuria.
  - Myoglobinuria.
  - Hematuria (rarely).

## Pathological Findings

- No characteristic gross or histopathological lesions.

## THERAPEUTICS

### Detoxification

- Wash wound off with water to remove residual venom on skin surface.
- Minimize animal movement and transport immediately to nearest veterinary facility for antivenom administration and supportive care.
- Pressure-immobilization bandaging is a compression pressure wrap of the bitten limb with ace-type bandage to retard lymph flow and reduce systemic venom distribution.
  - May be of benefit for coral snake bites.
  - Should only be considered in cases where there is a long period of time before veterinary care can be reached.

### Appropriate Health Care

- Do not wait for onset of clinical signs to initiate treatment.
- Treat signs as they develop.
- Hospitalize for a minimum of 48 hours.
- Clip and clean wound.
- Monitor respirations.
  - Be prepared to intubate.
  - If no antivenom, provide mechanical ventilation (2-4 days may be required).
  - Aspiration pneumonia may occur secondary to loss of swallowing reflex.
- ECG monitor.
- Cardiopulmonary resuscitation as needed.
- Blood pressure monitoring for hypotension.
- Sequential neurological evaluations for 48 hours post envenomation.
- Maintain renal function with fluids – do not fluid overload.

### Antivenoms

- North American coral snake antivenin (Wyeth Pharmaceuticals LLC), antivenin (*Micrurus fulvius*) (IgG equine origin) is FDA approved and available for human use in the United States. Product cost is a major consideration. Efficacy with Sonoran coral snake envenomation has not been established.
- Alternative coral snake antivenoms produced in other countries may sometimes be obtained from local zoos. Follow manufacturer's guidelines for preparation and administration.
- Protective cross-reactivity and para-specific coverage of North American coral snake (excluding the Sonoran coral snake) envenomation has been demonstrated with the following antivenoms.
  - Coralmyn® (polyvalent anti-coral fabotherapic (F(ab')2, equine origin); Instituto Bioclon, Mexico.
  - Anti-coral (elapid) antivenin (IgG equine origin), Costa Rican coral snake antivenin; Instituto Clodomiro Picado, Costa Rica.
  - Australian tiger snake (*Notechis scutatus*) antivenin; CSL Limited, Parkville, Victoria, Australia.
- Allergic reactions to antivenom are possible.
  - Anaphylaxis (type I hypersensitivity) should be treated with fluids and epinephrine.
  - Anaphylactoid reactions should be treated by stopping the antivenin administration, administering diphenhydramine (2–4 mg/kg PO or IM, lower dose for cats), waiting five minutes and resuming antivenin administration more slowly.

- Serum sickness-like reaction may occur 1–4 weeks after infusion and may be treated with corticosteroids and antihistamines.
- Pregnancy – antivenom has been used successfully in pregnant humans and should be considered for use in pregnant dogs or cats if deemed necessary.

## Drug(s) of Choice

- IV crystalloids to prevent dehydration and treat myoglobinuria and hematuria. Do not fluid overload.
- Blood products if anemia is severe.
- Broad-spectrum antibiotics for 7–10 days may be needed if local tissue damage with infection has occurred.
- Pain management.
  - Opioids.
    - Buprenorphine 0.005–0.03 mg/kg IM, IV or SQ q 6–12 hours.
    - Fentanyl transdermal patch appropriate for animal's weight or IV fentanyl.
    - Other opioids at the discretion of DVM.
- Diphenhydramine (2–4 mg/kg PO or IM, lower dose for cats) for anaphylactoid reaction to antivenom.
- Further therapy is symptomatic and supportive.

## Alternative Drugs

- Neostigmine – may be used if immediate restoration of neuromuscular transmission is needed until respiratory support can be implemented. This reversible cholinesterase inhibitor has been used successfully in human cases of coral snake envenomation. Will require repeated doses usually due to short half-life.

## Patient Monitoring

- Frequent monitoring of vital signs.
- Wound care if local tissue damage evident (rare with coral snake envenomation).
- Frequent turning in cases of paresis.

# COMMENTS

### Expected Course and Prognosis

- Prognosis is reasonably good with early intervention.
- Aspiration pneumonia worsens the prognosis.
- Marked clinical signs may last 1–1.5 weeks.
- Full recovery may take months as receptors regenerate.

### See Also

Chapter 64 Crotalids (Pit Vipers)

### Abbreviations

See Appendix 1 for a complete list.

### Suggested Reading

Alfaifi MS, Alotaibi AE, Alqahtani SA et al. Cobra snakebite mimicking brain death treated with a novel combination of polyvalent antivenom and anticholinesterase. *Am J Emerg Med* 2020;38:2490.e5–2490.e7.

Campos S, Allen-Durance AE, Schaer M et al. Retrospective evaluation of *Micrurus fulvius* (Eastern Coral Snake) envenomation and use of mechanical ventilation in dogs and a cat (2011–2016): 8 cases. *J Vet Emerg Crit Care* 2019;29:662–667.

Gold BS. Neostigmine for the treatment of neurotoxicity following envenomation by the Asiatic Cobra. Ann *Emerg Med* 1996;28:7–9.

Greene S, Ruha A-M, Campleman S et al., Tox IC Snakebite Study Group. Epidemiology, clinical features, and management of Texas Coral Snake (*Micrurus tener*) envenomations reported to the North American Snakebite Registry. *J Med Tox* 2021;17:51–56.

Maxwell K, Fraser B, Schaer M, Allen A. A retrospective evaluation of eastern coral snake envenomation and antivenom administration in cats: 30 cases (2012–2019). *Toxicon* 2021;191:38–45.

Perez ML, Fox K, Schaer M. A retrospective evaluation of coral snake envenomation in dogs and cats: 20 cases (1996–2011). *J Vet Emerg Crit Care* 2012;22:682–689.

**Authors**: Dominic Tauer, DVM, DABT, DABVT and Daniel E. Keyler, RPh, BS, Pharm D, FAACT
**Consulting Editor**: Lynn R. Hovda, RPh, DVM, MS, DACVIM

# Other Zootoxins (Venomous Lizards [Heloderma], Poisonous Salamanders [Newts], and Frogs

## DEFINITION/OVERVIEW

- Includes less common zootoxins including lizards of the genus *Heloderma*, salamanders (newts) of the genus *Taricha*, and *Notophthalmus*; frogs containing batrachotoxin are mentioned briefly.
- Species of the genus *Heloderma* are venomous, causing both local and systemic toxicity following bites. Specifically, the Gila monster (*H. suspectum* and *H. cinctum*) and Mexican beaded lizard (*H. horridum*).
  - Gila monster lizards are the only venomous lizard species native to North America and are geographically confined to the states of Arizona, New Mexico, southern California and Utah, and southwestern Nevada (Figure 66.1).
  - The Mexican beaded lizard is geographically distributed along the west coast of Mexico to Guatemala (Figure 66.2).

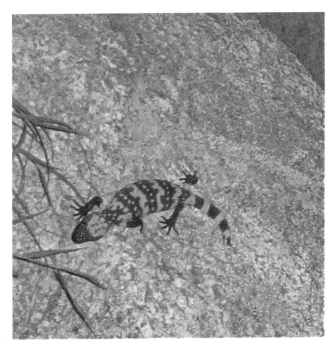

■ **Figure 66.1** Gila monster (*Heloderma suspectum*). Source: Courtesy of Daniel E. Keyler (co-author).

*Blackwell's Five-Minute Veterinary Consult Clinical Companion: Small Animal Toxicology*, Third Edition.
Edited by Lynn R. Hovda, Ahna G. Brutlag, Robert H. Poppenga, and Steven E. Epstein.
© 2024 John Wiley & Sons, Inc. Published 2024 by John Wiley & Sons, Inc.

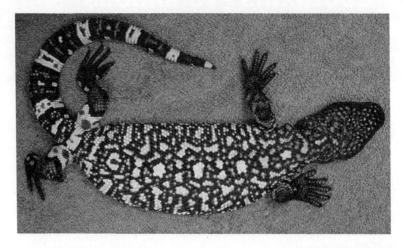

■ **Figure 66.2** Mexican beaded lizard (*Heloderma horridum*). Source: Courtesy of Daniel E. Keyler (co-author).

- The Gila monster is a protected species but in rare cases *Heloderma* species may be owned as pets, depending on state and local laws.
- Bites are typically tenacious and delivered with power, with the tendency to clamp down and hold on. However, rapid slashing bites with quick release occur.
- Venom is released from secretory glands located in the mandibles, elaborated onto the grooved teeth, and introduced into the victim via mastication with the bite.

■ Salamanders (newts) of the genus *Taricha* and *Notophthalmus* contain varying amounts of tetrodotoxin. Mammalian ingestion is not common due to the secretions from the newts being very distasteful. The amount of toxin present in the newts has both regional and species variations.

- There are four species of newts in the genus *Taricha* that carry tetrodotoxin. Their range stretches along the west coast from Alaska to the Sierra Nevada mountains.
- The eastern newt (*N. viridescens*) and its subspecies can be found east of the Mississippi River from Texas to Nova Scotia.
- The rough-skinned newt (*T. granulosa*) found in Oregon and northern California may contain more toxin than those found in other areas while newts of the same species found on Vancouver Island appear to be nontoxic. The eastern newt (*Notophthalmus viridescens*) also shows fluctuations in toxin levels across the eastern United States and Canada, ranging from nontoxic to toxic amounts. The origin of the tetrodotoxin in *Taricha* and *Notophthalmus* is either diet related or secreted from bacteria on the skin living in a symbiotic relationship.

■ Frogs of the genus *Phyllobates*, originating from Colombia, produce milky secretions from their skin containing batrachotoxin. Batrachotoxin is an antagonist to tetrodotoxin.

 ## ETIOLOGY/PATHOPHYSIOLOGY

### Mechanism of Action

■ Lizard venom comprises protein and nonprotein substances, and include bradykinin-releasing substance, hyaluronidase, phospholipase A, proteases, and serotonin.

- Phospholipase $A_2$, hyaluronidase, and proteases contribute to tissue destruction, allowing venom spread to tissues.

- Endogenous hydrolases are activated with third-spacing of fluids and edema develops.
- Gilatoxin is a serine protease that causes kallikrein-like and thrombin-activating activities.
  - Can cleave angiotensin I and trigger hypotensive effects.
  - May also potentiate the effects of venom hemorrhagic toxins.
- Tetrodotoxin is a sodium channel blocker. It binds to voltage-gated sodium channels in the nerve cell membrane, blocking the passage of sodium ions into the neuron. The result is a prolonged activation and propagation of action potential leading to an interruption in signals along the nervous system.
  - Tetrodotoxin also acts as a selective calcium channel blocker in dogs, leading to decreased cardiac function.
- Batrachotoxin binds to and irreversibly opens the sodium channel of nerve cells, preventing them from closing.

## Toxicokinetics

- Toxins that compose *Heloderma* venom all have their own individual toxicokinetics but may act collectively to enhance the absorption and distributions of specific toxins.
  - Multitoxin venom components make metabolism and elimination kinetics variable.
- Absorption of tetrodotoxin from the gastrointestinal tract can occur within minutes and severe clinical signs such as rapid weakness, paralysis of respiratory muscles and death can occur within 20–30 minutes but may be delayed up to 20 hours.
  - Metabolism of tetrodotoxin is rapid with no presence in the plasma after 24 hours. Excreted primarily from the kidneys unchanged in the urine.
- Batrachotoxin distributes though the body rapidly and can take effect within 15 minutes.

## Toxicity

### Heloderma

- Envenomation frequently results in hypotension due to the combined effects of fluid redistribution and gilatoxin-induced effects.
- Venom delivery route influences the time to effect (IV>IM>ID) and influences the level of systemic venom dosage (mg/kg BW).
- Teeth may be broken off in the process of biting or during lizard removal. Radiographs maybe needed.

### Tetrodotoxin

- Toxicity can occur at 0.25 mg/kg BW. *Taricha* newts can contain 0 to >3 mg/newt; *Notophthalmus* newts can contain 0–0.76 mg/newt.
- Reported death of an adult human male after ingestion of a rough-skinned newt (*Taricha granulosa*) in Oregon.
- SQ LD$_{50}$ in mice is 8 mcg/kg.
- Wild-caught newts fed commercial diets can lose tetrodotoxin after several years.

### Batrachotoxin

- An adult frog can contain 80 mcg of toxin.
- Toxicity at 0.1 mcg/kg BW.
- SQ LD$_{50}$ in mice is 2 mcg/kg.
- Clinical signs developed in mice with SQ injection at one minute with death at eight minutes.
- Wild-caught dart frogs have maintained batrachotoxin for up to six years after capture.
- Captive-bred dart frogs do not possess batrachotoxin.

## SIGNALMENT/HISTORY

- Veterinarians should be aware of the natural geographic distribution of venomous lizards and salamanders although private collections may exist in any part of the country.

### Risk Factors

- Animals with underlying health issues are at increased risk for medical complications. These factors may necessitate intensive medical management.
- Animals receiving medications for existing medical problems.
  - NSAIDS may predispose to clotting abnormalities in *Heloderma* bites.
  - Corticosteroids may decrease natural defenses, leading to infection with *Heloderma* bites.
- Aggressiveness and motivation of *Heloderma* lizards.
  - Rapid slashing bite delivers less venom.
  - Retracted bite delivers greater venom quantity.
  - Agonal bite – venom reservoirs may be depleted.

### Historical Findings

- If a *Heloderma* lizard is not observed biting the animal, puncture wounds from teeth can frequently be observed; may require clipping hair in affected areas.
- Ingestion of a newt containing tetrodotoxin may not be witnessed but sudden acute signs or respiratory distress or sudden weakness while in an area where the newts are present may indicate exposure.
- Exposure to a wild-caught dart frog should only occur when animal has access to a private collection.

### Location and Circumstances of Poisoning

- Owners may find their pet carrying around a dead lizard or newt.
- *Heloderma* lizards may still be attached to the patient.
- If exposure to a poison dart frog, confirm with owners if the frog is captive bred or wild caught as captive-bred frogs do not contain batrachotoxin. Wild-caught frogs can continue to carry the toxin six years after captivity.

 ## CLINICAL FEATURES

### Heloderma

- Nervous – generalized weakness, myokymia/fasciculations.
- Dermal – angioedema, puncture wounds, swelling, bleeding (epistaxis, gingival, hematuria, melena), erythema, ecchymosis, lymphangitis.
- Gastrointestinal – hypersalivation, vomiting, hematemesis, diarrhea.
- Respiratory – dyspnea.
- Cardiovascular – hypotension, tachycardia, shock.

### Tetrodotoxin

- Nervous – rapid generalized weakness.
- Ophthalmic – miosis noted in early stages, progressing to mydriasis at later stages.
- Gastrointestinal – hypersalivation, vomiting, nausea, diarrhea.
- Respiratory – dyspnea, acute respiratory failure.
- Cardiovascular – hypotension, bradycardia, dysrhythmia.

### Batrachotoxin

- Nervous – rapid paralysis of muscles, ataxia, loss of equilibrium, seizures.
- Respiratory – dyspnea, respiratory failure.
- Cardiovascular – bradycardia, hypotension, cardiac arrest.

 ## DIFFERENTIAL DIAGNOSIS

### *Heloderma*

- Animal bites – snakes, cats, rodents, shrews, etc.
- Hymenoptera venom-induced angioedema. When touched, these swollen areas are generally not significantly painful, in contrast to lizard envenomation.
- Trauma-induced puncture wounds (nails, barbed wire fence, etc.).

### Tetrodotoxin and Batrachotoxin

- Alpha-2 agonists such as imidazoline decongestants.
- Botulism.
- Bufo toad (*Rhinella marinus*).
- Strychnine.

 ## DIAGNOSTICS

- Obtain correct identification of the lizard, salamander or frog.
- Examine for puncture wounds, clip hair in affected area, examine for local tissue damage and ecchymosis.
- There are no laboratory tests for tetrodotoxin or batrachotoxin.

### Other Findings

- Radiographs if suspected ingestion of salamander and frog may show evidence of skeletal remains.

### Pathological Findings

- There are no characteristic gross or histopathological lesions associated with tetrodotoxin or batrachotoxin. Lizard envenomation will show evidence of localized edema near the bite wound.

 ## THERAPEUTICS

### Detoxification

- Lizards.
  - If a lizard is attached to a limb, it can be submerged in very warm water or very cold water for a brief period. A medical instrument can be used to apply force to the commissure of the mouth to aid in prying open the jaw. Do not hit the head of the lizard as this may cause more venom to be released into the patient. Wild lizards are under federal protection.
  - Gently wash wound area to remove any residual venom at the bite site.
- Newts or frogs.
  - Induction of emesis to remove any newt or frog ingested. Endoscopy or surgical retrieval may be indicated.

- Rinse out the mouth if ingestion of newt or frog. Wear gloves.
- Activated charcoal is most effective within 60 minutes of exposure for newt ingestion.

## Appropriate Health Care

- Observe for airway obstruction from swelling with lizard envenomation or respiratory paralysis from tetrodotoxin and be prepared to intubate.

## Antidotes

- No antivenom exists for treatment of lizard envenomation.
- No antidote for tetrodotoxin or batrachotoxin.

## Drug(s) of Choice

- IV crystalloid fluids for volume resuscitation.
- Appropriate pain management – PO or injectable depending on conditions.

## Precautions/Interactions

- *Heloderma* venom has potential for interactions with many drugs.
    - Corticosteroids have no documented value in the treatment of venomous lizard envenomation.
    - DMSO may enhance uptake and spread of lizard venom.
- With tetrodotoxin and batrachotoxin exposures, death may occur before support can be provided.

## Patient Monitoring

- For lizard envenomation, baseline laboratory values repeat as needed. Coagulation panel is not routinely preformed.
- Ensure all teeth fragments are removed from the patient and monitor for signs of infection.
- Monitor respiratory patterns in tetrodotoxin and batrachotoxin patients to see if intubation is required.

 # COMMENTS

### Expected Course and Prognosis

- Complete recovery should be anticipated with lizard envenomation.
- Tetrodotoxin and batrachotoxin have a favorable prognosis with limited oral exposure. Ingestion of a newt or frog carries risk for serious complications.

### Suggested Reading

Albuquerque EX, Daly JW, Witkop B. Batrachotoxin: chemistry and pharmacology: This novel steroidal alkaloid is a valuable tool for studying ion transport in electrogenic membranes. *Science* 1971; 172(3987):995–1002.

Hague MT, Avila LA, Hanifin CT. Toxicity and population structure of the Rough-Skinned Newt (*Taricha granulosa*) outside the range of an arms race with resistant predators. *Ecol Evolution* 2016;6(9):2714–2724.

Holstege SC, Baer AB. Eastern Newt (*Notophthalmus viridescens*). *Wild Env Med* 2021;32:130–131.

Hooker KR, Caravati EM. Gila monster envenomation. *Ann Emerg Med* 1994;24(4):731–735.

Kavoosi M, O'Reilly TE, Kavoosi M et al. Safety, tolerability, pharmacokinetics, and concentration-QTc analysis of tetrodotoxin: a randomized, dose escalation study in healthy adults. *Toxins* 2020;12(8):511.

Yotsu-Yamashita M, Gilhen J, Russell RW. Variability of tetrodotoxin and of its analogues in the red-spotted newt, *Notophthalmus viridescens* (Amphibia: Urodela: Salamandridae). *Toxicon* 2012;59(2):257–264.

## Acknowledgment

The author and editors acknowledge the prior contributions of Daniel E. Keyler, RPh, BS, Pharm D, FAAC, who authored this topic in the previous edition.

**Author**: Dominic Tauer, DVM, DABT, DABVT
**Consulting Editor**: Lynn R. Hovda, RPh, DVM, MS, DACVIM

# Chapter 67

# Scorpions

## DEFINITION/OVERVIEW

- Over 1500 species of scorpions are found in all parts of the world except Antarctica.
- Only one species in North America induces possibly life-threatening clinical signs after a venomous sting – the Arizona bark scorpion (*Centruroides exilicauda*, formerly *Centruroides sculpturatus*).
  - Natural range includes all counties of Arizona, part of western New Mexico, southern Utah, and southern Nevada.
  - This scorpion is light brown in color, nocturnal, ambushes its prey, and grows to about 8 cm (male) or 7 cm (female) (Figure 67.1).
  - It can be identified by the small tubercle under the stinger; magnification may be required to identify this (Figure 67.2).
- Most stings result only in localized pain or pruritus and usually resolve within 24 hours.

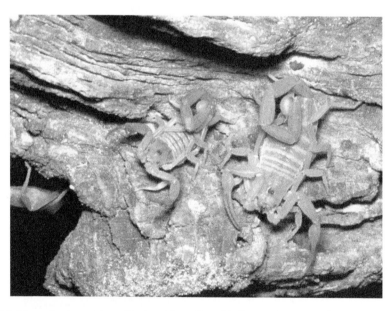

■ **Figure 67.1** Arizona bark scorpions (*Centruroides exilicauda*). Source: Courtesy of Arizona Poison and Drug Information Center, Tucson.

---

*Blackwell's Five-Minute Veterinary Consult Clinical Companion: Small Animal Toxicology*, Third Edition.
Edited by Lynn R. Hovda, Ahna G. Brutlag, Robert H. Poppenga, and Steven E. Epstein.
© 2024 John Wiley & Sons, Inc. Published 2024 by John Wiley & Sons, Inc.

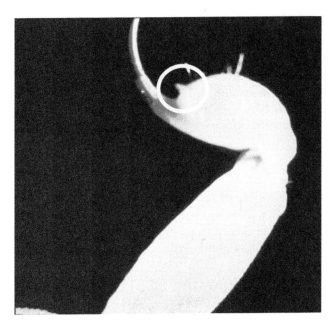

■ **Figure 67.2** The encircled tubercle located behind the stinger is characteristic of the bark scorpion. This tubercle may become less noticeable in some adults. Source: Courtesy of Arizona Poison and Drug Information Center, Tucson.

 # ETIOLOGY/PATHOPHYSIOLOGY

## Mechanism of Action

■ The venom is a complex mixture of polypeptides, proteins, and neurotoxins. The neurotoxins of the bark scorpion block or delay the opening of the sodium channels of cell membranes, inhibiting neuromuscular transmission.
■ Envenomation causes release of neurotransmitters, both sympathetic (causing tachycardia, hypertension, mydriasis) and parasympathetic (causing hypersalivation, bradycardia, hypotension).

## Toxicokinetics

■ Animal studies involving other species of scorpions showed a distribution half-life of 4–7 minutes.
■ Animal studies involving other species of scorpions showed an elimination half-life of 4.2–13.4 hours.

## Toxicity

There is little data available in veterinary medicine. Anecdotal information documents pain and pruritus with the initial sting, followed by hypertension either associated with the toxins or secondary to the pain and distress.

## Systems Affected

■ Nervous – numbness at the site, paresthesia (human beings), tremors, ataxia.
■ Cardiovascular – hypertension; tachycardia; possible hypotension, bradycardia.
■ Endocrine/metabolic – hyperglycemia.
■ Respiratory – rarely, pulmonary edema secondary to cardiovascular compromise.
■ Ophthalmic – nystagmus.
■ Gastrointestinal – salivation.

# SIGNALMENT/HISTORY

- No breed predilection.
- Diagnosis is based on history, clinical signs, and appropriate geographic environment.
- No specific studies have been done on dogs and cats. Anecdotally, cats seem to be seldom, if ever, affected. They have been known to hunt the scorpions without consequence. There are, however, a few documented cases in Arizona where clinical signs in cats have occurred.

## Risk Factors

- Geriatric or pediatric patients may be at higher risk of systemic involvement.

## Location and Circumstances of Poisoning

- The bark scorpion is primarily nocturnal, hiding under rocks or in clothes or shoes during the day. It will attack if threatened by an inquisitive animal or when disturbed or crushed during movement of bedding, clothing, etc.

# CLINICAL FEATURES

- Immediate pain at the site following the sting. Edema and pruritus may follow.
- Significant local tissue reaction rules out *C. exilicauda* envenomation.
- Hypertension may develop, especially in smaller animals. Whether this results from the venom itself or a pain response is unknown.
- Pulmonary edema may occur secondary to cardiovascular dysfunction.
- In humans, paresthesia and numbness have been documented at the site of the sting. Tremors and neuromuscular dysfunction were also noted.
- Other clinical features in dogs and cats reported by owners to the Arizona Poison and Drug Information Center (Tucson, AZ) include respiratory changes, gastrointestinal distress, CNS changes (restlessness and lethargy), sneezing, and a pain response as evidenced by vocalizing, limping, licking, pawing, and head shaking. Signs can persist for up to 24 hours but resolved on average at eight hours.
  - It should be noted these data reflect owners calling into a poison center and the species of scorpion involved is unknown.
  - 71% of cats, 39% of dogs under 33 pounds, and only 13% of dogs over 33 pounds exhibited clinical signs, which is consistent with the human experience (smaller size, greater signs) with bark scorpion envenomation.
  - 72 of the 84 cases responded to follow-up; no fatalities were reported.
  - Anecdotally local veterinarians reported 100% fatalities in ferrets.
  - The key finding, as in humans, is that the smaller the patient, the higher the risk of mortality.

# DIFFERENTIAL DIAGNOSIS

- Other venomous stings or bites (wasps, hornets, bees, spiders) causing pain or an allergic reaction.

# DIAGNOSTICS

- No specific diagnostics tests are recommended.
- Hyperglycemia due to decreased insulin production has been documented occasionally in human medicine.
- Identification of the scorpion, if possible, is the best diagnostic tool.

## Pathological Findings

- Rarely, the skin at the site of the envenomation may slough.

 # THERAPEUTICS

- The goal is to provide symptomatic and supportive care. This includes the use of analgesics or opioids for pain control, appropriate treatment for CNS and CV changes, careful monitoring of the skin at the envenomation site, and medications for allergic reaction to the venom should it occur.

### Detoxification

- Wash the sting area well and apply cool compresses as needed.
- If available, bind venom components with antivenom until cleared from body.

### Appropriate Health Care

- Cool compresses or ice may alleviate some of the local pain and swelling.
- Monitor the sting site for evidence of infection or skin sloughing.
- Frequent vital signs for first 24 hours to monitor for hypertension.
- Observe for onset of pulmonary edema and be prepared to intubate and provide oxygen as needed.
- Watch closely for local and systemic signs associated with a rare allergic reaction to venom.

### Antidotes and Drugs of Choice

- The use of scorpion antivenom (Anascorp®) is recommended in very small or geriatric patients with severe envenomation manifestations. The antivenom is very effective, but cost can be an issue. One vial should be sufficient.
- IV fluids as needed if hypotensive; caution required as many of these patients are hypertensive.
- Analgesics for pain.
  - NSAIDs.
    - Carprofen – dogs 2.2 mg/kg PO q 12–24 hours.
    - Robenacoxib 2 mg/kg SQ q 24 hours (maximum three days).
    - Other NSAIDs as determined by DVM.
  - Opioids.
    - Buprenorphine 0.005–0.02 mg/kg IM, IV or SQ q 6–12 hours.
    - Tramadol 4–10 mg/kg PO q 8–12 hours in dogs; 1–2 mg/kg PO q 12 hours in cats. Both are extra-label.
- Antihistamine.
  - Diphenhydramine 2–4 mg/kg IM or PO q 8–12 hours (dogs, cats).
- Hypertension
  - Acepromazine 0.01–0.03 mg/kg IV, IM, SQ (dogs, cats).

### Patient Monitoring

- Monitor hydration, pain level, blood pressure, heart rate, temperature, and development of hyperglycemia as needed based on degree of clinical signs being experienced.
- Monitor until clinical signs resolve.

 # COMMENTS

### Prevention/Avoidance

- Keep clothes picked up, shake out shoes and blankets prior to use; monitor pets' activities and keep them away from suspicious areas.

## Possible Complications

- Allergic reactions, pulmonary edema, CV collapse, coma, and death are rare complications.

## Expected Course and Prognosis

- Clinical signs generally resolve within 24 hours with no sequelae.

## Abbreviations

See Appendix 1 for a complete list.

## Suggested Reading

Gwaltney-Brant SM, Dunayer EK, Youssef HY. Terrestrial zootoxins. In: Gupta RC (ed.) *Veterinary Toxicology: Basic and Clinical Principles*, 2nd edn. New York: Elsevier, 2018; pp. 781–786.

Holzman D, Reilly L, McNally J et al. Dogs and cats with scorpion stings. Venom Week, June 1–4, 2009; Albuquerque, NM (Abstract).

Mebs D. Scorpions. In: Mebs D (ed.) *Venomous and Poisonous Animals*. Boca Raton: CRC Press, 2002; pp. 172–178.

**Author**: Michael E. Peterson, DVM, MS
**Consulting Editor**: Lynn R. Hovda, RPh, DVM, MS, DACVIM

# Chapter 68

# Toads

## DEFINITION/OVERVIEW

- Worldwide, there are more than 200 species of toads in the family Bufonidae, but six of them are a significant toxicity risk
- Two species in the family Bufonidae are of primary concern in the United States.
  - Colorado River toad or Sonoran Desert toad (*Incilius alvarius*, formerly *Bufo alvarius*). Found primarily in parts of California, New Mexico, southern Texas, and along the Colorado River between Arizona and California. Typically, smaller than the cane/marine toad.
  - Cane toad or marine toad (*Rhinella marina*, formerly *Bufo marinus*). Found primarily in Florida, Texas, Hawaii, and other tropical areas. Large toad that can grow up to 8 or 9 inches when mature (Figure 68.1).
- Other global species of concern include the following
  - Common or European toad (*Bufo bufo*). Present in Europe, NW Africa, western part of northern Asia.
  - Colombian giant toad or Blomberg toad (*Bufo blombergi*): in South America, specifically Colombia.
  - African common toad (*Amietophrynus regularis*, formerly *Bufo regularis*): primarily in Ethiopia
  - *Rhinella schineideri* (formerly *Bufo paracnemis*): found in Brazil.

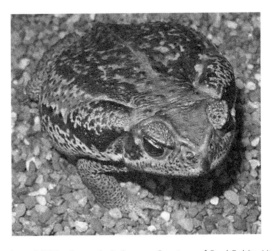

■ Figure 68.1 Marine (cane) toad (*Rhinella marina*). Source: Courtesy of Paul Eubig, University of Georgia.

*Blackwell's Five-Minute Veterinary Consult Clinical Companion: Small Animal Toxicology*, Third Edition. Edited by Lynn R. Hovda, Ahna G. Brutlag, Robert H. Poppenga, and Steven E. Epstein. © 2024 John Wiley & Sons, Inc. Published 2024 by John Wiley & Sons, Inc.

- Mouthing or ingestion of either can result in toxicity and death.
- Profuse salivation occurs within seconds of mouthing a toad.
- Cane toad is generally the most toxic of those found in US; may be fatal if left untreated.
- With prompt and appropriate treatment, outcome is typically very good.
- Other species of toads may cause mild ptyalism, gagging or pawing at the mouth with oral exposure but systemic toxicity is not expected.

 # ETIOLOGY/PATHOPHYSIOLOGY

### Mechanism of Action

- Venom components.
  - Bufadienolides or bufagenins and bufotoxins – cardioactive steroids like cardiac glycosides/ digitalis, inhibit Na/K ATPase pump in cardiac myocytes.
  - Bufotenins – pressor agents with hallucinogenic effect, found in Colorado River toad.
  - Catecholamines – epinephrine, norepinephrine, dopamine.
  - Indolealkylamines – compounds related to serotonin, may have hallucinogenic effect.

### Toxicokinetics

- Toxic secretions are in parotid glands (located just behind the eye) and skin; released by contraction of periglandular muscles.
- Secretions are rapidly absorbed across oral mucous membranes, open wounds, or conjunctiva. Buccal absorption bypasses first-pass metabolism.
- Toxicity may occur after mouthing or ingesting a toad. Toads sitting in a water dish for several hours may leave behind enough secretion/residue to intoxicate an average-size dog.
- Rapidly crosses blood–brain barrier.
- Rapidly excreted, short half-life.
- Signs may last up to 12–24 hours.

### Toxicity

- Toxicity depends on size of toad and dog and dose of secretions. Partoid glands of one average cane toad contain sufficient toxin to be lethal to a 10–15 kg dog.
- All *R. marina* and *I. alvarius* exposures should be treated as toxic.

### Systems Affected

- Gastrointestinal – rapid onset of hypersalivation in nearly all cases; occurs within seconds to minutes of mouthing or ingesting a toad; hyperemic/irritated mucous membranes (seem to be noted more often in dogs than cats), vomiting.
- Respiratory – increased respiratory rate and respiratory distress within 15 minutes. Rarely noncardiogenic nonpulmonary edema.
- Neurological – disorientation, agitation, ataxia, seizures within 30–60 minutes. CNS signs may be less common in cats.
- Cardiovascular – bradycardia or tachycardia with arrhythmias (first- or second-degree AV block, ventricular tachycardia or fibrillation), hypotension at any time.
- Hematological – hyperkalemia, acidosis.
- Miscellaneous – hyperthermia.

 # SIGNALMENT/HISTORY

### Risk Factors

- Primarily seen in dogs, reported also in cats.
- No age predilection.

- Geographically dependent, based on range of toad species. Toads are most active during periods of high humidity and warm weather. Exposures to the Colorado River toad occur most often during the late summer monsoon season in the desert southwest and for cane toads during the summer months in the southeast (though possible year round). Most encounters occur during the evening, night, or early morning hours.

### Historical Findings

- History of being outside and either seen ingesting/attacking a toad or found to have rapid onset of clinical signs. Owner may note salivation, pawing at the mouth, distress or disorientation. Owner may describe the dog as "foaming at the mouth."

# CLINICAL FEATURES

- Profuse hypersalivation within minutes.
- Vomiting and diarrhea.
- Respiratory distress – dyspnea, tachypnea, cyanosis within 15 minutes.
- Hyperexcitability, disorientation, vocalization; may progress to ataxia, seizures, collapse within 30–60 minutes.
- Brick-red buccal mucous membranes.
- Hyperthermia.
- Mydriasis.
- Brady- or tachycardia, cardiac arrhythmias.

# DIFFERENTIAL DIAGNOSIS

- Heat exhaustion.
- Toxicities.
  - Metaldehyde.
  - Caustic/corrosive agents, oral irritants.
  - Cardiac glycoside-containing plants/digoxin.
  - Organophosphate/carbamate intoxication.
- Underlying cardiovascular or CNS disease.

# DIAGNOSTICS

### Clinical Pathologic Findings

- CBC, chemistry, and urinalysis may show nonspecific findings.
- Hyperkalemia, acidosis, slight elevation in liver values may be seen.

### Other Diagnostics

EKG for arrhythmias.

# THERAPEUTICS

### Detoxification

- Rinsing the mouth/buccal lavage is the first line of therapy.
  - Have owner rinse out the mouth at home. Flush mouth with copious quantities of water for 10–15 minutes. Use a garden hose for larger dogs and put smaller ones in the sink. Tip nose forward to avoid choking or reingestion of the water.

- Rinse again in hospital. For cats, use a cotton swab soaked in room-temperature water to wipe buccal membranes for 10 minutes. If patient is seizing, use soaked gauze to wipe out mouth while airway is protected.
- Irrigate eyes with saline if ocular exposure.
- Emesis generally not recommended due to rapid onset of neurological signs.
- Single-dose activated charcoal with sorbitol may be given if patient is neurologically normal.
- Emesis or endoscopic removal will be needed in those patients that have swallowed an intact toad.

## Appropriate Health Care

- All patients with potential exposure to toxic toads should be evaluated in hospital after oral lavage at home.
- Rapid onset of clinical signs, monitor in hospital until asymptomatic.
- Monitor neurological status, heart rate, body temperature.
    - Actively cool if hyperthermic. As temperature falls below 103 °F (39.4 °C), stop measures. Do not overcool.
- EKG (continuous if symptomatic).
- IV fluid therapy at 1.5× maintenance, adjust as needed for hydration, hypotension.
- Oxygen therapy as needed if dyspneic or exhibiting noncardiogenic pulmonary edema.

## Antidote

- No specific antidote available.

## Drug(s) of Choice

- Antiemetics.
    - Maropitant 1 mg/kg SQ, IV q 24 hours.
    - Ondansetron 0.5–1 mg/kg IV q 12 hours for dogs; 0.1–01 mg/kg IV, SQ, IM q 6–12 hours for cats.
    - Dolasetron 0.6 mg/kg IV, SQ, PO q 24 hours.
- Atropine may resolve secretions but may worsen tachycardia and potentiate ventricular tachycardia. Use caution if giving to nonbradycardic patients.
- Seizures.
    - Diazepam 0.5–2.0 mg/kg IV may use CRI for persistent seizure activity; use diazepam with caution in cats. Midazolam may be used as an alternative.
    - If additional seizure control needed, use propofol CRI.
    - Longer acting agents such as phenobarbital typically not needed due to duration of clinical signs but may be used.
- Sinus tachycardia – beta-blocker.
    - Esmolol 0.05–0.1 mg/kg IV q 5 minutes for a maximum dose of 0.5 mg/kg.
    - Propranolol 0.02 mg/kg IV slowly over 2–3 minutes; repeat as needed for maximum dose of 0.1 mg/kg.
- Ventricular tachycardia – lidocaine.
    - Dogs 2 mg/kg IV slowly as a bolus; up to 4 mg/kg IV. If response is good, switch to CRI at 25–100 mcg/kg/min.
    - Lidocaine in cats should be used judiciously. 0.25–0.5 mg/kg IV slowly as bolus; repeat 0.15–0.25 mg/kg IV in 5–20 minutes. If response is good, switch to CRI at 10–20 mcg/kg/min.
- Sinus bradycardia – atropine 0.02–0.04 mg/kg IV PRN.
- For severe CV signs, Digibind® (digoxin FAB fragments, used for cardiac glycoside toxicity) has been used successfully. The exact dose for veterinary use has not been determined but may be as little as one vial.

- Corticosteroid for progressive CNS signs.
  - Dexamethasone 0.1–0.2 mg/kg IV or IM every 12 hours initially.
- If noncardiogenic pulmonary edema, treat with furosemide CRI (0.05–0.1 mg/kg/h) with cautious IVF therapy and $O_2$ until signs resolve.
- 20% lipid emulsion may be used to reduce bufadienolide toxicity (very lipophilic compound).
  - Use dedicated peripheral IV catheter.
  - Bolus 1.5 mL/kg of 20% ILE, IV over 1 minute, followed by 0.25 mL/kg/min × 30–60 minutes. Repeat bolus doses q 4–6 hours or start a CRI of 0.5 mL/kg/h. Check Hct tube for serum lipemia prior to repeat dosing.

### Precautions/Interactions

- Use beta-blockers, lidocaine with caution in patients with underlying cardiac disease. Esmolol may be preferred to propranolol, due to shorter duration of action.

### Patient Monitoring

- Recommend continuous EKG, temperature, and neurological monitoring until patient has fully recovered.

 **COMMENTS**

### Prevention/Avoidance

- Keep dogs and cats away from toads. Do not allow them to drink from water bowls that have been sitting outside where toads may be present.

### Expected Course and Prognosis

- No long-term sequalae expected if animal survives.
- Cane toads (*R. marina*) generally cause more severe toxicity than Colorado River toads (*I. alvarius*).
- Prognosis is excellent with aggressive decontamination and early treatment. Death may occur if exposure goes untreated.

### Abbreviations

See Appendix 1 for a complete list.

### Suggested Reading

Gowda RM, Cohen RA, Khan IA. Toad venom poisoning: resemblance to digoxin toxicity and therapeutic implications. *Heart* 2003;89(4):e14.

Johnnides S, Eubig P, Green T. Toad intoxication in the dog by *Rhinella marina*: the clinical syndrome and current treatment recommendations. *J Am Anim Hosp Assoc* 2016;52:1–8.

Leong OS, Padula AM, Webster RA et al. A retrospective study of cane toad (*Rhinella marina*) toxicity in 190 domestic cats in Southeastern Queensland: clinical presentations, treatments, and outcomes. *Aust Vet J* 2023;101:219–224.

Peterson ME, Roberts BK. Toads. In: Peterson ME, Talcott PA (eds) *Small Animal Toxicology*, 3rd edn. St Louis: Saunders, 2013; pp. 833–839.

Reeves MP. A retrospective report of 90 dogs with suspected cane toad (Bufo marinus) toxicity. *Aust Vet J* 2008;82(10):608–611.

**Author**: Ashley Smit, DVM, DABT
**Consulting Editor**: Lynn R. Hovda, RPh, DVM, MS, DACVIM

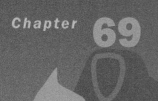
# Wasps, Hornets, and Bees

## DEFINITION/OVERVIEW

- Two important families in the order Hymenoptera.
  - Vespoidea (wasps, hornets, and yellow jackets) (Figure 69.1) and Apoidea (bees) (Figures 69.2 and 69.3).
- Except for killer bees, they are found worldwide.
  - Africanized killer bees/hybrid bees were introduced into Brazil and have made their way north. They are now found in Texas, Arizona, New Mexico, and southern California.
- Venom is injected through an adapted ovipositor.
  - Vespids do not have barbs on the stinger and can sting multiple times without dying.
  - Apids have a barbed stinger. After stinging, the barb and venom sac are left behind, allowing continued envenomation. This action is fatal to apids.
- Hymenoptera venoms are composed mainly of proteins.
  - Potent biologically active compounds.
  - Some act directly.
  - Others act indirectly by converting to active substances from host substrates.

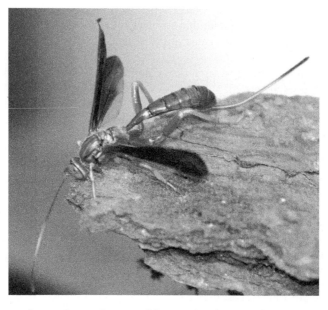

■ **Figure 69.1** Close-up of wasp. Source: Courtesy of C. Morgan Wilson, Hollins University, Roanoke, VA.

*Blackwell's Five-Minute Veterinary Consult Clinical Companion: Small Animal Toxicology*, Third Edition.
Edited by Lynn R. Hovda, Ahna G. Brutlag, Robert H. Poppenga, and Steven E. Epstein.
© 2024 John Wiley & Sons, Inc. Published 2024 by John Wiley & Sons, Inc.

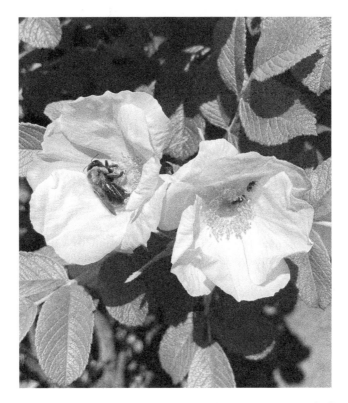

■ **Figure 69.2** Common eastern bumble bee (*Bombus impatiens*). Source: Courtesy of Alison Hodgkins Morse, Gloucester, MA.

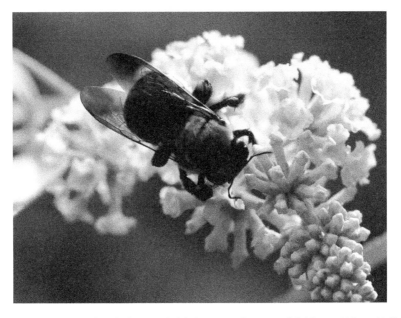

■ **Figure 69.3** Eastern carpenter bee (*Xylocopa virginica*). Source: Courtesy of C. Morgan Wilson, Hollins University, Roanoke, VA.

- Stings cause a variety of acute clinical signs, including decreased heart rate, decreased arterial blood pressure, respiratory depression, and elevation of plasma cortisol. In severe cases, anaphylactic shock, hemolysis, acute renal failure, acute lung injury/acute respiratory distress syndrome, and death may occur.

# ETIOLOGY/PATHOPHYSIOLOGY

## Mechanism of Action
- Vespid venom contains phospholipase A, hyaluronidase, biogenic amines, kinins, acid phosphatase, antigen 5, and mast cell degranulating peptide.
- Apid venom contains phospholipase A, hyaluronidase, mellitin, apamin, biogenic amines, acid phosphatase, mast cell degranulating peptide, and minimine.
  - Phospholipase A – disrupts cell membranes and causes release of pain-inducing agents.
  - Hyaluronidase – facilitates distribution and movement of the toxins through the tissues.
  - Mellitin – membrane-disrupting substance that increases a cell's susceptibility to attack by phospholipases. It also increases cell permeability and capillary blood flow, and causes pain and hemolysis. Most destructive part of Africanized bee venom.
  - Biogenic amines (histamine, serotonin, tyramine and catecholamines) – increase capillary permeability and induce itching and redness.
  - Kinins (bradykinin) – induce pain and cause smooth muscle contractions.
  - Mast cell degranulating peptide – release of biogenic amines.

## Toxicokinetics
- Absorption is immediate; first manifested as intense pain due to vasoactive compounds.
- Regional reactions are mediated by allergic mechanisms.
- Anaphylaxis may occur within minutes of the sting.
- Delayed hypersensitivity reactions occur within 3–14 days.

## Toxicity
- Most wasps inject about 17 mcg of venom per sting.
- Africanized killer bees can inject 94 mcg of venom per sting.
- Single stings may be toxic to susceptible animals but multiple stings result in serious consequences.
- Estimated lethal dose of honeybees in nonallergic mammals is 19 stings/kg.

## Systems Affected
- Skin/exocrine – pain, erythema, swelling/edema, wheals, pruritus.
- Cardiovascular – tachycardia, collapse secondary to anaphylaxis.
- Hemic/lymphatic/immune – hemolysis, clotting disorders such as DIC, spherocytosis.
- Renal/urological – acute renal failure, systemic rhabdomyonecrosis and acute tubular necrosis (severe cases).
- Respiratory – acute lung injury/acute respiratory distress syndrome (severe cases).
- Neuromuscular – ataxia, neural dysfunction (severe cases).

# SIGNALMENT/HISTORY

- Diagnosis is based on history (if available) and clinical signs.
- Certain breeds (American bull terrier, American Staffordshire terrier, boxer) appear to have a higher rate of reaction to Hymenoptera venom.

- Envenomation occurs more frequently in dogs kept outside, particularly when not monitored and allowed to wander and disturb nests or swarms (Figure 69.4).
- Stings are most common on the face (particularly around the muzzle, ears, eyes, and in the mouth), but can occur anywhere on the body (Figures 69.5–69.7).

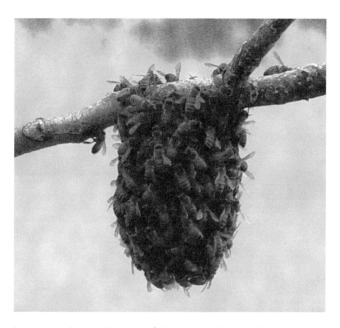

■ **Figure 69.4** Honeybee swarm. Source: Courtesy of C. Morgan Wilson, Hollins University, Roanoke, VA.

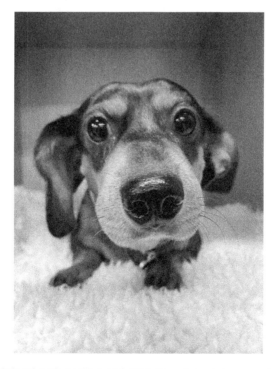

■ **Figure 69.5** Adult dachshund with swelling and respiratory compromise secondary to bee stings. Source: Courtesy Dr Steve Epstein, UC Davis, Davis, CA.

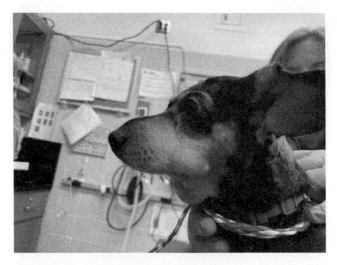

■ **Figure 69.6** Lateral view of the same dog with throat latch swelling. Source: Courtesy of Dr Steve Epstein, UC Davis, Davis, CA.

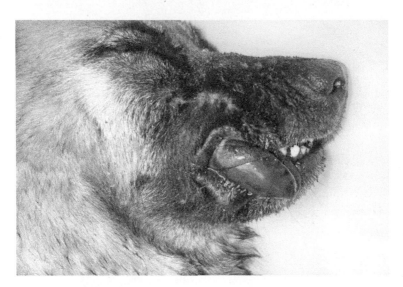

■ **Figure 69.7** Africanized killer bee strike in a dog. Note swollen face and tongue. Source: Courtesy of David Driemiere, UFRGS, Porto Alegre, RS.

## Risk Factors

■ Pediatric, geriatric, and sensitive individuals are at increased risk for more serious clinical signs and complications that may take longer to resolve.

## Historical Findings

■ Owner may or may not report witnessing the event or seeing bees/wasps/hornets.

## Location and Circumstances of Poisoning

■ Hornets and wasps prefer to live in shrubs and trees, attacking when provoked and stinging multiple times.

- Yellowjackets are ground dwellers and are aggressive when aggravated. An attack may occur if the nest is accidentally stepped on or disturbed.
- Honeybees often build their hives in hollow trees and other cavities. They are not typically aggressive and only sting when provoked.
- Africanized killer bees are very aggressive when disturbed. This problem is compounded by the fact that they tend to travel in swarms.

 # CLINICAL FEATURES

- There are four primary reactions seen after envenomation.
  - Local pain.
  - Regional reaction.
  - Anaphylactic response.
  - Skin rashes/serum sickness (unusual).
- Most stings simply result in localized edema and pain. The reaction is self-limiting and non-IgE mediated. These cases tend to resolve within 24 hours.
- Regional reactions can take up to 24 hours to manifest. During this time, the mast cells are degranulating and cellulitis is forming.
- Systemic anaphylaxis usually occurs within minutes. If it hasn't started within 30 minutes, it is unlikely to happen.
  - Signs in dogs include urination, vomiting, defecation, urticaria, pruritus, muscular weakness, depressed respiration, angioedema, cardiovascular compromise, and seizures.
  - Signs in cats include pruritus, vocalization, hypersalivation, ataxia, and collapse.
- Fatalities usually occur within an hour of the stinging event.
- Severe cases involving massive envenomation will be febrile and markedly lethargic.
- Hemolytic anemia and immune-mediated thrombocytopenia (IMTP) are reported with bee envenomation.
- Delayed hypersensitivity reactions include serum sickness, DIC, neuropathy, and renal damage, among others listed below in Possible Complications.

 # DIFFERENTIAL DIAGNOSIS

- Other venomous stings or bites. A third medically important family (Formicidae) of the order Hymenoptera includes fire ants which elicit similar clinical signs.
- Other causes of allergic reactions and anaphylaxis.

 # DIAGNOSTICS

- Laboratory analysis in severely affected animals should include a CBC, serum analysis, and coagulation tests as needed.
- Antiplatelet antibodies are the definitive diagnosis for IMTP.

## Pathological Findings

- No pathognomonic findings but stingers, insect parts, or entire bodies may be present at postmortem (Figure 69.8).
- The larynx is closely evaluated for evidence of hyperemia, edema, and hemorrhage.
- Findings consistent with anaphylaxis and DIC are supportive.

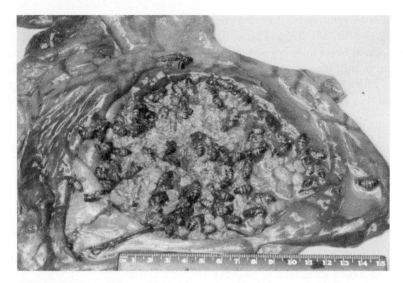

■ **Figure 69.8** Postmortem photo of dog's stomach filled with swallowed Africanized killer bees. Source: Courtesy of David Driemiere, UFRGS, Porto Alegre, RS.

 # THEREAPEUTICS

## Detoxification

- Prompt removal of the bee stinger and venom sac.
- Cold compresses and basic wound care.

## Appropriate Health Care

- Monitor for anaphylaxis and respiratory distress.
- In severe cases, intubation and oxygen may be required.

## Antidote

- No antidote available.

## Drug(s) of Choice

- IV fluids may be necessary if the patient is hypotensive secondary to cardiovascular compromise and hypovolemia. If hypotension persists after aggressive IV therapy (including colloids) and if the animal is well hydrated, consider adding the following.
  - Dopamine: 5–20 mcg/kg/min IV CRI.
  - Norepinephrine: 0.05–0.1 mcg/kg/min IV CRI.
  - Epinephrine: 0.05–0.4 mcg/kg/min IV CRI.
- Anaphylaxis.
  - Diphenhydramine 1–4 mg/kg IM or SQ; can be given IV but must be given very slowly and should be diluted.
  - Dexamethasone sodium phosphate 0.1–0.2 mg/kg IV q 12 hours.
  - Epinephrine 0.01–0.02 mg/kg IV, IM, SQ.
- Antiemetics if vomiting is severe or persists.
  - Maropitant 1 mg/kg SQ, IV q 24 hours.
  - Ondansetron 0.5–1 mg/kg IV q 12 hours for dogs; 0.1–1 mg/kg IV, SQ, IM q 6–12 hours for cats.

- Seizures.
  - Diazepam or midazolam 0.25–0.5 mg/kg IV PRN.
  - Phenobarbital 3–5 mg/kg IV PRN.
- Analgesics (do not use in combination with steroids).
  - Nonsteroidal anti-inflammatory drugs (NSAIDs).
    - Carprofen – dogs 2.2 mg/kg PO q 12–24 hours.
    - Meloxicam – cats 0.1 mg/kg PO q 24 hours. Limit dosing to two days.
    - Deracoxib 1–2 mg/kg PO q 24 hours (dogs).
    - Robenacoxib 1 mg/kg PO q 24 hours (cats). Limit dosing to three days.
  - Buprenorphine 0.005–0.03 mg/kg IM, IV or SQ q 6–12 hours (dogs, cats).

### Precautions/Interactions

- Animals should be monitored for at least 30–90 minutes due to the potential for an anaphylactic reaction.
- Beyond that, animals should be monitored at home by owners. Complications and delayed hypersensitivity reactions may occur.

### Patient Monitoring

- Monitor closely for signs of anaphylaxis and/or complications due to stings.
- Because of the risk of acute lung injury in severe cases, respiratory rate and effort should be monitored closely.

### Activity

- Patient should be kept quiet until clinical signs resolve.

 **COMMENTS**

### Prevention/Avoidance

- Avoid visible nests.
- Move away slowly if a nest is encountered when walking with a dog.

### Possible Complications

- Severe envenomation – hemolysis, spherocytosis, neural dysfunction, acute lung injury/acute respiratory distress syndrome (ALI/ARDS), secondary immune-mediated hemolytic anemia, IMTP, systemic rhabdomyonecrosis, acute tubular necrosis.

### Expected Course and Prognosis

- Excellent in uncomplicated cases with only a localized reaction.
- Fair to good in severe cases with anaphylaxis and further complications.

### Client Education

- Owners with animals at risk for reactions should keep diphenhydramine available.
- Those with known reactions should have epinephrine readily available.

### Abbreviations

See Appendix 1 for a complete list.

## Suggested Reading

Fitzgerald KT, Flood AA. Hymenoptera stings. *Clin Tech Small Anim Pract* 2006;21(4):194–204.

Nakamura RK, Fenty RK, Bianco D. Presumptive immune-mediated thrombocytopenia secondary to massive Africanized bee envenomation in a dog. *J Vet Emerg Crit Care* 2013;23(6):652–656.

Noble SJ, Armstrong PJ. Bee sting envenomation resulting in secondary immune-mediated hemolytic anemia in two dogs. *J Am Vet Med Assoc* 1999;214(7):1026–1027.

Oliveira EC, Pedroso PMO, Meirelles EWB et al. Pathological findings in dogs after multiple Africanized bee stings. *Toxicon* 2007;49(8):1214–1218.

Reed HC, Landolt PJ. Ants, wasps, and bees (Hymenoptera). In: Mullen GR, Durden LA (eds) *Medical and Veterinary Entomology*, 2nd edn. London: Academic Press, 2009; pp. 371–396.

Shimada AT, Nakai T, Morita T et al. Systemic rhabdomyonecrosis and acute tubular necrosis in a dog associated with wasp stings. *Vet Rec* 2005;156(10):320–322.

Walker T, Tidwell AS, Rozanski EA et al. Imaging diagnosis: acute lung injury following massive bee envenomation in a dog. *Vet Radiol Ultrasound* 2005;46(4):300–303.

**Author:** Sarah K. Jarosinski, DVM, DACVAA

**Consulting Editor:** Lynn R. Hovda, RPh, DVM, MS, DACVIM

# Foods

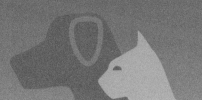

# Chapter 70

# Bread Dough

## DEFINITION/OVERVIEW

- Bread dough toxicosis occurs when yeast-containing dough products are ingested during the process of rising prior to baking or cooking.
- Toxicosis can occur with ingestion of any raw bread (including sourdough starters), pizza, bun, or pastry dough.
- The main concerns following bread dough ingestion are gastric distension with potential volvulus, gastrointestinal obstruction, and ethanol toxicosis.
- Even though bread dough toxicosis can occur at any time, most cases are reported during holidays like Easter and Christmas when more people bake at home.

## ETIOLOGY/PATHOPHYSIOLOGY

### Mechanism of Action

- Yeasts added to bread dough are live organisms that replicate and increase their cellular metabolism of fermentation when exposed to a moist, warm environment such as the gastrointestinal system at body temperature.
- During fermentation, sugars in the bread dough are converted into cellular energy while ethanol and carbon dioxide gases are produced as metabolic byproducts.
- The expanding dough mass and carbon dioxide gas can result in gastric distension that can progress to GDV, respiratory compromise, gastrointestinal obstruction, or gastric rupture.
- Ethanol absorption can lead to systemic alcohol toxicosis and its metabolites acetaldehyde and acetic acid can result in severe metabolic acidosis.
- Hypoglycemia can be present due to depleted glucose stores and inhibited gluconeogenesis by ethanol.

### Pharmacokinetics or Toxicokinetics – Absorption, Distribution, Metabolism, Excretion

- Ethanol is rapidly absorbed from the stomach and small intestine. It is metabolized in the liver by the enzyme alcohol dehydrogenase to form acetaldehyde and acetic acid.
- After further oxidation steps, acetic acids are excreted by the lungs and kidneys as carbon dioxide and water.

### Toxicity

- No $LD_{50}$ for bread dough or yeast ingestion exists in dogs or cats.
- $LD_{50}$ of 100% ethanol is 5.5 g/kg in dogs but ethanol content of unbaked bread varies widely and has not been well established.

---

*Blackwell's Five-Minute Veterinary Consult Clinical Companion: Small Animal Toxicology*, Third Edition. Edited by Lynn R. Hovda, Ahna G. Brutlag, Robert H. Poppenga, and Steven E. Epstein. © 2024 John Wiley & Sons, Inc. Published 2024 by John Wiley & Sons, Inc.

## Systems Affected

- Gastrointestinal – dough expansion: gastric distension, gastric rupture, GDV, gastrointestinal obstruction, abdominal distension, vomiting, nonproductive retching.
- Nervous – ethanol toxicosis: altered mentation ranging from excitation, to lethargy, stupor, or coma, vocalization, cranial nerve deficits, blindness, ataxia, weakness, recumbency, hypothermia, urinary incontinence.
- Cardiovascular – dough expansion: distributive or hypovolemic shock, tachycardia, weak pulses, pale or injected mucous membranes, tachyarrhythmias, hypo- or pain-associated hypertension. Ethanol toxicosis: bradycardia.
- Endocrine/metabolic – shock: hyperlactatemia, metabolic acidosis. Ethanol toxicosis: high anion gap metabolic acidosis, hypoglycemia.
- Respiratory – dough expansion: increased respiratory rate and effort, dyspnea, cyanosis, aspiration pneumonia and resulting hypoxemia, hypo- or hypercapnia. Ethanol toxicosis: respiratory depression.

# SIGNALMENT/HISTORY

### Risk Factors

- Although all species are susceptible, all reported cases of bread dough toxicosis have been in dogs.
- Dogs with indiscriminate eating habits are at higher risk of bread dough ingestion (e.g., Labrador retriever).

### Historical Findings

- Witnessed dough ingestion or missing bread dough prior to onset of clinical signs.
- Although owners may be aware of bread dough ingestion, they might not recognize its potential dangers and pets may present with advanced clinical signs.
- Evidence of dough in emesis.

# CLINICAL FEATURES

- Dough expansion: distended and tense abdomen, vomiting or retching, dyspnea, circulatory shock.
- Ethanol toxicosis: ataxia, vocalization, weakness, blindness, stupor, coma, reduced cranial nerve function, bradycardia, hypoventilation.

# DIFFERENTIAL DIAGNOSIS

- Abdominal distension – food bloat, GDV, gastrointestinal foreign body obstruction.
- High anion gap metabolic acidosis – ethylene glycol or salicylate toxicosis, uremia.
- Altered mentation – primary CNS disease such as meningitis, meningoencephalitis, cerebrovascular accidents, ingestion of other neurodepressants (e.g., benzodiazepines, opioids, muscle relaxants), hepatic encephalopathy.

# DIAGNOSTICS

- Point-of-care blood work should be performed upon presentation and include blood gas analysis, acid–base and electrolyte parameters, blood glucose and lactate concentration, and PCV/TP.

- Baseline bloodwork (CBC and serum biochemistry) and urinalysis should be performed to help rule out other differential diagnoses.
- Right lateral and orthogonal abdominal radiographs should be obtained to assess the extent of gastric dilation and identify potential gastric malpositioning.

### Clinical Pathological Findings

- High anion gap metabolic acidosis due to ethanol absorption.
- Hypoglycemia secondary to ethanol-induced reduced gluconeogenesis.
- Hyperlactatemia due to circulatory shock.
- Hypoxemia and hypocapnia with aspiration pneumonia, hypercapnia with severe gastric distension and hypoventilation.

### Other Diagnostics

- Blood ethanol concentrations may be obtained through specialized laboratories and can help verify the diagnosis and serve as a monitoring tool to guide therapy.
  - Blood ethanol concentrations of 2–4 mg/mL in dogs can result in clinical signs ranging from ataxia to coma.

### Pathological Findings

- Presence of dough in the stomach +/- small intestines.
- Gastric malpositioning, rupture, necrosis, septic peritonitis.
- Splenic congestion.

 # THERAPEUTICS

- The goals of therapy include the interruption of yeast fermentation and further dough expansion, removal of bread dough, reduction of further ethanol absorption, stabilization of the circulatory system, and supportive symptomatic or surgical interventions for gastrointestinal, metabolic, respiratory, and nervous system signs.

### Detoxification

- If ingestion occurred within 30 minutes and no clinical signs are present, emesis can be attempted in dogs.
  - Normoglycemia, appropriate mentation, and absence of GDV should be established prior to emesis induction.
- Patients with neurological signs and evidence of gastric material on radiographs should be placed under general anesthesia, orotracheally intubated to protect their airway, and undergo gastric lavage.
  - A large-bore orogastric tube is recommended for effective dough removal.
  - Cold water lavage may be effective at inhibiting further yeast fermentation, ethanol, and carbon dioxide production.
- Administration of activated charcoal in bread dough ingestion is controversial. It is ineffective in preventing ethanol absorption but if combined with a cathartic may aid in more rapid passage of residual dough.

### Appropriate Health Care

- Supportive care consisting of IV fluids is frequently sufficient for dogs that show no or mild clinical signs, and mild neurological signs are often self-limiting.
- Severe gastric distension can cause circulatory shock and IV fluids are indicated to establish normal perfusion and maintain hydration.

- For dogs in shock, isotonic crystalloids should be administered IV in 30 mL/kg increments over 10–20 minutes and the patient reevaluated to assess if a further bolus is indicated.
- Hypoglycemia (<60 mg/dL) should be treated with 0.5–1.0 mL/kg of 50% dextrose IV diluted 1:4 in saline and followed by a CRI of 2.5–5% dextrose in IV fluids as needed.
- Comatose dogs or those with absent gag reflex should be intubated to reduce aspiration risk. In cases with severe respiratory depression and hypercapnia ($PCO_2$ >60 mmHg), mechanical ventilation may be indicated.
- Severely ataxic or recumbent patients should be given dry, padded bedding, turned every four hours, and urinary catheterization should be considered.
- Hypothermic patients should be actively or passively warmed to maintain normothermia.
- In patients with reduced cranial nerve function, artificial tears should be applied every six hours to prevent corneal ulceration.

### Drug(s) of Choice

- In cases of severe CNS and respiratory depression, the administration of alpha-adrenergic antagonists such as yohimbine (0.1 mg/kg IV) or atipamezole (0.1 mg/kg IM) can be considered.
  - Ethanol has been shown to bind alpha-2-adrenergic receptors in the brain and alpha-adrenergic receptor antagonists can potentially antagonize ethanol effects.
  - Therapy should be reserved for severe cases where mechanical ventilation is not available or has been declined by the owners.

### Extracorporeal Therapy

- Referral for ethanol removal via hemodialysis can be considered in cases with severe neurological or cardiovascular compromise.

### Surgical Considerations

- In cases of confirmed GDV, gastric rupture, or complete mechanical obstruction of the gastric outflow or intestinal tract, patient stabilization followed by surgical intervention is indicated.
- Gastrotomy may be needed to remove large volumes of bread dough if gastric lavage is ineffective.

### Patient Monitoring

- Patient monitoring should include heart rate, pulse quality, mucous membrane color and capillary refill time, mentation, respiratory rate and effort, ECG, blood pressure, pulse oximetry, and point-of-care blood work every 2–6 hours depending on patient status.

### Diet

- Withhold food and water until mentation and gag reflex are appropriate.

 **COMMENTS**

### Prevention/Avoidance

- Educate owners on risks associated with bread dough ingestion.
- Supervise pets and remove them from the kitchen while yeast-containing doughs are rising.

## Possible Complications

- Monitor for aspiration pneumonia secondary to retching, vomiting, respiratory distress, and reduced gag reflex during CNS depression.

## Expected Course and Prognosis

- If left untreated, gastric distension and ethanol toxicosis from bread dough ingestion can progress to GDV, gastrointestinal obstruction or rupture, cardiovascular, respiratory, and metabolic compromise and can potentially be fatal.
- With prompt recognition and treatment, the prognosis for full recovery after bread dough ingestion is excellent.
- The incidence of fatal courses of bread dough toxicosis without therapeutic intervention versus medical or surgical therapies has not been established.

## Abbreviations

- CBC = complete blood count
- CRI = constant rate infusion
- CNS = central nervous system
- ECG = electrocardiogram
- GDV = gastric dilation volvulus
- IV = intravenous
- $LD_{50}$ = median lethal dose
- PCV/TP = packed cell volume/total protein

## Suggested Reading

Means C. Bread dough toxicosis in dogs. *J Vet Emerg Crit Care* 2003;13(1):39–41.

Suter RJ. Presumed ethanol intoxication in sheep dogs fed uncooked pizza dough. *Aust Vet J* 1992;69(1):20.

Thrall MA, Freemyer FG, Hamar DW et al. Ethanol toxicosis secondary to sourdough ingestion in a dog. *J Am Vet Med Assoc* 1984;184(12):1513–1514.

**Author**: Sabrina N. Hoehne, Dr. med. vet., DACVECC, DECVECC
**Consulting Editor**: Steven E. Epstein, DVM, DACVECC

# Chapter 71

# Chocolate and Caffeine

## DEFINITION/OVERVIEW

- Methylxanthines alkaloids originate from plants (e.g., cacao and coffee beans) and include theobromine, caffeine, and theophylline (not discussed in this chapter).
- Sources of theobromine: dark and milk chocolate, garden mulch with cacao bean shells.
- Sources of caffeine: dark and milk chocolate, guarana herbal supplements, caffeine tablets, coffee beans, tea, caffeinated soft drinks.
- Note that chocolate contains both theobromine and caffeine but has significantly more theobromine.
- Hallmark clinical signs include central nervous system (CNS) stimulation, tachycardia, and gastrointestinal (GI) signs.

## ETIOLOGY/PATHOPHYSIOLOGY

### Mechanism of Action

- Antagonizes cellular adenosine receptors which leads to CNS stimulation.
- Inhibits phosphodiesterase which increases intracellular cyclic adenosine monophosphate, leading to bronchial and GI smooth muscle dilation.
- Enhances release of catecholamines (e.g., norepinephrine) leading to tachycardia.
- Increases calcium entry into cells while inhibiting sequestration of calcium within the sarcoplasmic reticulum, enhancing skeletal and cardiac muscle contractility.

### Pharmacokinetics or Toxicokinetics – Absorption, Distribution, Metabolism, Excretion

- Caffeine is absorbed rapidly within 60 minutes (peak plasma levels within 1.5 hours), while theobromine is absorbed 10 times slower (peak plasma levels only at 5–10 hours).
- Methylxanthines are distributed throughout all body water compartments. They can cross the placenta and into the milk of lactating bitches.
- All methylxanthines undergo hepatic metabolism. Caffeine is first metabolized to theobromine.
- They are mostly excreted via the biliary system and undergo enterohepatic circulation.
- 10% of caffeine is also excreted unchanged in urine and can be reabsorbed from the urinary tract.
- Excretion of theobromine occurs more slowly than caffeine and accounts for its prolonged half-life in dogs (caffeine 4.5 hours vs theobromine 17.5 hours).

*Blackwell's Five-Minute Veterinary Consult Clinical Companion: Small Animal Toxicology*, Third Edition. Edited by Lynn R. Hovda, Ahna G. Brutlag, Robert H. Poppenga, and Steven E. Epstein. © 2024 John Wiley & Sons, Inc. Published 2024 by John Wiley & Sons, Inc.

## Toxicity

- Theobromine precipitates more clinical signs than caffeine due to its prolonged half-life.
- Clinical signs are related to the dose of methylxanthine exposure.
  - >20 mg/kg (mild): agitation, vomiting, diarrhea.
  - >40 mg/kg (moderate): cardiovascular effects (tachycardia, tachyarrhythmias, hypertension).
  - >60 mg/kg (severe): muscle stiffness, ataxia, tremors, seizures, coma.
- The reported minimum lethal dose is 110–200 mg/kg in dogs and 100–150 mg/kg in cats.
- To calculate dose exposure, see Tables 71.1 and 71.2 for the methylxanthine content in various products.

## Systems Affected

- Gastrointestinal: vomiting and diarrhea, due to GI smooth muscle relaxation and stimulation of gastric secretion.
- Nervous system: restlessness (with tachypnea + hyperthermia), hyperactivity, tremors, ataxia. Seizures and coma with severe toxicosis.
- Cardiovascular: sinus tachycardia, supraventricular tachycardia (SVT), ventricular tachycardia, hypertension, on occasion bradycardia.
- Musculoskeletal: muscle rigidity due to increased skeletal muscle contractility.
- Renal/urological: polyuria from diuresis.
- Respiratory: respiratory failure and noncardiogenic pulmonary edema have been reported but are rare.

**TABLE 71.1 Approximate methylxanthine content.**

| Chocolate type | Total methylxanthine (mg/oz) |
| --- | --- |
| Cacao beans | 300–1500 |
| Cacao bean mulch | 56–900 |
| Dry cocoa powder | 800 |
| Baker's chocolate (unsweetened) | 450 |
| Semisweet chocolate chips | 160 |
| Milk chocolate | 64 |
| White chocolate | Insignificant, low risk |

**TABLE 71.2 Approximate methylxanthine content in caffeine products.**

| Product | Content |
| --- | --- |
| Caffeine tablets | 200 mg/tablet |
| Coffee beans | 280–570 mg/oz |
| Coffee drip | 80–85 mg/5oz cup |
| Instant coffee | 30–90 mg/5oz cup |
| Cola soft drinks | 40–60 mg/8oz cup |

# SIGNALMENT/HISTORY

## Risk Factors

- Holiday periods with increased access to chocolates (e.g., Easter, Halloween, Christmas).
- Current medications of propranolol, erythromycin, corticosteroids, and cimetidine could decrease the metabolism of methylxanthines and prolong toxicosis.
- Dogs with CYP1A2 enzyme deficiency polymorphism may have higher risks of toxicosis from reduced metabolism of methylxanthines. This occurs across multiple breeds, but wolfhounds, whippets, beagles, Dalmatians and Australian shepherds are known to be homozygous for this mutation.

## Historical Findings

- Common owner-reported clinical signs include acute onset of vomiting, diarrhea, panting, restlessness, ataxia, tremors, seizures, and polyuria.

## Location and Circumstances of Poisoning

- Access to methylxanthine-containing food products (e.g., tabletop, pantry) leading to indiscriminate ingestion.
- Accidental feeding of dark chocolate to the pet by children.

# CLINICAL FEATURES

- Onset of clinical signs generally occurs within 2–4 hours after ingestion of a toxic dose.
- Restlessness, hyperthermia, and tachypnea with normal respiratory effort are frequent findings.
- Cardiovascular findings include tachycardia without pulse deficits and hypertension.
- Patients can present with muscle tremors +/– generalized ataxia and may also seizure.
- Patients are often dehydrated from GI losses and may have hypersalivation from nausea.
- Abdominal discomfort may be present on occasion due to gastroenteritis or pancreatitis.

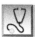

# DIFFERENTIAL DIAGNOSIS

- Other toxins that cause CNS stimulation, such as:
  - insecticides and molluscicides (pyrethrin, organophosphates, nicotine, strychnine, metaldehyde).
  - tremorgenic mycotoxins.
  - tricyclic antidepressants.
  - illicit drugs (cocaine, amphetamines, high doses of marijuana).
- Other toxins that cause tachycardia and tachyarrhythmias, such as:
  - pseudoephedrine.
  - beta-2 agonists.
  - digitalis.
- History of exposure and presence of chocolate in vomitus is the main way to identify a methylxanthine exposure.

# DIAGNOSTICS

## Clinical Pathological Findings

- Serum biochemistry may show hyperglycemia, a mild to moderate hypokalemia (36% of dogs), and/or a hepatopathy with mild increases in AST and ALT (41% of dogs).

- Complete blood count is usually unremarkable or may reflect a stress leukogram.
- Hyperlactatemia from increased muscle activity.

## Other Diagnostics

- Point-of-care ultrasound may show gastrointestinal ileus with fluid dilation and a normal to increased cardiac systolic function.
- Methylxanthine levels may be measured in stomach contents, plasma, serum, urine, and liver (biopsy/necropsy sample) to confirm the suspicion of methylxanthine toxicosis. Theobromine may be detected in serum 3–4 days post exposure. However, due to the lag time for results, this is not a practical diagnostic method.
- Electrocardiogram.
  - Typically, supraventricular tachycardia.
  - Ventricular arrhythmias are possible.

## Pathological Findings

- There are no specific necropsy lesions associated with methylxanthine toxicosis.
- Chocolate/coffee bean material or stimulant tablets may be found in the stomach, along with gastroenteritis and parenchymal organ congestion.

 **THERAPEUTICS**

## Detoxification

- Induce emesis if <4 hours from ingestion or 6–8 hours with large quantity exposure.
- Gastric lavage is rarely indicated and considered only in cases with lethal doses (e.g., caffeine tablets), severe clinical signs, and recent ingestion (<1–2 h). Most can be successfully managed with emesis.
- Activated charcoal 0.5–1 g/kg orally q 8–12 hours for 1–3 days due to enterohepatic recirculation.
- Forced diuresis of caffeine with intravenous fluid therapy at 1–2× maintenance fluid rates of an isotonic crystalloid for 12–24 hours.

## Appropriate Health Care

- *No clinical signs with successful emesis*: activated charcoal once, discharge for home monitoring.
- *Mild clinical signs (GI signs, mild hyperactivity)*: repeated activated charcoal doses, antiemetics, +/– subcutaneous fluids, monitor closely at home +/– 12 hours of in-hospital monitoring, frequent walks to reduce caffeine reabsorption from urinary tract.
- *Moderate to severe clinical signs (cardiac + neurological signs)*: hospitalization, antiemetics, +/– ECG monitoring for tachyarrhythmias, esmolol CRI for severe tachycardia or SVT, lidocaine CRI for ventricular tachycardia, blood pressure monitoring, active cooling for hyperthermia, anxiolytics (butorphanol, acepromazine), tremors or seizure control (diazepam, midazolam, phenobarbitone, levetiracetam), monitor electrolytes, frequent walks, +/– urinary catheterization for severe toxicosis.

## Drug(s) of Choice

- Arrhythmias.
  - Esmolol: 0.1 mg/kg loading dose then 10–200 mcg/kg/min IV CRI titrated to effect for SVT.
  - Lidocaine CRI: 2 mg/kg IV bolus over 1–2 mins, then 50–75 mcg/kg/min for ventricular arrhythmias.
- Sedatives.
  - Butorphanol: 0.2–0.5 mg/kg IV, q 2–4 hours as required.
  - Acepromazine: 0.02–0.05 mg/kg IV, q 4–6 hours as required.

- Antiepileptics.
  - Diazepam: 0.5 mg/kg IV, as required for seizures.
  - Midazolam: 0.25 mg/kg IV, as required for seizures.
  - Phenobarbital: 2–4 mg/kg IV, loading up to 16–20 mg/kg in 4–5 mg/kg doses q 4–6 hours as required.
  - Levetiracetam: 20 mg/kg IV, up to 60–80 mg/kg as required for seizures.
- Antiemetics.
  - Maropitant: 1 mg/kg IV/SQ q 24 hours.
  - Ondansetron: 0.5–1 mg/kg IV/SQ/IM q 8–12 hours.

### Precautions/Interactions

- Propranolol, as it may hinder the elimination of methylxanthines and has a long half-life.

### Alternative Drugs

- If esmolol is not available for severe tachycardia or SVT, oral atenolol and sotalol can be considered. Bear in mind that these have a longer duration of effect (e.g., up to 12 hours).

### Extracorporeal Therapy

- Hemodialysis in severe cases with lethal dose exposure.

### Diet

- Consider a digestible low-fat diet such chicken and rice, prescription GI diets (e.g., Hill's i/d) for 3–5 days for anticipated gastroenteritis.

 **COMMENTS**

### Prevention/Avoidance

- Keep chocolates and caffeine products out of reach.
- Increased awareness of risks of toxicosis during holiday periods.

### Possible Complications

- Gastroenteritis with vomiting and diarrhea lasting 3–7 days.
- Pancreatitis due to fat content from chocolate.
- Foreign body obstruction from concurrent large-quantity ingestion of candy wrappers.
- Aspiration pneumonia from protracted vomiting.

### Expected Course and Prognosis

- Prognosis is excellent even with moderate to severe clinical signs and fatalities are rare.
- Patients with successful emesis are mostly treated as outpatients with home monitoring.
- Patients with clinical signs of toxicosis are hospitalized for a median of two days, and up to four days for severe clinical signs or complications (e.g., pancreatitis, severe gastroenteritis).
- Methylxanthine-induced tachyarrhythmias generally resolve quickly, with discontinuation of antiarrhythmic therapy within a 12–24-hour period.

### Synonyms

Methylxanthines
Methylated xanthine alkaloids
Theobromine

## Abbreviations

- CNS = central nervous system
- GI = gastrointestinal
- CRI = continuous rate infusion
- SVT = supraventricular tachycardia

## Suggested Reading

Cortinovis C, Caloni F. Household food items toxic to dogs and cats. *Front Vet Sci* 2016;3:26.

Ooms TG, Khan SA, Means C. Suspected caffeine and ephedrine toxicosis resulting from ingestion of an herbal supplement containing guarana and ma huang in dogs: 47 cases (1997–1999). *J Am Vet Med Assoc* 2001;218(2):225–229.

Peterson ME, Talcott PA. *Small Animal Toxicology*, 3rd edn. St Louis: Elsevier Saunders, 2013.

Verschoor-Kirss M, Rozanski E, Rush JE. Use of esmolol for control of tachycardia in 28 dogs and cats (2003–2020). *J Vet Emerg Crit Care* 2022;32(2):243–248.

Weingart C, Hartmann A, Kohn B. Chocolate ingestion in dogs: 156 events (2015–2019). *J Small Anim Pract* 2021;62(11):979–983.

**Author:** Avalene W.K. Tan, BVSc, DACVECC
**Consulting Editor:** Steven E. Epstein, DVM, DACVECC

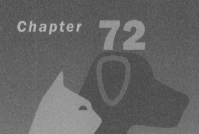

# Chapter 72

# Grapes and Raisins

## DEFINITION/OVERVIEW

- The *Vitis* genus includes grapes, raisins, zante currants, and sultanas. They have been associated with AKI in dogs. The fruits involved have been from both commercial and home cultivators and have been both organic and traditionally grown produce.

## ETIOLOGY/PATHOPHYSIOLOGY

- The toxic component in *Vitis* sp. is thought to be tartaric acid. Tartaric acid is an organic acid found in large amounts in grapes and raisins. The content varies with variety of fruit and stage of ripeness. This may explain the variable toxicity in some dogs.
- Dogs are uniquely sensitive as they lack renal (organic anion transporter) OAT-4 that would normally excrete organic acids into the renal lumen.

### Mechanism of Action

- Since dogs lack renal OAT-4, this allows significant proximal tubule cell accumulation of tartaric acid resulting in canine-specific nephrotoxicity. The mechanism by which tartaric acid causes renal tubular necrosis is not described in the literature. Other organic acids, such as maleic acid, are thought to cause depletion of ATP in the proximal tubules. It is possible that tartaric acid has similar mechanisms. A lack of ATP would lead to cellular death.

### Pharmacokinetics or Toxicokinetics – Absorption, Distribution, Metabolism, Excretion

- Tartaric acid is absorbed rapidly from the intestinal tract. Tissue metabolism is minimal and most is excreted unchanged in the urine. Tartaric acid is absorbed from the blood into the proximal tubule cells and then secreted into the lumen by OAT-4. In dogs, 50% is recovered in the urine within 12 hours.
- Vomiting usually begins within 2–24 hours and azotemia develops within 24–48 hours.

### Toxicity

- Decontaminate if more than 1 grape/raisin per 10 pounds (5 kg) of dog was ingested.
- Thermal decomposition of tartaric acid may explain the anecdotal observation that cooked raisins (raisin bread, cookies) are less likely to be implicated in cases of AKI, although the exact temperature and duration of the heating process for full decomposition were not located in the literature. Decontaminate at more than 2 raisins per 10 pounds (5 kg) of dog.

*Blackwell's Five-Minute Veterinary Consult Clinical Companion: Small Animal Toxicology*, Third Edition.
Edited by Lynn R. Hovda, Ahna G. Brutlag, Robert H. Poppenga, and Steven E. Epstein.
© 2024 John Wiley & Sons, Inc. Published 2024 by John Wiley & Sons, Inc.

## Systems Affected

- Gastrointestinal – vomiting, diarrhea, anorexia, abdominal pain.
- Renal/urological – acute proximal renal tubular necrosis, AKI, polyuria progressing to oliguria and anuria.
- Hepatobiliary – mild elevation in liver values.
- Endocrine/metabolic – hypercalcemia, hyperphosphatemia; metabolic acidosis if AKI occurs.
- Neuromuscular – weakness, ataxia (rare).

 # SIGNALMENT/HISTORY

- Dogs – any age, breed or sex.

## Risk Factors

- Preexisting renal disease.

## Historical Findings

- Witnessed ingestion of *Vitis* sp.
- Evidence of grapes or raisins in the vomitus or stool.

## Location and Circumstances of Poisoning

- Home or yard containing *Vitis* sp.

 # CLINICAL FEATURES

- Acute exposures will be normal.
- Dehydration, lethargy.
- +/– abdominal or renal pain.
- +/– uremic ulcers.

 # DIFFERENTIAL DIAGNOSIS

- Toxic – ethylene glycol, NSAIDs, *Lilium* (cats), cholecalciferol (vitamin D), aminoglycosides, heavy metals, amphotericin B, cisplatin.
- Nontoxic – leptospirosis, bacterial pyelonephritis, renal thromboembolism, hypovolemia, ischemia, acute pancreatitis, sepsis, MODS, hemoglobinuria/myoglobinuria.

 # DIAGNOSTICS

- CBC, biochemistry panel, urinalysis.
- Abdominal radiographs or ultrasound.

## Clinical Pathological Findings

- CBC – dehydration (elevated hematocrit and plasma protein).
- Serum biochemistry – azotemia (>12–24 h), hyperphosphatemia, hypercalcemia (>24 h), hyperkalemia, elevated liver values, elevated amylase and lipase.
- Urinalysis – isosthenuria, glucosuria, proteinuria, casts.

## Other Diagnostics

- Blood gases – decrease in bicarbonate concentration, metabolic acidosis.
- Ultrasound – renomegaly, hyperechoic renal cortices, renal pelvic dilation.
- Radiographs – renomegaly (rare), metastatic mineralization.

## Pathological Findings

- Moderate to severe mostly proximal renal tubular necrosis with intact basement membranes and renal epithelial regeneration.
- Proteinaceous and cellular debris in tubule lumens.
- Mineralization of necrotic cells and renal tubular basement membranes.
- Fibrinoid vascular necrosis, soft tissue mineralization.

# THERAPEUTICS

- Decontamination and fluid therapy are the most important parts of therapy to maintain urine output.

## Detoxification

- Emesis is recommended in asymptomatic animals; it may be rewarding up to 6–12 hours post exposure as tartaric acid delays gastric emptying. Further recommendations may change based on emesis results.
- Activated charcoal has shown no clinical benefit, but one dose can be given to large ingestions with lack of positive emesis results.

## Appropriate Health Care

- Hospitalization on fluids with monitoring of urine output is the best therapy.

## Antidote

- None.

## Drug(s) of Choice

- Isotonic crystalloid fluid therapy for 48 hours (longer if AKI develops) if dog is over a potential renal dose of grapes/raisins.
- Manage vomiting (maropitant 1 mg/kg SQ/IV) q 24 hours.
- Treat anuria/oliguria (mannitol 0.25–0.5 g/kg IV over 15–30 min once; furosemide 2–4 mg/kg IV up to 6 mg/kg if needed).
- Gastroprotectants if uremic gastritis (pantoprazole 0.7–1 mg/kg IV slow q 24 h).

## Precautions/Interactions

- If AKI develops, avoid potassium-sparing diuretics (spironolactone) and trimethoprim due to risk of hyperkalemia.
- Try to avoid nephrotoxic medications such as NSAIDs and aminoglycosides.

## Alternative Drugs

- If owner is unable to hospitalize, can monitor at home; any vomiting within the first 24 hours requires hospitalization on fluids.

## Extracorporeal Therapy

- Hemodialysis can help with AKI; it is unknown if it will remove tartaric acid.

## Surgical Considerations

- Consider gastrotomy to remove acute large ingestions that are refractory to emesis or gastric lavage.

## Patient Monitoring

- Renal values – baseline, 24 and 48 hours (longer if AKI).
- Urine output – hourly at first.
- Hydration status (body weight q 12–24 h).

## Diet

- Bland diet can be used if gastrointestinal signs are present.
- Consider renal diet if AKI develops.

# COMMENTS

- While grapes and raisins contain tartaric acid, commercial grape juice, wine, and jelly/jam are detartrated and are not a risk for renal failure.
- Spontaneous vomiting is common and is often the first sign of toxicosis.

## Prevention/Avoidance

- Do not feed grapes or raisins to dogs (client education).
- Keep all grapes and raisins away from dogs.

## Possible Complications

- Chronic renal failure, soft tissue mineralization, pancreatitis.

## Expected Course and Prognosis

- Prognosis for most dogs is good with appropriate decontamination and fluid therapy.
- Oliguria/anuria have a poor prognosis.

## Synonyms

*Vitis* intoxication.

## Abbreviations

- MODS = multiple organ dysfunction syndrome
- OAT = organic acid transporter

## Suggested Reading

Coyne SR, Landry GM. Tartaric acid induces toxicity in Madin-Darby Canine Kidney cells, but not Human Kidney-2 cells in vitro and is prevented by organic anion transporter (OAT) inhibition and human OAT-4 transfection. *J Vet Emerg Crit Care* 2023;33(3):298–304.

Eubig PA, Brady MS, Gwaltney-Brant SM et al. Acute renal failure in dogs after the ingestion of grapes or raisins: a retrospective evaluation of 43 dogs (1992–2002). *J Vet Intern Med* 2005;19:663–674.

Morrow CM, Valli VE, Volmer PA et al. Canine renal pathology associated with grape or raisin ingestion 10 cases. *J Vet Diagn Invest* 2005;17:223–231.

Wegenast CA, Meadows ID, Anderson RE et al. Acute kidney injury in dogs following ingestion of cream of tartar and tamarinds and the connection to tartaric acid as the proposed toxic principle in grapes and raisins. *J Vet Emerg Crit Care* 2022;32(6):812–816.

**Author:** Tina Wismer, DVM, MS, DABVT, DABT
**Consulting Editor:** Steven E. Epstein, DVM, DACVECC

# Chapter 73

# Hops

## DEFINITION/OVERVIEW

- *Humulus lupulus*, commonly known as hops, are a species of flowering vines that are part of the Cannainaceae family.
- Female hops plants contain cones which are most famously used during the beer brewing process to add bitterness and aroma. Hops also have potential medicinal properties for humans including antioxidant, antiinflammatory, antimicrobial, anticancer, and sedative effects.
- Hops can be ingested in several forms, including the plant itself, spent hops which are boiled and discarded as part of the beer brewing process, and commercially available dried hops pellets.
- Hops ingestion in dogs can cause a sometimes fatal malignant hyperthermia-like reaction. Commonly reported clinical signs include tachypnea/panting, hyperthermia, vomiting, and tachycardia. Several different forms of hops as listed above have caused toxicity in dogs.
- It is unknown if cats experience a similar toxicity to dogs.

## ETIOLOGY/PATHOPHYSIOLOGY

### Mechanism of Action

- The exact mechanism of action of this toxicity is unknown.
- Hops contain several bioactive compounds which could be responsible for the toxicity including volatile oils, alpha/beta acids, phenolic compounds, flavonoids, prenylflavonoids, phytoestrogens, essential oils, etc.

### Pharmacokinetics or Toxicokinetics – Absorption, Distribution, Metabolism, Excretion

- The absorption, distribution, metabolism and excretion are currently unknown.

### Systems Affected

- Respiratory – tachypnea, panting.
- Endocrine/metabolic – hyperthermia, metabolic acidosis, death.
- Gastrointestinal – vomiting, diarrhea.
- Cardiovascular – tachycardia.
- Nervous – agitation, lethargy.
- Renal/urological – polydipsia, myoglobinuria.
- Hemic/lymphatic/immune – DIC.

*Blackwell's Five-Minute Veterinary Consult Clinical Companion: Small Animal Toxicology*, Third Edition. Edited by Lynn R. Hovda, Ahna G. Brutlag, Robert H. Poppenga, and Steven E. Epstein.
© 2024 John Wiley & Sons, Inc. Published 2024 by John Wiley & Sons, Inc.

# SIGNALMENT/HISTORY

## Risk Factors

- There are no published risk factors. However, it is possible that breeds which have a predisposition to malignant hyperthermia, such as greyhounds, German shepherd dogs, Doberman pinschers, and Border collies, may be at a higher risk.

## Historical Findings

- Witnessed hops ingestion.
- Emesis containing hops plant material or packaging from commercially sold hops.
- Owners may report panting, vomiting, diarrhea, agitation, lethargy, or that dogs feel hot to the touch.

## Location and Circumstances of Poisoning

- Hops plants can grow throughout North America, but the majority are farmed from the Pacific Northwest. Dried hops pellets used for home brewing are sold everywhere.

# CLINICAL FEATURES

- Clinical signs often develop rapidly, most commonly within 2–8 hours of ingestion. Death has been reported to occur within 2–30 hour after ingestion.
- Initial clinical signs may include hyperthermia, tachypnea/panting, tachycardia, agitation, vomiting, and diarrhea.

# DIFFERENTIAL DIAGNOSIS

- Malignant hyperthermia, particularly if the patient has recently been under anesthesia or exposed to depolarizing skeletal muscle relaxants or volatile inhalants.
- Hyperthermia: heat stroke, exercise-induced hyperthermia, exogenous heat source.
- Fever: infectious, paraneoplastic, inflammatory, immune mediated.

# DIAGNOSTICS

## Clinical Pathological Findings

- CBC: thrombocytopenia if DIC develops.
- Biochemistry: elevated creatinine kinase, hyperkalemia, hypercalcemia, hyperphosphatemia, hypermagnesemia, elevated liver enzymes and azotemia secondary to hyperthermia injury.
- Coagulation testing: prolonged PT and aPTT and elevated D-dimers if DIC develops.
- Venous blood gas: metabolic acidosis, elevated or decreased $PCO_2$.
- Urinalysis: pigmenturia, myoglobinuria.

## Other Diagnostics

- Abdominal radiographs may show foreign material in the GI tract.
- Endoscopy may find plant material or dried hops within the stomach.

## Pathological Findings

- Rapid onset of rigor mortis.
- Hops material within the GI tract.
- Evidence of hyperthermia-induced organ damage or DIC.

## THERAPEUTICS

### Detoxification

- Emesis is recommended in asymptomatic patients with recent ingestion.
- In symptomatic patients, gastric lavage with an inflated endotracheal tube placed with the patient under heavy sedation or general anesthesia can be considered to remove hops from the stomach.
- Administration of a single dose of activated charcoal with a cathartic may prevent further absorption.

### Appropriate Health Care

- Evaluation by a veterinarian is recommended as some signs of toxicity, such as tachycardia and hyperthermia, will be more accurately detected by a veterinarian.
- IV fluid therapy to lower body temperature, prevent myoglobin-induced kidney injury, and maintain perfusion.
- Active cooling measures such as IV fluids, fans, cool water baths, use of ice packs over major vessels, wetting footpads with alcohol, cool water enemas, or cool water gastric lavage can be considered if severe hyperthermia develops. Cooling measures should be stopped when a temperature of 103 °F is reached to prevent rebound hypothermia.
- Mechanical ventilation and providing supplemental oxygen if $PCO_2$ is severely elevated.
- Supportive care as needed based on clinical signs which may include antiemetics or sedation if agitation is present.

### Antidote

- Dantrolene is a direct muscle relaxant that works by antagonizing intracellular calcium channels. It is the treatment of choice for traditional malignant hyperthermia, but effectiveness in treating this malignant hyperthermia-like reaction is unknown. If the IV form is available, it can be given at a dose of 3 mg/kg IV. Alternatively, it can be administered orally at 3.5 mg/kg. Rarely, hyperkalemia, sedation or hepatotoxicity may occur after use.

### Drug(s) of Choice

- Maropitant 1 mg/kg IV or SQ for vomiting and nausea.
- Acepromazine 0.02–0.04 mg/kg IV, IM, SQ q 4–6 hours as needed for sedation.

### Precautions/Interactions

- While it is unknown if patients who experience the malignant hyperthermia-like reaction after hops ingestion are predisposed to traditional malignant hyperthermia, avoiding known triggers of malignant hyperthermia (volatile anesthetics and depolarizing neuromuscular blocking drugs) should be considered.

### Alternative Drugs

- Cyproheptadine may be helpful to prevent serotonin syndrome. It is dosed at 1.1 mg/kg PO or rectally every 4–6 hours as needed.
- Methocarbamol may be used as a muscle relaxant if dantrolene cannot be obtained. It is a centrally acting muscle relaxant. It can be given IV at a dose of 40–50 mg/kg IV (not exceeding a cumulative dose of 330 mg/kg) or orally at a dose of 132 mg/kg/day divided into every 8 or 12 hours.

## Surgical Considerations

■ Gastrotomy to remove hops may be indicated if gastric lavage is unsuccessful in large ingestions.

## Patient Monitoring

■ Temperature should be monitored every 2–4 hours depending on patient status, especially if the patient is symptomatic or undergoing active cooling measures.
■ Frequent or continuous heart rate and rhythm monitoring.
■ Acid–base and electrolytes every 6–12 hours.
■ Urine color should be monitored for pigmenturia.

 # COMMENTS

### Prevention/Avoidance

■ Access to hops of any form should be avoided and owners (particularly home brewers) should be educated on the dangers of hops toxicosis.

### Possible Complications

■ Hyperthermia may lead to cellular damage including cardiac arrhythmias, acute kidney injury, hepatic injury, DIC, multiple organ dysfunction, and death.

### Expected Course and Prognosis

■ In two retrospective studies, survival rate was 77% and 95.2%. In both studies, all dogs who died developed hyperthermia.
■ If clinical signs develop, they usually resolve within 24–48 hours.

### Abbreviations

See Appendix 1 for a complete list.

### Suggested Reading

Becker J, Brutlag A, Hovda L, Rendahl A, Tart K. A retrospective evaluation of hops ingestion in 177 dogs (2005–2018). *J Vet Emer Crit Care* 2023;33:348–353.
Drobatz K. Heat stroke. In: Silverstein D, Hopper K (eds) *Small Animal Critical Care Medicine*, 2nd edn. St Louis: Elsevier, 2015; pp. 795–798.
Duncan K, Hare W, Buck W. Malignant hyperthermia-like reaction secondary to ingestion of hops in five dogs. *J Am Vet Med Assoc* 1997;210:51–53.
Pfaff A, Sobczak BR, Babyak JM et al. Retrospective analysis of hops toxicosis in dogs (2002–2014): 71 cases. *J Vet Emerg Crit Care* 2021;32:90–97.
Zanoli P, Zavatti M. Pharmacognostic and pharmacological profile of Humulus lupulus L. *J Ethnopharmacol* 2008;16:383–396.

**Author:** Jami Becker, DVM, DACVECC
**Consulting Editor:** Steven E. Epstein, DVM, DACVECC

# Chapter 74

# Macadamia Nuts

## DEFINITION/OVERVIEW

- Macadamia nuts are popular snack foods and are often incorporated into candies, cakes, and cookies.
- They are harvested from *Macadamia integrifolia* and *Macadamia tetraphyalla* trees (family Proteaceae).
- Macadamia nuts contain 75% fat and 6–8% sugar.
- All macadamia species accumulate very low concentrations of cyanogenic glycosides in their seeds.
- Macadamia nut toxicosis has only been reported in dogs.
- Ingestions as low as 0.7 g/kg of macadamia nuts have been associated with clinical signs, although signs are typically seen at doses greater than 2.2 g/kg.
- Common clinical signs include weakness, depression, vomiting, ataxia, pancreatitis, tremors, and hyperthermia.
- Prognosis for recovery is excellent with resolution of clinical signs within 24–48 hours.
- No fatalities have been reported to date with macadamia nut exposure.

## ETIOLOGY/PATHOPHYSIOLOGY

### Mechanism of Action

- The mechanism of action is currently unknown.
- Toxicity may involve the constituents of the nut themselves, contaminants from processing, mycotoxins, or other unidentified causes.

### Pharmacokinetics or Toxicokinetics – Absorption, Distribution, Metabolism, Excretion

- No pharmacokinetic studies have been reported in dogs.
- In dogs experimentally dosed with macadamia nuts, serum triglyceride levels peaked in 3–6 hours, suggesting a relatively rapid absorption.

### Toxicity

- Clinical signs have been reported at ingestions as low as 0.7 g/kg.
- Consistently toxicosis occurs at greater than 2.2 g/kg and as high as 62.4 g/kg.
- The median amount of macadamia nuts ingestion in dogs with naturally occurring toxicity was 11.7 g/kg.
- Signs of toxicity have been experimentally induced after administering 20 g/kg of commercially prepared roasted macadamia nuts to healthy dogs via stomach tube.

---

*Blackwell's Five-Minute Veterinary Consult Clinical Companion: Small Animal Toxicology*, Third Edition.
Edited by Lynn R. Hovda, Ahna G. Brutlag, Robert H. Poppenga, and Steven E. Epstein.
© 2024 John Wiley & Sons, Inc. Published 2024 by John Wiley & Sons, Inc.

## Systems Affected

- Endocrine/metabolic – hyperthermia, pancreatitis.
- Gastrointestinal – vomiting, abdominal pain, diarrhea.
- Musculoskeletal – hindlimb weakness, joint pain, muscle pain, muscle tremors, reluctance to rise.
- Nervous – CNS depression, absent conscious proprioception, ataxia, tremors.

# SIGNALMENT/HISTORY

## Risk Factors

- Any age or breed of dog may be affected.

## Historical Findings

- Witnessed ingestion of nuts or baked goods containing nuts.

## Location and Circumstances of Poisoning

- Patients are often affected at home after ingestion of human food including candies, cakes, cookies, etc.

# CLINICAL FEATURES

- Clinical signs have been reported as early as one hour after ingestion but generally develop within six hours of ingestion.
- Seventy-nine percent of dogs were noted to develop clinical signs within 12 hours of ingestion.
- Most common findings.
  - Weakness.
  - Depression.
  - Vomiting.
  - Ataxia.
  - Tremors.
  - Hyperthermia.
  - Joint/muscle pain.
  - Inability to rise.
- Clinical signs typically peak at 12 hours.
- Significant improvement in clinical signs expected within 24 hours with complete resolution in 48 hours.
- Experimentally affected dogs developed:
  - weakness – manifested by inability to rise.
  - mild depression.
  - vomiting.
  - hyperthermia.

# DIFFERENTIAL DIAGNOSIS

- Weakness/depression with hyperthermia – bromethalin, metaldehyde, ionophore poisoning, hops.
- Ataxia/hindlimb weakness and joint pain – spinal cord lesion (IVDD, FCE, trauma, neoplasia), tick paralysis, tick-borne disease, polyradiculoneuritis, immune-mediated joint disease.

## DIAGNOSTICS

### Clinical Pathological Findings

- With known history of ingestion, no confirmatory tests or advanced diagnostics needed.
- Complete blood count – no changes.
- Biochemistry profile – elevations in serum lipase and ALP have been noted transiently.

## THERAPEUTICS

- Treatment is symptomatic and supportive.

### Detoxification

- Consider induction of emesis in asymptomatic dogs with recent ingestion.
- Activated charcoal with a cathartic, one dose, may be administered to hasten the passage of nuts throughout the gastrointestinal tract.
- Efficacy of activated charcoal has not been established in this toxicity.

### Appropriate Health Care

- The majority of cases can typically be managed at home.
- Young or old dogs or those with significant preexisting health conditions may benefit from hospitalization and close monitoring.
- IV crystalloid fluid therapy as needed for hydration, perfusion, and as a cooling measure.
- Additional cooling measures (cool water baths, IV fluids, use of fans on the patient, and alcohol on the paw pads) may need to be instituted for patients with significant hyperthermia.

### Drugs(s) of Choice

- Antiemetics as needed for vomiting.
  - Maropitant 1 mg/kg SQ, IV q 24 hours.
  - Ondansetron 0.1–1.0 mg/kg SQ, IV slowly q 6–12 hours.

### Precautions/Interactions

- Dogs coingesting chocolate may require treatment for methylxanthine toxicosis.

### Patient Monitoring

- Symptomatic patients should be monitored for resolution of clinical signs for 24–48 hours.
- Body temperature should be measured every 4–8 hours and cooling measures instituted as needed.
- Recumbent patients should be given soft bedding and have their position switched every four hours.
- Patients may need assistance to stand to urinate and defecate; urinary catheterization may be needed.

### Diet

- Avoid high-fat diet due to risk of pancreatitis following ingestion.

## COMMENTS

### Prevention/Avoidance

- Client education about the toxicity of macadamia nuts and preventing access of pets to macadamia nuts and baked goods containing the nuts.

## Possible Complications

- Potential complications include pancreatitis, gastroenteritis, or intestinal obstruction (rare).

## Expected Course and Prognosis

- Resolution of clinical signs expected in 24–48 hours with minimal veterinary intervention.
- Prognosis is excellent.
- Dogs with preexisting diseases or those with coingestion of other toxicants may have slower recoveries.

## Abbreviations

See Appendix 1 for a complete list.

## Suggested Reading

Botha CJ, Penrith ML. Potential plant poisonings in dogs and cats in Southern Africa. *J S Afr Vet Assoc* 2009;80(2):63–74.

Gugler K, Piscitelli C, Dennis J. Hidden dangers in the kitchen: common foods toxic to dogs and cats. *Compendium* 2013;35(7):E1–E6.

Gwaltney-Brandt SW. Macadamia nuts. In: Peterson M, Talcott P (eds) *Small Animal Toxicology*, 3rd edn. St Louis: Saunders, 2013; pp. 625–628.

Hansen SR, Buck WB, Meerdink G et al. Weakness, tremors, and depression associated with macadamia nuts in dogs. *Vet Hum Toxicol* 2000;42:18–21.

**Author**: Rebecca A.L. Walton, DVM, DACVECC
**Consulting Editor**: Steven E. Epstein, DVM, DACVECC

# Chapter 75

# Mycotoxins (Aflatoxin)

## DEFINITION/OVERVIEW

- Aflatoxin is produced by some species of the mold genus *Aspergillus* (most commonly *A. flavus, A. parsiticus, A. nomius*).
- Four major types of aflatoxins (aflatoxin B1, aflatoxin B2, aflatoxin G1, and aflatoxin G2) are the best known and the most studied among more than 18 different types and metabolites presently identified, with B1 being the most common.
- The most common source of poisoning in small animals is from contaminated pet foods (often occurring in outbreaks; see Chapter 7, Pet Food) but can also occur by consuming moldy foods.

## ETIOLOGY/PATHOPHYSIOLOGY

### Mechanism of Action

- Aflatoxin B1 is metabolized by cytochrome P450 enzymes into the toxic metabolite AFB1-exo 8,9-epoxide which binds to DNA, RNA, and proteins in hepatocytes, interfering with cellular metabolism and protein synthesis.
- Aflatoxins also possess immunosuppressive and immunostimulatory properties, the mechanisms of which are unclear but currently under investigation.

### Toxicokinetics – Absorption, Distribution, Metabolism, Excretion

- Aflatoxins are absorbed rapidly from the intestinal tract into the portal circulation.
- There is widespread distribution of the toxin throughout the body, including milk in lactating animals.
- They are metabolized initially into toxic metabolites of which further metabolism can create other toxic metabolites.
- The major excretion route of aflatoxin B1 and its metabolites is the biliary pathway via feces, followed by the urinary system.

### Toxicity

- Oral $LD_{50}$ in dogs has ranged from 0.5 to 1.5 mg/kg and 0.5 mg/kg in cats.
- Clinical manifestations have been seen at doses greater than 60 g/kg of aflatoxin in dog food.

### Systems Affected

- Hepatobiliary – hepatic necrosis and dysfunction or failure.
- Gastrointestinal – vomiting, anorexia, diarrhea, melena.

---

*Blackwell's Five-Minute Veterinary Consult Clinical Companion: Small Animal Toxicology*, Third Edition. Edited by Lynn R. Hovda, Ahna G. Brutlag, Robert H. Poppenga, and Steven E. Epstein.
© 2024 John Wiley & Sons, Inc. Published 2024 by John Wiley & Sons, Inc.

- Hemic/lymphatic/immune – petechiae or ecchymosis.
- Renal/urological – acute kidney injury, bilirubinuria.
- Central nervous system – obtundation, seizures, encephalopathy.

# SIGNALMENT/HISTORY

### Risk Factors

- Toxicosis occurs in dogs most frequently from contamination of grain-containing foods.
- No clinical aflatoxin toxicosis cases have been reported in cats; however, aflatoxins have been found in commercial cat food.

### Historical Findings

- Lethargy, anorexia, vomiting, and diarrhea are commonly reported by owners.
- Icterus.
- Sudden death with no recognized antecedent illness is possible.
- Opening of a new bag of pet food in weeks prior to illness.
- Decreased interest in contaminated food has been reported.

### Location and Circumstances of Poisoning

- Most cases of canine aflatoxicosis are related to ingestion of contaminated dog food.

# CLINICAL FEATURES

- Vomiting, diarrhea, anorexia, and melena.
- Icterus.
- Ascites.
- Encephalopathy.
- In chronic toxicosis, weight loss, decreased appetite, rough haircoat, icterus, depression, abdominal distension due to ascites, and PU/PD have been reported.

# DIFFERENTIAL DIAGNOSIS

- Other hepatic toxicants: xylitol, blue-green algae, acetaminophen, carprofen, *Amanita* mushrooms, sago palm, etc.
- Leptospirosis or adenovirus.
- Chronic hepatitis.

# DIAGNOSTICS

### Clinical Pathological Findings

- Biochemistry panel – elevated ALT, AST, GGT, ALP, bilirubin or low cholesterol, albumin, BUN, globulin, and glucose concentrations.
- Elevated serum ammonia levels can be found.
- CBC – polycythemia or anemia, thrombocytopenia, or elevated WBC count.
- Coagulation testing – elevated PT, aPTT, decreased antithrombin, fibrinogen, and protein C. Hyperfibrinolysis may be found on viscoelastic testing.

## Other Diagnostics Findings

- Testing of pet food, urine, or liver samples for aflatoxin metabolites can be diagnostic and accomplished at many veterinary diagnostic laboratories.
- Abdominal ultrasound may find a hyperechoic liver, nodules in the liver or gall bladder wall thickening. Ascites may be present.

## Pathological Findings

- Histopathologic changes in acute hepatotoxicity include:
  - hepatic lipidosis.
  - acute hemorrhagic necrosis.
  - bile duct proliferation and stasis.
  - portal fibroplasia.
- Chronic aflatoxin exposure may present with:
  - cirrhosis with nodular degeneration and fibrosis.
  - hepatocellular carcinoma in humans.

 # THERAPEUTICS

- There is no specific therapeutic treatment for aflatoxicosis. Treatment is aimed at providing symptomatic care and treatments for liver failure.

## Detoxification

- Induction of emesis is typically not indicated unless recent ingestion of a moldy food substance has occurred.

## Appropriate Health Care

- Cases of suspected or diagnosed aflatoxin should be hospitalized for intensive care monitoring.
- Patients should have their mentation and vital signs closely monitored as well as evaluation for hemorrhage frequently.
- Evaluate electrolytes and blood glucose concentration every 2–8 hours.

## Drug(s) of Choice

- Fluid support to maintain intravascular volume with isotonic crystalloids is indicated.
  - Consider using lactate-free fluids (e.g., Plasma-Lyte-A®, Normosol-R®) when liver failure is present.
  - Supplemental potassium in fluids may be needed as plasma potassium concentration should be maintained in the reference interval to help minimize hepatic encephalopathy.
  - Supplemental dextrose in fluids is frequently needed to maintain euglycemia.
- Hepatic support.
  - N-acetylcysteine: 140 mg/kg IV (through filter) once, then 70 mg/kg IV or PO q 6 hours for 2–4 days. Dilution is required prior to administration.
  - S-adenosyl-methionine (SAMe)/silybin: 20–40 mg/kg PO in a dog, or 200–400 mg/cat (NOT mg/kg) PO daily for cats, on an empty stomach q 24 hours if oral medications are tolerated.
  - Lactulose: 0.1–0.5 mL/kg PO or lactulose retention enemas can be considered if hepatic encephalopathy is present.
  - Vitamin E: 10 IU/kg PO q 24 hours.

- Consider L-carnitine: 100–200 mg/kg PO q 8–12 hours in dogs, 250–500 mg/cat (NOT mg/kg) PO per day in cats.
- Coagulopathies.
    - Fresh frozen plasma: 10 – 20 mL/kg to treat elevated PT/aPTT if presence of hemorrhage or decreasing PCV is observed.
    - Vitamin K1: 1-2 mg/kg SC,PO bid.
- Antiemetics
    - Maropitant: 1 mg/kg IV/SC q 24 hr.
    - Ondansetron: 0.2-1.0 mg/kg IV,SQ, q 8-12 hr.
- GI protectants
    - Pantoprazole: 1 mg/kg IV q 24 hr.
    - Sucralfate: 0.25 – 1 g PO q 8 hr.
- Systemic antimicrobials
    - Ampicillin/sulbactam 30-50 mg/kg IV q 6-8hr for potential GI translocation

## Precautions/Interactions

- Consider dose reducing or avoiding other hepatically metabolized drugs.
- Avoid pyrethroid insecticides, which may potentiate aflatoxicosis experimentally.

## Alternative Drugs

- If S-Adenosyl-Methionine/Silybin is not available SAMe alone can be used.
- If pantoprazole is not available, omeprazole or famotidine can be used.

## Extracorporeal Therapy

- Hemadsorption has been shown to reduce mortality in experimental acutely exposed rats but is unlikely to be helpful when clinical signs are already present.

## Surgical Considerations

- Coagulation testing prior to invasive procedures and correction of elevated PT/aPTT is recommend.

## Patient Monitoring

- Blood glucose and electrolyte concentrations should be evaluated every 2-8 hours.
- CBC, biochemistry panel and coagulation testing daily.

## Diet

- Avoid feeding other asymptomatic pets in the household potentially contaminated food.

 # COMMENTS

## Prevention/Avoidance

- Report suspected cases associated with pet food to the manufacturer, FDA, and state regulatory agencies.
- Keep all food in clean containers in a cool, dry storage area.
- Keep garbage out of reach of pets.

## Possible Complications

- Chronic kidney disease.
- Hepatic cirrhosis.
- Hepatocellular carcinoma has been reported in humans.

## Expected Course and Prognosis

- Prognosis is poor dogs with mortality rates of 64-68%. Patients with liver failure likely have a worse prognosis.

## See Also

Chapter 115, Mushrooms
Chapter 79, Xylitol
Chapter 110, Blue-Green Algae (Cyanobacteria): Microcystins
Chapter 45, Acetaminophen

## Abbreviations

See Appendix 1 for complete list.
- SAMe: S-Adenyl Methionine

## Suggested Reading

Bates N. Aflatoxicosis in dogs. Companion Animal 2021; 26:8:197–202.

Bruchim Y, Segev G, Sela U, et al. Accidental fatal aflatoxicosis due to contaminated commercial diet in 50 dogs. Res Vet Sci 2012;93(1):279–87.

Dereszynski DM, Center SA, Randolph JF, et al. Clinical and clinicopathologic features of dogs that consumed foodborne hepatotoxic aflatoxins: 72 cases (2005–2006). J Am Vet Med Assoc. 2008; 232(9):1329–1337.

Martínez-Martínez L, Valdivia-Flores AG, Guerrero-Barrera AL, et al. Toxic Effect of Aflatoxins in Dogs Fed Contaminated Commercial Dry Feed: A Review. Toxins. 2021;13(1):65.

**Author:** Steven E. Epstein, DVM, DACVECC
**Consulting Editor:** Lynn R. Hovda, RPh, DVM, MS, DACVIM

# Chapter 76

# Mycotoxins (Tremorgenic)

## DEFINITION/OVERVIEW

- Penitrem A and roquefortine are tremorgenic mycotoxins responsible for producing toxicosis characterized by GI and neurological signs.
- Dogs and cats are most often exposed to tremorgenic mycotoxins through ingestion of moldy foods or after access to a compost pile.
- Although death can occur in severely affected animals, with early and appropriate treatment prognosis is generally good.

## ETIOLOGY/PATHOPHYSIOLOGY

### Mechanism of Action

- Mycotoxins are toxic secondary metabolites produced by fungi. Effects vary depending on chemical structure, concentration of the toxin in foods, and species affected.
- Penitrem A and roquefortine are the tremorgenic mycotoxins reported to affect dogs and cats. Both are produced by *Penicillium* spp.
- Mycotoxins are most commonly found in postharvest rot of crops, spoilage of moldy cheese, walnuts, dog food, bread, apples, and garbage.
- The exact pathophysiological mechanisms of toxicity are not well understood.
- Little is known about the mechanism of action of roquefortine.
- Penitrem A.
  - Inhibits calcium-regulated potassium channels, altering the spontaneous release of neurotransmitters such as glutamate, aspartic acid, and gamma-aminobutyric acid (GABA) in central and peripheral synapses.
  - In mice, acts as an antagonist to production of glycine which is an inhibitor neurotransmitter in the CNS. This action may facilitate transmission of impulses, leading to tremor activity.
  - In rats, may inhibit presynaptic transmission in the cerebellum, and has been shown to cause widespread necrosis and loss of Purkinje neurons.

### Pharmacokinetics or Toxicokinetics – Absorption, Distribution, Metabolism, Excretion

- Readily absorbed through the GI tract.
- Rapidly distributed, reaching main site of action in brain within 30 minutes to hours.
- Able to penetrate the blood–brain barrier.
- Metabolized in the liver and excreted in bile.

*Blackwell's Five-Minute Veterinary Consult Clinical Companion: Small Animal Toxicology*, Third Edition.
Edited by Lynn R. Hovda, Ahna G. Brutlag, Robert H. Poppenga, and Steven E. Epstein.
© 2024 John Wiley & Sons, Inc. Published 2024 by John Wiley & Sons, Inc.

## Toxicity

- The dose ingested is often difficult to determine, and toxicity of mycotoxins varies depending on species and exact toxin present.
- Experimentally, penitrem A has elicited tremors at doses of 0.125 mg/kg and death at 0.5mg/kg administered intraperitoneally.

## Systems Affected

- Neuromuscular – generalized muscle tremors, ataxia, weakness, hyperesthesia, agitation, stiff gait, seizures, stupor to coma in severe intoxications, hyperthermia secondary to tremors.
- Gastrointestinal – hypersalivation, nausea, vomiting, diarrhea presumptively from gastric irritation.
- Cardiovascular – tachycardia.
- Respiratory – panting, tachypnea, dyspnea; aspiration pneumonia is possible.
- Ophthalmic – blepharospasm, mydriasis, nystagmus due to neurotoxic effects.
- Renal/urological – pigmenturia if rhabdomyolysis occurs (uncommon).
- Hemic/lymphatic/immune – DIC secondary to prolonged muscle activity and hyperthermia.
- Hepatic – dose-related centrilobular hemorrhage and necrosis.

 # SIGNALMENT/HISTORY

- Species: dogs are most often affected due to their indiscriminate eating habits although cats may be affected.
- No breed, sex or age predilection.

## Risk Factors

- Animals that are exposed to moldy foods, including human foods, food in garbage cans, and moldy dog food.
- Animals that have access to compost piles or are allowed access outside unsupervised.

## Historical Findings

- Animals generally present for gastrointestinal (vomiting) or neuromuscular (tremors) signs.
- Owners may report that their dog is allowed to roam freely outdoors and may be unaware of toxin exposure.
- Dogs known to have indiscriminate eating habits and may have accessed trash or moldy food items.
- Feeding of dog food that has been exposed to moisture and may be moldy.

## Location and Circumstances of Poisoning

- Exposure generally occurs in the home, yard, or when allowed to roam unsupervised with access to molding organic material, garbage, or compost piles.

 # CLINICAL FEATURES

- Clinical signs most often develop with minutes to a few hours of toxin ingestion.
- Clinical signs most commonly include:
  - hypersalivation, vomiting, diarrhea.
  - generalized muscle tremors, ataxia, weakness, hyperesthesia, agitation, stiff gait, seizure.

- hyperthermia secondary to tremors.
- tachycardia, hyperemic mucous membranes.
- panting, tachypnea.

# DIFFERENTIAL DIAGNOSIS

- Intoxications – strychnine, methylxanthines, bromethalin, amphetamines, SSRIs, organophosphates/carbamates, organochlorides, metaldehyde, macadamia nuts, pyrethroids, cocaine, nicotine, paintballs, ethylene glycol, ivermectin, heavy metals (lead), hexachloraphene.
- Metabolic – hypoglycemia, hypocalcemia, hypo- or hypernatremia, hypomagnesemia, severe uremia, hepatic encephalopathy.
- Primary neurological disease – idiopathic epilepsy, encephalitis (inflammatory and infectious), trauma, neoplasia, idiopathic cerebellar disorders, idiopathic white shaker dog syndrome.

# DIAGNOSTICS

## Clinical Pathological Findings

- Complete blood count, biochemical profile including electrolytes, and urinalysis to obtain baseline values, assess patient status and differentiate from other causes of neurological signs.
- Degree of lab work changes depending on severity of clinical signs.
  - CBC – increased WBC count, elevated PCV (hemoconcentration).
  - Chemistry – mild to severe elevations in renal values, liver enzymes, creatine kinase.
  - Urinalysis – pigmenturia.
- Acid–base analysis – metabolic acidosis.
- Coagulation tests – prolonged PT/PTT, thrombocytopenia, increased FDPs, D-dimers (>24 hours from intoxication).

## Other Diagnostics

- Thoracic radiographs in animals with respiratory signs to evaluate for presence of aspiration pneumonia.
- Thin-layer chromatography or high-pressure liquid chromatography analysis of vomitus or gastric contents for penitrem A or roquefortine analysis is possible.

## Pathological Findings

- Pathological findings reported in dogs poisoned with penitrem A include the following.
  - Hemorrhagic lungs and urinary bladder with engorgement of renal capsular vessels.
  - Hemorrhage and edema of the small and large intestinal serosa.
  - Hepatic congestion with evidence of fatty degeneration.
  - Microscopic findings include marked vascular centrilobular hepatic congestion.

# THERAPEUTICS

- The objectives of treatment are decontamination to prevent further toxin exposure, controlling tremors/seizures, and providing supportive care.

## Detoxification

- Emesis induction in stable animals at low risk of aspiration.
- Gastric lavage in cases of ineffective emesis, presence of large amount of gastric material, or in patients exhibiting clinical signs due to the risk of aspiration. These patients should be heavily sedated or anesthetized to allow placement of a cuffed endotracheal tube.
- Single dose of activated charcoal with a cathartic administered orally in stable patients or via gastric tube after lavage has been performed.

## Appropriate Health Care

- If animals present acutely after ingestion and are successfully decontaminated, outpatient treatment may be possible.
- For those animals demonstrating clinical signs, hospitalization is recommended to allow for appropriate treatment until the patient is asymptomatic and stable.
- Temperature should be monitored frequently in symptomatic animals. For hyperthermic animals, active cooling measures can be instituted (tepid water bath, fan, intravenous fluids) but should cease once body temperature reaches 103 °F so as not to induce hypothermia.
- Intravenous crystalloids may be necessary to correct dehydration, maintain perfusion, and aid in thermoregulation.
- Heart rate and blood pressure should be monitored every 4–8 hours while symptomatic.
- Respiratory rate and effort should be monitored frequently. Oxygen supplementation may be necessary in hypoxemic animals.
- Animals with severe respiratory compromise or those that are unresponsive/comatose may require mechanical ventilation.

## Drug(s) of Choice

- Intralipid emulsion (ILE) 20% solution.
  - Given its lipid solubility and widespread distribution, ILE could be considered to act as a lipid sink/shuttle.
  - In a large case series in dogs, the median time to clinical improvement was four hours after ILE administration. However, other treatments were administered concurrently, so the component responsible for clinical improvement is unknown.
  - CRI of 0.25 mL/kg/min over 30–60 minutes.
  - Repeat every 2–4 hours as necessary to control clinical signs unless lipemia occurs.
- For control of muscle tremors: methocarbamol 55–220 mg/kg IV to effect administered at a rate of ≤2 mL/min PRN to effect, not to exceed 330 mg/kg/day.
- For control of seizures.
  - Diazepam 0.5–1 mg/kg IV; studies have shown that mycotoxin-induced seizures are less responsive to benzodiazepine.
  - Phenobarbital 2–4 mg/kg IV q 30 minutes to effect, not to exceed 18–20 mg/kg.
  - Levetiracetam 30–60 mg/kg IV slow bolus.
  - Propofol 2–8 mg/kg IV slow bolus, followed by CRI of 0.1–0.4 mg/kg/min.
- Antiemetics as needed.
  - Maropitant 1 mg/kg IV, SQ q 24 hours.
  - Ondansetron 0.1–0.3 mg/kg IV, SQ q 8–12 hours.

## Precautions/Interactions

- Activated charcoal can bind to oral medications so consideration must be given to timing of dosing.

- ILE may interfere with the action of lipid-soluble medications so consideration must be given to timing of dosing.

### Alternative Drugs

- If IV methocarbamol is unavailable, oral methocarbamol can be given crushed and administered rectally.

### Patient Monitoring

- Heart rate and body temperature should be monitored every 2–4 hours in symptomatic patients.
- Pulse oximetry should be monitored every 4–8 hours in patients showing respiratory signs.

 **COMMENTS**

### Prevention/Avoidance

- Owners should be warned of the dangers of allowing their pets to roam freely unsupervised.
- Clients should be warned about the toxic potential of moldy foods.
- Compost piles should be enclosed to restrict animal access.

### Possible Complications

- If patients vomit, aspiration pneumonia may occur which alters treatment and prognosis.
- In cases with severe or prolonged hyperthermia, secondary organ dysfunction can occur (rhabdomyolysis, kidney injury, liver damage, DIC).

### Expected Course and Prognosis

- In cases of mild toxin exposure or those treated appropriately early in the clinical course, signs generally resolve in 24–48 hours with no long-term clinical effects.
- With severe intoxications or in cases with treatment delays, clinical signs may persist for days, prolonging hospitalization.
- Patients suffering from toxicosis generally respond well to IV methocarbamol. In patients that are unresponsive, persistent presence of gastric toxin or other toxins should be considered as a cause for clinical signs.
- Rare reports of dogs with persistent neurological signs several months to years after toxin ingestion.
- Some cases can be fatal if large amounts of toxin are consumed before decontamination and treatment can be instituted.
- Animals that develop complications (aspiration pneumonia, DIC) may require prolonged hospitalization and carry a more guarded prognosis.

### Abbreviations

- ALT = alanine aminotransferase
- AST = aspartate aminotransferase
- CK = creatinine kinase
- DIC = disseminated intravascular coagulation

### Suggested Reading

Boysen SR, Rozanski EA, Chan DL et al. Tremorgenic mycotoxicosis in four dogs from a single household. *J Am Vet Med Assoc* 2002;221(10):1441–1444.

Eriksen GS, Jaderlund KH, Moldes-Anaya A et al. Poisoning of dogs with tremorgenic *Penicillium* toxins. *Med Mycol* 2010;48:188–196.

Kormpou F, O'Sullivan Aoife, Troth L, Adamantos S. Use of intravenous lipid emulsion in dogs with suspected tremorgenic mycotoxicosis: 53 cases. *Vet Evidence* 2018;3(2): doi: 10.18849/ve.v3i2.166.

Walter SL. Acute penitrem A and roquefortine poisoning in a dog. *Can Vet J* 2002;43:372–374.

Young KL, Villar D, Carson TL et al. Tremorgenic mycotoxin intoxication with penitrem A and roquefortine in two dogs. *J Am Vet Med Assoc* 2003;222:52–53.

**Author:** Julie Schildt, DVM, DACVECC
**Consulting Editor:** Steven E. Epstein, DVM, DACVECC

# Onions and Garlic

## DEFINITION/OVERVIEW

- The genus *Allium* includes onions (*A. cepa*), leeks (*A. porrum*), garlic (*A. sativum*), and chives (*A. schoenoprasum*). Toxicosis occurs after oral ingestion of fresh or dried plant material, dietary supplements, or food preparations.
- The disulfides and thiosulfates in *Allium* spp. are metabolized to compounds that can cause oxidative damage to erythrocytes, leading to Heinz body production, methemoglobinemia, and hemolytic anemia.
- Treatment involves early decontamination and supportive care; prognosis is generally good.

## ETIOLOGY/PATHOPHYSIOLOGY

### Mechanism of Action

- Several toxic compounds have been identified in *Allium* spp., including *n*-propyl disulfide and 3 sodium alk(en)yl thiosulfates (onion-induced toxicosis), and sodium *n*-propylthiosulfate (garlic-induced toxicosis).
- Metabolism of these compounds causes oxidative damage to hemoglobin, resulting in sulfhemoglobin and precipitation of hemoglobin (eccentrocytes), Heinz body formation, and oxidation of the heme ion (methemoglobinemia).
  - Sulfhemoglobin aggregates and forms Heinz bodies and eccentrocytes.
  - Heinz bodies and eccentrocytes increase RBC fragility and hemolysis may occur.
  - Direct oxidative damage to the cell membrane and sodium-potassium pump may contribute to cell lysis.
  - Methemoglobin may cause a left shift of the Hb-oxygen dissociation curve, resulting in impaired oxygen delivery to tissues.
  - *n*-Propyl disulfide reduces glucose-6-phosphate dehydrogenase activity in RBCs, and interferes with reduced glutathione regeneration, which is needed to prevent oxidative denaturation of hemoglobin.
  - Allicin and ajoene, active agents in garlic, are cardiac and smooth muscle relaxants, vasodilators, antithrombotics, and hypotensive agents, and may exacerbate effects of anemia and impaired oxygen transportation.

*Blackwell's Five-Minute Veterinary Consult Clinical Companion: Small Animal Toxicology*, Third Edition.
Edited by Lynn R. Hovda, Ahna G. Brutlag, Robert H. Poppenga, and Steven E. Epstein.
© 2024 John Wiley & Sons, Inc. Published 2024 by John Wiley & Sons, Inc.

## Pharmacokinetics or Toxicokinetics – Absorption, Distribution, Metabolism, Excretion

- Toxicosis most commonly occurs after oral consumption, with rapid absorption from the GI tract.
- Metabolism occurs in the liver and RBCs.
- Excretion is thought to occur through GI tract and kidneys.

## Toxicity

- Fresh, cooked, boiled, dried, liquid, and dehydrated forms are all toxic.
- Acute $LD_{50}$ values for dogs and cats have not been published.
- Dogs – hematological changes have been reported with ingestion of 15–30 g/kg of onions.
- Cats – toxicosis has been reported with ingestion of 5 g/kg of onions.
- Toxicosis consistently noted in animals that ingest >0.5% of body weight (kg) in onions.
- Cats fed a diet of 3% onion powder added to canned diet developed nearly 100% Heinz body anemia and a significant decrease in PCV within a week.
- Garlic can be up to five times more toxic than onions.

## Systems Affected

- Cardiovascular – tachycardia secondary to anemia and methemoglobinemia, hypotension.
- Gastrointestinal – diarrhea, vomiting, abdominal pain, mucosal erosions.
- Hemic/lymphatic/immune – Heinz body anemia, methemoglobinemia.
- Renal/urological – hemoglobinuria, hemoglobin (possibly hemosiderin) urinary casts.
- Respiratory – tachypnea, hypoxemia secondary to anemia and methemoglobinemia.

 # SIGNALMENT/HISTORY

- Dogs may present more often due to indiscriminate eating habits.
- Cats are more sensitive due to increased hemoglobin sulfhydryl groups and reduced methemoglobin reductase activity.
- Japanese breeds (Akita, shiba inu) or those with hereditary high reduced glutathione and elevated intracellular RBC potassium concentrations have been shown to be more susceptible to oxidant injury.

## Risk Factors

- No age or sex predilections have been reported.
- Animals fed home-made diets containing *Allium* spp.
- Animals with concurrent diseases causing oxidative stress (diabetic ketoacidosis, hepatic lipidosis) or preexisting anemia may manifest more severe toxicosis.

## Historical Findings

- History of recent or chronic ingestion of *Allium* spp.
- Owners may note lethargy, weakness, anorexia, exercise intolerance, pale or icteric gums, diarrhea/vomiting, discolored urine.

## Location and Circumstances of Poisoning

- Toxicosis most commonly occurs following oral consumption of a single large quantity of fresh plant material, juice, dietary supplements, powdered preparations, dehydrated material, or food preparations containing *Allium* spp.

- Chronic toxicosis may occur with long-term exposure when onions or garlic are added to the diet or treats.

 ## CLINICAL FEATURES

- Clinical signs of vomiting and diarrhea may appear within one day of consumption, but signs of anemia typically lag by several days to a week.
- The toxic signs produced by onions/garlic mainly represent the effects on RBCs.
- Clinical signs and physical examination findings most commonly noted include the following.
  - Depressed mentation.
  - Pale, icteric, or cyanotic mucous membranes.
  - Tachypnea.
  - Tachycardia.
  - Abdominal pain.
  - Pigmenturia.

 ## DIFFERENTIAL DIAGNOSIS

- Other toxicoses: brassicaceous vegetables, naphthalene, propylene glycol, acetaminophen, benzocaine, vitamin $K_3$, dl-methionine, zinc, and copper.
- Other causes of Heinz body formation in cats: diabetes mellitus, hepatic lipidosis, hyperthyroidism, neoplasia, repeated propofol infusions.
- Other causes of hemolytic anemia: immune-mediated hemolytic anemia, infectious agents (*Mycoplasma*, *Anaplasma*, *Babesia*), pyruvate kinase or phosphofructokinase enzyme deficiencies, hypophosphatemia, neoplasia, or envenomation.

 ## DIAGNOSTICS

### Clinical Pathological Findings

- CBC and blood smear – regenerative anemia, decreased hemoglobin, Heinz bodies, eccentrocytosis (major feature of garlic toxicity), leukocytosis. Monitor for several days, as nadir may occur several days following ingestion.
- Biochemical profile: hyperbilirubinemia, elevated liver enzymes secondary to hypoxic injury, hemolytic or icteric serum.
- Urinalysis – hemoglobinuria, bilirubinuria, hemoglobin/hemosiderin casts.

### Other Diagnostics

- CO-oximeter blood gas analysis to assess methemoglobin concentration; typically performed at veterinary specialty centers or human hospitals. Methemoglobin levels can be measured poin-of-care with pulse CO-oximetry (Masimo rainbow®).
- Blood pressure monitoring to assess for hypotension in cases of garlic ingestion.
- Abdominal radiographs may be useful to help rule out other causes of hemolysis (zinc, neoplasia).
- Abdominal ultrasound may be normal or may reveal hepatomegaly or splenomegaly secondary to extramedullary hematopoiesis.

## Pathological Findings

▪ Postmortem findings are consistent with hemolytic anemia and include hemosiderin deposition in liver, spleen, and renal tubular epithelium; renal tubular pigment necrosis; nephrotubular casts.

 **THERAPEUTICS**

Treatment objectives are decontamination to prevent further toxin exposure in those animals presenting acutely in stable condition, and stabilization and aggressive supportive care in those patients exhibiting clinical signs.

### Detoxification

▪ Induce emesis if recent ingestion (previous 1–2 hours) and asymptomatic.
▪ Administer a single dose of activated charcoal with carthartic.

### Appropriate Health Care

▪ Patients presenting after acute ingestion can be decontaminated and treated as outpatients.
  • Baseline blood work and PCV monitoring should be performed up to one week post ingestion.
▪ Animals presenting with clinical signs may require hospitalization and supportive care.
▪ Intravenous crystalloid fluid administration may be indicated in patients with vomiting/diarrhea, hemoglobinuria, or hypotension.
▪ Packed red blood cell transfusion should be considered if patients are showing clinical signs of anemia.

### Drug(s) of Choice

▪ For control of vomiting, consider:
  • Maropitant 1 mg/kg IV or SQ q 24 hours.
  • Ondansetron 0.1–0.3 mg/kg IV q 8–12 hours.
▪ Antioxidants may be beneficial.
  • N-acetylcysteine – 140 mg/kg IV initial dose, followed by 70 mg/kg IV q 4 hours for six additional doses. Can be given orally but has an unpleasant taste.
  • Ascorbic acid (vitamin C) 30 mg/kg PO, SQ, IV q 6 hours.
  • Vitamin E anecdotally used at 50–600 units PO once daily.

### Precautions/Interactions

▪ Increased susceptibility with concurrent treatment with drugs that induce erythrocyte oxidative injury (e.g., propofol, propylene glycol, dl-methionine, sulfonamides, benzocaine, acetaminophen).

### Alternative Drugs

▪ Whole blood transfusion may be given when packed RBCs are not available.

## Patient Monitoring

- Animals presenting after *Allium* spp. ingestion should have an initial CBC or minimally a PCV measured to obtain a baseline values. Recheck in 5–7 days as nadir may occur several days following ingestion.
- Clients should be educated about clinical signs to monitor at home (weakness, pale gums, inappetence, pigmenturia) and blood work should be evaluated immediately in patients exhibiting these signs.

## Diet

- Avoid semimoist diets that contain propylene glycol.
- Discontinue use of any diet containing *Allium* spp.

 **COMMENTS**

### Prevention/Avoidance

- Clients should be educated about the toxicity of onions/garlic and should avoid feeding of all forms of *Allium* spp. to dogs and cats.

### Possible Complications

- In patients with significant anemia, a blood transfusion may be necessary which may require transfer to a veterinary facility that can provide blood products.

### Expected Course and Prognosis

- Prognosis is good with early decontamination and supportive care.
- Frequent rechecks may be necessary to assess RBC count and monitor for development of anemia.
- In patients presenting with severe anemia, hospitalization for several days may be necessary until clinical signs have resolved and anemia has stabilized.
- Prognosis is guarded for severely affected patients without aggressive care.

### Abbreviations

- CBC = complete blood count
- GI = gastrointestinal
- Hb = hemoglobin
- PCV = packed cell volume
- RBC = red blood cell

### Suggested Reading

Cope RB. *Allium* species poisoning in dogs and cats (Toxicology Brief). *Vet Med* 2005;August:562–566.

Harvey JW, Rackear D. Experimental onion-induced hemolytic anemia in dogs. *Vet Pathol* 1985;22:387–392.

Hill AS, O'Neill S, Rogers QR et al. Antioxidant prevention of Heinz body formation and oxidative injury in cats. *Am J Vet Res* 2001;62:370–374.

Guitart R, Mateu C, Agullo AL, Alberola J. Heinz body anaemia in two dogs after Catalan spring onion ("calcot") ingestion: a case reports. *Veterinarni Medicina* 2008;53(7):392–395.

Lee K, Yamato O, Tajima M et al. Hematologic changes associated with the appearance of eccentrocytes after intragastric administration of garlic extract to dogs. *Am J Vet Res* 2000;11:1446–1450.

Tang X, Xia Z, Yu J. An experimental study of hemolysis induced by onion (*Allium cepa*) poisoning in dogs. *J Vet Pharmacol Ther* 2007;31:143–149.

Yamato O, Kasai E, Katsura T et al. Heinz body hemolytic anemia with eccentrocytosis from ingestion of Chinese chive (*Allium tuberosum*) and garlic (*Allium sativum*) in a dog. *J Am Anim Hosp Assoc* 2005;41:68–73.

**Author**: Julie Schildt, DVM, DACVECC
**Consulting Editor**: Steven E. Epstein, DVM, DACVECC

# Chapter 78

# Salt (Sodium Chloride)

## DEFINITION/OVERVIEW

- Elevated serum sodium concentrations (hypernatremia) can be caused by either sodium gain or water loss.
- Common sources of sodium include ingestion of table salt, rock salt used to deice roads, homemade play dough, paintballs, sea water, inappropriately mixed formula or feed, administration of sodium phosphate enemas.
- Clinical signs include gastrointestinal signs such as vomiting and diarrhea and neurological signs such as altered mentation, tremors, and seizures.

## ETIOLOGY/PATHOPHYSIOLOGY

### Mechanism of Action

- Enteral intake or parenteral administration of sodium increases serum sodium concentration and serum osmolarity, and causes fluid shifts across body water compartments.
  - Increases in serum osmolarity lead to fluid shifts from the intracellular space (with relatively lower sodium concentration) to the intravascular space according to the sodium concentration gradient.
  - Fluid shifts out of the intracellular space have the most critical effect on the CNS where cellular dehydration can lead to brain shrinkage, detachment from the meninges, and hemorrhage from meningeal vessels.
  - Increases in serum osmolarity can damage the vascular endothelium, lead to increased endothelial permeability, and cause cerebral edema in later stages.
  - Hypervolemia develops as a consequence of fluid shifts into the intravascular space.
- After 4–7 days of hypernatremia, CNS cells begin to form idiogenic osmoles to increase intracellular osmolarity and protect themselves from further cell shrinkage.
  - If hypernatremia is corrected too rapidly (e.g., free access to oral water or rapid IV replacement of free water deficit), fluids shift from the intravascular into the intracellular space, causing cerebral edema and demyelination.
- With enteral intake, high doses of salt can cause gastroenteritis due to a direct mucosal irritant effect.
- The amount of salt ingested, external circumstances (e.g., access to water), and patient comorbidities all influence the severity of developing hypernatremia, severity of clinical signs, and prognosis.

*Blackwell's Five-Minute Veterinary Consult Clinical Companion: Small Animal Toxicology*, Third Edition.
Edited by Lynn R. Hovda, Ahna G. Brutlag, Robert H. Poppenga, and Steven E. Epstein.
© 2024 John Wiley & Sons, Inc. Published 2024 by John Wiley & Sons, Inc.

## Pharmacokinetics or Toxicokinetics – Absorption, Distribution, Metabolism, Excretion

- After enteral intake, sodium is rapidly absorbed from the small intestines and clinical signs of salt toxicosis frequently occur within three hours of ingestion.
- Sodium directly deposited in the bloodstream following IV administration can result in clinical signs being observed faster.
- Sodium is excreted renally, and this can be impaired in patients with preexisting renal disease.

## Toxicity

- NaCl ingestion (table salt): lethal dose is 4 g/kg and signs of toxicity can occur after ingestion of 2–3 g/kg.
  - One tablespoon contains approximately 17.85 g of NaCl.
- Homemade play dough: ingestion of 1.9 g/kg can be toxic as the sodium content can be as high as 8 g/tablespoon.
- $NaHCO_3$ ingestion (baking soda): signs of salt toxicosis can occur after ingestion of 10–20 g/kg.
- Clinical signs vary with the severity of hypernatremia and are generally not observed until serum sodium concentrations reach $\geq$170 mEq/L.

## Systems Affected

- Gastrointestinal – most commonly with oral intake: anorexia, vomiting, diarrhea.
- Endocrine/metabolic – hypernatremia, hyperosmolarity, ± hyperchloremia, metabolic acidosis with NaCl ingestion, metabolic alkalosis with $NaHCO_3$ ingestion.
- Nervous – CNS dehydration or edema, altered mentation ranging from lethargy to coma, ataxia, cranial nerve deficits, blindness, tremors, seizures.
- Cardiovascular – hypervolemia, tachycardia, arrhythmias.
- Respiratory – pulmonary edema or pleural effusion secondary to hypervolemia.
- Musculoskeletal – rigidity, myoclonus.
- Renal/urological – acute tubular necrosis, polyuria, polydipsia, azotemia.
- Hepatobiliary – hepatic necrosis.

 # SIGNALMENT/HISTORY

## Risk Factors

- There are no reported species, breed or sex predilections.
- Lack of or limited access to free water (e.g., frozen water bowl) can worsen hypernatremia and predispose to clinical signs.

## Historical Findings

- Witnessed ingestion of table salt, home-made play dough, salt dough Christmas ornaments, sea water, or paintballs.
- Administration of salt to induce emesis or over-the-counter enemas.
- Recent winter walks or play on roads using deicing salts.

## Location and Circumstances of Poisoning

- A thorough medical history is needed to determine whether hypernatremia was caused by solute gain or water loss.

# CLINICAL FEATURES

- Anorexia, vomiting, and diarrhea.
- Neurological signs vary with severity of hypernatremia.
- Interstitial dehydration despite hypervolemia.
- Tachypnea, tachycardia, cardiac arrhythmias.
- Increased respiratory rate and effort, dyspnea, and pulmonary crackles in case of pulmonary edema secondary to hypervolemia.

 # DIFFERENTIAL DIAGNOSIS

- Hypernatremia can be due to either solute gain (hypervolemic hypernatremia) or water loss (hypovolemic or euvolemic hypernatremia).
  - Pure water loss (euvolemic hypernatremia): central or renal diabetes insipidus, heat stroke, severe burn wounds, inadequate access to water.
  - Hypotonic fluid loss (hypovolemic hypernatremia): gastrointestinal losses, vomiting, diarrhea, renal losses, diabetes mellitus, diuretic administration.
- Altered mentation: primary intracranial disease (e.g., meningitis, meningoencephalitis, cerebrovascular accidents), metabolic disease (e.g., hepatic or uremic encephalopathy), ingestion of neurodepressants (e.g., benzodiazepines, opioids, muscle relaxants).

 # DIAGNOSTICS

## Clinical Pathological Findings

- Serum sodium concentrations above institutional reference intervals confirm hypernatremia but are not specific for any underlying cause.
- Serum biochemistry panels in severe cases may reveal azotemia or elevated liver enzymes.

## Other Diagnostics

- CSF sodium concentrations >160 mEq/L are supportive of salt toxicosis.

## Pathological Findings

- Gross pathological findings in severe hypernatremia: retraction of the brain from the calvarium, meningeal vascular trauma and hematoma formation. In cases with enteral salt intake: gastric, small intestinal, and colonic hemorrhage.
- Histopathological changes: cerebral edema, widened extracellular spaces, vascular congestion and necrosis of vessel walls, renal and hepatic necrosis.
- Cerebral tissue sodium concentrations of >1800 ppm are supportive of salt toxicosis.

 # THERAPEUTICS

- The goal of therapy is to lower the serum sodium concentration slowly and safely at a rate not exceeding 1.0–2.0 mEq/L/h in acute hypernatremia (<48 h duration) and not exceeding 0.5–1.0 mEq/L/h in chronic hypernatremia (>48 h duration). Calculation of the free water deficit and frequent sodium monitoring help guide therapy. Animals with worsening neurological signs after initiation of therapy may have developed cerebral edema and will require additional interventions.

## Detoxification

- If salt ingestion was recent, mentation is appropriate, and serum sodium concentrations are normal, emesis induction or gastric lavage can be attempted.
- The use of activated charcoal is contraindicated as it does not reliably bind sodium ions and can contribute to hypernatremia by causing free water losses.

## Appropriate Health Care

- Patients with moderate to severe hypernatremia (>170 mEq/L) should be hospitalized to ensure a controlled decrease of serum sodium concentrations by free water administration.
- With recent/unknown time of ingestion that presents with a normal serum sodium concentration, monitoring sodium concentration for four hours after presentation to determine need for hospitalization is indicated.
- Frequent monitoring of serum sodium concentrations and for development of cerebral edema is imperative.
- Severely ataxic or recumbent patients should be given dry, padded bedding, turned every four hours, and urinary catheterization should be considered.
- If cerebral edema develops, the head should be elevated 15–30° to decrease intracranial pressure and jugular venous compression should be avoided.

## Drug(s) of Choice

- "Free water" is administered to the patient intravenously as dextrose 5% in water (D5W) or enterally as tap water in patients willing to drink.
- The amount of water to be administered to correct hypernatremia is determined by calculating the free water deficit.
    - Water deficit (liters) = (body weight in kg) × (0.6) × [(current sodium concentration/desired sodium concentration) − 1].
    - For example, a 10 kg patient with a current sodium concentration of 180 mEq/L and desired concentration of 145 mEq/L has a free water deficit of 1.45 L.
- Deficits should be replaced ensuring a serum sodium decrease of no more than 1.0–2.0 mEq/L/h for acute and 0.5–1.0 mEq/L/h for chronic hypernatremia.
    - For example, in the above patient, lowering the sodium concentration by 35 mEq/L (180–145) at a rate of 1.0 mEq/L/h would take 35 hours. The hourly rate of IV D5W would be 1450 mL/35 h = 41 mL/h.
- Furosemide (2 mg/kg IV q 8–24 hours) is indicated if patients develop pulmonary edema and may aid in sodium excretion.
- Antiemetic/antinausea.
    - Maropitant 1 mg/kg SQ/IV q 24 hours.
    - Ondansetron 0.2–1.0 mg/kg IV q 6–12 hours.
- Anticonvulsants.
    - Midazolam 0.25 mg/kg IV PRN.
    - Phenobarbital 4 mg/kg IV q 6–12 hours.
    - Levetiracetam 20–30 mg/kg IV q 8 hours.
- If neurological signs worsen and cerebral edema is suspected, mannitol 0.5–2 g/kg IV over 20 minutes should be administered, and free water therapy discontinued.

## Precautions/Interactions

- Do not lower serum sodium concentrations by more than 1.0–2.0 mEq/L/h for acute (<48 h) or 0.5–1.0 mEq/L/h for chronic (>48 h) hypernatremia.

## Alternative Drugs

- If D5W for IV free water replacement is unavailable, a nasogastric tube can be placed and enteral water administered slowly.
- Due to its hypoosmolar nature and the risk of hemolysis, sterile water for injection **cannot** be used for IV administration in place of D5W.

## Patient Monitoring

- Monitor serum sodium concentration every 2–6 hours depending on severity of hypernatremia and adjust fluid type and administration rates accordingly.
- Monitor respiratory rate and effort in patients with cardiac comorbidities as they may develop congestive heart failure secondary to hypervolemia.
- Consider repeat biochemistry panel to monitor for signs of renal or hepatic necrosis in 24–48 hours.

## Diet

- To avoid decreasing serum sodium concentrations too rapidly, oral water should be withheld while parenteral water replacement is ongoing, or the amount of oral water offered must be strictly measured and subtracted from the calculated daily parenteral water requirements.
- Due to gastrointestinal effects of oral salt intake, a bland and soft diet may be indicated for 5–7 days.

 **COMMENTS**

### Prevention/Avoidance

- Owner education on salt sources and importance of ensuring unlimited access to water.
- Avoid the use of salt for emesis induction.
- Supervise pets to prevent ingestion of homemade play dough, paintballs, and table salts.
- Wipe paws after winter walks with exposure to deicing salts.

### Possible Complications

- Cerebral edema if hypernatremia is corrected too rapidly.
- Renal and hepatic necrosis.
- Rarely CNS demyelination.

### Expected Course and Prognosis

- Prognosis depends on the severity of hypernatremia and success of slow correction.
- Both sustained and severe hypernatremia and its rapid correction can cause cerebral edema and potentially be fatal.
- Symptomatic hypernatremic patients should be hospitalized for correction of serum sodium concentrations.

### Synonyms

Hypernatremia, paint balls, play dough.

### Abbreviations

- CNS = central nervous system
- CSF = cerebrospinal fluid
- D5W = dextrose 5% in water
- IV = intravenous

- NaHCO$_3$ = sodium bicarbonate salt
- NaCl = sodium chloride salt

## Suggested Reading

Adrogué HJ, Madias NE. Hypernatremia. *N Engl J Med* 2000;342:1493–1499.

Barr JM, Safdar AK, McCullough, SM et al. Hypernatremia secondary to homemade play dough ingestion in dogs: a review of 14 cases from 1998 to 2001. *J Vet Emerg Crit Care* 2004;14:196–202.

Pouzot C, Descone-Junot C, Loup J et al. Successful treatment of severe salt intoxication in a dog. *J Vet Emerg Crit Care* 2007;17:294–298.

Ueda Y, Hopper K. Sodium and Water Balance. In: Drobatz KJ, Hopper K, Rozanski E, Silverstein DC (eds) *Textbook of Small Animal Emergency Medicine*. Hoboken: Wiley Blackwell, 2019.

**Author**: Sabrina N. Hoehne, Dr. med. vet., DACVECC, DECVECC

**Consulting Editor**: Steven E. Epstein, DVM, DACVECC

# Chapter 79

# Xylitol

## DEFINITION/OVERVIEW

- Xylitol is a naturally occurring, five-carbon sugar alcohol used most commonly as a sweetener. It is present in many sugar-free gums, mints, candy, nicotine gum, weight loss food products, liquid or chewable medications, compounded medications, over-the-counter supplements, nasal sprays, and baked goods. Additional food products include sugar-free or low-sugar peanut butters, puddings, ice cream and protein bars, to name a few. Xylitol is also available as a granulated powder for cooking and baking.
- Due to its humectant effect and antifermentation/molding properties, xylitol may be included in nonfood products including diapers, skin gels, lotion, and deodorants, as well as others, though less common and typically in lower amounts than in food products.
- Its anticariogenic properties make it a popular addition for toothpaste, mouthwash, dental floss, and other oral health care products.
- Other sugar alcohols including erythritol, maltitol, and sorbitol have not shown negative effects in animals.

## ETIOLOGY/PATHOPHYSIOLOGY

- Xylitol poisoning has two clinical manifestations: hypoglycemia and acute hepatic necrosis. The clinical syndrome typically depends on the amount of xylitol ingested as well as the timing between exposure and intervention.

### Mechanism of Action

- Xylitol stimulates pancreatic insulin secretion, resulting in hypoglycemia in dogs.
- The large insulin release causes an intracellular shift of potassium, resulting in hypokalemia. Hypokalemia is not expected to occur in the absence of hypoglycemia.
- Two proposed theories for hepatic necrosis exist.
  - Depletion of ATP may result in the inability of hepatocytes to perform necessary cellular functions, resulting in cellular necrosis.
  - Metabolism of xylitol results in high concentrations of cellular nicotinamide adenine dinucleotide, which produces reactive oxygen species, causing cellular damage and death of hepatocytes.

*Blackwell's Five-Minute Veterinary Consult Clinical Companion: Small Animal Toxicology*, Third Edition.
Edited by Lynn R. Hovda, Ahna G. Brutlag, Robert H. Poppenga, and Steven E. Epstein.
© 2024 John Wiley & Sons, Inc. Published 2024 by John Wiley & Sons, Inc.

## Pharmacokinetics or Toxicokinetics – Absorption, Distribution, Metabolism, Excretion

- Rapidly absorbed from stomach, with peak plasma levels within 30 minutes after ingestion.
- Liver is primary site of metabolism, with lesser amounts in lungs, kidneys, myocardium, fat stores, and erythrocytes.

## Toxicity

- Hypoglycemia may occur at doses ≥0.1 g/kg.
- Hepatic failure may occur at doses ≥0.5 g/kg. Risk for hepatic failure increases as ingested doses are closer to and exceeding 1 g/kg, with secondary coagulopathy possible due to hepatic failure.

## Systems Affected

- Endocrine/metabolic – insulin secretion, hypoglycemia, hypokalemia.
- Gastrointestinal – vomiting, diarrhea.
- Hemic/lymphatic/immune – coagulopathy.
- Hepatobiliary – acute hepatic necrosis, elevated hepatic enzymes, icterus.
- Musculoskeletal – weakness.
- Nervous – behavioral changes, ataxia, tremors, seizures.

 **SIGNALMENT/HISTORY**

- Any age or breed of dog can be affected.
- Cats and ferrets are not expected to be affected.

### Risk Factors

- Ingestion of xylitol or xylitol-containing products.

### Historical Findings

- Witnessed ingestion or finding of chewed packages of xylitol-containing products.
- Acute onset of weakness, lethargy, vomiting, seizures.
- Evidence of xylitol-containing product in vomitus.

### Location and Circumstances of Poisoning

- Exposure typically occurs in the home or vehicle.
- Pets often find xylitol-containing products left in areas of easy access.

 **CLINICAL FEATURES**

- Vomiting may develop within 15–30 minutes of exposure.
- Hypoglycemia may develop in as little as two hours after ingestion with signs including progressive lethargy, weakness, ataxia, collapse, and seizures.
- Hypokalemia may develop if hypoglycemia is present due to transcellular shifts.
- Hepatic failure with signs of icterus as well as possible hemorrhage including petechiae, ecchymosis as well as gastrointestinal and abdominal bleeding may be seen within 24–48 hours after ingestion.
- Hypoglycemia may not occur prior to onset of hepatic failure.

# DIFFERENTIAL DIAGNOSIS

- Hypoglycemia.
  - Insulin overdose.
  - Sulfonylurea antihyperglycemic agents.
  - Insulinoma (pancreatic beta-cell tumor).
  - Sepsis.
- Acute hepatic failure.
  - Acetaminophen.
  - Sago palm (*Cycad* spp.).
  - Aflatoxin.
  - Cyanobacteria (microcystin).
  - *Amanita* and similar hepatoxic mushrooms.
  - Iron.
  - Leptospirosis.

# DIAGNOSTICS

## Clinical Pathological Findings

- Serum chemistry: hypoglycemia, hypokalemia, hypophosphatemia. If hepatic necrosis occurs, elevated ALT, hyperbilirubinemia.
- PT/aPTT: use if evidence of hepatic failure is present to monitor for development of secondary coagulopathy resulting in prolonged values.

## Other Diagnostics

- Radiographs and ultrasound may offer evidence of pleural or thoracic effusion in cases where coagulopathy is present.

## Pathological Findings

- Severe acute periacinar and midzonal hepatic necrosis with periportal vacuolar degeneration.
- Cavitary, joint, pericardial bleeding suggestive of secondary coagulation abnormalities.

# THERAPEUTICS

## Detoxification – Ingestion

- Emesis up to 1–2 hours post ingestion is ideal in most situations, except for liquid products only having benefit from emesis in the first 15–20 minutes after ingestion.
- If hypoglycemia is present upon presentation, emesis can be performed once patient is stabilized and hypoglycemia is addressed.
- Emesis up to six hours post ingestion is valid for gum exposures if patient is stable.

## Appropriate Health Care – Hospitalize

- Monitor blood glucose every 2–4 hours for hypoglycemia, if hypoglycemia is present, and correct as needed.
- Monitor hepatic enzymes every 12 hours for 48 hours with ingestions ≥0.5 g/kg.
  - Hypophosphatemia typically self-corrects and is not generally monitored unless patient is not responding to general care.

- For exposures at and near the 0.1 g/kg ingested dose, monitoring at home and offering small snacks every 2–4 hours may be appropriate and sufficient care.

## Antidote

- No true antidote.

## Drug(s) of Choice

- Dextrose: 0.25–0.5 g/kg IV bolus for hypoglycemia, followed by addition of 2.5–5% dextrose to isotonic crystalloid fluids at a maintenance rate. Consider starting for ingestions >1 g/kg for hepatoprotection even if normoglycemic.
- Potassium chloride: supplement in fluids if potassium concentration <2.5 mmol/L.
- N-acetylcysteine: if hepatic enzyme elevations occur; 140 mg/kg PO or IV (extra-label) followed by 70 mg/kg q 6 hours × 7–17 doses, depending on degree of hepatic enzyme changes.
- SAM-e: PO daily for ingestions >0.5 g/kg. Administer for two weeks if no to mild hepatic enzyme elevations occur and continue for four weeks if significant elevations occur.
- Fresh frozen plasma: 10–20 mL/kg IV given over four hours, may be necessary if a secondary coagulopathy develops.
- Vitamin $K_1$: 1.0 mg/kg q 12 hours PO given with food if a secondary coagulopathy develops from liver failure.

## Alternative Drugs

- If hospitalization is not possible, a small meal may be fed, or honey/syrup can be given along the gums to patient up to every few hours to help minimize hypoglycemia.
- N-acetylcysteine may be purchased over the counter, but there are current efforts being made to make this a prescription-only product.
- SAM-e products may be purchased over the counter. Ensure no xylitol is present.

## Patient Monitoring

- Monitor blood glucose concentrations for at least 8–10 hours post ingestion, up to 24–48 hours if hypoglycemia is present.
- Monitor hepatic enzymes for 48 hours. If hepatic failure is evident, continue to monitor until concentrations begin to decline and again four weeks post ingestion.
- Monitor for evidence of bleeding/bruising and consider evaluating PT/aPTT every 24 hours if hepatic failure is evident, or as needed based on patient's clinical status.

## Diet

- Patient can be fed small, frequent meals in the first 24 hours after ingestion to potentially minimize degree of hypoglycemia.

 **COMMENTS**

- Chewed xylitol-containing gum has a significantly decreased xylitol content; after five minutes of chewing by a human, approximately 4% of xylitol remains in gum and after 15 minutes of chewing by a human, approximately 0.6% of xylitol remains. Therefore, gum chewed for at least five minutes carries an extremely low risk for poisoning unless a very large amount of gum was ingested.
- Xylitol content varies significantly from product to product. It is imperative to attempt to determine the amount of xylitol in the specific product ingested for proper assessment and to ensure the most appropriate therapies are determined.

- Making exposure assessments from packaging of product is recommended as internet searches and company websites may fail to provide the most accurate and up-to-date ingredient information.
- Pharmacists and human medical specialists are often not aware of the concern of xylitol in dogs. It is important to ensure that compounded medications or other medications/supplements intended for humans do not contain xylitol before using in dogs.

### Prevention/Avoidance

- Keep xylitol-containing products up and out of reach of pets.
- Do not allow dogs to be alone in a vehicle with xylitol-containing gum or candy packages accessible.

### Expected Course and Prognosis

- Prognosis good to excellent for uncomplicated hypoglycemia with mild to moderate elevations of ALT; guarded to poor if severe hepatic necrosis occurs and early intervention is not initiated.
- Patients who recover are not expected to have long-term negative effects.

### Synonyms

Birch sugar, birch bark extract, wood sugar.

### See Also

Chapter 45 Acetaminophen
Chapter 110 Blue-green Algae: Microcystins
Chapter 115 Mushrooms
Chapter 75 Mycotoxins (Aflatoxin)
Chapter 118 Sago Palm (Cycads)

### Abbreviations

See Appendix 1 for a complete list.
- SAM-e = S-adenosyl-methionine

### Suggested Reading

Jerzsele A, Karancsi Z, Paszti-Gere E et al. Effects of p.o. administered xylitol in cats. *J Vet Pharmacol Ther* 2018;41(3):409–414.
Rajapaksha SM, Gerken K, Archer T et al. Extraction analysis of xylitol in sugar-free gum samples by GC-MS with direct aqueous injection. *J Anal Methods Chem* 2019;2019:1690153.
Schmid RD, Hovda LR. Acute hepatic failure in a dog after xylitol ingestion. *J Med Toxicol* 2016;12:201–205.

**Author:** Renee D. Schmid, DVM, DABT, DABVT
**Consulting Editor:** Steven E. Epstein, DVM, DACVECC

# Foreign Objects

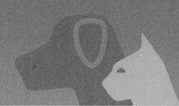

# Chapter 80

# Foreign Objects

## DEFINITION/OVERVIEW

- Many substances pose toxic risks to pets, but dogs and cats may also ingest nontoxic foreign objects. Owners are often uncertain of the risk for toxicity or other complications and might contact veterinarians or poison control centers to discuss the appropriate course of action. Familiarity with common nontoxic substances is helpful for this reason.
- This chapter addresses frequently encountered foreign bodies that are considered nontoxic or of low risk (e.g., potentially mild GI signs).
- For treatment purposes, GI foreign objects that are nontoxic and small may require no intervention. However, foreign bodies may still pose a risk for mechanical obstruction, and further assessment may be required.

## ETIOLOGY/PATHOPHYSIOLOGY

- The toxicity of foreign bodies is dependent on the composition of the material ingested. Many types of materials (plastic, paper, fabric, wood, sticks, gravel/rocks) are nontoxic but may still present a risk for mechanical obstruction. Foreign objects may be more likely to result in mechanical consequences if they are large, sharp, linear, or capable of absorbing liquid. Even if material is nonobstructive, there remains the potential for irritation of the GI tract and resultant gastroenteritis.
- If the risk for mechanical obstruction is low, nontoxic foreign bodies ingested by dogs and cats may result in minimal harm.

### Common Nontoxic Foreign Bodies

- Ant and roach traps.
  - Bait traps contain multiple active ingredients but at very low concentrations that are unlikely to harm pets. Most common insecticides include boric acid, sulfluramid, fipronil, avermectin, hydramethylnon, and indoxacarb.
  - Exposure to these traps typically requires no decontamination or treatment. Mild GI signs may be seen uncommonly.
  - For rare circumstances of large ingestions, it may be worthwhile to check ingredients and ensure no concern for foreign body obstruction.
- Bandages (e.g., Band-Aids® or other adhesive bandages) – medicated.
  - Medicated bandages contain minimal medication and are nontoxic if consumed.
  - Large quantities of bandage material could be a risk for obstruction, but minimal risk is expected even with multiple Band-Aids.

---

*Blackwell's Five-Minute Veterinary Consult Clinical Companion: Small Animal Toxicology*, Third Edition.
Edited by Lynn R. Hovda, Ahna G. Brutlag, Robert H. Poppenga, and Steven E. Epstein.
© 2024 John Wiley & Sons, Inc. Published 2024 by John Wiley & Sons, Inc.

- Cat litter – clumping.
  - Small ingestions may result in no clinical signs or mild GI signs.
  - Large ingestions have more potential to result in mechanical obstruction.
- Charcoal/barbeque briquettes.
  - Ingredients can include charcoal, coal, sawdust, limestone, starch, sodium nitrate, borax, and other additives. Used briquettes may be covered in dried food or grease, increasing palatability.
  - These are considered nontoxic but could result in mild GI signs. Activated charcoal granules have been reported to cause obstruction in a dog.
- Coins.
  - Pennies minted in the US after 1982 are made primarily of zinc and can result in zinc toxicosis (see Chapter 105).
  - Other coins are made of metals such as copper, nickel, and manganese and present minimal risk. Depending on the quantity ingested and size of the animal, they could result in mechanical obstruction.
- Crayons, markers, pens, pencils.
  - Most are nontoxic and of minimal concern. Crayons are generally made of wax and pigment, pencil "lead" is inert graphite, and pens or markers are typically constructed from plastic, small amounts of metal, pigment/dye, and potentially other chemicals. Some inks contain glycol or glycol ethers but in insufficient quantities to cause concern.
  - Small ingestions are unlikely to cause clinical signs.
  - Large ingestions might result in mild GI signs or, less likely, obstruction.
- Ear buds.
  - Headphones or ear buds are composed of nontoxic materials, typically combinations of plastic, silicone, foam, and very small quantities of metal (often aluminum).
  - Ingestion of small or chewed-up pieces likely presents minimal risk.
  - If whole ear buds are ingested by small pets, the main risk is obstruction.
- Firestarter logs (e.g., Duraflame® logs).
  - Logs are generally constructed from compressed sawdust, agricultural fibers, and non-petroleum waxes and oils. They do not pose a toxicosis risk but also do not break down readily in the stomach, increasing the risk for obstruction with large ingestions. Small ingestions may result in mild GI signs.
  - Rarely, firestarter logs contain heavy metals to provide a sparkle effect. Assessment of the label may be warranted but concentrations are typically small.
- Magnets.
  - A single small magnet is unlikely to result in toxic or obstructive consequences.
  - If multiple magnets are ingested, they can attract each other from different segments of bowel, causing tissue entrapment, pressure necrosis, obstruction, and perforation. Surgical intervention should be considered for multiple magnets.
- Mulch or bark chips.
  - Most garden mulch and bark chips are nontoxic and of minimal cause for concern.
  - One exception is cocoa bean mulch, which has become increasingly popular in landscaping. Toxic components include theobromine and caffeine. Cocoa bean hulls used in mulch typically contain <1% theobromine. However, significant intake can lead to methylxanthine toxicosis, characterized by GI, cardiovascular, and CNS signs (see Chapter 71).
- Oxygen absorbers.
  - These absorb oxygen and are found in medications and foods susceptible to oxidation. Most commonly, they are a mixture of sodium chloride, iron powder, and activated charcoal. Iron binds to oxygen once it is exposed (converting it to ferric oxide/rust), so the iron in these packets is typically inert and nontoxic if eaten.

- Large ingestions can potentially cause iron toxicity (see Chapter 103), though this is rare. If very large quantities are consumed, measurement of serum iron levels 2–3 hours and again 5–6 hours following ingestion could be considered.
- Pool water.
  - The chemicals in pool water are sufficiently diluted to prevent harm to pets. No intervention is necessary for ingestion of small to moderate volumes of pool water.
  - Large intake of pool water is uncommon except in drowning cases with inadvertent swallowing of larger volumes. These patients are at risk for serum sodium abnormalities and aspiration pneumonia.
- Silica gel packets.
  - Silica gel is a desiccant that manufacturers place in packets to keep moisture from damaging clothes, shoes, medications, and foods.
  - The product itself is biologically and chemically inert, though large ingestions could potentially lead to vomiting, inappetence, osmotic diarrhea, or obstruction.

## Systems Affected

- Gastrointestinal – vomiting, nausea, inappetence, diarrhea, abdominal discomfort.

 # SIGNALMENT/HISTORY

### Risk Factors

- Any pet could ingest a foreign body. Younger animals prone to dietary indiscretion may be more likely to ingest foreign material.

### Historical Findings

- History may include witnessed ingestion of specific items, evidence of chewed foreign objects, disrupted garbage cans, or vomitus containing foreign material.
- Owners might report no clinical signs or potentially GI signs depending on the material and quantity ingested.

 # CLINICAL FEATURES

- Dogs and cats with nontoxic, nonobstructive GI foreign bodies are likely to have no clinical signs and require no interventions.
- Mild GI signs such as nausea, diarrhea, or decreased appetite may result from irritation caused by the passage of small amounts of foreign material. Signs are likely to occur within several hours of ingestion.
- Animals with persistent or severe GI signs (including vomiting, hematemesis, regurgitation, or marked abdominal pain), lethargy/weakness, dehydration, or other non-GI symptoms should be evaluated by a veterinarian, as these may indicate the potential for an obstructive foreign body, ingestion of a toxic substance, or other underlying systemic disease.

 # DIAGNOSTICS

- Abdominal radiographs or ultrasound may be utilized to evaluate the quantity of ingested material, its location, and the potential for mechanical obstruction.
- A CBC and biochemistry can be used to assess the patient's systemic health or evaluate for other differentials, but clinicopathological abnormalities are not generally expected for the nontoxic foreign bodies discussed (unless mentioned above for specific items).

## THERAPEUTICS

### Detoxification

- Induction of emesis may be considered if an ingested foreign body is known to be toxic or of a size/shape to potentially result in GI obstruction. Additional therapy would depend on the specific material ingested.

### Appropriate Health Care

- In general, no therapy is needed for nontoxic, nonobstructive foreign bodies.
- Subcutaneous crystalloid fluids can be considered for mild to moderate dehydration.
- Antinausea medication can be administered as needed and if obstructive GI foreign material has been ruled out.

### Patient Monitoring

- For nontoxic foreign bodies with no obstructive risk, no monitoring is required.
- If mechanical obstruction remains a potential, patients should be monitored closely for persistent or worsening GI signs (such as vomiting or abdominal pain). The patient's stool may also be examined to assess for passage of foreign material.
- Repeat abdominal radiographs or ultrasound may be required to assess for movement of foreign material through the GI tract or for development of obstruction.

### Diet

- If a pet requires monitoring for signs of obstruction, it may be advisable to withhold food.
- If an object is considered nontoxic and of no risk for obstruction, no dietary limitations are necessary. If mild gastroenteritis is present, a bland diet could be considered.

 ## COMMENTS

### Prevention/Avoidance

- It is important to educate clients generally about preventing access to foreign bodies that might be of interest to pets. While it is impossible to prevent dogs and cats from having contact with all potential foreign objects, removal of the most enticing options is warranted. This may include small items, substances that smell or taste appealing, or objects that pets have previously shown interest in eating.
- For repeat offenders, owners might consider crate training, muzzle training, or other behavioral modification.
- Clients should be educated about common toxic (and nontoxic) household items and provided with resources in case of questions or emergencies.

### Expected Course and Prognosis

- Prognosis for nontoxic or minimally toxic foreign bodies is excellent.
- Prognosis may be complicated by foreign bodies that result in mechanical obstruction.

### Suggested Reading

Brutlag AG, Flint CT, Puschner B. Iron intoxication in a dog consequent to the ingestion of oxygen absorber sachets in pet treat packaging. *J Med Toxicol* 2012;8(1):76–79.

Farrell KS, Burkitt-Creedon JM, Osborne LG, Gibson EA, Massie AM. Gastrointestinal obstruction secondary to activated charcoal granule impaction in a dog. *J Vet Emerg Crit Care* 2020;30(4): 461–466.

Hansen S, Trammel H, Dunayer E et al. Cocoa bean mulch as a cause of methylxanthine toxicosis in dogs. *Clin Toxicol* 2003;41(5):720.

Hayes G. Gastrointestinal foreign bodies in dogs and cats: a retrospective study of 208 cases. *J Small Anim Pract* 2009;50:576–583.

Kiefer K, Hottinger H, Kahn T, Ngo M, Ben-Amotz R. Magnet ingestion in dogs: two cases. *J Am Anim Hosp Assoc* 2010;46(3):181–185.

**Author**: Kate S. Farrell, DVM, DACVECC

**Consulting Editor**: Steven E. Epstein, DVM, DACVECC

# Garden, Yard, and Farm Chemicals

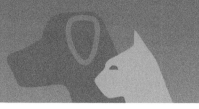

# Chapter 81

# Bone and Blood Meal

## DEFINITION/OVERVIEW

- Bone meal and blood meal (Figure 81.1) are by-products from the meatpacking industry that are widely utilized as soil amendment products, fertilizer components, and as deer, rabbit, and wildlife repellants.
- Bone meal may also be a component in calcium and phosphorus mineral supplements.
- In general, these meals are considered a low-level toxicity concern; they can result in GIT irritation and less commonly foreign body obstruction (FBO) and pancreatitis when ingested.
- Old fertilizers may become contaminated with mold, which may lead to risk of tremorgenic mycotoxicosis.
- Bone meal or blood meal may be added to other products (pesticides, herbicides, fertilizers), resulting in additional toxicity.

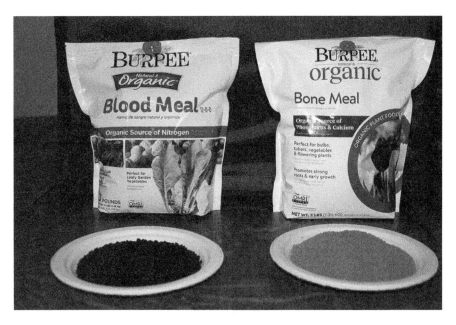

■ Figure 81.1 Blood and bone meal. Source: Courtesy of Lynn R. Hovda (book author).

*Blackwell's Five-Minute Veterinary Consult Clinical Companion: Small Animal Toxicology*, Third Edition. Edited by Lynn R. Hovda, Ahna G. Brutlag, Robert H. Poppenga, and Steven E. Epstein. © 2024 John Wiley & Sons, Inc. Published 2024 by John Wiley & Sons, Inc.

# ETIOLOGY/PATHOPHYSIOLOGY

## Mechanism of Action

- Direct irritation to the GI tract and potential for FBO.

## Toxicokinetics

- Bone meal and blood meal are poorly absorbed through gastrointestinal and dermal routes.

## Toxicity

- Bone meal and blood meal are generally considered low-level toxins.
- Large ingestions of bone meal or blood meal can congeal or solidify in the stomach, resulting in a gastric FBO.

## Systems Affected

- Gastrointestinal – GI irritation (vomiting, diarrhea, drooling, anorexia, abdominal discomfort) FBO, and pancreatitis.

# SIGNALMENT/HISTORY

## Risk Factors

- No breed or sex predilection.
- Outdoor dogs may have more opportunity for exposure, and young dogs may be more prone to dietary indiscretion.

## Historical Findings

- History of exposure to bone or blood meal.
- GIT signs with bone or blood meal, soil, or plant material visualized in vomitus or feces.

## Location and Circumstances of Poisoning

- Access to containers or spilled bone or blood meal in the garage, shed, or other storage facility.
- Access to recently fertilized crops, garden, lawn, or other plants.
- Organic lawn and gardening products more commonly contain bone or blood meal and may lead to increased exposure opportunities for animals.
- The scent of bone and blood meal may entice dogs to ingest newly planted toxic bulbs/plants as well.

# CLINICAL FEATURES

- Clinical signs usually occur within 2–10 hours of ingestion and GIT signs usually resolve within 12–24 hours.
- GIT signs including vomiting, diarrhea, anorexia, bloating, and abdominal discomfort.
- Blood meal ingestion can result in vomiting of partially digested blood and mucoid, foul-smelling diarrhea containing digested blood.
- GI FBO can rarely occur. Risk is higher with large ingestions.

# DIFFERENTIAL DIAGNOSIS

Toxicosis from ingestion of other GI irritants.

- Dietary indiscretion.
- Gastroenteritis.
- Foreign body obstruction.

- Pancreatitis.
- Inflammatory bowel disease.
- Metabolic disease – liver or renal disease, Addison disease.

 ## DIAGNOSTICS

### Clinical Pathological Findings

- No specific or diagnostic features.
- Diagnostics are not usually necessary for minor exposures.
- Evaluation of hydration (based on PCV/TS) and electrolytes may be assessed if GIT signs are prolonged.

### Other Diagnostics

- Abdominal radiographs to rule out FBO with large exposures. Bone meal is radiopaque (bone density).
- Other advanced diagnostics may need to be performed to rule out other differential diagnoses.

### Pathological Findings

- Evidence of bone or blood meal within the GIT.

 ## THERAPEUTICS

### Detoxification

- Emesis within 2–4 hours if:
  - spontaneous emesis has not already occurred.
  - evidence of foreign material within the stomach.
  - ingestion was a significant amount.
  - patient is susceptible or has a prior history of pancreatitis.
- Unsuccessful emesis with large ingestion of blood meal – consider gastric lavage if no change in stomach contents with supportive care and time. Bone meal can be difficult to remove via gastric lavage.
- Activated charcoal is not indicated for bone or blood meal exposures.

### Appropriate Health Care

- Small exposures may be monitored by the pet owner at home.
- Hospitalization may be necessary if pancreatitis or GI FBO develops.

### Antidote

- No antidote.

### Drug(s) of Choice

- Antiemetics if vomiting is persistent.
  - Maropitant 1 mg/kg SQ or IV q 24 hours.
  - Ondansetron 0.1–0.5 mg/kg IV q 8–12 hours.
- Antidiarrheals if diarrhea is persistent.
  - Bland diet will suffice in most cases as diarrhea is typically self-limiting.
  - Probiotics as needed.
  - Metronidazole 10–15 mg/kg PO q 12 hours may be considered if hemorrhagic diarrhea occurs.
- Fluids – IV or SQ depending on patient's level of dehydration.
- Analgesics as needed, especially if pancreatitis develops. Avoid NSAIDs if GI signs are present.

- GI protectants if needed.
  - H$_2$-blockers.
    - Famotidine 0.5–1 mg/kg PO, SQ, IM, IV q 12 hours.
  - Omeprazole 0.5–1 mg/kg PO q 12–24 hours.
  - Sucralfate 0.25–1 g PO q 8 hours.

### Precautions/Interactions

- Avoid use of NSAIDs if GI signs are present.

### Extracorporeal Therapy

- Extracorporeal therapy is not indicated.

### Surgical Considerations

- Surgical removal of material may be necessary if gastrointestinal obstruction develops.

### Patient Monitoring

- Monitor for resolution of clinical signs and passage of material.

### Diet

- Bland diet until GI signs have resolved. Low-fat diet if pancreatitis develops.

    COMMENTS

### Prevention/Avoidance

- Prevent access to bone and blood meal, especially to containers or other large quantities.

### Possible Complications

- Aspiration pneumonia may rarely occur in vomiting patients.
- Rare FBO may necessitate surgical removal with risk of surgical and anesthetic complications concordant with any other abdominal exploratory procedure.

### Expected Course and Prognosis

- Small exposures can typically be managed at home with only mild, self-limiting GI signs expected.
- Larger exposures may require supportive care, but prognosis is good. Clinical signs often resolve within 24 hours.

### See Also

Chapter 83 Fertilizers
Chapter 76 Mycotoxins (Tremorgenic)

### Abbreviations

See Appendix 1 for a complete list.

### Suggested Reading

Means C. Treating fertilizer ingestions? As easy as N-P-K. *Today Vet Pract* 2016; May/June:49–52.
Plumlee K. *Clinical Veterinary Toxicology*. Philadelphia: Mosby, 2004; pp. 408–409.

**Author:** Charlotte Flint, DVM, DABT, DABVT
**Consulting Editor:** Lynn R. Hovda, RPh, DVM, DACVIM

# Chapter 82

# Diquat and Paraquat

## DEFINITION/OVERVIEW

- Diquat (6,7-dihydrodipyrido[1,2-a:2′,1′-c] pyrazinediium dibromide; $C_{12}H_{12}Br_2N_2$) is a bipyridyl herbicide.
  - General use nonselective contact herbicide, algicide, desiccant, and defoliant available as aqueous solutions (15–25% w/v) or water-soluble granules (2.5%); many trade names.
  - Moderately toxic but considerably less so than paraquat.
  - Concentrated diquat is corrosive to the skin, eyes, GI tract.
  - Typically causes GI signs, but large exposures may lead to more severe systemic toxicity.
- Paraquat (1,1′-dimethyl-4,4′-bipyridinium dichloride; $C_{12}H_{14}Cl_2N_2$) is an herbicide with use restricted to licensed applicators.
  - Technical products – concentrated liquids (20–50%).
  - As of 2021 in the USA, paraquat is a restricted-use pesticide (licensed applicators only). There are no homeowner uses/products, although some 0.04–0.44% products may still be found in storage.
  - In the USA, products are often colored blue, have a noxious odor added to prevent accidental consumption, contain an emetic to induce vomiting once consumed, and potentially a natural alginate that causes the product to form a gel in the stomach along with magnesium sulfate, an osmotic purgative.
  - Paraquat is one of the most selective pulmonary toxins known.
  - Toxicity can be severe – GI signs, respiratory distress, multiorgan failure.

## ETIOLOGY/PATHOPHYSIOLOGY

### Mechanism of Action

#### Diquat

- Potent oxidation-reduction cycler, readily generates free radicals, leads to lipid peroxidation of cell membranes and cell death.

#### Paraquat

- Cyclic reduction-oxidation reactions in the lung generate reactive oxygen species and free radicals and deplete antioxidants (superoxide dismutase, NADPH).
- Membrane damage, cell injury, and multiorgan damage ensue. In the lungs, cell wall injury and necrosis of type II pneumocytes occur, leading to pulmonary fibrosis.

*Blackwell's Five-Minute Veterinary Consult Clinical Companion: Small Animal Toxicology*, Third Edition.
Edited by Lynn R. Hovda, Ahna G. Brutlag, Robert H. Poppenga, and Steven E. Epstein.
© 2024 John Wiley & Sons, Inc. Published 2024 by John Wiley & Sons, Inc.

## Toxicokinetics

### Diquat

- Absorption – poor cutaneous absorption; 10–20% absorbed within six hours after oral administration (dogs).
- Distribution – no accumulation in lungs; highest concentrations found in the kidneys.
- Metabolized into mono- and dipyridones, both of which are less toxic than diquat itself.
- Excretion – majority (approx. 89%) of ingested diquat is excreted in feces due to poor absorption from GIT (monopyridone); dipyridone is excreted in urine.
- Minimal enterohepatic recirculation.
- Half-life of parent compound and metabolites is less than 24 hours.

### Paraquat

- Absorption after oral ingestion is 25–28% and is rapid, with peak plasma levels within 75 minutes.
- Systemic absorption via inhalation or through intact skin is poor and causes a less severe reaction, typically more of a problem with chronic exposure.
- Distribution – selectively accumulates in type I and II alveolar cells and Clara cells, as well as renal proximal tubule epithelium.
- At four hours, lung concentrations are 10 times higher than other sites; by 4–10 days post exposure, concentrations in lungs are 30–80× higher than in plasma.
- Metabolism – considerable cyclic reduction-oxidation reactions in sequestered tissues, but a large amount of paraquat is excreted mostly unchanged in urine.
- Excretion – absorbed paraquat is rapidly excreted by the kidneys: 80–90% excreted within six hours, almost 100% within 24 hours (in absence of paraquat-induced renal disease). Unabsorbed paraquat is excreted unchanged in feces (can be detected up to seven days post ingestion in rodents).
- As renal damage progresses with toxicosis, renal clearance decreases and plasma T½ increases from <12 hours to >120 hours (Figure 82.1).

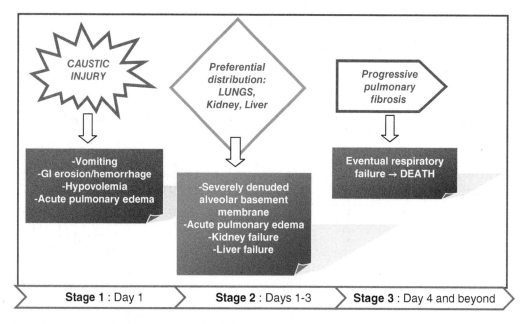

■ Figure 82.1 Pathophysiology of paraquat toxicity.

## Toxicity

- Diquat generally has a low to moderate level of toxicity with household use.
- Paraquat is highly toxic and often fatal.
- $LD_{50}$ varies by species (Table 82.1).

## Systems Affected

### Diquat

- Gastrointestinal – vomiting, diarrhea, GI ulceration, GI hemorrhage, abdominal pain, drug-induced paralytic ileus.
- Renal – azotemia, acute renal failure (rare).
- Respiratory – upper airway irritation, laryngeal edema, pulmonary edema, pneumonia, ARDS.
- Cardiovascular – ventricular dysrhythmias, subendocardial hemorrhage (rare).
- Hepatic – mild liver enzyme elevations, hepatic necrosis (rare).
- Neurological – depression, lethargy, collapse, disorientation, decreased reflexes, restlessness, decreased PLR, miosis, coma, death (rare).
- Dermal – irritation and corrosive injury (concentrated products).
- Ocular – irritation, corneal and conjunctival ulceration.

### Paraquat

- Gastrointestinal – vomiting, diarrhea, aphagia, oral and abdominal pain, severe esophageal or gastric ulceration, pancreatitis.
- Respiratory – respiratory distress, pulmonary edema, ARDS, pulmonary fibrosis.
- Cardiovascular – hypertension, cor pulmonale, cardiovascular collapse.
- Renal – azotemia (prerenal and renal), acute tubular necrosis, glomerulonephritis, oliguria/anuria.
- Neurological (rare) – hyperexcitability, depression, decreased motor activity, ataxia, hindlimb paresis, seizures, cerebral edema.
- Dermal – irritation, ulceration, erythema, blistering.
- Ocular – eye irritation, corneal and conjunctival ulceration.

 # SIGNALMENT/HISTORY

- No breed, sex or age predilections; both diquat and paraquat are toxic to all mammals.

## Historical Findings

- Owners with high-risk jobs (pesticide industry, agriculture).
- Exposure to agricultural areas where pesticides have been sprayed recently.
- Observed ingestion or finding malicious baits intended for pets.

## Location and Circumstances of Poisoning

- Primarily accidental exposure.
- Skin absorption from concentrated formulations or chronic exposure.
- Animals exposed to concentrated products (agricultural centers, etc.).
- Paraquat has not been readily available since the 1960s but may still be stored in numerous places, including homes, garages, storage sheds, barns.

 # CLINICAL FEATURES

### Diquat

- Primarily mild to moderate toxicity – gastrointestinal signs (oral/pharyngeal irritation or burning sensation, nausea, vomiting, diarrhea, abdominal pain, ulceration), potential for renal impairment.

**TABLE 82.1 Comparative toxicity (oral LD$_{50}$) of paraquat in selected species.**

| | Dog | Cat | Human | Monkey | Cow | Sheep | Pig | Rat | Chicken | Turkey | Rabbit | Guinea pig | Mouse |
|---|---|---|---|---|---|---|---|---|---|---|---|---|---|
| LD$_{50}$ (mg/kg) | 25–50 | 35–50 | 3–5 | 50–70 | 35–50 | 8–10 | 75 | 100–344 | 262 | 290 | 50 | 22–30 | 290–360 |

- Rarely severe toxicity – GI ulceration, paralytic ileus, pulmonary edema, acute renal and hepatic failure, neurological signs, dysrhythmias, coma and death within 24–48 hours.
- Neurological signs can be progressive over 72–96 hours in severe cases.

### Paraquat

- Salivation, vomiting, diarrhea, and abdominal pain develop quickly due to caustic nature of paraquat, and are typically the first signs to develop.
- Dose dependent but often fatal.
- High-dose ingestion – rapid multiorgan failure, severe pulmonary edema, ARF, hepatic damage, death within 1–4 days.
- Moderate or subacute dose ingestion – slower onset of multiorgan failure, but eventual death from pulmonary edema and respiratory failure.
- Low dose and/or chronic exposure ingestion – death may be delayed for several weeks and is typically secondary to pulmonary fibrosis and respiratory failure.
- Chronic skin exposure or via inhalation – typically less severe clinical signs and less commonly fatal.
- Acute renal failure can occur within 1–3 days post injury.

 # DIFFERENTIAL DIAGNOSIS

### Diquat and Paraquat

- Gastrointestinal disease.
  - Ingestion of strongly alkaline or acidic compounds, zinc phosphide rodenticide, inorganic arsenic, zinc, mercury or lead.
  - Gastroenteritis/infectious agents.
  - Pancreatitis.
- Primary renal or hepatic disease.

### Paraquat Only

- Primary cardiac disease.
- Primary or secondary pulmonary disease.
  - Pneumonia/pneumonitis.
  - Canine distemper.
  - Asthma.
  - Bronchitis.
  - *Pneumocystis* infection.
  - Pulmonary interstitial fibrosis.

 # DIAGNOSTICS

### Diquat

#### Clinical Pathological Findings

- Serum chemistry – azotemia, elevated liver enzymes.
- Urinalysis – isosthenuria.

#### Other Diagnostic Tests

- Thoracic radiographs in patients with respiratory distress.
- Serum or urine diquat level (thin-layer or high-performance liquid chromatography, spectroscopy or spectrofluorometry) – not routinely available or performed.
  - Must store specimens in plastic containers – diquat binds to glass.

- Urine qualitative colorimetric test (adding sodium bicarbonate or hydroxide, followed by sodium dithionite powder) may detect diquat in urine (production of green color); however, this test is not specific, color can be mistaken for paraquat in some cases.

### Pathological Findings
- Oral, esophageal, and/or gastric erosion, ulceration, hemorrhage.
- Upper airway irritation, laryngeal, and/or pulmonary edema.
- Acute renal tubular necrosis.

## Paraquat
### Clinical Pathological Findings
- Serum chemistry – elevated lipase, azotemia, elevated liver enzymes.
- Urinalysis – isosthenuria, tubular casts.
- Arterial blood gas – hypoxemia, acidosis.

### Other Diagnostic Tests
- Monitor serial chest radiographs for the first 1–3 days following exposure.
  - May see pulmonary infiltrates, pneumomediastinum, bronchial changes, pleural effusion, pneumothorax, subcutaneous emphysema.
  - Urine dithionite colorimetric test (1% aqueous sodium dithionite in 0.1 N sodium hydroxide) may detect paraquat in urine (blue color) – may be easy method for early diagnosis.
  - Serum paraquat levels – most predictive of severity and prognosis but not readily available in veterinary laboratories.
  - Spectroscopic or high-performance liquid chromatography of urine paraquat levels.
  - Paraquat detection in stomach contents, vomitus, tissues, organs (spectrophotometry, gas/liquid chromatography, radioimmunoassay).

### Pathological Findings
- Gross lesions – erosive stomatitis/esophagitis, interstitial pneumonia, fulminating pulmonary edema/hemorrhage, pneumomediastinum, atelectasis, bronchodilation.
- Microscopic lesions – necrosis of alveolar type II pneumocytes denuding alveolar basement membrane with severe pulmonary edema and/or fibroplasia; proximal renal tubular degeneration, focal centrizonal hepatic degeneration.

 # THERAPEUTICS

### Detoxification
- Early emesis or careful gastric lavage (<1 hour of ingestion).
  - Concentrated forms are highly corrosive so emesis may not be advised in some cases.
- Activated charcoal with cathartic (one dose), Fuller's Earth or bentonite clay (if activated charcoal is not available).
- Paraquat – charcoal hemoperfusion and hemodialysis are considered the most efficient extracorporeal procedures to decrease plasma concentrations if initiated early; peritoneal dialysis is not effective.
- Ocular exposure – flush eyes for at least 15 minutes; fluorescein stain, slit lamp examination, and/or ophthalmology consultation as needed.
- Dermal exposure – bathe in mild dish soap for 15 minutes, rinse well (wear appropriate personal protective equipment).

## Appropriate Health Care

- Treatment is symptomatic and supportive.
- IV fluid therapy to increase renal excretion; adjust therapy as indicated based on degree of fluid losses, perfusion parameters, etc.
- Diuretics have not been shown to increase renal excretion of paraquat.
- Antiemetics, GI protectants (proton pump inhibitors or $H_2$-blockers, sucralfate).
- Treat seizures with benzodiazepines, phenobarbital, levetiracetam or propofol.
- Bronchospasm may require treatment with inhaled beta-2-adrenergic agonists and systemic corticosteroids.
- Hemodialysis for oliguric renal failure can be considered.
- Corneal ulceration – topical lubricants and antibiotics; topical and/or oral pain medication as indicated.

### Paraquat

- Early oxygen therapy is contraindicated as it may lead to increased oxygen free radical formation and oxidative damage. However, it may be useful in patients with respiratory compromise and progressive lung failure.
- Cautious IV crystalloid fluid therapy titrated to effect to avoid worsening pulmonary edema.
- Antioxidant therapy with N-acetylcysteine (Mucomyst®) and/or glutathione has been recommended (unknown clinical benefit).
  - High-dose vitamin C (ascorbic acid) is no longer recommended as studies have shown the risk of worsening cellular damage/death.
- In human medicine, treatment consists of gastric lavage via NG tube, one dose of activated charcoal with cathartic, hemoperfusion, and pulse immunosuppressive therapy (cyclophosphamide and steroids) in attempt to limit pulmonary fibrosis.
  - Lung transplantation in patients with severe pulmonary fibrosis has also been used, but this is not practical in veterinary medicine.

## Antidote

- There is no antidote for diquat or paraquat.

## Precautions/Interactions

- Emesis and potentially gastric lavage may further damage esophagus and/or stomach if concentrated solutions are ingested.
- Paraquat – oxygen therapy is contraindicated initially due to enhancement of oxidative damage (not indicated in human medicine until $PaO_2$ is <50 mmHg).

## Patient Monitoring

- In symptomatic patients, monitor electrolytes, renal and hepatic enzymes q 24 hours; closely monitor urine output in patients with renal compromise.
- Severely affected patients should also have ECG, BP, and $SpO_2$ monitored.

## Extracorporeal Therapy

- Paraquat – charcoal hemoperfusion and hemodialysis are considered the most efficient extracorporeal procedures to decrease plasma concentrations if initiated early; peritoneal dialysis is not effective.

# COMMENTS

## Prevention/Avoidance

- Avoid access to concentrated products or treated yards.

## Expected Course and Prognosis

### Diquat

- Mild toxicity – good prognosis with recovery expected within 24 hours with supportive care.
- Severe toxicity – may be guarded to poor prognosis with GI ulceration, cardiac arrhythmias, and organ damage.

### Paraquat

- Prognosis is poor with resultant organ damage and respiratory failure typically within days of exposure.

## Abbreviations

See Appendix 1 for a complete list.

## Suggested Reading

Chen K, Kuo Y, Li YC et al. Thoracic radiographic features of fatal paraquat intoxication in eleven dogs. *Vet Quarterly* 2021;41(1):217–225.

Donaldson C. Paraquat, In: Talcott P, Peterson M (eds) *Small Animal Toxicology*, 3rd edn. St Louis: Elsevier, 2013; pp. 731–739.

Magalhães N, Carvalho F, Dinis-Oliveira R. Human and experimental toxicology of diquat poisoning: toxicokinetics, mechanisms of toxicity, clinical features, and treatment. *Human Exp Toxicol* 2018; 37(11):1131–1160.

Marrs TC, Adjei A. Paraquat, In: *Pesticide Residues in Food – 2003: Toxicological Evaluations*. Geneva: WHO, 2003; pp. 203–266.

Williams JH, Whitehead Z, Van Wilpe E. Paraquat intoxication and associated pathological findings in three dogs in South Africa. *J S Afr Vet Assoc* 2016;87(1):e1–e9.

**Authors:** Pamela S. Kloepfer, DVM and Colleen M Almgren, DVM, PhD, DABT, DABVT
**Consulting Editor:** Lynn R. Hovda, RPh, DVM, MS, DACVIM

# Fertilizers

## DEFINITION/OVERVIEW

- Fertilizers are soil amendment products used in agriculture, lawn and garden care, and indoor plant applications to enhance plant growth.
- Fertilizers are composed of organic and inorganic material containing varying percentages of nitrogen, phosphorus, and potassium (potash), as indicated by the three numbers on the packaging (e.g., 30-10-10).
- Fertilizers may also contain the following micronutrients: iron, sulfur, calcium, magnesium, copper, zinc, boron, manganese, and molybdenum.
- In general, fertilizer ingestions are of low-level toxicity and symptoms are primarily limited to mild and self-limiting gastrointestinal irritation. Iron-containing fertilizers, especially in large ingestions of high concentration products, may rarely cause iron toxicity.
- Ingestion of fertilizers containing Milorganite®, a sewage-based fertilizer, carries increased risk of toxicosis with potential for gastrointestinal signs, muscle pain, and stiffness. The iron in Milorganite is insoluble, so iron toxicosis is not expected to develop.

## ETIOLOGY/PATHOPHYSIOLOGY

- The widespread use of lawn and garden fertilizers results in frequent exposure opportunities for animals.

### Mechanism of Action

- Fertilizer exposure generally results in a low level of toxicity due to poor gastrointestinal and dermal absorption.
- Methemoglobinemia may occur if nitrates convert to nitrites in the intestine or colon, but this occurs rarely in dogs, cats, and other monogastric animals.
- Industrial fertilizers containing anhydrous ammonia have the potential to cause corrosive injury to skin and mucous membranes, and potentially lung injury.
- The mechanism of action of toxicosis with Milorganite fertilizer is unknown.
- Some fertilizers may also contain other additives such as fungicides, insecticides, and herbicides, which may produce additional toxic effects.
- Old fertilizers may become contaminated with mold and bacteria, which may lead to risk of tremorgenic mycotoxicosis and increased risk of gastroenteritis.

### Toxicokinetics

- Fertilizers generally have poor gastrointestinal and dermal absorption.
- Metabolism is minimal except as indicated above for nitrates.

*Blackwell's Five-Minute Veterinary Consult Clinical Companion: Small Animal Toxicology*, Third Edition.
Edited by Lynn R. Hovda, Ahna G. Brutlag, Robert H. Poppenga, and Steven E. Epstein.
© 2024 John Wiley & Sons, Inc. Published 2024 by John Wiley & Sons, Inc.

## Systems Affected

- Gastrointestinal – vomiting, diarrhea, drooling, anorexia, and abdominal discomfort.
- Musculoskeletal – myalgia and stiffness with Milorganite ingestion.

 # SIGNALMENT/HISTORY

### Risk Factors

- No breed or sex predilection.
- Outdoor or farm dogs may have more opportunity for exposure, and young dogs may be more prone to dietary indiscretion.

### Historical Findings

- History of exposure to fertilizer.
- GIT signs with possible fertilizer, soil, or plant material visualized in vomitus or feces.

### Location and Circumstances of Poisoning

- Access to garage, shed, or other storage facility containing fertilizer or spilled fertilizer.
- Access to recently fertilized crops, garden, lawn, or other plants.

 # CLINICAL FEATURES

- Clinical signs usually occur within 2–10 hours of ingestion and resolve within 12–24 hours.
- GIT signs including salivation, vomiting, diarrhea, abdominal discomfort, anorexia.
- Muscle pain and stiffness may occur with Milorganite ingestion, in addition to potential for GIT signs. Iron toxicosis is not expected.
- Corrosive injury and potentially lung injury can occur with direct exposure to industrial fertilizers containing anhydrous ammonia.

 # DIFFERENTIAL DIAGNOSIS

- Toxicosis from ingestion of other GI irritants.
- Dietary indiscretion.
- Gastroenteritis.
- Pancreatitis.
- Foreign body obstruction.
- Inflammatory bowel disease.
- Metabolic disease – liver or renal disease, Addison disease.
- Orthopedic conditions with Milorganite myalgia.

 # DIAGNOSTICS

### Clinical Pathological Findings

- No specific or diagnostic features.
- Typically, clinical signs are self-limiting and diagnostics are not necessary for most patients.
- Evaluation of hydration (based on PCV/TS) and electrolytes may be assessed if GIT signs are prolonged.

## Other Diagnostics

■ Abdominal radiographs and other advanced diagnostics may need to be performed to rule out other differential diagnoses.

## Pathological Findings

■ Evidence of fertilizer within the GIT.

# THERAPEUTICS

## Detoxification

■ Emesis within two hours with large-volume ingestions if spontaneous emesis has not occurred.
  • Small ingestions do not require emesis induction.
  • Do not induce emesis with ingestion of corrosive fertilizers or liquid products containing xylene or toluene solvents.
■ Activated charcoal is not recommended as it binds poorly to fertilizer components. It is contraindicated with corrosive exposures.
■ Rinse skin and mucous membranes copiously with water and irrigate eyes with eye wash or water if exposed to corrosive fertilizers.
■ Milk of magnesia (5–10 mL/dog) q 8–12 hours may be considered in cases of large ingestions of iron-containing fertilizer if the elemental iron dose is considered to be >20 mg/kg.

## Appropriate Health Care

■ Small ingestions and asymptomatic patients may be monitored by the pet owner at home.
■ Symptomatic patients can usually be treated as an outpatient. Hospitalization is rarely necessary.

## Antidote

■ No antidote.

## Drug(s) of Choice

■ Antiemetics if vomiting is persistent.
  • Maropitant 1 mg/kg SQ or IV q 24 hours.
  • Ondansetron 0.1–0.5 mg/kg IV q 8–12 hours.
■ Antidiarrheals if diarrhea is persistent.
  • Bland diet will suffice in most cases as diarrhea is typically mild and self-limiting.
  • Probiotics as needed.
  • Metronidazole 10–15 mg/kg PO q 12 hours may be considered if hemorrhagic diarrhea occurs.
■ Fluids – IV or SQ depending on patient's level of dehydration.
■ GI protectants as needed.
  • $H_2$-blockers.
      ○ Famotidine 0.5–1 mg/kg PO, SQ, IM, IV q 12 hours.
  • Omeprazole 0.5–1 mg/kg PO q 12–24 hours.
  • Sucralfate 0.25–1 g PO q 8 hours.
■ Analgesics as needed for muscle soreness associated with Milorganite ingestions; may want to avoid NSAIDs if GI signs are present.

## Precautions/Interactions

- Avoid use of NSAIDs if GI signs are present, especially with ingestion of corrosive fertilizers.

## Extracorporeal Therapy

- Extracorporeal therapy is not indicated.

## Surgical Considerations

- Surgical removal of material may be necessary in rare instances of gastrointestinal obstruction.

## Patient Monitoring

- Monitor for resolution of clinical signs.

## Diet

- Bland diet until GI signs have resolved.

 **COMMENTS**

### Prevention/Avoidance

- Prevent access to stored, concentrated, and industrial fertilizers.

### Possible Complications

- Aspiration pneumonia may rarely occur in vomiting patients.

### Expected Course and Prognosis

- Prognosis is good with minimal supportive treatment in most cases. Coingestions may cause additional toxicity requiring more aggressive treatment.

### See Also

Chapter 81 Bone and Blood Meal
Chapter 90 Alkalis
Chapter 84 Herbicides
Chapter 103 Iron
Chapter 76 Mycotoxins (Tremorgenic)

### Abbreviations

See Appendix 1 for a complete list.

### Suggested Reading

Albretsen JC. Fertilizers. In: Plumlee KH (ed.) *Clinical Veterinary Toxicology*. St Louis: Mosby, 2004; pp. 154–155.
Campbell A, Chapman M. *Handbook of Poisoning in Dogs and Cats*. Ames: Blackwell Science, 2000; pp. 133–134.
Gerken DF. Lawn care products. In: Bonuagura JD (ed.) *Kirk's Current Veterinary Therapy XII*. Philadelphia: WB Saunders, 1995; pp. 248–249.
Levengood JM, Beasley VR. Principles of ecotoxicology: environmental contaminants. In: Gutpa RC (ed.) *Veterinary Toxicology: Basics and Clinical Principles*. New York: Elsevier, 2007; pp. 693–694.
Means C. Treating fertilizer ingestions? As easy as N-P-K. *Today Vet Pract* 2016;May/June:49–52.

**Author:** Charlotte Flint, DVM, DABT, DABVT
**Consulting Editor:** Lynn R. Hovda, RPh, DVM, MS, DACVIM

# Herbicides

## DEFINITION/OVERVIEW

- Herbicides are chemicals used to control or kill unwanted plants.
- Herbicide-containing products for use around the home have a low risk of toxicity in animals.
- Herbicides are the largest class of pesticides used; exposures are common, toxicoses are not.
- Clinical signs are typically of low severity and self-limiting, requiring minimal supportive care.
- Herbicides mixed with insecticides, fungicides, surfactants, etc. can be more toxic to pets.
- Specific herbicidal compounds are numerous, so this chapter will focus on the most common based upon the most recent EPA "Pesticide Industry Sales and Usage Report."
  - Phenoxy acid derivatives (2,4-D, MCPP, MCPA).
  - Dinitroanilines (pendimethalin).
  - Phosphonomethyl amino acids (glyphosate).
  - Benzoic acids (dicamba).

## ETIOLOGY/PATHOPHYSIOLOGY

- Animal exposures to lawns after application of herbicides are unlikely to result in toxicity.
- Exposure to concentrated products meant for dilution prior to application is more significant.
- Vomiting after eating treated grass is not enough to establish an herbicide as the cause.
- Reported toxicoses from herbicide exposure are uncommon.

### Mechanism of Action

Not precisely described for herbicides in general.
- 2,4-D, MCPP, MCPA.
  - Depress ribosome nuclease synthesis and uncouple oxidative phosphorylation.
  - In dogs, the myotonia is attributed to altered potassium and chloride conductance on the membranes of myocytes.
- Glyphosate – not reported in animals.
  - Clinical signs are more attributed to the anionic surfactants present rather than the herbicidal compound itself.
- Pendimethalin.
  - Stimulates respiration and uncouples oxidative phosphorylation.
- Dicamba – not reported in animals.

*Blackwell's Five-Minute Veterinary Consult Clinical Companion: Small Animal Toxicology*, Third Edition.
Edited by Lynn R. Hovda, Ahna G. Brutlag, Robert H. Poppenga, and Steven E. Epstein.
© 2024 John Wiley & Sons, Inc. Published 2024 by John Wiley & Sons, Inc.

## Toxicokinetics

- 2,4-D, MCPP, MCPA.
  - Oral absorption is rapid and complete.
  - Dermal absorption varies by product and species.
  - Widely distributed to tissues, does not accumulate in fat.
  - Readily excreted in urine; excretion can be saturated, leading to extended half-life in some species like dogs.
- Glyphosate.
  - Toxicokinetics not well described in dogs or cats.
  - Poor oral and dermal absorption.
  - Unlikely to result in toxicosis.
- Pendimethalin.
  - Poor absorption and excreted, largely unchanged, in feces.
- Dicamba.
  - Rapidly absorbed with oral exposure.
  - Readily excreted in the urine, 80–90% in the first 24 hours.

## Toxicity

- Additional toxicity data are listed in Table 84.1.
- 2,4-D.
  - Acute ingestion of 2,4-D has a reported $LD_{50}$ of 100 mg/kg.
  - All dogs exposed to 200 mg/kg lived; overt clinical signs were appreciated at 175 and 220 mg/kg.
  - Dogs were confined to grass treated at 4× the maximum recommended application rate 30 minutes after application; no adverse effects were noted at any time.
  - Dietary inclusion of 500 ppm (25 mg/kg bodyweight) for two years caused no adverse effects in dogs.
- MCPP.
  - 64 mg/kg bodyweight PO caused decreased rate of gain and decreased hematocrit in dogs.
- MCPA.
  - Dogs receiving >20 mg/kg for four weeks had a dry haircoat and mild changes in liver and kidney values.
- Glyphosate.
  - Dogs receiving 500 mg/kg bodyweight PO for a year did not exhibit toxic effects.

**TABLE 84.1 Toxicity data for the most commonly used herbicides in the US adapted from the EPA Pesticide Industry Sales and Usage report (2008–2012).**

| Rank | Compound | Toxicity designation | Acute oral $LD_{50}$ in rats |
| --- | --- | --- | --- |
| 1 | 2,4-D | Slight to moderate | 375–666 mg/kg |
| 2 | Glyphosate | Practically nontoxic | 5600 mg/kg |
| 3 | MCPP | Low | 930–1210 mg/kg |
| 4 | Pendimethalin | Slight to practically nontoxic | 1050–5000+ mg/kg |
| 5 | Dicamba | Slightly toxic | 757–1707 mg/kg |
| 6 | MCPA | Slightly toxic | 700–1160 mg/kg |

Adapted from herbicide-specific pages at http://extoxnet.orst.edu/pips/ghindex.html.

- Pendimethalin.
    - Dogs receiving 200 mg/kg bodyweight PO for two years had microscopic liver lesions and a dose-related increase in alkaline phosphatase.
- Dicamba.
    - Dogs fed dicamba for two years at 50 ppm in the diet showed no observable effects.
    - 250 ppm in the diet for two years cause mild hepatic discoloration.

## Systems Affected

- Gastrointestinal – vomiting, diarrhea.
- Musculoskeletal – rigidity, posterior weakness, ataxia.
- Nervous – seizures rarely reported.
- Neuromuscular – tremors.
- Ophthalmic – irritation, epiphora, conjunctivitis.
- Renal/urological – azotemia.
- Skin/exocrine – irritation, erythema.

 # SIGNALMENT/HISTORY

## Risk Factors

- Pets exposed to agricultural and home-use concentrates are more at risk.
- No breed or sex predilections.
- Typically, not reported during winter months.
- Preemergent products are used early in the growing season.

## Historical Findings

- Recent use of herbicides on the property.
- History of pets getting loose during times of high use (spring and fall).
- Signs and observations often reported by the owner: vomiting, diarrhea, ocular irritation, depression.

## Location and Circumstances of Poisoning

- Reported after application of products to lawns.

 # CLINICAL FEATURES

- 2,4-D, MCPP, MCPA.
    - Clinical signs expected within a few hours.
    - Vomiting, diarrhea, melena.
    - Depression, reluctance to move, ataxia, posterior weakness.
    - Skin or eye irritation if exposed.
    - Poisoning uncommon.
- Glyphosate.
    - In humans, oral exposure resulted in fluid and electrolyte loss causing renal tubular necrosis, attributed to the anionic surfactant rather than glyphosate.
    - Eye irritation if exposed.
    - Poisoning uncommon.
- Pendimethalin.
    - Skin or eye irritation if exposed.
    - Inhalation of dusts may be physically irritating to the upper respiratory tract.
    - Poisoning uncommon.

- Dicamba.
  - Anorexia, vomiting, urinary incontinence.
  - Muscle weakness, tremors, shortness of breath, cyanosis.
  - Upper respiratory tract irritation if inhaled.
  - Eye irritation if exposed, can be severe if concentrated.
  - Poisoning uncommon.

 # DIFFERENTIAL DIAGNOSIS

- Gastrointestinal signs – corrosive toxin ingestion, numerous plants, primary GI disease, metabolic disease.
- Muscular signs – stimulant compound exposure, tremorgenic compound exposure, neuropathy, myelopathy.
- Ocular signs – any irritant contact with the eye, foreign body, conjunctivitis.

 # DIAGNOSTICS

## Clinical Pathological Findings

- CBC, serum chemistry, urinalysis should be used to rule out other causes of clinical signs.
- 2,4-D, MCPP, MCPA – elevations in CK, ALP, LDH.
- Glyphosate – no specific abnormalities, dehydration/electrolyte abnormalities due to surfactant.
- Pendimethalin – no specific abnormalities.
- Dicamba – expected similar to 2,4-D.

## Other Tests

- Serum – can be used to confirm/rule out exposure to most herbicides.
  - Likely cost-prohibitive and many are excreted so rapidly that biological samples need to be obtained within 24 hours of exposure.
- Urine – can be used to confirm exposure to those excreted in the urine.

## Pathological Findings

- Gross lesions are nonspecific and not well characterized for any herbicide; list is for exposure to concentrated products.
  - Oral ulceration, gastritis, friable liver, renal congestion.

 # THERAPEUTICS

- The objective of therapy is decontamination and supportive care.

## Detoxification

- Ingestion – induce vomiting, followed by activated charcoal if exposure was recent.
- Oral – rinse mouth with water, provide fresh water.
- Topical – bathe with dish soap and warm water; pendimethalin will stain hair and skin a yellow-orange color.
  - Staff should consider PPE.
- Inhalation – provide access to fresh air.
- Ocular – flush eyes with isotonic saline or tap water for 10–15 minutes.

## Appropriate Health Care

- Typically, signs will be mild and self-limiting.
- Supportive care for any clinical signs.
- Fluid therapy.

## Antidote

- There are no specific antidotes for any herbicides.

## Drug(s) of Choice

- Apomorphine to induce emesis in dogs: 0.03 mg/kg IV, 0.04 mg/kg IM.
- Dexmedetomidine to induce emesis in cats: 5–10 mcg/kg IM.
  - Antidote is Antisedan® at equal volume.
- Xylazine to induce emesis in cats: 0.44 mg/kg IM.
  - Antidote is yohimbine 0.25–0.5 mg/kg IM.
- Activated charcoal with sorbitol cathartic: 1–3 mL/kg PO.
- Antiemetics.
  - Maropitant 1 mg/kg IV or SQ q 24 hours.
  - Ondansetron 0.5–1 mg/kg IV q 12 hours.

## Precautions/Interactions

- Many herbicides are acids, so acidification of the urine should be avoided in order to not limit the excretion of those acidic compounds.
- Many herbicides are mixed with other pesticides or fertilizers and these other compounds may enhance the toxicity of herbicides.

## Extracorporeal Therapy

- Extracorporeal therapy has not reportedly been used; it is likely cost-prohibitive given the poor absorption and rapid excretion of these compounds.

## Patient Monitoring

- 2,4-D, MCPP, MCPA: hydration status, CK, LDH, ALP.
- Glyphosate: hydration, electrolyte balance.
- Pendimethalin: hydration.
- Dicamba: similar to 2,4-D.

## Diet

- A bland diet should be offered for animals with gastrointestinal signs.
- Alkalinizing diets may increase excretion of acidic compounds.

 **COMMENTS**

- This is a common topic for pet owners to question their veterinarian about. These compounds are very common in urban and rural settings alike. Clinical signs appearing temporally near the application of these compounds cause much concern about herbicide involvement. In most cases, herbicides used in their diluted form are not expected to result in toxicity. The recent class action lawsuit involving Round-up® may cause a decrease in glyphosate use in the home and garden setting.

## Prevention/Avoidance

- Pets should not be allowed access to areas where concentrates are stored/mixed.
- Pets should not be allowed on treated lawns for 24–48 hours after treatment, or at least until the product has dried.

## Expected Course and Prognosis

- Clinical signs should be expected to occur within a few hours and the self-limiting GI signs to resolve in 24–48 hours.
- Herbicide exposure usually has a good prognosis.

## Synonyms

Weedkiller.

## See Also

Chapter 82 Paraquat and Diquat
Chapter 83 Fertilizers
Section on Insecticides and Molluscicides

## Abbreviations

See Appendix 1 for a complete list.
- 2,4-D = 2,4 dichlorophenoxyacetic acid
- MCPA = 2-methyl-4-chlorophenoxyacetic acid
- MCPP = 2-(4 chloro-methylphenoxy) propionic acid
- PPE = personal protective equipment

## Suggested Reading

Arnold EK, Lovell RA, Beasley VR et al. 2,4-D toxicosis. III: an attempt to produce 2,4-D toxicosis in dogs on treated grass plots. *Vet Hum Toxicol* 1991;33(5):457–461.

Beasely VR, Arnold EK, Lovell RA et al. 2,4-D toxicosis. I: a pilot study of 2,4-dichlorophenoxyacetic acid and dicamba-induced myotonia in experimental dogs. *Vet Hum Toxicol* 1991;33(5):435–440.

Gupta PK. Toxicity of herbicides. In: Gupta RC (ed.) *Veterinary Toxicology: Basic and Clinical Principles*, 3rd edn. San Diego: Elsevier, 2018; pp. 553–567.

Talcott PA. Miscellaneous herbicides, fungicides, and nematocides. In: Peterson ME, Talcott PA (eds) *Small Animal Toxicology*. St Louis: Saunders, 2013; pp. 401–408.

Welch SL. Glyphosate herbicides. In: Plumlee KH (ed.) *Clinical Veterinary Toxicology*. St Louis: Mosby, 2004; pp. 162–163.

**Author:** Scott A. Fritz DVM, DABVT
**Consulting Editor:** Lynn R. Hovda, RPh, DVM, MS, DACVIM

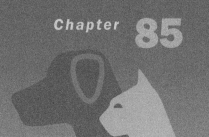
# Methionine

## DEFINITION/OVERVIEW

- Methionine is a sulfur-containing essential amino acid/nutrient, a urine acidifier, and treatment for fatty liver in choline deficiency.
- It is the primary ingredient in products designed to prevent urine-induced lawn damage.
- It is used in veterinary medicine for urine acidification and reduction of urine odor and is available OTC to decrease dog urine damage to lawns.
  - Therapeutic dose for dogs 100 mg/kg PO q 12 hours.
  - Therapeutic dose for cats 1000–1500 mg/cat PO per day.
- May also be present in human dietary supplements.
- It may be used to treat hepatopathies including acetaminophen toxicosis and chronic hepatitis.
- Clinical signs of toxicosis in dogs include gastrointestinal upset, neurological signs, and metabolic acidosis.
- Clinical signs of toxicosis in cats include gastrointestinal upset, methemoglobinemia, and Heinz body anemia.

## ETIOLOGY/PATHOPHYSIOLOGY

### Mechanism of Action

- Unknown mechanism of action.
- Methionine overdose may cause the production of toxic mercaptans, including homocysteine, which have been demonstrated to act synergistically with ammonia to produce signs of hepatic encephalopathy.
- After methionine is metabolized, sulfate is excreted in the urine as sulfuric acid.
- Metabolites lead to the development of oxidative injury and subsequent development of Heinz body anemia and methemoglobinemia, especially in cats.

### Pharmacokinetics

- Pharmacokinetic data are limited in veterinary species.
- Methionine is absorbed from the intestinal tract.
- Metabolism occurs in the liver and can follow two metabolic pathways.
  - Transsulfuration appears to be the primary route.
  - With high levels/toxicity, increased transamination occurs, leading to the production of mercaptans.

*Blackwell's Five-Minute Veterinary Consult Clinical Companion: Small Animal Toxicology*, Third Edition.
Edited by Lynn R. Hovda, Ahna G. Brutlag, Robert H. Poppenga, and Steven E. Epstein.
© 2024 John Wiley & Sons, Inc. Published 2024 by John Wiley & Sons, Inc.

## Toxicity

- Dogs
    - Previously healthy dogs have experienced toxicity at doses as low as 22.5 mg/kg.
    - Doses less than 200 mg/kg have been reported to cause mild, self-limiting gastrointestinal upset.
    - Doses greater than 400 mg/kg may result in signs of hepatic encephalopathy, especially in patients with underlying conditions (e.g., liver disease, kidney disease, pancreatitis).
- Cats
    - Doses >0.5 g/kg/day or 0.75 g/cat have resulted in methemoglobinemia, increased Heinz body formation, cyanosis, and hemolysis, especially in kittens.

## Systems Affected

- Dogs
    - Gastrointestinal – vomiting, salivation, diarrhea.
    - Renal/urological – aciduria.
    - Neurological – postural abnormalities/ataxia, hindlimb weakness, CNS depression/coma, seizures.
- Cats
    - Gastrointestinal – anorexia, vomiting, diarrhea.
    - Hematological – methemoglobinemia, Heinz body anemia.
    - Neurological – ataxia.
    - Respiratory – cyanosis, tachypnea.

# SIGNALMENT/HISTORY

- All species and breeds are affected.
- Dogs will more commonly ingest larger amounts of supplements.
- Kittens have been noted to be particularly sensitive and may develop signs at low doses.

## Risk Factors

- Animals with documented liver disease, kidney disease, or pancreatitis may be more predisposed to toxicosis.

## Historical Findings

- Recent exposure or administration.
- Owners may report vomiting with large exposures.

# CLINICAL FEATURES

- Dogs
    - Signs typically develop within 3–4 hours of ingestion.
    - Gastrointestinal signs include drooling, vomiting, and abdominal pain.
    - Neurological signs include ataxia, posterior paresis, anxiety, hyperactivity, restlessness, panting, seizures.
- Cats
    - Vomiting, anorexia, and ataxia.
    - Signs of hemolytic anemia secondary to Heinz body formation have been noted within days of administration: pale mucous membranes, tachycardia, tachypnea, weakness, lethargy.

- Signs of methemoglobinemia may also be noted: muddy mucous membranes, cyanosis, tachypnea.

# DIFFERENTIAL DIAGNOSIS

- Heinz body anemia – onions/garlic, acetaminophen, zinc, naphthalene.
- Neurological disease – inflammatory, infectious, trauma, degenerative, structural disease, other neurological toxins.
- Metabolic disease – renal disease, liver disease, other causes of acidosis such as lactic acidosis, diabetic ketoacidosis, ethylene glycol toxicity, aspirin toxicity.
- Gastrointestinal disease – dietary indiscretion, gastroenteritis, pancreatitis, biliary obstruction.

# DIAGNOSTICS

## Clinical Pathological Findings

- Complete blood count – Heinz body formation, regenerative anemia.
- Chemistry profile – increased liver enzymes, findings consistent with hepatic insufficiency.
- Serum ammonia – normal to elevated.
- Venous blood gas analysis – metabolic acidosis.
- Urinalysis – aciduria.

## Pathological Findings

- Splenomegaly, splenic hemosiderosis.
- Erythrophagocytosis.

# THERAPEUTICS

## Detoxification

- Induction of emesis in asymptomatic patients.
- Due to potential adverse effects of repeated activated charcoal administration and the new understanding regarding methionine metabolism, activated charcoal administration is no longer recommended.

## Appropriate Health Care

- Intravenous fluids for maintenance of hydration and perfusion.
- For severe metabolic acidosis (pH <7 or $HCO_3$ <10 mEq/L), consider sodium bicarbonate administration.
  - mEq bicarbonate = bodyweight (kg) × base deficit (mEq/L) × 0.3; administer 25% of this dose in intravenous fluids over 30 minutes and give the remainder over 4–6 hours.
  - Ensure appropriate patient ventilation prior to administration.

## Antidote

- No specific antidote.

## Drug(s) of Choice

- Antiemetics as needed for vomiting.
  - Maropitant 1 mg/kg SQ or IV q 24 hours.
  - Ondansetron 0.1–1 mg/kg IV slowly q 6–12 hours.
  - Metoclopramide 0.2–0.5 mg/kg IV, IM, or PO q 6–8 hours.

- GI protectants as needed.
  - Famotidine 0.5–1.0 mg/kg PO, IV, SQ or IM q 12 hours.
  - Pantoprazole 0.5–1 mg/kg IV q 12 hours.
- Seizure control as needed.
  - Diazepam 0.5 mg/kg IV.
  - Midazolam 0.1–0.25 mg/kg IV or IM.
  - Phenobarbital 10–20 mg/kg IV to effect.
- Control of agitation.
  - Acepromazine 0.02–0.1 mg/kg IM, IV or SQ PRN.
  - Trazodone 2–5 mg/kg PO for dogs PRN.
- Hematological support.
  - Patients with signs of severe cardiovascular collapse and anemia may require blood transfusions.
  - Oxygen therapy may be needed in severely affected patients.

## Extracorporeal Therapy

- Not reported/described.

## Patient Monitoring

- Severely affected patients may need monitoring of BP, ECG, respiratory rate, and effort.
- Monitor complete blood count and chemistry profile q 24 hours for resolution of abnormalities.

## Diet

- Discontinue supplementation.
- Bland diet until resolution of gastrointestinal upset.
- Protein-restricted diet in patients with evidence of hepatic insufficiency.

 **COMMENTS**

### Prevention/Avoidance

- Client education regarding the potential palatability of methionine supplements and preventing access of pets to methionine supplements.

### Possible Complications

- No long-term complications are anticipated.

### Expected Course and Prognosis

- Prognosis is good for most exposures, with full recovery within 24–48 hours.
- Dogs with preexisting conditions may have more severe clinical signs and a slower recovery.
- No deaths reported.

### Abbreviations

See Appendix 1 for a complete list.

### Suggested Reading

Branam JE. Suspected methionine toxicosis associated with a portocaval shunt in a dog. *J Am Vet Med Assoc* 1982;181:929–931.

Hickey M, Son T, Wismer T. Retrospective evaluation of methionine intoxication associated with urinary acidifying products in dogs: 1,525 cases (2001–2012). *J Vet Emerg Crit Care* 2015;25(5):640–645.

Maede Y, Hoshino T, Inaba M et al. Methionine toxicosis in cats. *Am J Vet Res* 1987;48:289–292.

Plumb DC. *Plumb's Veterinary Drug Handbook*, 9th edn. Ames: Wiley-Blackwell, 2018.

Villar D, Carson T, Osweiler G et al. Overingestion of methionine tablets by a dog. *Vet Hum Toxicol* 2003;45:311–312.

**Author**: Rebecca A.L. Walton, DVM, DACVECC:
**Consulting Editor**: Lynn R. Hovda, RPh, DVM, MS, DACVIM

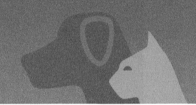

# Herbals

# Chapter 86

# Ephedra (Ma Huang)

## DEFINITION/OVERVIEW

- *Ephedra sinica*, common name ephedra or ma huang, is an herbal sympathomimetic used primarily as a weight loss aid, decongestant, and recreational drug known as herbal ecstasy.
- Overdoses cause hyperactivity, tachycardia, hypertension, tremors, seizures, hallucinations, and serotonin syndrome.
- The FDA banned dietary supplements containing ephedra from the market in 2004. Ephedra may still be obtained through various channels, including internet sales. Veterinarians should be aware that most products containing ephedra will not be manufactured with quality controls, standardization, or regard for purity and dosage. Some products will contain ingredients not listed on the label.
- As of 2023, *Ephedra sinica* is still illegal in the United States.

## ETIOLOGY/PATHOPHYSIOLOGY

### Mechanism of Action

- Ephedra contains ephedrine and pseudoephedrine. These alkaloids are structurally similar to amphetamines.
- Ephedra stimulates alpha- and beta-adrenergic receptors and releases endogenous catecholamines at synapses in the brain and heart. This results in peripheral vasoconstriction and cardiac stimulation.
- The clinical effects are increased blood pressure, tachycardia, mydriasis, ataxia, and restlessness. Central nervous system effects include tremors, seizures, agitation, and serotonin syndrome.
- Serotonin syndrome is the overstimulation of serotonin receptors in the nervous system, gastrointestinal tract, cardiovascular, and respiratory system. Clinical signs associated with serotonin syndrome seen in ephedra toxicosis include tremors and seizures, hyperesthesia, hyperthermia, hypersalivation, and death.

### Pharmacokinetics or Toxicokinetics – Absorption, Distribution, Metabolism, Excretion

- Ephedra is absorbed orally.
- It is metabolized in the liver and excreted in the urine.
- Ephedra excretion is enhanced if the urine is acidified.

*Blackwell's Five-Minute Veterinary Consult Clinical Companion: Small Animal Toxicology*, Third Edition. Edited by Lynn R. Hovda, Ahna G. Brutlag, Robert H. Poppenga, and Steven E. Epstein. © 2024 John Wiley & Sons, Inc. Published 2024 by John Wiley & Sons, Inc.

## Toxicity

- Clinical signs may be seen at 5–6 mg/kg.
- Death has been seen at 10–12 mg/kg.

## Systems Affected

- Nervous – hyperactivity, hallucinations, tremors, seizures, head bobbing, serotonin syndrome.
- Cardiovascular – tachycardia, hypertension.
- Metabolic – hyperthermia.
- Musculoskeletal – rhabdomyolysis (sequela to prolonged seizure activity and hyperthermia).
- Hemic – DIC (sequela to prolonged seizure activity and hyperthermia).
- Renal – myoglobinuria.

 # SIGNALMENT/HISTORY

- Dogs are the most common species to be affected by ephedra although any species may develop toxicity if a sufficient dose is ingested.
- Younger dogs may be more likely to "counter-surf" or get into purses and thus have exposure to a supplement.
- Diagnosis is based on history and clinical signs.

### Risk Factors

- Animals with preexisting cardiovascular disease (including hypertension) or seizure disorders may develop more severe clinical signs.

### Historical Findings

- Witnessed ingestion.
- Access to herbal decongestants, diet products, and/or recreational drugs.
- Owners frequently report restlessness, pacing, vocalizing, hyperactivity, panting, apparent hallucinations, head bobbing, and tremors or seizures.

### Location and Circumstances of Poisoning

- Most animals will ingest supplements in a home or car.

 # CLINICAL FEATURES

- Clinical signs can develop within 30 minutes to eight hours post exposure.
- The duration of clinical signs is 24–72 hours.
- The most common signs are mydriasis, hyperactivity, panting, hyperthermia, nervousness, and tachycardia, followed by collapse.
- Hypertension, muscle tremors, and/or seizures may be noted on exam.
- Head bobbing has been associated with increased mortality.
- Death is usually due to cardiovascular collapse.

 # DIFFERENTIAL DIAGNOSIS

- Clinical signs are similar to the ingestion of pseudoephedrine found in cold and sinus medications, as well as amphetamine ingestion (attention deficit disorder drugs such as methylphenidate and dextroamphetamine) and illicit substances.

# DIAGNOSTICS

## Clinical Pathological Findings

- Serum chemistry– hyperglycemia and hypokalemia may be noted.

## Other Diagnostics

- OTC drug tests will test positive for amphetamines if ephedra is ingested. Most OTC tests require urine.

## Pathological Findings

- No specific gross or histopathological findings have been reported.

# THERAPEUTICS

- The treatment plan goals are to prevent further absorption, stabilize the cardiovascular system, control CNS signs, and provide supportive care.

## Detoxification

- Induce emesis only in asymptomatic animals within one hour of ingestion.
- One dose of activated charcoal may be given within four hours of ingestion in an asymptomatic animal who has ingested a high dose of ephedrine.

## Appropriate Health Care

- IV fluids as needed for supportive care in symptomatic animals.

## Antidote

- None.

## Drug(s) of Choice

- Acepromazine, 0.05–1.0 mg/kg IM or IV, to control restlessness and agitation. Start lowend of range and increase as needed.
- Propranolol, 0.02–0.06 mg/kg, slow IV to effect, for tachycardia. Propranolol is also a serotonin antagonist and may help reduce some clinical signs associated with serotonin syndrome.
- Cyproheptadine, 1.1 mg/kg PO or crush in saline and give rectally q 6–12 hours for dogs, 2–4 mg/cat q 6–12 hours, for serotonin syndrome. Maximum 2–3 doses cyproheptadine is a specific serotonin antagonist. It should only be given if appropriate clinical signs of serotonin syndrome are present.

## Precautions/Interactions

- Diazepam can potentially cause increased CNS excitation resulting in crying, head bobbing, and death.
- If ingested with other sympathomimetic agents (pseudoephedrine, phenylpropanolamine), methylxanthines (chocolate or caffeine), MAO inhibitors (selegiline), or tricyclic antidepressants, toxicity may be enhanced.

## Alternative Drugs

- If propranolol is unavailable, or if an animal is hypertensive and tachycardic, a specific beta-1 antagonist may be preferred.
  - Esmolol 0.05–0.1 mg/kg IV boluses up to 0.5 mg/kg, or an infusion of 50–200 mcg (0.05–0.2 mg)/kg/min in dogs. A loading dose of 200–500 mcg/kg IV over 1 minute followed by a CRI of 10–200 mcg/kg/min can be used in cats.

- Atenolol 0.2–1.5 mg/kg PO q 12–24 hours for dogs, 2 mg/kg or 6.25–12.5 mg PO *total* (not mg/kg) q 24 hours for cats.
- Metoprolol 0.2 mg/kg PO q 12 hours for dogs, 2–15 mg PO q 8 hours for cats.
■ Dexmedetomidine (2 mcg/kg IV bolus followed by 0.5 mcg/kg/h IV CRI has been used successfully in a cat to treat stimulatory signs.

### Patient Monitoring

■ Frequency of monitoring will vary with severity of clinical syndrome.
  - Hydration parameters.
■ Electrolytes.
■ Heart rate.
■ Blood pressure.
■ Heart rhythm (ECG).
■ Body temperature.
■ Minimize sensory stimulation.

 **COMMENTS**

### Prevention/Avoidance

■ Make sure the environment is safe for the pet before releasing to go home. Owners should check crates, blankets, under beds, etc. to make sure all pills or capsules have been removed.
■ Owners should be educated about keeping medications out of reach of pets.
■ Discuss "counter-surfing," keeping purses, briefcases, etc. out of pet's reach. Discuss use of training aids like scat mats for pets constantly getting items off counters.

### Possible Complications

■ DIC, rhabdomyolysis, and myoglobinuria (with subsequent renal failure) are possible if prolonged, untreated tremors/seizures or hyperthermia present.

### Expected Course and Prognosis

■ Clinical signs generally resolve within 24–72 hours.
■ Prognosis is generally good.
■ If head bobbing, myoglobinuria, or DIC present, prognosis is poor.

### Synonyms

■ Ephedra/ma huang is also known as yellow horse or sea grape.
■ There are several *Ephedra* species, but *Ephedra sinica* is the plant used in manufacturing of supplements.
■ *Sida cordifolia*, also known as Indian common mallow, is another plant containing pseudoephedrine and ephedrine alkaloids sometimes used in herbal supplements.
■ *Ephedra nevadensis*, common name Mormon Tea, does not contain ephedrine. It is sold as both a beverage and folk medication. Mormon Tea is sometimes used in alternative medicine practices.

### See Also

Chapter 15 Amphetamines
Chapter 49 Decongestants (Pseudoephedrine, Phenylephrine)
Chapter 40 Methamphetamine

## Abbreviations

See Appendix 1 for a complete list.

- CRI = constant rate infusion
- DIC = disseminated intravascular coagulation
- MAO = monoamine oxidase
- OTC = over the counter

## Suggested Reading

DerMarderosian A, Beutler JA. *The Review of Natural Products*, 3rd edn. St Louis: Facts and Comparisons, 2002; pp. 265–266.

Fugh-Berman A. *The 5-minute Herb and Dietary Supplement Consult*. Philadelphia: Lippincott Williams & Wilkins, 2003; pp. 116–117.

Means C. Selected herbal toxicities. *Vet Clin North Am Small Anim Pract* 2002;32:367–382.

Norkus CL, Keir I, Means C. Dexmedetomidine to control signs associated with lisdexamfetamine dimesylate toxidrome in a cat. *Can Vet J* 2017;58(3):261–264.

Ooms TG, Khan SA, Means C. Suspected caffeine and ephedrine toxicosis resulting from ingestion of an herbal supplement containing guarana and ma huang in dogs: 47 cases (1997–1999). *J Am Ved Med Assoc* 2001;218:225–229.

**Author**: Charlotte Means, DVM, MLIS, DABVT, DABT
**Contributing Editor**: Ahna G. Brutlag, DVM, MS, DABT, DABVT

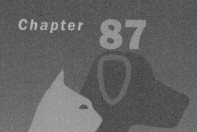

# Essential Oils and Liquid Potpourri

## DEFINITION/OVERVIEW

- Essential oils are organic volatile components extracted by distillation or cold pressing from a range of plants.
- Over 3000 essential oils have been identified, with 300 in common usage.
- There is worldwide distribution in aromatherapy, herbal remedies, insect repellants, insecticides, fragrances, flavorings, cosmetics, and as preservatives.
- Essential oils have scent, flavor, antioxidant, antiaging, antimicrobial, and antiviral properties.
- Essential oil toxicity and clinical signs vary widely depending on type and concentration. In general, essential oils at low concentrations have a wide margin of safety.
- Exposure is common and occurs from application of essential oils on pets, accidental dermal exposure, oral exposure (directly or from grooming of dermal products), inhalation, and ocular exposure.
- Tea tree oil (melaleuca oil) and phenols are discussed in separate chapters.
- Liquid potpourri can contain cationic detergents, essential oils, and sometimes alcohol. Ingredient information is often not available from the manufacturer.
- Liquid potpourri is often contained in simmer pots, liquid plug-in diffusers, and nonheated reed diffusers.

## ETIOLOGY/PATHOPHYSIOLOGY

### Mechanism of Action

- Limited data is available and varies by oil.
- Wintergreen and birch oil contain methylsalicylate. This is related to aspirin and has the same toxicity concerns.
- Pennyroyal oil contains pulegone which causes hepatotoxicity, hepatic necrosis, GI involvement, and potential fatalities.
- Citrus oil contains D-limonene and linalool; causes GI ulcerations, phototoxicity, and rarely toxic epidermal necrolysis (TENS) in cats with massive doses.
- Peppermint oil contains menthol and pulegone; large doses cause GI ulceration, hepatotoxicity, and seizures.
- Cinnamon and clove oils contain eugenol; cause GI irritation at low doses; at high doses may cause metabolic acidosis, hepatic damage, seizures.
- Cinnamon and cassia oils contain cinnamaldehyde; oregano, savory, and thyme oil contain carvacrol; thyme and oregano oil contain thymol, all of which can cause GI irritation.

*Blackwell's Five-Minute Veterinary Consult Clinical Companion: Small Animal Toxicology*, Third Edition. Edited by Lynn R. Hovda, Ahna G. Brutlag, Robert H. Poppenga, and Steven E. Epstein.
© 2024 John Wiley & Sons, Inc. Published 2024 by John Wiley & Sons, Inc.

- Hyssop oil (pinocamphone); wormwood, sage, and thuja oils (thujone); and eucalyptus oil (eucalyptol) can result in neurological signs.
- Bitter almond can contain prussic acid; this is removed in most commercial products and labeled Free From Prussic Acid (FFPA).

## Pharmacokinetics or Toxicokinetics – Absorption, Distribution, Metabolism, Excretion

- The majority of pharmacokinetic and toxicity information is derived from human and laboratory animal studies.
- Essential oils are generally small, nonpolar, and lipophilic molecules that are well absorbed via dermal, mucosal, respiratory, and oral exposures. Onset of signs is typically within eight hours.
- Lipophilic molecules have a large volume of distribution.
- Hepatic metabolism and the potential for enterohepatic recirculation are present for most essential oils with known pharmacokinetics.
- Excretion is primarily renal, with some hepatic and pulmonary involvement.

## Toxicity

- Toxicity varies greatly depending on essential oil type, concentration, route of exposure, and dose.

## Systems Affected

- Gastrointestinal – vomiting, diarrhea, hypersalivation, and anorexia may occur with oral exposure.
  - Risk for corrosive injury, especially with liquid potpourri (largely from other ingredients including cationic factors). Greater risk in cats.
- Skin/exocrine – prolonged contact and higher concentrations of essential oils are associated with increased dermal irritation.
  - Idiopathic dermal reactions including toxic epidermal necrolysis in cats after large dermal exposure to citrus oils.
  - Phototoxicity may develop; associated with citrus oils, bergamot, fig leaf, angelica root, and verbena.
  - Reports of allergic contact dermatitis in humans, typically following repeated exposures.
- Respiratory – irritation following respiratory exposure.
  - Risk for aspiration secondary to vomiting.
- Neuromuscular – lethargy, ataxia, weakness, tremors, seizures.
  - Seizures have been associated with exposure to pinocampone, thujone, pulegone, methylsalicylate, and eucalytol.
- Hepatobiliary – hepatocellular enzyme elevations and hepatic necrosis following exposure to pennyroyal, calamint, buchu, birch tar, cassia bark, and cinnamon oil.
- Ophthalmic – blepharospasm, tearing, and corneal ulceration following ocular exposure.
- Renal/urological – rarely acute kidney injury.
- Cardiovascular – rarely tachycardia, bradycardia, hypertension, or hypotension.
- Hemic/lymphatic/immune – hypersensitivity reactions.

 # SIGNALMENT/HISTORY

### Risk Factors

- Cats are at increased risk due to decreased glucuronyl transferase activity.
- Liquid potpourri is often placed on counters and other areas where cats have greater access than dogs, increasing their risk of exposure.

- Dogs are at increased risk due to their propensity for dietary indiscretion.
- Animals with underlying respiratory disease, such as asthma, may have increased risk following respiratory exposure.

## Historical Findings

- History of known or suspected exposure.
- Clinical signs noted by owners can vary significantly depending on exposure type. Early signs may include presence/odor of the product on the animal's skin/fur, dermal irritation, hypersalivation, vomiting, hiding, lethargy, cough, and tachypnea.

 **CLINICAL FEATURES**

- Onset of signs may be noted immediately or up to eight hours post exposure in most cases.
- Exposure route, type, and amount, individual variation, and species impact progression of clinical signs.
- Initial clinical signs are largely related to the irritant nature of many essential oils. In mild cases, signs do not progress beyond this point.
    - If an oral exposure, or grooming of a dermal exposure occurred, signs may be GI in nature including hypersalivation, vomiting.
    - Dermal exposures may result in pruritus and erythema.
    - Ocular exposures may result in tearing and blepharospasm.
- Depending on the essential oil type, concentration, and amount of exposure, clinical signs may progress.
- Further clinical signs, as listed previously under Systems Affected, have been reported.
- Mild cases resolve within a few hours. Clinical signs may persist for days in severe cases.

 **DIFFERENTIAL DIAGNOSIS**

- GI irritation: dietary indiscretion, parasitic, and infectious causes.
- GI ulceration: ingestion of caustic/corrosive materials (drain cleaners, phenols, and batteries), NSAIDs, aspirin; neoplasia; infection.
- Respiratory irritation: exposure to other respiratory irritants or asphyxiants; infection.
- Hepatic involvement: ingestion of xylitol, acetaminophen, NSAIDs, mycotoxins, cycad palms, cyanobacteria, and oral benzodiazepines (cats); hepatitis; leptospirosis.
- Neurological signs including seizures: ingestion of amphetamines, SSRI medications, mycotoxins, xylitol, cyanobacteria, 5-fluorouracil, baclofen, albuterol, bromethalin, metaldehyde, phosphides, ethylene glycol; infection; trauma; neoplasia.

 **DIAGNOSTICS**

### Clinical Pathological Findings

- Varies depending on type and amount of essential oil.
- CBC/electrolytes: hemoconcentration and electrolytes changes associated with dehydration.
- Serum chemistry: hepatic elevations due to hepatotoxins or hepatic lipidosis in anorexic cats.

### Other Diagnostics

- Radiology, ultrasound, and/or endoscopy (use cautiously) may be used to assess severity of GI ulcerations and for sequela such as perforation.

## Pathological Findings

- No pathognomonic findings. Changes consistent with clinical progression.
- Hepatic necrosis associated with pennyroyal oil.
- Dermal, ocular, and GI mucosal irritation or injury.

 **THERAPEUTICS**

- Varies greatly depending on details of exposure; largely supportive and symptomatic.

## Detoxification

- Dermal exposure – bathe with degreasing liquid dish soap or follicle stripping shampoo.
- Inhalation exposure – provide fresh air or oxygen/humidified air if clinically necessary.
- Oral exposure – do not induce emesis due to risk of aspiration and/or corrosive injury.
  - Activated charcoal is not typically required.
  - In severe cases at risk for systemic toxicity (including hepatotoxicity), consider single or multiple doses of activated charcoal if patient can protect their airway and is not hypernatremic.

## Appropriate Health Care

- Treatment depends on type and concentration of essential oils as well as clinical signs.
- If exposure to low concentration product(s) and signs are mild, home monitoring is often appropriate.
- If significant neurological, hepatic, or other clinical signs develop, hospitalize as needed.
- Monitor vitals, blood pressure, and neurological status; frequency depends on clinical status.

## Antidote

- None available.

## Drug(s) of Choice

- Note: Dosages provided are for dogs, unless otherwise specified. Appropriate drugs and dosages should be confirmed for other species.
- Fluid therapy: SQ or IV balanced crystalloid fluids as needed to maintain hydration, perfusion, and aid with excretion. Adjust as needed.
- Antiemetic agents: maropitant 1 mg/kg SQ or IV (slowly over 1–2 min) q 24 hours or others.
- GI protectants.
  - Proton pump inhibitor (omeprazole 0.5–1 mg/kg PO q 12 hours).
  - Sucralfate (0.5–1 g/dog [not mg/kg] PO q 8 hours. Dissolve in water to form slurry).
- Anticonvulsant agents.
  - Benzodiazepines (diazepam 0.5–1 mg/kg IV or per rectum; midazolam 0.25–0.5 mg/kg IV). Continue with either intermittent boluses or CRI IV depending on clinician preference and response to treatment. Adjust doses as needed.
  - Barbiturates (phenobarbital 4–8 mg/kg IV PRN).
  - Levetiracetam (30–60 mg/kg IV slow bolus over 5–15 minutes).
- Antitremorgenic agent: methocarbamol 55–220 mg/kg IV. Recommend not to exceed total dose of 330 mg/kg/day as may cause sedation.
- Hepatoprotectants if hepatotoxicity is a concern or hepatic elevations present.
  - S-adenosyl-methionine (SAM-e) 40 mg/kg PO on day 1, then 20 mg/kg PO q 24 hours for 2–4 weeks.

- N-acetylcysteine (NAC) dilute to 5% or less solution. 140 mg/kg IV or PO on day 1, then 70 mg/kg IV or PO q 6 hours × 7–17 doses.
- Other treatments.
  - In cases with severe signs, intravenous lipid emulsion (ILE) (1.5 mL/kg IV initial bolus of 20% ILE followed by 0.25 mL/kg/min IV CRI for 30–60 minutes). Repeat boluses every 4–6 hours, if needed, once serum is no longer lipemic.

## Precautions/Interactions

- In cases with significant hepatic impairment, use medications with hepatic metabolism cautiously.

## Alternative Drugs

- Treatment is supportive and symptomatic. Other drugs can be substituted as needed depending on supply and expense logistics.

## Extracorporeal Therapy

- Extracorporeal therapy has not been researched with exposure to essential oils.

## Surgical Considerations

- Cardiovascular, respiratory, and neurological status should be evaluated and treated accordingly if anesthesia is required.

## Patient Monitoring

- Monitor vitals, blood pressure, and neurological status. Frequency depends on clinical status.
- Monitor hepatic values if significant exposure to hepatotoxic product such as pennyroyal oil.

## Diet

- For essential oils that pose a risk for significant GI irritation or ulceration, encourage additional water consumption to dilute product within the GI tract.
- Discontinue oral intake if patients cannot protect their airway.

 **COMMENTS**

### Prevention/Avoidance

- Avoid application of potentially toxic essential oils on animals. Secure concentrated essential oils out of reach of pets and educate owners on their risks.

### Possible Complications

- Scarring and stricture formation upon healing of significant caustic/corrosive GI injury.

### Expected Course and Prognosis

- Prognosis varies depending on type and amount of exposure, but overall is good.
- Poor prognosis with significant pennyroyal exposure.

### See Also

Chapter 95 Phenols and Pine Oils
Chapter 96 Soaps, Detergents, Fabric Softeners, Enzymatic Cleaners, and Deodorizers
Chapter 88 Tea Tree Oil (Melaleuca Oil)

## Abbreviations

See Appendix 1 for a complete list.

- FFPA = free from prussic acid
- TENS = toxic epidermal necrolysis

## Suggested Reading

De Groot AC, Schmidt E. *Essential Oils. Contact Allergy and Chemical Composition*. Boca Raton: CRC Press, 2016.

Moss MJ. Salicylate toxicity from ingestion of an oil of wintergreen containing insecticide. *Clin Toxicol* 2020;58(3):219–220.

Nejad SM, Özgüneş H, Başaran N. Pharmacological and toxicological properties of eugenol. *Turk J Pharmaceut Sci* 2017;14(2):201.

Pelkonen O, Abass K, Wiesner J. Thujone and thujone-containing herbal medicinal and botanical products: toxicological assessment. *Regulat Toxicol Pharmacol* 2013;65(1):100–107.

Wojtunik-Kulesza KA. Toxicity of selected monoterpenes and essential oils rich in these compounds. *Molecules* 2022;27(5):1716.

**Author:** Sarah R. Alpert, DVM, DABT
**Consulting Editor:** Ahna G. Brutlag, DVM, MS, DABT, DABVT

# Chapter 88

# Tea Tree Oil (Melaleuca Oil)

## DEFINITION/OVERVIEW

- An essential oil produced from the Australian tea tree, *Melaleuca alternifolia*.
- Tea tree oil is also known as melaleuca oil.
- Known antibacterial and antifungal properties; possible antipruritic and antiinflammatory properties.
- Found in gels and body lotions, shampoos, conditioners, toothpastes, balms, insect repellants, and other household cleaning products, ranging from <1% to 100% oil.
  - Marketed for use on dogs, cats, ferrets, and horses.
- Intoxication most commonly results from 100% oil applied as external parasite repellant.
  - As little as seven drops of 100% oil have caused clinical toxicosis.
  - Toxicosis generally produces CNS dysfunction, muscular tremors, and hypothermia. May also result in hepatic injury.

## ETIOLOGY/PATHOPHYSIOLOGY

- Toxicosis results from dermal application or oral ingestion.
- Prevalence of intoxication may increase as pet owners' interest grows in "natural" therapies.
- Toxicosis is similar to other essential oils, such as pine oil, eucalyptus, and d-limonene.
- Composed of 50–60% terpenes, 6–8% cineole, and other alcohols.
- Terpinen-4-ol is the main antimicrobial and antifungal agent.
- Cineole produces irritation of mucous membranes and skin.

### Mechanism of Action

- Exact mechanism of action is unknown. Presumed similar to turpentine and other essential oil toxicities.

### Pharmacokinetics or Toxicokinetics – Absorption, Distribution, Metabolism, Excretion

- Transdermal and GI absorption is rapid due to highly lipophilic nature.
- Terpene metabolism is largely hepatic.
- Phase I and phase II biotransformation via cytochrome P450 enzymes.
- Conjugated to glycine or glucuronide in the liver.
- Undergoes enterohepatic recirculation.
- Urinary excretion of metabolites takes 2–3 days; small amount via fecal elimination.

*Blackwell's Five-Minute Veterinary Consult Clinical Companion: Small Animal Toxicology*, Third Edition.
Edited by Lynn R. Hovda, Ahna G. Brutlag, Robert H. Poppenga, and Steven E. Epstein.
© 2024 John Wiley & Sons, Inc. Published 2024 by John Wiley & Sons, Inc.

## Toxicity

- Exact toxic doses are not established.
- Oral $LD_{50}$ (various species) = 1.9–5 g/kg or 1.9–2.6 mL/kg.
- Poisoning is most often seen with direct application of 100% oil. Products with low concentrations (i.e., shampoo, conditioner, toothpaste) are generally not considered toxic.
- Clinical toxicities reported following 7–8 drops of 100% oil applied to the skin.
- Applications of approximately 10 mL of 100% oil has resulted in toxicosis in cats and dogs.
- Three cats with dermal flea bite lesions received 20 mL each of concentrated oil and suffered severe toxicosis (3) and death (1).

## Systems Affected

- Nervous – target system of toxicity resulting in CNS depression/coma (similar to other terpenes).
- Hepatobiliary – elevated liver enzymes secondary to induction of microsomal P450.
- Skin – possible contact irritation, especially of the mucous membranes.
- Musculoskeletal – unknown MOA; possible direct effect of toxic metabolites.
- Cardiovascular – peripheral vasodilation following all routes of absorption.
- Respiratory – primary or secondary affects due to CNS depression.
- Gastrointestinal – vomiting and/or ptyalism likely from oral irritation, secondary from hepatic effects, shock.

 # SIGNALMENT/HISTORY

- There are no reported breed, sex, or age predilections.
- Cats may be more sensitive due to metabolism (glucuronidation).

### Risk Factors

- Animals with underlying CNS or hepatic disease may exhibit more severe clinical signs or suffer toxicity at lower doses.
- Juveniles and smaller animals may be more sensitive due to poor metabolism and lower body surface area.

### Historical Findings

- Well-intentioned but misinformed owners may admit to administering tea tree oil directly to the pet.
- There may be a characteristic and strong odor (minty) associated with the pet.
- Oily/greasy fur on the neck/back/ear canals from topical application.
- Owners may report CNS depression, unresponsiveness, difficulty or inability to walk, shaking or tremors.
- Witnessed ingestions/discovery of chewed tea tree oil containers.

### Location and Circumstances of Poisoning

- Given the heightened interest in "natural remedies," the incidence of misuse may increase.

 # CLINICAL FEATURES

- Onset of clinical signs is 1–2 hours after application (up to 12 hours).
- Signs slowly resolve over 2–4 days. Mild cases may resolve within hours.

- The most common clinical signs are mild-to-moderate hypothermia, weakness, CNS depression, ataxia, and generalized muscle tremors.
- Less common signs include skin/mucous membrane irritation, vomiting, salivation, bradypnea, bradycardia, hypotension secondary to shock or CNS depression, unresponsive pupils, paralysis, and coma.

 **DIFFERENTIAL DIAGNOSIS**

- Cardiovascular – shock (sepsis, hypovolemia, hemorrhagic), primary cardiac disease, other toxins (e.g., narcotics, benzodiazepine overdose).
- Neuromuscular – focal or diffuse primary CNS disease (e.g., neoplasia, distemper, other infectious disease), ethylene glycol, hypocalcemia, hepatic or uremic encephalopathy, IVDD, FCE, other neurotoxins.
- Respiratory – primary respiratory disease (e.g., allergic and parasitic airway disease, fungal or bacterial pneumonia), congestive heart failure, pain, sedative/narcotic overdose.
- Integument – drug eruption/reaction, sunburn, thermal burn, vasculitis, contact dermatitis, pyoderma, insect/arthropod bite, parasitic, other primary skin disease may be suspected based upon location of lesion.
- Gastrointestinal – primary gastrointestinal disease (e.g., parasite, foreign body, infectious, inflammatory), other toxin, primary neuropathy, secondary gastrointestinal (neoplasia, pancreatitis, hepatobiliary disease, renal disease, endocrinopathy).

 **DIAGNOSTICS**

### Clinical Pathological Findings

- Chemistry profile— possible increase in AST, ALP, and ALT (primarily reported in cats).

### Other Diagnostics

- Confirmation of terpinen-4-ol in urine by GC-MS (concentration will decrease with IV fluid therapy, so pretreatment samples should be obtained).

### Pathological Findings

- No specific findings expected.

 **THERAPEUTICS**

### Detoxification

- Bathe with liquid hand dishwashing detergent to remove excess oils and reduce dermal absorption.
- Induction of emesis is not usually recommended following ingestion of the liquid/oil formulation due to rapid systemic absorption and onset of clinical signs. It is unlikely to prevent intoxication and should be considered *only* if the patient is asymptomatic and the ingestion was within 15–30 minutes.
- Repeated doses of activated charcoal (PO q 6–8 hours over 24 hours) due to enterohepatic recirculation if no risk of aspiration and GI motility is normal. Give first dose with a cathartic (e.g., sorbitol) and subsequent doses without.
- If mucous membrane/oral irritation is present, consider flushing the oral cavity.

## Appropriate Health Care

- IV fluid therapy to maintain hydration and tissue perfusion. The use of colloid therapy for persistent hypotension may be necessary (i.e., Hetastarch).
- Body temperature regulation and heat support PRN, as hypothermia is common.
- Other supportive measures are largely related to nursing care dependent upon the CNS status of the patient.
- With severe CNS depression, intubation and mechanical ventilation may be needed.

## Antidote

- No antidote available.

## Drug(s) of Choice

- Hepatoprotectants if indicated based on lab results (e.g., SAMe, loading dose 40 mg/kg q 24 hours × 2–4 days, maintenance dose 18–20 mg/kg PO q 24 hours × 2–3 weeks).
- Methocarbamol 25–250 mg/kg, IV, as needed; administer slowly to effect; may be administered as a constant rate infusion (cats).
- Benzodiazepines.
    - Diazepam may be administered IV, rectally, or intranasally. General dosage range is 0.5–2 mg/kg (dogs) and 0.3–2 mg/kg (cats), depending on route and concomitant medications. Repeat dosing may be required. Consult a veterinary drug formulary for specifics.
    - Midazolam may be administered IV, IM, or intranasally. General dosage range is 0.1–0.5 mg/kg (dogs) and 0.2–0.5 mg/kg (cats), depending on route and concomitant medications. Repeat dosing may be required. Consult a veterinary drug formulary for specifics.
- Maropitant 1 mg/kg, SQ or IV (over 1–2 minutes) q 24 hours, if needed for vomiting or prior to activated charcoal.
- Atropine 0.02–0.04 mg/kg IV, IM, or SQ as needed, for severe bradycardia.
- Vasopressors, e.g., dopamine 2–20 **mcg**/kg/min IV CRI or dobutamine for persistent hypotension.

## Precautions/Interactions

- Do not administer oral medications/activated charcoal to animals with CNS depression unless the airway is protected.
- Monitor serum sodium closely if administering activated charcoal (risk of hypernatremia).

## Patient Monitoring

- Monitor during use of warming therapies to prevent hyperthermia or burns.
- If severe CNS signs:
    - monitor TPR every 5–15 minutes until stable.
    - rotate body position to prevent atelectasis or thermal burns.
    - monitor blood pressure closely until stable.
- Daily renal values should be evaluated while in hospital until normal.
- Hepatic values may not normalize and appropriate short-term monitoring is needed.
    - Recheck liver enzymes q 5–7 days until clinical signs and liver enzymes return to normal.
    - PRN monitoring of vital parameters until stabilized, then 3–4 times daily.

### Diet

- Typically, no changes are needed.
- With severe CNS depression, withhold feeding until stable.

## COMMENTS

### Prevention/Avoidance

- Provide appropriate client education on the use of herbal or "natural" remedies.
- Urge clients to consult with veterinarian prior to use of any alternative therapies.
- Appropriate dilutions of tea tree oil can be used, but clients should consult with veterinarian prior to use; the use of 100% oil is never recommended.
- Owners should be aware that concentrated tea tree oil is also toxic to humans if ingested. Poisoning has been reported in children and adults.

### Possible Complications

- Severe and unresponsive CNS depression leading to bradycardia, hypoperfusion, and coma.

### Expected Course and Prognosis

- Good with appropriate treatment and no underlying health problems.

### Synonyms

Tea tree oil is also called melaleuca oil (from *Melaleuca alternifolia*, the tea tree).

### See Also

Chapter 87 Essential Oils/Liquid Potpourri Phenols and Pine Oils

### Abbreviations

See Appendix 1 for a complete list.
- FCE = fibrocartilaginous emboli
- GC-MS = gas chromatography-mass spectrometry
- IVDD = intervertebral disc disease
- SAMe = s-adenosyl-methionine

### Suggested Reading

Bischoff K, Fessesswork G. Australian tea tree (Melaleuca alternifolia) oil poisoning in three purebred cats. *J Vet Diagn Invest* 1998;10:208–210.

Khan SA, McLean MK, Slater MR. Concentrated tea tree oil toxicosis in dogs and cats: 443 cases (2002–2012). *J Am Vet Med Assoc* 2014;244:95–99.

Villar D, Knight M, Hansen S, Buck W. Toxicity of melaleuca oil and related essential oils applied topically on dogs and cats. *Vet Hum Toxicol* 1994;36:139–142.

**Author**: Seth L. Cohen, DVM
**Consulting Editor**: Ahna G. Brutlag, DVM, MS, DABT, DABVT

# Home Care and Recreational Products

# Chapter 89

# Acids

## DEFINITION/OVERVIEW

- Acids are chemical compounds that act as proton donors. They have a pH less than 7.0. The most common harmful acids encountered include hydrochloric (muriatic), sulfuric, nitric, phosphoric, and oxalic acids.
- Exposures can be oral, dermal, ocular, or inhalational. Oropharyngeal and esophageal burns are most common.
- Immediate pain occurs on contact with strong acids, which can serve to limit injury.
- Treatment is focused on mitigating tissue injury and managing clinical signs.
- Severe sequelae such as esophageal stricture, aspiration pneumonia, and GI perforation are possible.
- Prognosis is usually good with prompt treatment. Prognosis is guarded if stricture, GI perforation, or aspiration pneumonia develops.

## ETIOLOGY/PATHOPHYSIOLOGY

- Acid exposures are usually accidental and rarely malicious. Oral exposures are most common, but ocular, dermal, and inhalational exposures can occur. Sources include the following:
  - Household cleaners such as toilet and drain cleaners.
  - Automotive batteries (also commonly contain lead in addition to sulfuric acid).
  - Metal or rust cleaners.
  - Pool cleaners and sanitizers.
  - Industrial cleaners and stain removers.

### Mechanism of Action

- Acids cause rapid protein coagulation and necrosis upon contact with body tissues. The proton donated from the acid joins with a water molecule from tissue to form hydronium ions ($H_3O^+$). This leads to protein desiccation and denaturation. Inflammatory cytokines are released, and cellular necrosis and eventually mucosal sloughing occur. The precipitation of the proteins forms an eschar, which can be protective to underlying tissues.

### Pharmacokinetics or Toxicokinetics – Absorption, Distribution, Metabolism, Excretion

- Systemic absorption of acids is not typically a concern (except hydrofluoric acid – see Chapter 13).
- Rarely, acidemia may result from systemic absorption through injured tissue.

*Blackwell's Five-Minute Veterinary Consult Clinical Companion: Small Animal Toxicology*, Third Edition.
Edited by Lynn R. Hovda, Ahna G. Brutlag, Robert H. Poppenga, and Steven E. Epstein.
© 2024 John Wiley & Sons, Inc. Published 2024 by John Wiley & Sons, Inc.

- Ions such as hydrogen, chloride (hydrochloric acid), or sulfate (sulfuric acid), if systemically absorbed, are well distributed and may disrupt normal metabolic function.

## Toxicity

- Acids with pH 2.0 or lower have the potential to cause corrosive injury to the gastrointestinal mucosa and epidermis.
- The corneal epithelium can be damaged by acids with a pH of 3.5 or lower.
- Specific chemical, concentration, and pH can usually be found in any accompanying Safety Data Sheets.
- Generally, the longer the contact and the more concentrated the acid, the greater the injury.

## Systems Affected

- Gastrointestinal – oropharyngeal, esophageal, gastric, and duodenal mucosal irritation, edema, ulceration, and necrosis can occur. Perforation and stricture are possible sequelae. Oropharyngeal and esophageal injury is most common.
- Skin/exocrine – dermal erythema and burns with infection, eschar, and scarring as possible sequelae.
- Ophthalmic – corneal and conjunctival ulceration and necrosis can occur. Corneal perforation and scarring as well as visual impairment are possible sequelae.
- Respiratory – bronchospasm, pulmonary edema, and pneumonitis are common after inhalational exposure. Aspiration pneumonia can develop subsequent to pharyngeal and gastrointestinal injury. Pharyngeal edema can cause airway obstruction.
- Cardiovascular – in severe cases, hypovolemic or distributive shock is possible, resulting in hypotension and tachycardia.

 **SIGNALMENT/HISTORY**

## Risk Factors

- Companion animal species are at highest risk due to close living proximity to cleansers and sanitizers.

## Historical Findings

- Product is often spilled, and packaging often found damaged or chewed. Presenting complaints are based on the route of exposure. They are described with the clinical features below.

 **CLINICAL FEATURES**

- Physical exam findings based on route of exposure.
  - Oral – white, gray, or black lesions of the lips, mouth, and pharynx; ptyalism, dysphagia, oropharyngeal pain and edema; tongue protrusion, lip licking, pawing or rubbing the face or mouth, vomiting, hematemesis, regurgitation, difficulty eating or anorexia, lethargy, abdominal pain, nausea, depression, pyrexia, tachycardia (pain). Stridor can be present if pharyngeal edema is severe.
  - Dermal – pain, self-mutilation, skin erythema, ulceration, blanching, or eschar; evidence of self-mutilation of affected area, lameness may be present if the feet are affected. Pyrexia and tachycardia are also common findings.
  - Ocular – blepharospasm, pain, epiphora, corneal ulceration or perforation, chemosis, conjunctival ulceration, lethargy, pawing or rubbing of the eye, ocular discharge.

- Inhalation – sneezing, coughing, stridor, dyspnea, tachypnea, pallor or cyanosis, pulmonary crackles or wheezes. Pyrexia and tachycardia are also common findings.

# DIFFERENTIAL DIAGNOSIS

- Alkali exposure.
- Cationic detergent exposure.
- Thermal injury.
- Electrical injury.
- Trauma.

# DIAGNOSTICS

- Typically diagnosed based on history and compatible physical examination findings.

## Clinical Pathological Findings

- CBC – may be normal or show neutrophilia acutely. Decompensated patients may show anemia, and neutrophilia or neutropenia with a left shift.
- Serum chemistry – no characteristic changes expected.

## Other Diagnostics

- Thoracic and abdominal radiographs – may show pulmonary edema, pneumothorax, pneumoperitoneum or pleural or peritoneal effusions if GI perforation is present.
- Ultrasound – may help detect GI perforation or pulmonary edema.
- Endoscopy – considered the best tool for initial diagnosis and evaluation of GI integrity. Must be done very carefully as tissue may be delicate, and scope should not be passed beyond any severe lesions. Avoid endoscopy during the subacute phase of tissue healing (days 3–14) as this is when risk of perforation is highest.
- Fluorescein stain – to evaluate corneal integrity.
- Abdominocentesis – if septic peritonitis is suspected.

## Pathological Findings

- Lesions are consistent with coagulative necrosis. Acutely, edema and inflammation predominate. Polymorphoneclear leukocytes infiltrate injured areas and granulation tissue may begin to develop.
- Depending on the severity of the injury, inflammation may extend through muscularis and serosa. After several days, edema decreases and fibroblasts proliferate. Eventually, collagen deposition and neovascularization will occur in healing tissue.

# THERAPEUTICS

- The goals are to mitigate tissue injury, manage signs, and monitor for sequelae.

## Detoxification

- Oral – dilution with water or milk should be performed immediately. Induction of emesis and gastric lavage are contraindicated. Activated charcoal is NOT recommended.
- Dermal – affected area should be flushed copiously with water and then bathed with a liquid hand dish-washing detergent.
- Ocular – ocular irrigation with tepid water for a minimum of 20 minutes.
- Inhalational – return pet to fresh air, provide oxygen if necessary.

## Appropriate Health Care

- Patients exposed to concentrated acids should always be evaluated by a veterinarian.
- Patients exposed to weak or dilute acids (pH 2–4) may be able to be treated at home with decontamination (dilution, bath, or ocular irrigation) and then only presented to the veterinarian if clinical signs develop.
- Patients with systemic signs or persistent anorexia or adipsia should be hospitalized. After decontamination, provide symptomatic and supportive care based on patient's clinical status.

## Antidote

- None.

## Drug(s) of Choice

- Antiemetics – standard care for any oral exposure.
  - Maropitant 1 mg/kg SC or IV (over 1–2 min) q 24 hours.
  - Ondansetron 0.2–1 mg/kg IV (slow) q 8–12 hours.
- Gastrointestinal protectants – standard care for any oral exposure to acid with pH less than 2.0.
  - Pantoprazole 1 mg/kg IV q 12 hours × 14 days or until resolution of ulcerations.
  - Omeprazole 1 mg/kg PO q 12 hours × 14 days or until resolution of ulcerations.
  - Sucralfate slurry 0.25–1 g PO q 6–8 hours × 14 days or until resolution of ulcerations.
- Analgesics.
  - Opioids are recommended for analgesia: buprenorphine 10–30 mcg/kg IV q 4–8 hours.
  - Topical lidocaine-based mouthwashes (use with caution in cats as lidocaine overdose can cause methemoglobinemia as well as CNS and cardiovascular depression).
  - Topical 1% atropine for ocular cycloplegia.
- Crystalloid fluid therapy – as needed to maintain perfusion and hydration.
- Antibiotics – indicated if there is concern for secondary infection or GI perforation.
  - Ampicillin/sulbactam 22–30 mg/kg IV q 8 hours.
  - Enrofloxacin.
    - 10–20 mg/kg IV q 24 hours (dogs).
    - 5 mg/kg IV q 24 hours (cats).
  - Topical ophthalmic broad-spectrum antibiotic for corneal ulcers.
- Oxygen – for patients with respiratory compromise or shock.
- Intubation – may be indicated with severe upper airway edema.
- Blood products – fresh whole blood or packed RBCs may be needed for patients with severe GI hemorrhage.
- Corticosteroids – use is controversial as they can reduce inflammation and fibroblastic activity but can also increase risk for infection and perforation. A single dose or short course is only recommended where potential benefits outweigh the risks (e.g., severe airway edema) in the first 48 hours after an exposure. A broad-spectrum antibiotic should be started if corticosteroids are utilized.
  - Dexamethasone SP 0.1–0.2 mg/kg IV q 24 hours.

## Precautions/Interactions

- Neutralization of burns by application of an alkaline substance is **contraindicated**. The reaction creates heat and worsens the injury.

## Surgical Considerations

- Exploratory thoracotomy/laparotomy is indicated as soon as GI perforation is suspected. Placement of gastrostomy or jejunostomy tube is recommended.
- Conjunctival grafts may be necessary to repair severe corneal ulceration.
- Dermal grafting may become necessary to repair large areas of dermal necrosis.

## Patient Monitoring

- Overall patient clinical status and appearance of lesions are best indicators of treatment effectiveness.
- Temperature, HR, RR, and pain score should be monitored at least four times daily in hospitalized patients.
- CBC and electrolytes should be monitored daily in hospitalized patients or if there is acute patient clinical decline.
- Venous or arterial blood gas should be monitored in patients with respiratory compromise or if hypoxemia is suspected.

## Diet

- A soft, bland diet is recommended for patients with oral or GI lesions that are still eating.
- Gastrotomy or jejunostomy tube placement and enteral nutrition are recommended for patients with persistent anorexia.

 **COMMENTS**

- The absence of oral lesions on physical exam does not rule out the possibility of esophageal or gastric lesions.
- In theory, ingestion of large quantities of oxalic acid can lead to hypocalcemia, neurological signs, and renal injury. However, with immediate pain upon contact, consumption is limited and there is not enough oxalic acid distributed systemically to cause these signs.

## Prevention/Avoidance

- All cleaning products, sanitizers, and batteries should be sealed and kept out of reach of curious pets. Do not use the laundry or utility space to confine pets.

## Possible Complications

- Aspiration pneumonia.
- Esophageal, pyloric, or duodenal strictures (weeks to months after initial exposure).
- Visual impairment or blindness.
- Dermal scarring and contracture.

## Expected Course and Prognosis

- After corrosive injury, there are three phases to tissue declaration and healing.
  - 1–7 days: inflammatory phase, characterized by cellular necrosis and thrombotic events in the vasculature.
  - 3–14 days: granulation phase, highest risk of perforation.
  - 14 days+: fibrous phase, scarring and possible stricture formation may occur.
- With prompt treatment, prognosis is generally good. If pulmonary edema, aspiration pneumonia, infection, perforation, or stricture develops, prognosis is guarded.

## See Also

Chapter 90 Alkalis
Chapter 95 Phenols and Pine Oils
Chapter 13 Hydrofluoric Acid
Chapter 96 Soaps, Detergents, Fabric Softeners, Enzymatic Cleaners, and Deodorizers

## Suggested Reading

Calello DP. Caustics. In: Brent J (ed.) *Critical Care Toxicology Diagnosis and Management of the Critically Poisoned Patient*, 2nd edn. Cham: Springer International, 2017; pp. 2005–2019.

Gwaltney-Brant SM. Miscellaneous indoor toxicants. In: Peterson ME, Talcott PA (eds) *Small Animal Toxicology*, 3rd edn. St Louis: Elsevier, 2013; pp. 294–295.

Richardson J. Acids and alkalis. In: Plumlee KH (ed.) *Clinical Veterinary Toxicology*. St Louis: Mosby, 2005; pp. 139–140.

**Author:** Renee Tourdot, DVM, DABT, DABVT
**Consulting Editor:** Ahna G. Brutlag, DVM, MS, DABT, DABVT

# Chapter 90

# Alkalis

## DEFINITION/OVERVIEW

- Alkaline substances have a pH of greater than 7, are proton acceptors and come in a variety of solid and liquid forms. Commonly encountered alkalis include sodium hydroxide, sodium hypochlorite, potassium hydroxide, and calcium hydroxide.
- Exposures can be oral, dermal, ocular, or via inhalation. Mucosal injuries to the oropharyngeal tissues, esophagus, and stomach are the most common.
- Extent of caustic injury is dependent on concentration, viscosity, pH, and duration of contact.
- Treatment following exposure includes efforts to reduce caustic injury, management of clinical signs, and monitoring for sequelae.
- Prognosis is good in most exposures with prompt intervention.
- Prognosis is guarded if severe sequelae such as esophageal stricture or perforation, GI perforation, aspiration pneumonia or pneumonitis develop.

## ETIOLOGY/PATHOPHYSIOLOGY

- Exposures are generally via accidental oral ingestion and/or dermal contact. Splash ocular contact or inhalation exposures can be seen when chemicals, such as those for pools, are mixed improperly.
- Commonly encountered alkalis.
  - 4–6% sodium hypochlorite as in household bleach (pH 11–12).
  - 10–15% sodium hypochlorite as in pool chemicals (pH 13).
  - 20–36% potassium hydroxide as in batteries (pH 13–14).
  - 2–4% sodium hydroxide as in chemical hair straighteners (pH 12).
  - 3.75% calcium hydroxide as in uncured cement (pH 12–13).

### Mechanism of Action

- Alkalis are proton acceptors and produce tissue damage through liquefactive necrosis.
- The caustic injury begins with edema and inflammation, then progresses to thrombosis, necrosis, and ulceration. No eschar is formed to limit depth of injury, and the saponification of fats and proteins softens tissues, allowing for deeper wounds. Nerve endings are damaged, delaying pain responses and potentially allowing longer contact time.
- Additionally, the body's attempt to neutralize the hydroxide ion (OH-) formed during contact is exothermic, only adding to the injury.

---

*Blackwell's Five-Minute Veterinary Consult Clinical Companion: Small Animal Toxicology*, Third Edition. Edited by Lynn R. Hovda, Ahna G. Brutlag, Robert H. Poppenga, and Steven E. Epstein.
© 2024 John Wiley & Sons, Inc. Published 2024 by John Wiley & Sons, Inc.

## Pharmacokinetics or Toxicokinetics – Absorption, Distribution, Metabolism, Excretion

- Systemic absorption of alkalis is not typically concerning, and systemic alkalosis is not expected.
- Exception: large ingestions of chlorine bleach may cause hyperchloremic acidosis and hypernatremia.

## Toxicity

- Exposures that involve prolonged contact time, concentrated alkalis or those with pH >12 carry a higher risk for ulceration and perforation.
- Weak (pH <11) or diluted alkalis tend to cause irritation rather than ulceration.
- OSHA Safety Data Sheets can be referenced for physical and chemical properties, including pH, concentration, and any hazard classifications.

## Systems Affected

- Gastrointestinal – oropharyngeal, esophageal, gastrointestinal mucosal caustic injury and ulceration. Sequelae may include stricture, perforation, sepsis.
- Skin/exocrine – mild irritation to severe contact burns. Sequelae may include cellulitis, infection, contraction, slow healing wounds.
- Ocular – irritation to ulceration. Sequelae may include vision loss, corneal malacia, and perforation.
- Respiratory – mild upper respiratory irritation to dyspnea. Sequelae may include laryngeal edema, aspiration pneumonia, pneumonitis, hypoxemia.
- Cardiovascular – hypotension and tachycardia may be associated with hypovolemic (blood loss) or vasodilatory (sepsis) shock.

 ## SIGNALMENT/HISTORY

## Risk Factors

- Any animal could be at risk, but companion animals are by far the most commonly exposed. This is likely due to in-home access to chemicals, degreasers, and detergents.

## Historical Findings

- Witnessed or discovered evidence of chewed, ripped, or spilled alkaline products. Reported clinical signs would vary based on route of exposure but could include the following.
  - Oral – drooling, pawing at mouth, retching, vomiting, bloody vomit, inappetence, and lethargy.
  - Dermal – redness, swelling, dermal sores, licking at wounds, lethargy, and a change in posture or gait.
  - Ocular – blepharospasm, conjunctivitis, tearing, ocular discharge, face rubbing, and lethargy.
  - Respiratory – head shaking, sneezing, panting, coughing, wheezing, lethargy, inappetence.

## Location and Circumstances of Poisoning

- Any area in which the animal has access to products such as chemical hair straighteners, dishwasher detergents, oven cleaners, drain openers, bleach, lye, or alkaline batteries – home, garage, shed, place of work.

# CLINICAL FEATURES

- Physical exam findings are based on route of exposure. Patients with caustic injury from any route may be painful, lethargic, febrile, and tachycardic.
  - Oral – lesions can be seen on the tongue and surfaces of the oral and pharyngeal cavities. Other findings include ptyalism, oropharyngeal pain and edema, esophagitis, abdominal pain, stridor (laryngeal edema), and depression.
  - Dermal – erythema, swelling, ulceration, full-thickness burns. Posture or gait changes if ulcerations on feet or legs.
  - Ocular – blepharospasm, pain, chemosis, conjunctival inflammation to ulceration, and corneal ulceration, malacia, or perforation.
  - Inhalation – sneezing, coughing, tachypnea, dyspnea, stridor, cyanosis, respiratory distress.

# DIFFERENTIAL DIAGNOSIS

- Acid exposure.
- Cationic detergent exposure.
- Thermal or electrical injury.
- Trauma.

## Clinical Pathological Findings

- CBC: often normal to mild inflammatory leukogram in mild cases. May see neutropenia with left shift and/or anemia in severe cases.
- Serum chemistry: see Patient Monitoring.

# DIAGNOSTICS

- Thoracic and abdominal radiographs: may see aspiration pneumonia, pneumonitis, pulmonary edema, pleural or peritoneal effusion, pneumomediastinum or pneumoperitoneum. Can also visualize any batteries remaining in the GIT.
- Endoscopy: used to assess the extent of injury and integrity of esophagus/upper GIT. Any endoscopic examinations should be done with care as the tissues will be delicate and prone to perforation. The esophagus will be most friable in the necrotic and granulation phases of injury (days 3–12).
- Abdominal ultrasound: may aid in diagnosis of GI perforation +/- abdominocentesis.
- Fluorescein stain: to determine the extent of corneal injury.
- Culture and sensitivity: indicated when infection and/or sepsis are present.

# THERAPEUTICS

- Goals are to reduce caustic tissue injury, manage clinical signs, support patient, and monitor for sequelae.

## Detoxification

- Oral exposures.
  - Emesis, gastric lavage, and activated charcoal are **contraindicated**.
  - Dilution (milk or water) within three hours is standard of care in patients not actively vomiting.

- Ophthalmic exposures.
  - Ocular irrigation with water or saline for 20 minutes, flushing behind nictitans gland. Topical ophthalmic proparacaine +/- sedation of the patient may be needed.
- Dermal exposures: bathe using a mild liquid hand dishwashing detergent.
- Inhalation exposures: move patient to fresh air, wipe nares free of residue, and provide oxygen as indicated.

### Appropriate Health Care

- Encounters with concentrated alkalis warrant a veterinary exam.
- Patients exposed to diluted or weak alkalis may be candidates for at-home decontamination and monitoring initially, taking in for exam if clinical signs develop.
- Patients with anorexia, lethargy, fever, or other signs of systemic illness require hospitalization.
- Treatment is symptomatic and supportive based on clinical picture.

### Drug(s) of Choice

- Antiemetics – standard of care for any oral exposure.
  - Maropitant 1 mg/kg SQ or IV (over 1–2 min) q 24 hours.
  - Ondansetron 0.2–1 mg/kg IV (slow) q 8–12 hours.
- GI protectants – standard of care for any oral exposure to alkalis with pH >11.
  - Sucralfate slurry 0.25–1 g PO q 6–8 hours × 14 days or until resolution of ulcerations.
  - Proton pump inhibitor × 14 days or until resolution of ulcerations.
    - Omeprazole 1 mg/kg PO q 12 hours.
    - Pantoprazole 1 mg/kg IV q 12 hours.
- Analgesia.
  - Opioids such as
    - Buprenorphine for moderate to severe pain: dog/cat 5–30 mcg/kg IV q 4–8 hours; cat (Simbadol® 1.8 mg/mL) 0.24 mg/kg SQ q 24 hours × 1–3 days.
    - Tramadol for mild pain: dog 4–10 mg/kg PO q 8 hours; cat 2–4 mg/kg PO q 12 hours.
  - Lidocaine-diphenhydramine-MgOH/AlOH mouthwashes. Must use with caution in cats due to risk of lidocaine toxicosis.
  - Ophthalmic cycloplegics such as atropine or tropicamide may reduce pain from ciliary spasm.
- Crystalloid fluids as needed to maintain hydration and ensure adequate perfusion.
- Antibiotics if signs of secondary infection or GI perforation.
  - For minor infections, consider cephalosporins such as cefpodoxime 5 mg/kg PO q 24 hours for 5–7 days, or 2–3 days beyond resolution.
  - For severe infections, consider potentiated penicillin beta-lactamase inhibitors such as ampicillin/sulbactam 22–30 mg/kg IV q 8 hours.
  - Dermal application of silver sulfasalazine cream.
  - Ophthalmic triple antibiotic ointment.
- Oxygen as needed for respiratory signs or patients in shock +/- intubation if upper airway obstruction from laryngeal/pharyngeal edema.
- Blood products may be needed in patients with significant GI hemorrhage.
- Other therapies.
  - Topical ophthalmic application of autogenous serum can be considered in cases of corneal malacia.
  - Respiratory therapies for sequelae such as pneumonia may include nebulization, coupage, and bronchodilators (e.g., terbutaline 0.01 mg/kg IM, SQ, or slow IV q 8–12 hours).

- Steroids are controversial. They can reduce inflammation and may reduce risk of stricture, but also increase the risk of infection and perforation. A single dose or short course could be considered in the first 48 hours when the benefit outweighs the risk. A broad-spectrum antibiotic should be used if steroids are implemented.
    o Dexamethasone SP 0.1–0.2 mg/kg IV q 24 hours.

## Precautions/Interactions

- NSAIDs and steroids can increase the risk of perforation.
- Following ingestion, emesis, gastric lavage, and activated charcoal are **contraindicated**.
- Neutralization by application of an acidic substance is **contraindicated**. The reaction creates heat and worsens the injury.

## Surgical Considerations

- Placement of feeding tube for nutritional support (gastrostomy or jejunostomy).
- Exploratory celiotomy if GI perforation is suspected.
- Dermal necrotic tissue debridement. Skin grafting in large areas of dermal necrosis.
- For upper airway obstruction with severe laryngeal or pharyngeal edema where intubation is not possible, tracheostomy should be performed.
- Temporary tarsorrhaphy to protect the corneal surface or a conjunctival graft for melting ulcers or perforations.

## Patient Monitoring

- Indicators of treatment effectiveness include patient clinical status and lesion appearance.
- Hospitalized patients should have frequent pain score evaluations. HR/BP/RR and temperature should be monitored 3–4 times daily, or as needed based on clinical picture.
- Severe cases and any patients with an acute decline should have daily labs (CBC, BUN/creatinine, urine output, albumin, total protein, electrolytes, acid–base, +/- coagulation profile).

## Diet

- Enteral nutrition is preferred to parental nutrition. A soft, bland diet should be fed to patients with oral/GI lesions that are still able to eat. Feeding tube (gastrostomy or jejunostomy) placement may be needed in patients with persistent anorexia.

 # COMMENTS

- The absence of oral lesions *does not* rule out the presence of esophageal or GI injury.
- Signs of pain/injury can be delayed for hours with less caustic alkalis, while viscous, concentrated alkalis may cause severe acute necrosis.
- Caustic injury from alkalis is often deeper and more severe than corrosive injury from acids.

## Prevention/Avoidance

- All detergents, chemicals, and batteries should be kept out of reach of animals.

## Possible Complications

- Esophageal perforation or stricture, altered esophageal motility, GI perforation, and septic peritonitis.
- Aspiration pneumonia,
- Slow healing, deep wounds,
- Melting corneal ulcers, corneal perforation, vision loss,

## Expected Course and Prognosis

- See Chapter 89 Acids for phases of tissue healing.
- Prognosis is good in most exposures with prompt intervention. Prognosis is guarded if severe sequelae such as perforation, stricture, or aspiration pneumonia develop.

## See Also

Chapter 89 Acids
Chapter 91 Batteries
Chapter 96 Soaps, Detergents, Fabric Softeners, Enzymatic Cleaners, and Deodorizers

## Suggested Reading

Calello DP. Caustics. In: Brent J (ed.) *Critical Care Toxicology Diagnosis and Management of the Critically Poisoned Patient*, 2nd edn. Cham: Springer International, 2017; pp. 2005–2019.

Gwaltney-Brant SM. Miscellaneous indoor toxicants. In: Peterson ME, Talcott PA (eds) *Small Animal Toxicology*, 3rd edn. St Louis: Elsevier, 2013; pp. 294–295.

Methasate A, Lohsiriwat V. Role of endoscopy in caustic injury of the esophagus. *World J Gastrointest Endosc* 2018;10(10):274–282.

Richardson J. Acids and alkalis. In: Plumlee KH (ed.) *Clinical Veterinary Toxicology*. St Louis: Mosby, 2005; pp. 139–140.

**Author**: Ginger Watts Brown, DVM, DABT, DABVT
**Consulting Editor**: Ahna G. Brutlag, DVM, MS, DABT, DABVT

# Chapter 91

# Batteries

## DEFINITION/OVERVIEW

- Exposure commonly occurs after access to remote controls and electronic toys.
- Clinical signs include drooling, frequent swallowing, pawing at mouth, refusal to eat, regurgitation, abdominal pain, and, rarely, death.
- Multiple battery types: alkaline dry cell and lithium ion button/disc are most common and have differing mechanisms of action and management considerations.
  - Disc/button batteries.
    - ○ Lithium ion batteries were responsible for 91% of human pediatric esophageal perforations and are the most common variety of disc or button batteries. Other varieties include alkaline, zinc air, and manganese.
    - ○ Noncorrosive but cause electrochemical burns in the GI tract within 15 minutes.
    - ○ Entrapment within the esophagus is life-threatening.
    - ○ Irrigation: honey, sucralfate (ideal) or tap water (less effective) will slow damage.
  - Dry cell batteries.
    - ○ Most common household batteries categorized based on size (e.g., AAA or D; come in many shapes).
    - ○ Create a pH gradient across which ions flow.
    - ○ Contain corrosive alkaline compounds such as potassium or sodium hydroxide.
    - ○ Sharp metal casing can injure tissues.
- General treatment includes tissue irrigation, locating the battery, and removal by endoscopy, surgery or natural passage, followed by supportive care.
- Prognosis is good. Rarely see severe complications if the battery exits the GI tract within 24 hours.

## ETIOLOGY/PATHOPHYSIOLOGY

**Mechanism of Action**

- Disc/button.
  - Lithium batteries contain no corrosive compounds but when both sides of the battery are in contact with the lining of the esophagus or GIT, electric current is generated, causing deep ulcers and, potentially, perforation.
- Dry cell.
  - Battery casing that is chewed or degraded by stomach acid leaks alkaline (potassium hydroxide or sodium hydroxide) or acidic (ammonium chloride or magnesium dioxide) contents.

---

*Blackwell's Five-Minute Veterinary Consult Clinical Companion: Small Animal Toxicology*, Third Edition. Edited by Lynn R. Hovda, Ahna G. Brutlag, Robert H. Poppenga, and Steven E. Epstein.

- Acid dry cell batteries cause coagulation necrosis and alkaline dry cell batteries trigger liquefaction necrosis.
- As the acid or alkaline contents react with local tissues, the contents become nonreactive and systemic absorption does not typically occur.
- If the battery remains lodged in the gastrointestinal tract for a prolonged period, the heavy metals in the casing (lead, mercury, zinc, cobalt, cadmium) may cause toxicosis.

## Toxicity

- Disc/button.
  - One 20 mm, 3-volt battery can cause tissue necrosis after only 15 minutes of tissue contact.
  - Only 2% of pediatric esophageal perforations occur less than 24 hours after ingestion.
  - Most are passed unchanged in the stool.
  - Heavy metal toxicity is not a described sequela (see Expected Course and Prognosis).
- Dry cell.
  - Puncture/ingestion of just one battery poses risk for tissue damage.
  - If the battery remains lodged in the gastrointestinal tract for a prolonged period, the heavy metals in the casing (lead, mercury, zinc, cobalt, cadmium) may cause toxicosis.

## Systems Affected

### Gastrointestinal

- Disc: ulceration and potentially perforation of the esophagus and trachea leading to tracheoesophageal fistulas.
- Dry cell: traumatic injury from chewed casings to oral cavity, esophagus, stomach, and small intestine. Necrosis from contact with battery contents if casing is punctured. Ulceration may lead to GIT perforation, secondary peritonitis, and tracheoesophageal fistulas.

### Skin/Exocrine

- Disc: none.
- Dry cell: traumatic injury to the muzzle from sharp edges of the chewed battery casing.

### Respiratory

- Disc: secondary to esophageal ulceration/tracheoesophageal fistulas.
- Dry cell: stridor from pharyngeal ulceration. Dyspnea from airway obstruction. Chemical pneumonitis if corrosive material inhaled.

### Hepatobiliary/Nervous

- Disc/dry cell: possible hepatic injury secondary to lead, mercury, zinc, cobalt or cadmium heavy metal toxicity if the casing of a dry cell battery breaks down due to prolonged exposure to stomach acid. See chapters on lead (104), zinc (105) and Appendix 4 Other Metallic Toxicants.

### Hemic/Lymphatic/Immune

- Disc: ulceration of the GIT may lead to fistulization into major vessels, and massive hemorrhage/exsanguination.
- Dry cell: intravascular hemolysis may develop secondary to heavy metal toxicosis if batteries are retained in the GIT. See chapters on lead (104), zinc (105) and Appendix 4 Other Metallic Toxicants.

# SIGNALMENT/HISTORY

## Risk Factors

- No breed or sex predilection. Anecdotally, exposure occurs more frequently in young dogs.

## Historical Findings

- Owner reports witnessing the ingestion or finding the partially ingested battery or battery-containing device.
- Owners may report hypersalivation, pawing at the mouth, anorexia, or vomiting. Signs typically begin 2–12 hours after ingestion.

# CLINICAL FEATURES

- Oral cavity may be erythematous, with ulcers on the gums, tongue, and larynx/pharynx.
- Occlusal surfaces of the teeth may be black or gray from exposure to dry cell battery contents.
- Hypersalivation.
- Frequent swallowing.
- Abdominal pain, free abdominal fluid, and distension could occur.
- Other clinical signs (e.g., evidence of hemolysis) may develop if heavy metal toxicosis is present.

# DIFFERENTIAL DIAGNOSIS

- There are multiple other conditions that can cause acute gastroenteritis with ulceration and possible perforation. NSAID toxicosis, foreign body ingestion, pancreatitis, corrosive chemical ingestion, and endotoxemia ("garbage gut") can present with similar clinical signs.

# DIAGNOSTICS

## Clinical Pathological Findings

- No changes expected initially.
- PCV/TS or CBC to assess blood loss, hydration, inflammation, or infection.
- Serum biochemistry prior to anesthesia or if ingestion occurred more than 24 hours earlier.

## Other Diagnostics

- Radiographs: determine the battery location. Include the back of the mouth and esophagus. Disc batteries can easily be mistaken for coins.
- Endoscopy to characterize ulcerations and potentially remove lodged batteries.

# THERAPEUTICS

- The goal is to stop further ulcerative damage, safely remove the battery, then provide supportive therapy for ulcerations.

## Detoxification

- Do not induce vomiting or give activated charcoal. Emesis may increase the potential for corrosive injury or esophageal entrapment of the battery. Activated charcoal will not bind to battery contents and increases risk of vomiting.
- Dilution: initiate immediately in patients less than 12 hours post ingestion.
  - Disc/button: give 10 mL honey or 10 mL of sucralfate slurry every 15 minutes until the battery is no longer in the esophagus or patient is 12 hours post ingestion. Owner can substitute 20 mL tap water in place of honey or sucralfate until arrival at the clinic.
  - Dry cell: irrigate the oral cavity and exposed skin for 10–15 minutes with tap water to remove or dilute any remaining caustic material.
- Battery removal.
  - Select the appropriate removal strategy based on the battery type, location on radiographs, and condition of the casing.
    - Disc/button: endoscopic removal from the esophagus and stomach. Allow natural passage of battery in the stomach and small intestine. Monitor stools and perform serial radiographs q 1–2 day to ensure passage within four days.
    - Intact dry cell: endoscopic removal from the esophagus. Allow natural passage of batteries in the stomach and small intestine. Monitor stools and perform serial radiographs q 1–2 day to ensure passage within four days.
    - Ruptured dry cell: endoscopic removal from the esophagus and surgical removal from the stomach and small intestine.

## Appropriate Health Care

- After battery removal, care will depend on the extent of the injury. Patients may benefit from a short course of supportive care while injury to their oral cavity, esophagus or stomach heals.

## Antidote

- None.

## Drug(s) of Choice

- Acid reduction.
  - Proton pump inhibitors (e.g., omeprazole 0.5–1 mg/kg PO q 24 hours, pantoprazole 0.7–1 mg/kg IV slowly q 24 hours).
  - Sucralfate slurry 0.25–1 g PO q 8 hours, on an empty stomach.
- Antiemetic/promotility agents.
  - Metoclopramide 0.2–0.5 mg/kg IM, IV, SQ or PO q 6–8 hours or 1–2 mg/kg delivered as a CRI over 24 hours.
  - Maropitant 1 mg/kg SQ or IV (over 1–2 minutes) or PO q 24 hours.
- Antimicrobials (if necessary).
  - Cefazolin 10–30 mg/kg IV q 8 hours and enrofloxacin 5–20 mg/kg IV q 12–24 hours (dogs).
  - Metronidazole 15 mg/kg PO q 12 hours.
- Pain relief.
  - Buprenorphine 0.005–0.01 mg/kg IV, IM, SQ or sublingual q 8 hours.
  - Topical analgesia (oral cavity only): Magic Mouthwash (multiple options – consult veterinary drug formulary) applied to affected areas of the mouth 3–4 times daily at least 30 minutes before or after eating.

### Precautions/Interactions

- Sucralfate should be given separately from other drugs.

### Patient Monitoring

- Monitor for esophageal stricture.
- Educate the pet owner on emesis vs regurgitation and monitoring for esophageal stricture.

### Diet

- Small quantities given frequently (unless fasting prior to surgery).
- NG or EG tube if voluntary intake is inadequate.
- Consider highly palatable, bioavailable, and calorie-dense diets such as RC Recovery, Hill's Prescription Diet a/d or Hill's Prescription Diet ONC Care, or Purina ProPlanRx Recovery Diet.

 **COMMENTS**

### Prevention/Avoidance

- Prevent access to batteries by disposing of them immediately and avoiding chew toys that contain batteries.

### Expected Course and Prognosis

- Less than 0.2% of children ingesting button batteries had complications.
- In case reviews of children, esophageal perforation took more than 10 hours to develop, occurring less than 24 hours after ingestion in less than 2% of cases.
- Once in the stomach, human button battery management is controversial. *In vitro* studies show that simulated gastric acids degrade the battery, releasing heavy metals, but toxicosis has not been reported. Most allow passage without intervention.
- 75% of child-ingested batteries pass in the stool within four days.
- Esophageal stricture may develop weeks after ingestion. Difficulty swallowing, drooling, loss of appetite, and regurgitation are common.

### Synonyms

Button battery, disc battery, alkaline battery, dry cell battery.

### See Also

Chapter 89 Acids
Chapter 90 Alkalis
Chapter 80 Foreign Objects
Chapter 104 Lead
Chapter 105 Zinc
Appendix 4 Other Metallic Toxicants

### Suggested Reading

Anfang RR, Jatana KR, Linn RL, Rhoades K, Fry J, Jacobs IN. pH-neutralizing esophageal irrigations as a novel mitigation strategy for button battery injury. *Laryngoscope* 2019;129:49–57.

Rebdandl W, Steffan I, Schramel P et al. Release of toxic metals from button batteries retained in the stomac: an in vitro study. *J Pediatr Surg* 2002;37:87–92.

Soto E, Reid N, Litovitz T. Time to perforation for button batteries lodged in the esophagus. *Am J Emerg Med* 2019;37:805–809.

Tanaka J, Yamashita M, Yamashita M, Kajigaya H. Esophageal electrochemical burns due to button type lithium batteries in dogs. *Vet Hum Toxicol* 1998;40(4):193–196.

Varga A, Kovács T, Saxena A. Analysis of complications after button battery ingestion in children. *Pediatr Emerg Care* 2018;34(6):443–446.

**Author**: Catherine Angle, DVM MPH

**Consulting Editor**: Ahna G. Brutlag, DVM, MS, DABT, DABVT

# Chapter 92

# Matches and Fireworks

## DEFINITION/OVERVIEW

- Matches contain potassium chlorate and possibly phosphorus sesquisulfide. The chlorates are the biggest concern for toxicosis. Animals exposed to chlorates can develop methemoglobinemia. Wooden matches can potentially be a foreign body.
- In fireworks, chlorates and barium are the toxins of most concern. They can cause methemoglobinemia, cardiovascular effects, and renal failure (see Table 92.1 for other possible ingredients). Used fireworks can have a different composition from unused, and the kinetics and toxicity can vary (increased or decreased bioavailability).
- Most match ingestions only cause GI signs, while serious toxicosis can result with firework ingestions.
- Poisoning by matches and fireworks is not common.

## ETIOLOGY/PATHOPHYSIOLOGY

### Mechanism of Action

- Barium: causes severe systemic hypokalemia by blocking the exit channel for potassium in skeletal muscle cells. Barium also stimulates skeletal, smooth, and cardiac muscle, causing violent peristalsis, arterial hypertension, and arrhythmias.
- Chlorates: locally irritating and potent oxidizing agents. The irritation leads to vomiting and diarrhea while oxidation of red blood cells causes hemolysis and methemoglobin formation. Chlorates are directly toxic to the proximal renal tubules, producing cellular necrosis and renal vasoconstriction. Hemoglobinemia and methemoglobin catalysis also contribute to the renal effects.

### Pharmacokinetics or Toxicokinetics – Absorption, Distribution, Metabolism, Excretion

- Barium: oral absorption of barium is generally rapid but depends on the solubility of the barium salt. Peak serum concentrations are reached within two hours after ingestion. Barium is distributed into the bone, with an estimated half-life of 50 days. The main route of excretion of barium is fecal (less than 3% is excreted renally).
- Chlorates: chlorates are well absorbed orally and are slowly excreted unchanged by the kidney.

### Toxicity

- Barium: $LD_{LO}$ (oral) human = 11 mg/kg.
- Barium chloride: $LD_{50}$ (oral) rat = 220 mg/kg.

*Blackwell's Five-Minute Veterinary Consult Clinical Companion: Small Animal Toxicology*, Third Edition.
Edited by Lynn R. Hovda, Ahna G. Brutlag, Robert H. Poppenga, and Steven E. Epstein.
© 2024 John Wiley & Sons, Inc. Published 2024 by John Wiley & Sons, Inc.

**TABLE 92.1 Toxicological information on the ingredients commonly found in fireworks.**

| Ingredient | Fireworks usage/toxicity information |
| --- | --- |
| Aluminum | Silver and white flames and sparks (common in sparklers)<br>Poor oral absorption; little risk of toxicity |
| Antimony (antimony sulfide) | Glitter effects<br>Poor oral absorption; poisoning is very rare |
| Barium (barium chlorate, barium nitrate) | Green colors and can help stabilize other volatile elements<br>Gastrointestinal, cardiac, neurological, and electrolyte issues can occur |
| Beryllium | White sparks<br>Poor oral absorption; inhalation can cause lung cancer |
| Calcium (calcium chlorate) | Orange coloring and used to deepen other colors<br>Oral irritation/corrosive injury |
| Cesium (cesium nitrate) | Indigo colors<br>Toxicity is of minor importance |
| Chlorine | Component of many oxidizers in fireworks |
| Copper (copper chloride, copper halides) | Blue colors<br>Copper salts are locally corrosive |
| Iron | Gold sparks (see Chapter 103 Iron) |
| Lithium (lithium carbonate) | Red color<br>Gastrointestinal signs |
| Magnesium | White sparks and improves brilliance |
| Phosphorus | Glow-in-the-dark effects and may be a component of the fuel<br>Red phosphorus (safety matches) is an insoluble substance that is nontoxic in oral ingestions. White phosphorus (fireworks) can cause severe gastroenteritis and cardiotoxic effects |
| Potassium (potassium nitrate, potassium perchlorate) | Violet color, black powder explosive and used to oxidize firework mixtures<br>Animals with normal renal function have minimal toxicity consisting of GI signs |
| Rubidium (rubidium nitrate) | Violet color |
| Sodium (sodium nitrate) | Gold or yellow colors<br>Nitrates can cause methemoglobinemia |
| Strontium (strontium carbonate) | Red color and used to stabilize firework mixtures<br>Gastrointestinal signs |
| Sulfur (sulfur dioxide) | Component of black powder<br>Vomiting and diarrhea are common following sulfur ingestion |
| Titanium | Silver sparks<br>Poor oral absorption; heavy dust exposures can cause coughing and dyspnea |
| Zinc | Smoke effects |

- Chlorates: $LD_{50}$ (oral) dog = 1000 mg/kg.
- Potassium chlorate: $LD_{50}$ (oral) rat = 1870 mg/kg.
- Sodium chlorate: $LD_{50}$ (oral) mouse = 596 mg/kg; rat = 1200 mg/kg.
- Methemoglobinemia (chlorate) can be seen with ingestions of more than one match per pound in dogs or 0.5 matches per pound of cat.

## Systems Affected

- Gastrointestinal – vomiting (possibly bloody), diarrhea, hypersalivation.
- Skin/exocrine – dermal burns.
- Nervous – lethargy.
- Hemic/lymphatic/immune – hemolysis, methemoglobinemia (chlorates).
- Cardiovascular – arrhythmias, hypertension.
- Respiratory – tachypnea, dyspnea.
- Endocrine/metabolic – hyperkalemia (chlorates), hypokalemia (barium).
- Renal/urological – renal failure (rare, chlorates).
- Musculoskeletal – weakness, paresis (rare, barium).

 # SIGNALMENT/HISTORY

## Risk Factors

- Animals that ingest wooden matches are at risk for developing a GI foreign body.
- Dogs are more likely than cats to ingest matches and fireworks.
- Roaming animals are more likely to ingest fireworks.

## Historical Findings

- Vomiting, lethargy, diarrhea, bloody diarrhea.
- Owners may report matches or fireworks in vomitus.

## Location and Circumstances of Poisoning

- Matches are most commonly found in the household but may also be found outside near grills or firepits.
- Fireworks may be found in the house (before using), outside in the yard, or in large fields used for public firework shows.

 # CLINICAL FEATURES

- Vomiting, lethargy, diarrhea, hypersalivation, and hematemesis are most common.
- Tachycardia, hemolysis, hyperkalemia, methemoglobinemia, and nephropathy have also been reported.
- Barium: ingestion can cause vomiting, diarrhea, salivation, cyanosis, bradycardia, and dyspnea within 10–60 minutes after exposure. Later signs (2–3 hours) include tremors, seizures, paralysis, mydriasis, severe hypokalemia, hypertension, arrhythmias, tachypnea, respiratory failure, and cardiac shock. If no signs within 6–8 hours, none are expected to develop.
- Chlorates: vomiting, tachycardia, hemolysis, hyperkalemia, methemoglobinemia, and nephropathy can be seen in sodium chlorate toxicosis. Methemoglobinemia may not develop for 1–10 hours after exposure.

 # DIFFERENTIAL DIAGNOSIS

- Methemoglobinemia – acetaminophen, 3-chloro-p-toluidine hydrochloride (Starlicide®), phenols (cats; should also have oral lesions), garlic, onions, aniline dyes, naphthalene (usually smells like mothballs), phenazopyridine (bright orange urine).

- Hemorrhagic gastroenteritis – arsenic ("rice water" diarrhea), parvoviral enteritis (ELISA or PCR), acute hemorrhagic diarrhea syndrome (high PCV).
- History is important in differentiating many other causes as there are no pathognomonic lesions or lab work.

 # DIAGNOSTICS

### Clinical Pathological Findings

- CBC: methemoglobin level (chlorates), hematocrit (chlorates).
- Chemistry panel and electrolytes.
  - Renal panel (chlorates).
  - Potassium (barium, chlorates).
- Urinalysis: hemoglobinuria (chlorates).
- Blood gases (barium).
- Chlorate levels: blood or urine (rarely performed due to lag time for results).

### Other Diagnostics

- ECG: QRS or QTc interval changes (barium).

### Pathological Findings

- Chocolate-colored blood and tissues (methemoglobinemia), dark kidneys, renal tubular necrosis (chlorates).
- Oral, esophageal, GI ulcers (corrosive salts).

 # THERAPEUTICS

- With firework ingestion, it is common that the exact composition is unknown and treatment is tailored to the clinical signs.

### Detoxification

- Emesis if asymptomatic and only if noncorrosive agents were ingested (weigh risk of esophageal damage with wooden matches).
- Dilution with milk or water for corrosive agents.
- Gastric lavage: only if noncorrosive agents ingested and large amount of material.
- Barium: magnesium sulfate will precipitate barium in the GI tract and prevent further absorption.
- Chlorates: mineral oil gastric lavage may prevent further GI absorption of chlorates and help speed unabsorbed chlorate through the intestinal tract. It may be mixed with 1% sodium thiosulfate for increased efficacy.

### Appropriate Health Care

- Intravenous fluids to maintain normal blood pressure and urine production.

### Antidote

- None.

### Drug(s) of Choice

- Oxygen if cyanotic.
- Saline diuresis to increase excretion (barium).

- Silver sulfadiazine topically for burns.
- Gastroprotectants.
  - Sucralfate (0.25–1 g PO q 6–8 hours) for gastric irritation (corrosive salts).
  - Omeprazole (0.5–1 mg/kg PO q 24 hours) or other proton pump inhibitor.
- Sodium bicarbonate (1–2 mEq/kg IV, titrate up as needed) to shift potassium intracellularly (chlorates).
- Potassium chloride (do not exceed 0.5 mEq/kg/h IV) to correct hypokalemia, cardiac arrhythmias, and diarrhea (barium).
- Methylene blue (1–1.5 mg/kg IV slowly over several minutes, as a 1% solution) to convert methemoglobin to hemoglobin (chlorates).
- Sodium thiosulfate is thought to convert chlorate ions to the less toxic chloride ion. Administer 250 mg/kg slow IV over 15–30 minutes; dilute each mL of the 25% solution 1:1 with sterile water for injection to decrease its isotonicity.

## Precautions/Interactions

- Activated charcoal does not bind to chlorate or heavy metals and, with the risk of aspiration, it should be avoided. Activated charcoal should also not be given if corrosive agents were ingested.

## Alternative Drugs

- Ascorbic acid (10–20 mg/kg IV, SQ, PO q 4 hours) to aid in the conversion of methemoglobin to hemoglobin (chlorates).

## Extracorporeal Therapy

- Plasma exchange has been the most successful treatment in human chlorate intoxication.

## Patient Monitoring

- Monitor $SPO_2$ to evaluate oxygenation (monitor continuously until normal).
- Liver and renal function – baseline, 24, 48, and 72 hours.
- Urine output – daily.

## Diet

- NPO while symptomatic; may need an esophagostomy or gastrostomy tube if severe oral or esophageal burns are evident.

 # COMMENTS

- Poisoning is rare.

## Prevention/Avoidance

- Keep all matches and fireworks away from pets. Do not allow pets into municipal firework pits.

## Expected Course and Prognosis

- Most animals will recover within 24–72 hours with supportive care. Barium and chlorate ingestion carries a more guarded prognosis.

## See Also

Chapter 103 Iron
Chapter 105 Zinc
Chapter 129 Smoke Inhalation
Appendix 4 Other Metallic Toxicants

## Abbreviations

- $LD_{50}$ = median lethal dose
- $LD_{LO}$ = lowest lethal dose

## Suggested Reading

DiBartola SP. *Fluid Therapy in Small Animal Practice*, 4th edn. New York: W.B. Saunders, 2011.

Gahagan P, Wismer T. Toxicology of explosives and fireworks in small animals. *Vet Clin North Am Small Anim Pract* 2018;48(6):1039–1051.

Means C. Illuminating the toxicity of fireworks. *Today Vet Pract* 2016;July/Aug:65–69.

Sheahan BJ, Pugh DM, Winstanley EW. Experimental sodium chlorate poisoning in dogs. *Res Vet Sci* 1971;12:387–389.

**Author:** Tina Wismer, DVM, MS, DABVT, DABT
**Consulting Editor:** Ahna G. Brutlag, DVM, MS, DABT, DABVT

# Chapter 93

# Mothballs

## DEFINITION/OVERVIEW

- The two primary toxic ingredients in moth repellants are naphthalene and paradichloroben-zene (PDB). Camphor is also used in some countries.
- Moth repellants are sold as flakes, crystals, cakes, scales, powder, cubes, and spheres ("mothballs").
- Naphthalene is a dry, white, solid crystalline material with a classic "mothball odor."
  - Historically, naphthalene has been used as an antiseptic, expectorant, anthelmintic, and insecticide (in dusting powders), and as a treatment for intestinal and dermal diseases.
- PDB is an organochlorine insecticide.
  - Found in deodorizers for diaper pails, urinals, and bathrooms.
  - PDB is considered less toxic than naphthalene.
- Mothballs may take several days to completely dissolve in the GIT.
- GI signs are most common. Hepatic, renal, and neurological signs have also been reported.

## ETIOLOGY/PATHOPHYSIOLOGY

- Ingestion, inhalation, and dermal contact with mothballs can lead to intoxication.
- Majority of poisonings are due to ingestion.

### Mechanism of Action

- Local GI, dermal, and ocular effects are likely secondary to irritant properties.
- Depletes cellular glutathione, impeding ability to counteract oxidative damage.
- Metabolites cause oxidant stress resulting in methemoglobinemia, Heinz body formation, Heinz body anemia, and hemolysis.

### Pharmacokinetics – Absorption, Distribution, Metabolism, Excretion

- Absorption.
  - Readily soluble in oils and fats. Dermal absorption is increased if oils/lotions have been applied or if ingested with fatty meals.
  - Rapid uptake by the lungs with inhalational exposure.
  - GI absorption can be delayed as mothballs may be slow to dissolve in the GIT.

*Blackwell's Five-Minute Veterinary Consult Clinical Companion: Small Animal Toxicology*, Third Edition.
Edited by Lynn R. Hovda, Ahna G. Brutlag, Robert H. Poppenga, and Steven E. Epstein.
© 2024 John Wiley & Sons, Inc. Published 2024 by John Wiley & Sons, Inc.

- Distribution.
  - Greatest affinity for adipose tissue. High concentrations also found in lungs, kidneys, and liver.
  - Can enter placental blood supply and affect the fetus.
- Metabolism.
  - Naphthalene is metabolized in the liver by microsomal P450 enzymes and conjugated to glutathione, glucuronide, sulfate, or mercapturate.
  - PDB's major metabolite is 2,5-dichlorophenol, which can cause oxidative damage to liver, kidneys, lungs, and CNS. PDB is oxidized to phenolic compounds prior to conjugation with sulfate and glucuronide.
  - Detoxification depends on glucuronide conjugation in the liver.
  - Glutathione depletion may result secondary to oxidative damage.
  - Metabolite oxidation of Hb to MetHb. Results in Heinz body formation and erythrolysis.
- Excretion.
  - Excreted almost exclusively via the kidneys (up to 91–97%). PDB is eliminated via the urine in five days.
  - Small amounts may be eliminated in bile/stool and breast milk.
  - Half-life of naphthalene in guinea pig blood is 10.4 hours and decay is biphasic in other tissues.

## TOXICITY

- PDB is less toxic than naphthalene (approximately by one-half).
- PDB.
  - Rat (oral) $LD_{50}$ = 3.8 g/kg.
  - Dogs ingesting 1.5 g/kg developed no clinical signs.
  - Rats receiving 770–1200 mg/kg for five days showed CNS signs.
- Naphthalene.
  - Rat oral $LD_{50}$ = 1.8 g/kg.
  - Hemolytic anemia reported in one dog from single 1.525 g/kg dose.
  - Hemolytic anemia reported in one dog from 263 mg/kg/day over seven days.
  - Lowest reported canine oral lethal dose = 400 mg/kg.
- Mothballs typically weigh 2.7–4 g; rarely 5 g/mothball.

### Systems Affected

- Gastrointestinal – vomiting, diarrhea due to irritant properties.
- Neuromuscular – CNS stimulation followed by depression (with PDB).
- Hemic/lymphatic/immune – oxidation of Hb to MetHb; Heinz body formation; hemolysis; depletion of glutathione.
- Hepatobiliary – direct injury via oxidative damage; secondary to hemolysis or metabolism of toxin.
- Respiratory – cellular damage via direct inhalation or secondary to anemia.
- Skin – local irritation if absorbed/contacted.
- Renal – primary or secondary damage, likely secondary to hemolysis. With chronic toxicity of PDB, kidney is primary organ injured.
- Ophthalmic – metabolized in the lens causing free radical damage.
- Cardiovascular – secondary to hematological effects/hemorrhagic shock.

# SIGNALMENT/HISTORY

## Risk Factors

- Cats may be more sensitive to toxic effects based on metabolism (glucuronidation).
- There is no known breed, age, or sex predilection.

## Historical Findings

- Witnessed ingestion, inhalation or contact with substance.
- Discovery of ingested material in the emesis.
- Mothball-scented breath.
- Owner may notice signs of intoxication from mothballs, including vomiting, lethargy, trembling, depression, weakness, anorexia, seizures.

## Location and Circumstances of Poisoning

- Exposure will often occur in the home or yard (some people may use mothballs to repel outdoor pests).
- Not confined to mothballs – active ingredients are found in cake deodorizers used in diaper pails, urinals, and bathrooms.
- Pet owner may find cat playing with mothballs.

# CLINICAL FEATURES

- Clinical signs typically begin within minutes to hours of exposure.
- Duration of signs is based on effect and dose (may last for days).
- Gastrointestinal – dehydration, nausea/hypersalivation, anorexia, vomiting, abdominal pain.
- CNS – depression, trembling, tremors, ataxia, seizures, stimulation.
- Cardiovascular – mucous membrane pallor/icterus/brown discoloration, tachypnea, tachycardia, weakness, hypotension.
- Respiratory – tachypnea, dyspnea, hypoxemia.
- Integument – dermal abrasions/irritation if contacted, jaundice.

# DIFFERENTIAL DIAGNOSIS

- Gastrointestinal signs.
  - Primary or secondary GI diseases.
  - Intoxications – NSAIDs, aspirin, iron, soaps/detergents, etc.
- Neurological signs.
  - Primary CNS disease – inflammatory, infectious, neoplasia, epilepsy.
- Anemia.
  - Blood loss – melena, neoplasia, coagulopathy, DIC, cavital bleed, anticoagulant rodenticide poisoning.
  - Lack of production – bone marrow disease, aplastic anemia.
  - Destruction – immune- and nonimmune-mediated disease/causes for hemolysis, toxicants such as acetaminophen, garlic onions, zinc; Heinz body anemia.
- Primary metabolic disease – renal, hepatic, hypoadrenocorticism, hypoglycemia; other hepatic toxicants – acetaminophen, *Amanita* mushroom, blue-green algae (cyanobacteria), xylitol.

- Dermatological signs.
  - Infectious – pyoderma, insect/arthropod bite, parasitic.
  - Inflammatory – drug eruption/reaction, vasculitis.
- Other – sunburn, thermal burn, contact dermatitis.

# DIAGNOSTICS

## Clinical Pathological Findings

- CBC – anemia, Heinz bodies, evidence of hemolysis.
- Chemistry – azotemia, liver enzyme elevation, hyperbilirubinemia.
- Venous blood gas analysis – metabolic acidosis, electrolyte abnormalities from vomiting.
- Urinalysis – pigmenturia, hemoglobinuria, isosthenuria if underlying renal injury.

## Other Diagnostics

- To help differentiate naphthalene from PBD mothballs, float mothballs in plain water and 100 mL of 50% dextrose.
  - Camphor floats in water and 50% dextrose.
  - Napthalene sinks in water; floats in 50% dextrose.
  - PDB sinks in water and in 50% dextrose.
- Alternatively, make a saturated salt solution. Mix 4 ounces tepid water with three heaping tablespoons (~45 g) table salt. Stir vigorously (minimum 45 seconds) until salt will not further dissolve.
  - In this solution, napthalene floats; PDB sinks; camphor floats.
- Radiographs – PDB mothballs are densely radiopaque; naphthalene mothballs are radiolucent or faintly radiopaque.
- Urine can be submitted to a laboratory for isolation of naphthalene and metabolites using TLC or HPLC and identification using GC-MS.

# THERAPEUTICS

## Detoxification

- Stabilize symptomatic animals prior to decontamination.
- Induce emesis in asymptomatic patients (due to slow dissolution, emesis may be effective many hours after ingestion). Emesis is **contraindicated** in animals exhibiting CNS signs (i.e., depression, ataxia, tremors, seizures).
- Gastric lavage if emesis is nonproductive or in cases of massive ingestions.
- Activated charcoal with a cathartic (e.g., sorbitol) may be given once within 24 hours of ingestion.
- Decontaminate dermal exposures by bathing the area (see Chapter 1 Decontamination and Detoxification of the Poisoned Patient).
- Irrigate exposed eyes with eyewash solution, tap water, or isotonic saline for 10–15 minutes.
- Animals exposed to naphthalene fumes should be removed from the source of exposure.

## Appropriate Health Care

- Immediate patient assessment and stabilization are extremely important.
- Treatments are supportive and symptomatic, based upon the clinical signs of the patient.
- Dyspneic patients should receive supplemental oxygen if needed.

- Patients with signs of hemorrhagic shock (i.e., hypotension, tachycardia, anemia, severe hemolysis or MetHg) should be volume resuscitated and transfused, if needed.

## Antidote

- None.

## Drug(s) of Choice

- IV fluid therapy with a balanced, isotonic crystalloid should be used for all symptomatic animals.
- GI signs may be treated with the following.
  - Antiemetics.
    - ○ Maropitant 1 mg/kg, SQ or IV (over 1–2 min) q 24 hours.
    - ○ Ondansetron 0.1–1 mg/kg IV, PO (canine); 0.1–1 mg/kg IV (slow), 0.5 mg/kg PO (feline).
  - Sucralfate 0.25–1 g, PO q 8 hours.
  - H$_2$ antagonist (e.g., famotidine 0.5–1.0 mg/kg, PO, SQ, IM, or IV q 12–24 hours).
  - Proton pump inhibitor (e.g., pantoprazole 0.5–1 mg/kg q 24 hours IV; omeprazaole 0.5–1.5 mg/kg PO q 24 hours).
- Anticonvulsant therapy.
  - Benzodiazepines.
    - ○ Diazepam may be administered IV, rectally, or intranasally. General dosage range is 0.5–2 mg/kg (dogs) and 0.3–2 mg/kg (cats), depending on route and concomitant medications. Repeat dosing may be required. Consult a veterinary drug formulary for specifics.
    - ○ Midazolam may be administered IV, IM, or intranasally. General dosage range is 0.1–0.5 mg/kg (dogs) and 0.2–0.5 mg/kg (cats), depending on route and concomitant medications. Repeat dosing may be required. Consult a veterinary drug formulary for specifics.
  - Phenobarbital 4 mg/kg, IV q 4–6 hours × 4 doses. Use higher doses if needed. If refractory, may add midazolam CRI IV at 0.05–0.5 mg/kg/h.
  - Levetiracetam.
    - ○ Dogs: 30 – 60 mg/kg IV over 5–15 minutes.
    - ○ Cats: 20 mg/kg IV.
- MetHb can be treated with ascorbic acid and/or methylene blue.
  - Ascorbic acid reduces MetHb to Hb, but is a slow conversion.
    - ○ 20 mg/kg, PO, IM, SQ q 6 hours.
  - Methylene blue converts to leukomethylene blue to rapidly reduce MetHb to Hb.
    - ○ Dogs 1–4 mg/kg IV, slow infusion given once.
    - ○ Cats 1–1.5 mg/kg IV, slow infusion given once. This drug can also cause Heinz body anemia in cats so should be used cautiously.

## Precautions/Interactions

- Methylene blue can induce further MetHb.
- Cats are at greater risk for adverse effects from methylene blue.

## Alternative Drugs

- N-acetylcysteine (NAC) may be useful to maintain glutathione and sulfate concentrations.
  - 10% or 20% solutions should be diluted to a 5% solution prior to IV administration.
  - Initial loading dose of 140 mg/kg, then 70 mg/kg PO q 6 hours for 7–17 treatments.

- Oral formation may be given IV (off-label) slowly over 15–20 minutes through a 0.2 micron bacteriostatic filter.
- S-adenosyl-methionine (SAMe), 18–20 mg/kg, PO q 24 hours on an empty stomach, may help with glutathione production and maintenance.

### Extracorporeal Therapy

- No data are available for companion animals. In human medicine, extracorporeal rherapy is not routinely recommended; however, exchange transfusion or hemodialysis may help enhance elimination.

### Patient Monitoring

- Proper monitoring and nursing care should be provided accordingly as it pertains to the symptoms of each patient (TPR, oxygenation).
- Patients with CNS depression and/or sedated from anticonvulsants should have appropriate nursing care and be monitored carefully.
- PCV should be assessed at a minimum twice daily in anemic patients.
- Hepatic and/or renal values should be monitored daily in affected patients.
- Blood assessment for resolving MetHb or presence of hemolysis as needed.
- CBC and chemistry values should be monitored to ensure return to normal.

 **COMMENTS**

### Prevention/Avoidance

- Clients should be made aware of the potential for mothball intoxication and advised to use them in secure locations in/around the home/yard.

### Possible Complications

- Acute kidney injuries have potential for chronic changes.
- Patients could require transfusions due to secondary hemolysis.

### Expected Course And Prognosis

- Good, provided treatment is initiated early and there is no underlying hepatic or renal impairment.

### See Also

Chapter 87 Essential Oils and Liquid Potpourri
Chapter 95 Phenols and Pine Oils

### Abbreviations

See Appendix 1 for a complete list.
- Hb = hemoglobin
- MetHb = methemoglobin
- NAC = N-acetylcysteine
- PDB = paradichlorobenzene
- TLC = thin-layer chromatography
- HPLC = high-performance liquid chromatography
- GC-MS = gas chromatography–mass spectrometry

## Suggested Reading

DeClementi C. Moth repellant toxicosis. *Vet Med* 2005;100:24.

Desnoyers M, Hebert P. Heinz body anemia in a dog following naphthalene ingestion. *Vet Clin Pathol* 1995;24(4):124–125.

Gwaltney-Brant SM. Miscellaneous indoor toxicants. In: Peterson ME, Talcott PA (eds) *Small Animal Toxicology*, 3rd edn. St Louis: Saunders, 2013; p. 304.

Moss M, Maskell K, Hieger M, Wills B, Cumpston K. An algorithm for identifying mothball composition. *Clin Toxicol* 2017;55:919–921.

Tang KY, Chan CK, Lau FL. Dextrose 50% as a better substitute for saturated salt solution in mothball float test. *Clin Toxicol* 2010;48:750–751.

**Author**: Seth L. Cohen, DVM

**Consulting Editor**: Ahna G. Brutlag, DVM, MS, DABT, DABVT

# Chapter 94

# Paintballs

## DEFINITION/OVERVIEW

- Paintball toxicosis is uncommon in dogs and is reported rarely in cats and ferrets. The ingredients in paintballs are nontoxic. However, the components are osmotically active and can draw free water into the GIT, causing diarrhea and electrolyte abnormalities.
- Common paintball components include glycerol, glycerin, polyethylene glycol (PEG), sorbitol, gelatin, propylene glycol, wax, mineral oil, and dye. The exact ingredients vary by manufacturer (Figure 94.1).
- Common clinical signs include vomiting, diarrhea, ataxia, and tremors.
- Treatment includes decontamination of the GIT, management of hypernatremia and neurological complications, and supportive care.

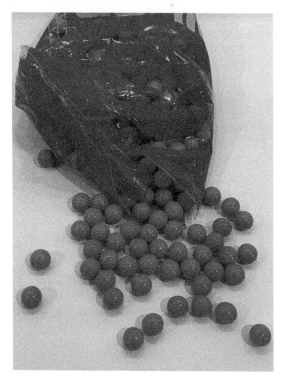

■ **Figure 94.1** An example of commercially available paintballs, size and appearance, and original packaging.

*Blackwell's Five-Minute Veterinary Consult Clinical Companion: Small Animal Toxicology*, Third Edition. Edited by Lynn R. Hovda, Ahna G. Brutlag, Robert H. Poppenga, and Steven E. Epstein. © 2024 John Wiley & Sons, Inc. Published 2024 by John Wiley & Sons, Inc.

■ Clinical reports of paintball toxicosis are very limited in veterinary medicine, yet the prognosis appears to be good with appropriate supportive care and monitoring.

 **ETIOLOGY/PATHOPHYSIOLOGY**

### Mechanism of Action

■ The ingredients in paintballs are nontoxic (see Definition/Overview).
■ After the paintballs are ingested, the osmotically active ingredients (e.g., sorbitol, glycerol, propylene glycol, and PEG) draw water from the interstitial fluid compartment into the GIT. The result is an overall loss of free water, which causes an increase in plasma osmolality and hypernatremia. Neurological effects are secondary changes in osmolality and serum sodium concentrations due to loss of water from the CNS tissues.
■ Large volumes of free water within the GIT, in addition to the osmotically active ingredients of the paintballs themselves, can cause vomiting and diarrhea.

### Pharmacokinetics – Absorption, Distribution, Metabolism, Excretion

■ The osmotically active ingredients within paintballs remain in the GIT until the patient vomits or they are excreted through the feces. They are not absorbed from the GIT or metabolized by other organs.

### Toxicity

■ None of the commonly used components of paintballs are toxic. Toxicosis results from the fluid and electrolyte shifts caused by the osmotically active nature of many of the ingredients used.
■ As few as 5–10 paintballs have caused signs in a 30 kg dog.

### Systems Affected

■ Gastrointestinal.
 • Direct irritation of the esophageal or gastric mucosa may cause vomiting.
 • Free water movement into the stomach, with secondary gastric distension, and intestines may result in vomiting and diarrhea.
 • Polydipsia may occur because of hypernatremia and stimulation of central osmoreceptors.
■ Nervous.
 • Movement of free water into the GIT leads to increased serum osmolality via hypernatremia and hyperchloremia.
 • Acute increases in serum sodium result in increased serum osmolality, causing dehydration, free water shifts, and eventually cerebral cellular dehydration and cell shrinkage. Cerebral and meningeal vessels may tear with cellular shrinkage and lead to cerebral and subarachnoid hemorrhage, which may exacerbate neurological signs.
■ Renal/urological – prerenal azotemia secondary to dehydration can occur.
■ Endocrine/metabolic.
 • Antidiuretic hormone (ADH) may be released secondary to significant free water shifts/loss.
 • Metabolic acidosis can result from hyperchloremia (secondary to free water loss), bicarbonate loss through diarrhea, prerenal azotemia, and lactic acidosis if perfusion is compromised.

- Cardiovascular – hypovolemia may occur secondary to significant fluid losses, resulting in tachycardia (compensatory), vasoconstriction, decreased pulse quality, poor perfusion, and hypotension.
- Neuromuscular – weakness may occur secondary to electrolyte imbalances, dehydration, hypovolemia, and neurological impairment.
- Ophthalmic– cerebral cellular shrinkage may cause central blindness.

 ## SIGNALMENT/HISTORY

- There are no breed, sex, or age predilections.
- Paintball toxicosis has been reported in dogs, cats, and ferrets; however, dogs represent the majority of animals affected.
- No mean age has been reported. Younger animals are likely more frequently affected due to their increased incidence of ingesting foreign objects (Figure 94.2).

### Risk Factors

- Animals living in homes or areas where paintballs are stored.
- Animals that have access to outdoor areas where paintballs are fired.
- Animals with underlying diseases that cause increased water loss (such as renal, metabolic, or gastrointestinal disease) could be at increased risk of more severe consequences with paintball ingestion.

### Historical Findings

- Witnessed ingestion.
- Discovery of damaged/chewed packaging or spilled paintballs.
- Owners may see paint on the pet's coat or face and may witness vomiting (which may or may not contain paint or paintball pieces), diarrhea (+/- paint), and CNS changes.

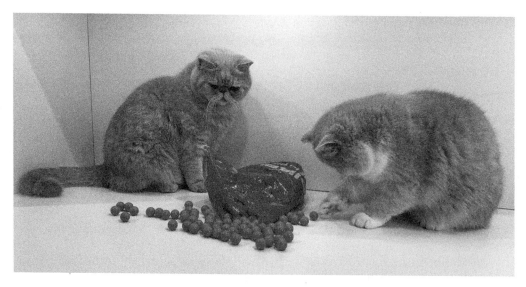

■ **Figure 94.2** The author's cats who were very interested in the fun little pink balls.

## CLINICAL FEATURES

■ The onset of clinical signs can occur quickly (within one hour) due to rapid shifting of free water from the interstitial space into the GIT.

■ The severity of clinical signs is dependent upon the number of paintballs consumed and any underlying disease process predisposing to fluid loss (see earlier). Packages may contain up to 2000 paintballs and the exact amount ingested is often unknown, making it difficult to predict the severity of signs that will result (Figure 94.1).

   • Gastrointestinal – hypersalivation, vomiting, diarrhea, gastric distension.
   • Renal/urological – polydipsia, polyuria.
   • Nervous – depression, ataxia, stupor, coma, hyperexcitability, seizures.
   • Cardiovascular – tachycardia, poor pulse quality, prolonged CRT, hypotension.
   • Neuromuscular – weakness.
   • Ophthalmic – central blindness.
   • Skin/exocrine – paint on the skin or haircoat.

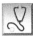 ## DIFFERENTIAL DIAGNOSIS

■ Diabetes insipidus.
■ Salt toxicosis (e.g., sea water ingestion, home-made play dough, salt emetic).
■ Ethanol ingestion.
■ Ethylene glycol toxicosis – early clinical signs of ethylene glycol toxicosis are similar to those seen with paintball toxicosis. Several common paintball components, including sorbitol, glycerol, and propylene glycol, can react with the chemicals used in blood ethylene glycol tests to produce false-positive results. For more information on ethylene glycol toxicosis, see Chapter 9.

 ## DIAGNOSTICS

■ There are no specific diagnostic tests.

### Clinical Pathological Findings

■ Serum sodium concentration and other electrolytes should be determined at presentation and monitored frequently (q 2–4 hours during hospitalization).

### Other Diagnostics

■ To distinguish true ethylene glycol toxicosis from other chemicals that cross-react with ethylene glycol tests, high-performance liquid chromatography is needed.

### Pathological Findings

■ There are no characteristic gross or histopathological lesions.
■ Gross necropsy findings may include paintball paint and remnants within the alimentary tract, edema of the intestinal wall, and increased fluid content within the GIT. If hypernatremic patients have a necropsy performed prior to fluid therapy, there may be gross signs of brain shrinkage and retraction of the meninges and attachments to the calvarium. If necropsy is performed after aggressive fluid therapy for hypernatremia, there may be signs of cerebral edema such as herniation of the cerebellum or brainstem.
■ Histopathology may reveal edema of the gastrointestinal mucosa and submucosa, cerebral cellular shrinkage, torn meninges and meningeal vessels, or cerebral cellular swelling.

# THERAPEUTICS

- Treatment includes aggressive decontamination if the patient is presented soon after ingestion and neurologically normal, electrolyte and neurological monitoring, fluid therapy, and supportive care.

## Detoxification

- In asymptomatic animals, emesis should be induced as quickly and as safely as possible.
- The use of activated charcoal is **contraindicated** (see Precautions/Interactions).
- Induction of emesis is **contraindicated in neurologically inappropriate patients.** Initial treatment should be aimed at managing neurological signs, such as seizure control. Appropriate sedation, intubation (to protect the airway), and gastric lavage should be considered.
- Warm water enemas (2–4 mL/kg) may be considered to help evacuate the osmotically active paintball remnants from the large intestine and decrease free water loss into the GIT. The frequency will depend on the patient's serum sodium concentration and clinical signs. Given the large absorptive capacity of the colon for water, the enemas may provide an additional source of free water. Close monitoring of serum sodium concentrations is important since colonic absorption may be unpredictable, resulting in rapid sodium concentration changes.

## Appropriate Health Care

- When managing hypernatremia, the duration of time for which the electrolyte was increased is imperative information. If this information is not known, hypernatremia must be assumed to be chronic and therefore treated slowly.
  - **Acute hypernatremia** (<18 hours) may be treated aggressively to normalize the sodium level, and sodium levels can be dropped relatively quickly with IV fluids with *acute* toxicosis.
  - **Chronic hypernatremia** (>18 hours) must be treated slowly. The sodium should not be decreased more than 0.5 mEq/L per hour (12 mEq/L per day) due to the presence of idiogenic osmoles that can osmotically draw fluid into cerebral cells. The isotonic crystalloid's sodium content should be selected so that it is closest to the patient's current serum sodium concentration, which could require making a custom sodium concentration fluid – see Drug(s) of Choice.
    - For patients with chronic hypernatremia who have a rapid decrease in serum sodium and develop signs of depressed mentation, decreased PLR, decreased responsiveness, or seizures, cerebral edema should be suspected and treated appropriately.
- Patients often require intensive nursing care and neurological monitoring every 2–4 hours.
  - Care for recumbent patients should be provided, including frequent turning, passive range of motion, bladder and colon care, and eye and oral care.
- For patients with seizures and concerns for cerebral edema, a board under the head and neck, positioned at a 15–30° angle, can help decrease intracranial pressure. Compression of the jugular veins (especially for venipuncture), sneezing, coughing, and hyperthermia should be avoided. Mannitol (0.25–2 g/kg, IV, to effect) can be considered for increased intracranial pressure but may contribute to hyperosmolality and should therefore be used judiciously.

## Antidote

- None.

## Drug(s) of Choice

- Fluid choice.
  - In patients with both acute and chronic hypernatremia that require fluid boluses, 0.9% NaCl should be used, as this isotonic crystalloid will have the least impact on serum sodium concentration compared with other crystalloids.
  - Once hydration is restored, D5W (5% dextrose in sterile water) or 0.45% NaCl may be used to provide free water to compensate for GIT losses and manage hypernatremia. This therapy should be used with caution in patients with chronic or unknown duration of hypernatremia, as rapid decreases in serum sodium concentration may result. D5W and 0.45% NaCl are hypotonic fluids and should **never** be administered as a bolus.
  - Hypertonic saline (7.5%) should be avoided for the management of hypovolemia, as this will perpetuate interstitial dehydration and hypernatremia. Hypovolemia should be treated prior to attempting to safely manage dehydration and hypernatremia.
  - Serum sodium levels should be monitored every 2–4 hours to ensure safe, gradual decreases in serum sodium concentration. Blood glucose should also be monitored for patients receiving D5W therapy.
- For patients that develop seizures secondary to fluid shifts from paintball toxicosis, as well as iatrogenically from fluid therapy and rapid serum sodium concentration decrease, seizures should be controlled with diazepam (0.5–1 mg/kg IV) or midazolam (0.2–0.5 mg/kg IV). Mannitol (0.25–2 g/kg) may be considered for management of cerebral edema but should be used with caution due to concerns for worsening of free water losses via osmotic diuresis.
  - Seizures must be aggressively controlled to prevent cerebral edema, noncardiogenic pulmonary edema, and aspiration of GIT contents. Intubation should be considered in any patient that has questionable ability to protect its airway.
- Antiemetic therapy should be used in any nauseated or vomiting patient to prevent further fluid losses, electrolyte derangements, and to decrease the risk of aspiration pneumonia. Options for antiemetic therapy include:
  - ondansetron 0.1–0.2 mg/kg IV q 8–12 hours.
  - dolasetron 0.6–1 mg/kg IV/SQ q 24 hours.
  - metoclopramide CRI 1–2 mg/kg/day or 0.2–0.4 mg/kg SQ/IM q 6–8 hours.
  - maropitant 1.0 mg/kg SQ/IV slowly q 24 hours.

## Precautions/Interactions

- Treatment with activated charcoal with a cathartic, such as sorbitol, is contraindicated, as the cathartic will exacerbate fluid flux into the GIT and contribute to hypernatremia.
  - Since none of the components of paintballs are toxic, administration of activated charcoal is of little value anyway.
- Warm water enemas are contraindicated in patients with chronic hypernatremia due to unpredictable rate of water absorption and changes in serum sodium concentration.

## Patient Monitoring

- Careful monitoring of hydration parameters (e.g., patient weight, physical exam, UOP, urine specific gravity, PCV/TS) should be performed.
- Serum electrolytes (e.g., sodium, potassium, chloride), PCV/TS, and blood glucose should be obtained at presentation and monitored at least every 2–4 hours initially, depending on

the extent of electrolyte derangements and fluid losses. Once electrolyte derangements have stabilized, monitor every 4–6 hours.

- In neurologically impaired patients, serum potassium and blood glucose should be monitored and appropriately supplemented as needed. Hyperglycemia should be avoided.

### Diet

- For patients with neurological compromise, vomiting, regurgitation, or those that are sedated, oral food and water should be withheld until the patient is neurologically appropriate and GIT signs have resolved.
- Due to gastric irritation from vomiting, a bland diet may be considered for 3–5 days before gradual transition back to the normal diet over another 3–5 days.

 **COMMENTS**

### Prevention/Avoidance

- Proper storage of paintballs in an area inaccessible to pets will help prevent exposure. Those involved with paintball sports should be advised of the risks to pets, and pets should not be allowed access to areas where paintball games are played. Any paintball remnants in the environment should be disposed of properly.

### Possible Complications

- In most patients, a full recovery is made after appropriate monitoring and supportive care.

### Expected Course and Prognosis

- A toxic dose of ingested paintballs is not known, therefore every exposure beyond a taste/lick should be monitored closely.
- Between 2012 and 2022, Pet Poison Helpline managed more than 600 cases involving paintball ingestion by dogs and cats. Euthanasia or death was extremely rare.
- The overall prognosis for paintball toxicosis is good to excellent with appropriate monitoring and treatment.

### Synonyms

Paintball ingestion, paintball toxicity, paintball toxicosis.

### See Also

Chapter 27 Diuretics
Chapter 9 Ethylene Glycol and Diethylene Glycol

### Abbreviations

See Appendix 1 for a complete list.
- ADH = antidiuretic hormone
- D5W = dextrose in water
- PEG = polyethylene glycol

### Suggested Reading

DiBartola SP. Disorders of sodium and water: hypernatremia and hyponatremia. In: DiBartola SP (ed.) *Fluid, Electrolyte, and Acid–Base Disorders in Small Animal Practice*, 4th edn. St Louis: Elsevier, 2012; pp. 45–79.

Donaldson CW. Paintball toxicosis in dogs. *Vet Med* 2003;98(12):995–998.
Howard J. Paintball toxicosis. *Vet Tech* 2007;28(5):336–337, 340.
King JB, Grant DC. Paintball intoxication in a pug. *J Vet Emerg Crit Care* 2007;17(3):290–293.

**Author**: Dana L. Clarke, VMD, DACVCC
**Contributing Editor**: Ahna G. Brutlag, DVM, MS, DABT, DABVT

# Chapter 95

# Phenols and Pine Oils

## DEFINITION/OVERVIEW

- Phenol, phenolic compounds, and pine oil are used in household cleaning products, disinfectants, medicated shampoos, scents, and, rarely, insecticides.
- **Phenol** is an aromatic alcohol derived from coal tar.
  - Phenols are highly corrosive in all species and can cause neurological, renal, and liver disease.
- **Phenolic derivatives** include creosote, creosol, hexachlorophene (Phisohex®), phenylphenol, chlorophenol, dinitrophenol, alkyl phenols, phenolic resins and epoxy (bisphenol A), and others (see Synonyms).
  - Phenolic disinfectants may contain chlorophenols (3–8%), phenyl phenol (2–10%) or pure phenol (20–50%).
  - Phenolic derivatives are generally less corrosive than phenol.
- **Pine oil** is an essential oil derived from pine trees. Pine oil contains alpha-terpineol, terpene ethers, and phenolic compounds.
  - Pine Sol formerly contained up to 20% pine oil. Many recent products no longer contain pine oil; always confirm the labeled ingredients of the product.
  - Pine oil is a gastric irritant, but in large amounts, in high concentrations, or if ingested by cats, it can cause GI signs followed by changes in mentation, respiratory depression, ataxia, anemia, and nephritis.
- Cats are very sensitive to these chemicals due to their limited glucuronyl transferase activity.
- Toxicosis can follow all routes of exposure.

## ETIOLOGY/PATHOPHYSIOLOGY

### Mechanism of Action

- Pine oils are a direct irritant to the mucous membranes. The mode of action is poorly understood.
- Phenols are corrosive to the skin and mucous membranes. The true mode of action is unknown.
- Phenolic derivatives have a similar MOA as phenols but are less corrosive.

*Blackwell's Five-Minute Veterinary Consult Clinical Companion: Small Animal Toxicology*, Third Edition. Edited by Lynn R. Hovda, Ahna G. Brutlag, Robert H. Poppenga, and Steven E. Epstein.

## Pharmacokinetics – Absorption, Distribution, Metabolism, Excretion

- Pine oil.
  - Absorbed across the skin and from the GIT.
  - Well distributed with highest concentrations in the brain, lungs, and kidneys.
  - Metabolized via the epoxide pathway, oxidized in the liver by cytochrome P450, and conjugated with glucuronic acid.
  - Excreted in the urine.
- Phenol and phenolic derivatives.
  - Rapidly absorbed following oral, dermal, or inhalation exposures. Absorption begins within five minutes and is complete within a few hours.
  - Distributed to all tissues with peak concentration within one hour of ingestion and 6–10 hours of dermal exposure. The highest concentrations are found in the liver.
  - Metabolized by glucuronyl and sulfotransferases. The metabolites are excreted via the kidneys in 24–72 hours.

## Toxicity

- Toxicity is dependent upon the concentration, the volume ingested/applied, and the amount of exposed body surface area.
- Cats are more sensitive than dogs (limited glucuronyl transferase activity).
- Pine oil.
  - Cat $LD_{50}$ (oral)= 1–2.5 mL/kg.
  - Severe toxicosis develops at much lower doses.
  - One cat which ingested 100 mL of undiluted Pine Sol containing 20% pine oil died within 12 hours.
- Phenol.
  - Cat $LD_{50}$ (unknown route) = 80 mg/kg.
  - Dog $LD_{50}$ (oral) = 500 mg/kg.
  - Mouse and rat $LD_{50}$ (oral) = 270–317 mg/kg.
  - Rat $LD_{50}$ (dermal) = 669 mg/kg.
  - Concentrations 1–5%: expect tissue irritation. May result in dermal burns.
  - Concentrations 5–10%: dermal burns possible. May result in oral/GI burns.
  - Concentrations >10%: expect corrosive damage to all tissues.

## Systems Affected

- Gastrointestinal – ulcerations at high concentrations. Salivation, emesis, diarrhea, laryngeal edema, and esophageal strictures may result.
- Skin/exocrine – deep caustic burns to the dermis with prolonged exposure. Burns may not be painful initially due to local anesthetic properties of some phenols.
- Nervous – ataxia, tremors, CNS stimulation or depression, seizures, or coma.
- Hepatobiliary – hepatic failure as early as 12 hours post exposure.
- Renal – renal failure as early as 12 hours post exposure.
- Respiratory – respiratory depression and panting (in dogs) followed by pulmonary edema and cardiac muscle damage. Aspiration pneumonia and chemical pneumonitis (secondary to gastric absorption and deposition in lung tissue).
- Cardiovascular – prolonged CRT with pale to muddy mucous membranes.
- Hemic – methemoglobinemia, hemoglobinemia, and Heinz body anemia (especially cats).
- Ophthalmic – ulcers with direct exposure to the cornea.

**SIGNALMENT/HISTORY**

**Risk Factors**

- Cats develop toxicosis at lower doses than dogs due to their limited glucuronyl transferase activity.

**Historical Findings**

- Witnessed ingestion of pine oil/phenol-based products.
- Chewed mop heads after phenol-based cleaners were used. (Water evaporates faster than phenols, resulting in a potentially corrosive concentration of phenols.)
- Pine oil/phenol products applied directly to pets (often by children).

**Location and Circumstances of Poisoning**

- Exposure usually occurs within the home and is rarely intentional.

 **CLINICAL FEATURES**

- May create deep, penetrating ulcers. Phenols have anesthetic properties that may render the injury initially painless.
- Common clinical signs following oral exposure include drooling, gagging, or vomiting.
- Inhalation may cause tissue irritation/damage leading to dyspnea, panting, and increased respiratory effort.
- CNS abnormalities may develop within five minutes of ingestion and one hour of dermal exposure.
    - Ataxia, mydriasis, muscle tremors, CNS stimulation or depression, seizures, or coma.
- Hepatic or renal failure may develop within 12–24 hours.
- Animals that remain asymptomatic for six hours or more following exposure are not expected to develop clinical signs.

 **DIFFERENTIAL DIAGNOSIS**

- Corrosive injury from acid or alkaline products.
- Dermal or GI exposures to other essential oils/liquid potpourri.
- Ethylene glycol toxicosis (expect metabolic acidosis with crystalluria)
- Mothballs.
- Primary renal failure.

 **DIAGNOSTICS**

**Clinical Pathological Findings**

- CBC, UA, chemistry panel, and acid–base analysis should be performed and repeated 12–24 hours after the exposure.
    - CBC – hemolysis, Heinz body formation, hemolytic anemia, and methemoglobinemia.

- UA – the urine may have a dark green to black discoloration from phenolic intermediates or due to methemoglobinemia, hematuria, and albuminuria.
- Chemistry panel – elevation of liver enzymes, BUN, and creatinine may develop 12–24 hours after exposure.
- Acid–base status – metabolic acidosis or a respiratory alkalosis.

## Other Diagnostics

- Cautious endoscopic examination to evaluate for ulceration or stricture.
- If ocular or respiratory exposure, diagnostics may include corneal stain/slit lamp examination, thoracic radiographs, or bronchoscopy.

## Pathological Findings

- Enlarged, congested, and friable liver with hepatocellular necrosis; severe renal proximal tubular and cortical necrosis; pulmonary edema and congestion; a hyperemic gastrointestinal tract; or edema of the cerebral cortices.

 **THERAPEUTICS**

### Detoxification

- Use protective gear when treating to avoid dermal contact.
- Dermal.
  - Blot visible material.
  - Use polyethylene glycol (PEG) 300 or 400 to dilute and remove the product. (*Water may increase dermal absorption and is not recommended.*) Followed by washing with a mild liquid hand dishwashing detergent and then rinse with water.
  - If PEG is not available, isopropyl alcohol can be used on small areas. Alternatively, use liquid dishwashing detergents and copious amounts of water.
- GI.
  - Do not induce emesis (risk of corrosive injury and aspiration).
  - Activated charcoal – some benefit for phenols but not effective for pine oil.
  - Pine oil – gastric lavage if large ingestion and within one hour. Confirm no tissue damage is present first.
  - Phenol – gastric lavage may increase risk perforation due to phenols being highly corrosive. The decision to lavage should be based on the amount ingested and the concentration of product. If gastric lavage is not indicated, dilute the product with water or saline and prevent emesis.
  - Some sources recommend oral mineral oil (10 mL/kg lavage) to dilute (vs water).
- Ocular – flush the eye for 20 minutes with tepid water or saline.

### Appropriate Health Care

- Stabilize.
  - Balanced electrolyte solution IV.
  - Evaluate body temperature.

### Antidote

- None.

## Drug(s) of Choice

- Support the liver and kidney.
- Liver protectants.
  - o SAMe.
  - o N-acetylcysteine – loading dose of 140 mg/kg PO or IV as a 5% solution, then 70 mg/kg q 4–6 hours.
- Treat ulcerations.
  - Antibiotics for gastrointestinal or dermal lesions.
  - GI ulcerations.
    - o Omeprazole (0.5–1 mg/kg PO q 24 hours) or other proton pump inhibitor.
    - o Sucralfate (0.25–1 g PO q 6–8 hours).
  - Consider antiinflammatory therapy but **use cautiously** and weigh against risk of worsening GI ulcerations and renal function.
    - o Carprofen 2.2 mg/kg PO or SQ q 12 hours (dog).
    - o Prednisone 0.5 mg/kg PO or dexamethasone equivalent SQ or IV. **Use is controversial**.
- Analgesia.
  - Buprenorphine 0.005 mg/kg IV or IM q 4–6 hours.
  - Tramadol 4–10 mg/kg PO q 6–8 hours (dog); 1–2 mg/kg PO q 12 hours (cat).
- Correct acid–base imbalances. For metabolic acidosis, sodium bicarbonate administration if pH is less than 7.2.
- Methemoglobinemia.
  - Methylene blue 1–4 mg/kg slowly IV in dogs or 1–1.5 mg/kg slowly IV in cats one time. Use cautiously.

## Precautions/Interactions

- Methylene blue – may affect accuracy of urinalysis due to green/blue discoloration of urine. May also increase Heinz body formation. **Use is controversial**.

## Alternative Drugs

- Ascorbic acid (10–20 mg/kg IV, SQ, PO q 4 hours) to aid in the conversion of methemoglobin to hemoglobin.

## Extracorporeal Therapy

- No evidence of benefit.

## Surgical Considerations

- Endoscopy may be needed to evaluate esophageal damage and should be done carefully as tissues may be fragile and risk of perforation is high.
- Surgical correction of gastrointestinal perforation may be needed.

## Patient Monitoring

- Monitor body temperature, especially after bathing.
- Recheck liver and kidney values q 24–48 hours while hospitalized or until the patient is stable.
- Esophageal ulcers may take weeks to heal. Evidence of esophageal stricture may take weeks to months to develop. Repeat endoscopy is recommended to follow progress.

## Diet

- NPO for up to 72 hours after ingestion if oropharyngeal damage is severe. Obese cats should not be fasted for greater than 24 hours. Consider feeding a liquid diet and stomach tube placement.

 **COMMENTS**

- Animals that remain asymptomatic for six hours or more following exposure are not expected to develop clinical signs. Their prognosis is excellent.

### Prevention/Avoidance

- Do not prescribe pine oil-based insecticides to cats, and caution owners not to use canine products on cats.
- Do not allow pets to have access to products that contain phenol or pine oil.
- Secure used mops or mop water out of the reach of children and pets. Rinse mops well before drying.

### Possible Complications

- Liver failure/necrosis, renal failure/necrosis, methemoglobinemia, metabolic acidosis, esophageal strictures, GI perforation, and aspiration pneumonia.

### Expected Course and Prognosis

- Prognosis for cats exposed to phenol/phenolic derivatives is poor; pine oil guarded. Small ingestions can quickly result in rapidly progressive signs and require aggressive treatment.
- Most dogs recover uneventfully.

### Synonyms

- **Pine oil**: alpha-terpineol, arizole, terpentinoel.
- **Phenol**: benzenol, carbolic acid, fenosmolin, hydroxybenzene, monophenol, oxybenzene, phenic acid, phenol alcohol, phenyl alcohol, phenyl hydroxide, phenylic acid, phenylic alcohol.
- **Phenolic derivatives**: cade oil, chlorinated phenols, creosote, creosol, coal tar, cresolic acid, hexachlorophene, hydroquinone, resorcin, resorcinol, xylenol.

### See Also

Chapter 89 Acids
Chapter 90 Alkalis
Chapter 87 Essential Oils and Liquid Potpourri
Chapter 88 Tea Tree Oil (Melaleuca Oil)

### Abbreviations

- SAMe = S-adenosyl-L-methionine

### Suggested Reading

Brook MP, McCarron MM, Mueller JA. Pine oil cleaner ingestion. *Ann Emerg Med* 1989;18(4):391–395.
Chan TY, Sung JJ, Crichley JA. Chemical gastro-oesophagitis, upper gastrointestinal haemorrhage and gastroscopic findings following Dettol poisoning. *Hum Exp Toxicol* 1995;14:18–19.
Gieger TL, Correa SS, Taboada J et al. Phenol poisoning in three dogs. *J Am Anim Hosp Assoc* 2000;36(4):317–321.

Gwaltney-Brant SM. Miscellaneous indoor toxicants. In: Peterson ME, Talcott PA (eds) *Small Animal Toxicology*, 3rd edn. St Louis: Elsevier, 2013; p. 297.

Monteiro-Riviere NA, Inman AO, Jackson H, Dunn B, Dimond S. Efficacy of topical phenol decontamination strategies on severity of acute phenol chemical burns and dermal absorption: in vitro and in vivo studies in pig skin. *Toxicol Ind Health* 2001;17(4):95–104.

Rousseax CG, Smith RA. Acute pinesol toxicity in a domestic cat. *Vet Hum Toxicol* 1986;28:316–317.

Vearrier D, Jacobs, D, Greenberg MI. Phenol toxicity following cutaneous exposure to Creolin®: a case report. *J Med Toxicol* 2015;11:227–231.

Welker JA, Zaloga GP. Pine oil ingestion: a common cause of poisoning. *Chest* 1999;116:1822–1826.

**Author**: Dominic Tauer, DVM, DABT, DABVT

**Consulting Editor**: Ahna G. Brutlag, DVM, MS, DABT, DABVT

# Chapter 96

# Soaps, Detergents, Fabric Softeners, Enzymatic Cleaners, and Deodorizers

## DEFINITION/OVERVIEW

- Soaps, detergents, fabric softeners, and enzymatic cleaners are composed mainly of anionic, cationic, nonionic, or amphoteric surfactants (Table 96.1). Some also contain builders such as complex phosphates, sodium carbonate, and sodium silicate or enzymes such as proteases, amylases, or lipases. Deodorizers and soaps contain perfume oils, and some products contain alcohol(s) (e.g, ethanol or isopropanol).
- Toxicity with these products is generally low except with cationic detergents and automatic dishwashing detergents (ADWD), which can be caustic.
- Signs of intoxication following ingestion may include nausea, vomiting, diarrhea, and drooling. More serious complications include CNS depression, renal injury, GI burns or bleeds, convulsions, aspiration pneumonitis, and coma.

### TABLE 96.1 Common surfactants.

**Anionic**

- Alkyl sodium sulfate
- Alkyl sodium sulfonate
- Dioctyl sodium sulfosuccinate
- Linear alkyl benzene sulfonate
- Sodium lauryl sulfate
- Tetrapropylene benzene sulfonate

**Nonionic**

- Alkyl ethoxylate
- Alkyl phenoxy polyethoxy ethanol
- Polyethylene glycol stearate

**Cationic**

- Quaternary ammonium compounds: benzalkonium chloride, benzethonium chloride
- Pyridinium compounds: cetylpyridinium chloride
- Quinolinium compounds: dequalinium chloride

**Amphoteric**

- Imidazolines
- Betaines

*Blackwell's Five-Minute Veterinary Consult Clinical Companion: Small Animal Toxicology*, Third Edition.
Edited by Lynn R. Hovda, Ahna G. Brutlag, Robert H. Poppenga, and Steven E. Epstein.
© 2024 John Wiley & Sons, Inc. Published 2024 by John Wiley & Sons, Inc.

# ETIOLOGY/PATHOPHYSIOLOGY

## Mechanism of Action

- The surfactants in soaps and detergents reduce water surface tension, allowing surfaces to wet more efficiently.
- Builders emulsify grease and oil while reducing water hardness. High concentrations of certain builders (e.g, trisodium phosphate) bind calcium and may cause hypocalcemia.
- Enzymatic cleaners break down organic stains to enhance cleaning efficacy, but can also release bradykinin and histamine, resulting in dermal irritation and possible bronchospasm.
- Biting and rupturing a laundry detergent pod (LDP) can lead to rapid detergent expulsion and potential aspiration due to its high-pressure packaging.

## Pharmacokinetics or Toxicokinetics – Absorption, Distribution, Metabolism, Excretion

- Amphoteric and cationic detergents are well absorbed after ingestion and typically peak within one hour, whereas nonionic and anionic detergents are poorly absorbed.
- Topical absorption is very minimal but can occur through defects in the skin surface. Dermal irritation can occur immediately.
- Surfactants are metabolized in the liver and resulting metabolites are excreted mainly in the urine and minimally in feces.

## Toxicity

- Cationic detergents are the most toxic, especially in concentrations >7.5% in dogs and >1% in cats, where they become corrosive. Although pH <2 and pH >12 are hallmarks for corrosivity, pH cannot be a determining factor as there are some pH-neutral yet corrosive cationic detergents.
- Anionic, nonionic, and amphoteric surfactants are usually mild irritants. Many personal care soaps, hand dishwashing soaps, regular liquid laundry detergents, deodorizers, and enzymatic cleaners may cause nausea, vomiting, and diarrhea from tissue irritation.
- Builders are irritants at low concentrations but corrosive at high concentrations.
- Perfume oils and alcohols cause irritant effects and drying/defatting of skin.

## Systems Affected

- Gastrointestinal – nausea, vomiting, diarrhea, gastritis, drooling, dysphagia, and GI burns.
- Nervous – lethargy, CNS depression, seizures (cationic detergents).
- Respiratory – cough, stridor, dyspnea, and acute lung injury.
- Ophthalmic – conjunctive erythema, pain, tearing, and potential corneal damage.
- Skin/exocrine – dryness, irritation, hair loss, chemical burns.
- Endocrine/metabolic – metabolic acidosis (with severe GI signs).
- Cardiovascular – hypotension and shock (severe cationic detergent exposures).

# SIGNALMENT/HISTORY

## Historical Findings

- It is common to directly witness exposure to these products or discover spilled or chewed products.

# CLINICAL FEATURES

- Ingestion: rapid onset of drooling, nausea, vomiting, or diarrhea. Exposure to cationic detergents may lead to lethargy, stridor, dysphagia, or oral/esophageal burns. Serious, but uncommon systemic signs include restlessness, CNS depression, renal insufficiency, and coma.
- Inhalation/aspiration of powdered products: coughing, shortness of breath, and drooling initially, which can progress to respiratory depression or airway compromise.
- Ocular: irritation, redness, and tearing initially. Cationic detergents and corrosive products can lead to corneal damage if there is a delay in treatment.
- Dermal: irritation, pruritus, erythema, and even dermal necrosis with concentrated products.
- Fatalities are usually associated with respiratory failure, aspiration, asphyxia, and corrosive GI injuries.

# DIFFERENTIAL DIAGNOSIS

- Toxicities.
  - Pesticides (organophosphates).
  - Bleaches.
  - Other corrosive products.

# DIAGNOSTICS

- Diagnosis should be made based on patient history, physical examination, signs, and clinical suspicion. No specific laboratory testing is useful in confirming the diagnosis.

## Other Diagnostics

- Endoscopy should be performed within 12–24 hours of cationic surfactant ingestion if signs of tissue injury are present (drooling, stridor, anorexia, etc.).
- Animals with respiratory signs should be evaluated with thoracic radiographs.

# THERAPEUTICS

- Goals of treatment include removal from exposure site, prevention of further absorption, and providing necessary supportive and symptomatic care.
- Exposures to most soaps, hand dishwashing soaps, detergents, and deodorizers can be treated at home.
- Exposures to cationic surfactants, LDPs, and ADWD should be carefully evaluated.
  - Minimal exposures to low concentrations of cationic detergents (<7.5%) can be handled similarly to hand dishwashing soaps and laundry detergents.
- Ingestions may require a proton pump inhibitor and liquid sucralfate. If lesions are present, start analgesia and a soft food diet.
- Admit a patient that has severe signs, such as respiratory compromise.

## Detoxification

- Oral exposure: emesis, gastric lavage, and administration of activated charcoal are not generally indicated, especially with cationic detergents, due to risk of further corrosive exposure.
- Ocular exposures should be flushed with buffered eye wash or tepid water if at home for 15–20 minutes until the pH of the conjunctival sac is 8 or less (for alkaline exposures).

If ocular irritation persists for >2 hours, if the product's pH is >12, if cationic concentration is >2% or if an ADWD is involved, the animal should be referred to an ophthalmic specialist.

▪ Dermal exposures should be irrigated with tepid water for 15–20 minutes.

## Appropriate Health Care

▪ Protect the airway, supply oxygen, and provide respiratory supportive care as needed.
▪ Aggressively monitor and replace fluids and electrolytes when necessary.
▪ Ingestions
  • Oral dilution with water.
  • Monitor for GI bleeding.
  • If excessive vomiting and/or diarrhea occur, consider an antiemetic or antidiarrheal as needed.
  • Liquid GI protectant, such as sucralfate or a proton pump inhibitor.
  • Analgesia and softened diet if lesions occur.
  • In cases with a significant potential for gastritis, corrosive injury, or GI bleeding, NSAIDs should be avoided.
▪ Inhalation of powder or deodorizer mist
  • No treatment usually necessary other than monitoring for development of signs.
  • Oral or IV corticosteroids (e.g, prednisone 0.5–1 mg/kg PO q 24 hours or equivalent doses of dexamethasone, dogs) and inhaled beta-2 agonists (e.g, albuterol 0.05 mg/kg PO q 8 hours, dogs) may help control bronchospasm.
  • Analgesic administration as needed following exposure (e.g, buprenorphine 0.005–0.03 mg/kg IV, IM q 6–12 hours).

## Precautions/Interactions

▪ Do not try to neutralize the exposure with additional chemicals as this can create an exothermic reaction and cause thermal burns.
▪ Do not orally dilute with large volumes of water post ingestion as this may increase the risk of vomiting, "sudsing," and aspiration.
▪ Avoid topical oil-based creams, lotions, or ointments if exposed to potentially corrosive products as this may "trap" the product against the skin.
▪ Do not induce emesis or administer activated charcoal if you suspect ingestion of a corrosive product (cationic concentration >7.5% or ADWD) or if vomiting has already occurred.
▪ Be alert to interactions with strong oxidizers, strong reducing agents, strong acids, and metals.

## Alternative Drugs

▪ Magic Mouthwash for ingestions – there are numerous recipes, usually consisting of liquid antacid, diphenhydramine, sucralfate, and viscous lidocaine. Gently syringe a small amount into the oral cavity 3–4 times daily.
▪ Sevelamer or another oral phosphate-binding medication if electrolyte abnormalities occur after phosphate-containing products are ingested. Monitor phosphorus, magnesium, and calcium blood levels.
▪ Calcium gluconate 10% solution (0.5–1.5 mL/kg IV, slowly over 15–30 min) or calcium chloride 10% (0.15–0.50 mL/kg IV, slowly) for hypocalcemia following ingestion of builder-containing detergents.
▪ Benzodiazepines (diazepam 0.5–2 mg/kg IV bolus) for seizures.

### Surgical Considerations

- Surgical resection of damaged tissue in cases of severe corrosive damage.
- Severely injured patients may need nasoesophageal or percutaneous feeding tube placement for nutritional support.

### Patient Monitoring

- Monitor electrolytes, hydration, and acid–base status post ingestion if severe signs are present.
- Monitor 6–8 hours post-vomiting for signs of aspiration, coughing, gagging, or stridor.
- Monitor serum calcium levels following significant ingestion of detergents containing builders.
- Monitor respiratory signs for up to 12 hours post inhalation.

### Diet

- If the animal is vomiting or unconscious, keep NPO until signs resolve.

 ## COMMENTS

### Prevention/Avoidance

- Prevent access to products in the home, particularly while cleaning or doing laundry.

### Possible Complications

- Aspiration post-vomiting.
- Irreversible ocular damage, changes in vision.
- Development of esophageal or intestinal strictures.

### Expected Course and Prognosis

- Prognosis depends mainly on the specific ingredients, product pH, concentration, quantity, viscosity, and route of exposure.
- For animals with exposure to personal care soap, hand dishwashing detergent, laundry detergent, deodorizers, enzymatic cleaners, and other noncorrosive products, the prognosis is generally excellent and the course uneventful.
- For animals with clinical signs such as hypotension, CNS depression, coma, seizures, necrosis, GI bleeds, metabolic acidosis, or dysphagia, the prognosis is guarded. The animal should be monitored for stricture development.

### Synonyms

Air fresheners, surfactants, builders.

### See Also

Chapter 8 Alcohols
Chapter 87 Essential Oils and Liquid Potpourri
Chapter 89 Acids
Chapter 90 Alkalis
Chapter 95 Phenols and Pine Oils

## Abbreviations

- ADWD = automatic dishwashing detergent
- LDP = laundry detergent pod

## Suggested Reading

Berny P, Caloni F, Croubels S et al. Animal poisoning in Europe. Part 2: Companion animals. *Vet J* 2010;183(3):255–259.

Bertero A, Fossati P, Caloni F. Indoor poisoning of companion animals by chemicals. *Sci Total Environ* 2020;733:139366.

Bertero A, Rivolta M, Davanzo F, Caloni F. Suspected environmental poisoning by drugs, household products and pesticides in domestic animals. *Environ Toxicol Pharmacol* 2020;80:103471.

Day R, Bradberry S, Thomas S, Vale J. Liquid laundry detergent capsules (PODS): a review of their composition and mechanisms of toxicity, and of the circumstances, routes, features, and management of exposure. *Clin Toxicol* 2019;57(11):1053–1063.

Handley HG, Hovda LR. Risks of exposure to liquid laundry detergent pods compared to traditional laundry detergents in dogs. *J Vet Emerg Crit Care* 2021;31(3):396–401.

**Authors:** Anna Folska, PharmD and Heather Handley, DVM
**Consulting Editor:** Ahna G. Brutlag, DVM, MS, DABT, DABVT

# Insecticides and Molluscicides

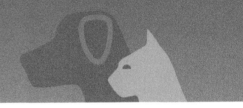

# Chapter 97

# Amitraz

## DEFINITION/OVERVIEW

- Amitraz is a formamidine derivative insecticide that is used as an acaracide and miticide in veterinary medicine.
- Amitraz is available in various formulations and concentrations, including powders, collars, sprays, dips, and topicals for companion animal, livestock, and industrial use. Common trade names include Certifect®, Francodex®, Mitaban®, Mitac®, Mitacur®, Ovasyn®, Preventic®, Taktic®, Triatix®, and Triatox®.
- Amitraz collars contain 9% amitraz (90 mg/g), so each 27.5 g collar contains 2500 mg of amitraz.
- Animal exposures resulting in toxicosis are often due to ingestion of amitraz-containing collars or from amitraz product misuse.
- Clinical signs range from transient sedation lasting from 48 to 72 hours and topical overdose to depression, head pressing, ataxia, seizures, coma, ileus, diarrhea, vomiting, hypersalivation, polyuria, hypothermia, bradycardia, hyper- or hypotension, and mydriasis from oral exposure.

## ETIOLOGY/PATHOPHYSIOLOGY

### Mechanism of Action

- Amitraz is a diamide topical parasiticide with a poorly understood mechanism of action.
- Amitraz primarily acts as a CNS alpha-2-adrenergic agonist and a weak monoamine oxidase inhibitor (MAOI). Other suspected actions include mild serotoninergic, antihistaminic, and antiplatelet effects.

### Pharmacokinetics or Toxicokinetics – Absorption, Distribution, Metabolism, Excretion

- Rapidly absorbed orally; peak plasma levels occur approximately 1.5–6 hours following ingestion, and the elimination half-life in dogs is approximately 12 hours.
- Dermal absorption is minimal.
- Tissues accumulating the highest concentrations of amitraz are bile, liver, eye, and intestines.
- Metabolized in the liver to active and inactive metabolites. The main metabolite in dogs is 4-amino-3-methylbenzoic acid, which is inactive.
- Metabolites are excreted primarily in urine; some fecal excretion occurs.

*Blackwell's Five-Minute Veterinary Consult Clinical Companion: Small Animal Toxicology*, Third Edition.
Edited by Lynn R. Hovda, Ahna G. Brutlag, Robert H. Poppenga, and Steven E. Epstein.
© 2024 John Wiley & Sons, Inc. Published 2024 by John Wiley & Sons, Inc.

## Toxicity

- Some dogs exposed to topical amitraz develop toxicosis in spite of poor dermal absorption.
- Oral $LD_{50}$ in dogs is 100 mg/kg.
- 4 mg/kg/day PO for 90 days in beagles resulted in CNS depression, ataxia, hypothermia, hyperglycemia, and increased pulse rates. No dogs died during the study.
- Cats are very sensitive to toxicosis and develop signs at much lower dosages than dogs.
- Toxicosis associated with ingestion of amitraz-containing collars is significant in all species studied.
  - Ingestion of a 2-inch portion of an amitraz collar (estimated dose 10 mg/kg) resulted in moderate lethargy, mydriasis, bradycardia, and hypotension in a dog.
  - Ingestion of a 3.5-inch portion of an amitraz collar (estimated dose 23 mg/kg) resulted in profound depression, recumbency, mydriasis, profound bradycardia, and distended abdomen in a dog.

## Systems Affected

- Nervous – depression, ataxia, seizure, and/or coma due to alpha-2-adrenergic stimulation.
- Gastrointestinal – hypersalivation, vomiting, diarrhea, bloat or ileus secondary to anticholinergic effects.
- Cardiovascular – hypertension or hypotension, bradycardia secondary to alpha-2-adrenergic receptor activity.
- Endocrine/metabolic – hyperglycemia via adrenergic inhibition of insulin release. Hypothermia due to peripheral vasodilation. Hyperthermia due to increased muscle activity from tremors or seizures.
- Respiratory – respiratory depression due to depression of the respiratory center of the brain.
- Ophthalmic – mydriasis due to alpha-2-adrenergic receptor activity.
- Renal/urological – polyuria may result at higher overdoses due to suppression of ADH.
- Hemic/lymphatic/immune – DIC can occur secondary to severe hyperthermia.
- Skin/exocrine – improperly diluted concentrates can cause skin irritation; as with all topical products, idiosyncratic dermal hypersensitivity is possible.

 # SIGNALMENT/HISTORY

### Risk Factors

- All ages, sexes, and breeds of dogs are affected. Toy breeds are reported to be more susceptible to the CNS effects.
- Amitraz is contraindicated for use on cats and canine patients ≤4 months of age.
- Geriatric and debilitated animals are at greater risk of toxicosis even at normal doses.
- Animals with severe skin inflammation may be at higher risk for dermal absorption, leading to systemic toxicosis.
- Amitraz is not suitable for patients with seizure disorders as it may potentially lower the seizure threshold.
- Amitraz can interact with several classes of drugs, including corticosteroids and other immune-suppressing drugs (e.g., azathioprine, cyclophosphamide), MAOIs (e.g., selegiline) and those with MAOI-like activity, tricyclic antidepressants (e.g., amitriptyline and clomipramine), SSRIs (e.g., fluoxetine and fluvoxamine), atypical antipsychotic agents (e.g., quetiapine, risperidone), and anesthetic drugs with known adrenergic activity (e.g., xylazine or medetomidine).

## Historical Findings

- History of exposure, which may be witnessed. Pet owners may find chewed amitraz collars in the household, along with symptomatic pets if enough time has elapsed.
- Owners may cause toxicosis in their pets when canine or livestock products are inadvertently or inappropriately applied to pets.

## Location and Circumstances of Poisoning

- Exposures generally occur in the home due to unsecured products or via direct application.
- There is risk for exposure in the farm environment due to the use of amitraz in livestock and agricultural products.

 # CLINICAL FEATURES

- Onset of signs generally occurs within 30 minutes to two hours after ingestion although delay up to 10–12 hours is possible.
- Patients may present with CNS depression, tremors, ataxia, mydriasis, hypotension or hypertension, bradycardia, and gastrointestinal signs (including vomiting, hypersalivation, gastrointestinal stasis). Hypothermia or hyperthermia may be present. Dehydration, tachypnea, and dyspnea are less commonly reported.
- Some patients may present seizing or with an owner history of having seized. Other patients may present minimally responsive or comatose.
- The duration of clinical signs is generally quite long (3–7 days) if reversal agents are not used.

 # DIFFERENTIAL DIAGNOSIS

- Intoxications.
  - Alpha-2-adrenergic agents (e.g., xylazine, dexmedetomidine, tizanidine).
  - Anticholinesterase insecticides.
  - Antidepressants (e.g., SSRIs, TCAs).
  - Benzodiazepines.
  - Ethanol, methanol, isopropanol.
  - Ethylene glycol.
  - Macrocyclic lactone parasiticides (e.g., ivermectin, milbemycin).
  - Marijuana.
  - Nicotine.
  - Tremorgenic mycotoxins.
- Primary or secondary neurological disease.
- Primary metabolic disease (e.g., hepatic encephalopathy, uremic encephalopathy, diabetes mellitus).

 # DIAGNOSTICS

## Clinical Pathological Findings

- Baseline chemistry and CBC.
- Monitor blood glucose levels frequently, especially for those patients that are known to be diabetic.

## Other Diagnostics

- ECG and blood pressure monitoring for bradycardia and hypotension.
- Gas chromatography-mass spectrometry of gastric contents, plasma, and hair can be used to detect exposure, but long turn-around times make this of little value in emergent cases.

## Pathological Findings

- No specific gross or microscopic pathological lesions are expected.

 ## THERAPEUTICS

- The goals of treatment are to manage serious or life-threatening clinical signs, administer reversal agent if appropriate, remove the source of the intoxication, monitor for development of complications, and provide supportive care until signs have resolved.

## Detoxification

- If the patient is asymptomatic following amitraz collar ingestion, induction of emesis may be attempted. Do not use xylazine or medetomidine.
  - 3% hydrogen peroxide 2 mL/kg PO up to maximum of 45 mL; feeding small, moist meals may improve efficacy.
  - Apomorphine (dogs only): 0.02–0.04 mg/kg IV, SQ, IM; can cause CNS depression, so use with care.
  - Ropinirole (dogs only): 3.75 mg/m$^2$ topically into conjunctival sac; follow product dosing chart for appropriate number of drops.
- Induction of emesis is not recommended in animals with clinical signs.
- If incomplete retrieval of collar in asymptomatic or mildly symptomatic patient, consider activated charcoal and cathartics.
  - Activated charcoal 1–3 g/kg PO q 12 hours until collar is retrieved or eliminated in the stools.
  - Nonoily laxative (e.g., sorbitol); when using osmotic diuretics, monitor closely for signs of hypernatremia.
  - Enema to evacuate colon may aid in decreasing intestinal transit time.
  - Bulky diet may aid in decreasing intestinal transit time.
- If the patient is stable and if exposure was topical, bathe with warm water and liquid dish detergent to remove the product.

## Appropriate Health Care

- Patients displaying mild sedation may require no specific treatment beyond monitoring for worsening signs.
- Provide thermoregulation as needed, especially after bathing.
- Crystalloid IV fluids can maintain hydration and treat hypotension. Diuresis does not speed amitraz elimination, but fluids do help to support the cardiovascular system.
- If the patient remains hypotensive, additional therapy may be necessary, including colloid and/or vasopressor therapy.

## Drug(s) of Choice

- Alpha-2-adrenergic antagonists can be helpful in reversing the CNS depression, hyperglycemia, and cardiovascular effects of amitraz.
- Atipamezole 50 mcg/kg IM; may need to repeat if collar remnants remain in GI tract and signs persist.

■ Yohimbine 0.1–0.2 mg/kg IV; start with lower end of dose; may need to repeat due to short half-life and/or if collar remnants remain in GI tract and signs persist.

## Precautions/Interactions

■ Do not use xylazine or medetomidine as emetic agents as these will exacerbate the effects of amitraz.
■ Atropine is contraindicated for treatment of bradycardia as it may exacerbate/precipitate hypertension and/or GI stasis.
■ Insulin is contraindicated to treat hyperglycemia; administration of alpha-2-adrenergic antagonist will restore euglycemia.

## Surgical Considerations

■ Ingested collars or collar pieces may need to be removed via endoscopy or surgery.

## Patient Monitoring

■ Frequent monitoring of vital signs is essential in symptomatic patients: heart rate, blood pressure, body temperature, respiratory rate (if comatose).
■ Monitor urine production.
■ Monitor blood glucose.
■ Monitor for and manage ileus as needed.
■ Observation may be required for 24–72 hours, or up to 5–7 days in severe cases.

## Diet

■ Return to normal diet at discharge in uncomplicated cases.
■ Patients experiencing ileus or GI irritation may require dietary alterations until these signs have resolved.

# COMMENTS

## Prevention/Avoidance

■ Secure all pesticides/medications where they cannot be accessed by pets.
■ Always use pesticide products per label directions based on dog age and/or weight.
■ Never apply/administer a product labeled for dogs only to other species; never use products intended for livestock on pets.
■ Manufacturer warnings state that amitraz may alter an animal's ability to maintain homeostasis following topical treatment, so treated animals should not be subjected to stress for at least 24 hours following amitraz treatment.

## Possible Complications

■ Patients with prolonged periods of tremoring, seizure, or hypothermia may develop myoglobinuric renal failure or DIC.
■ Gastrotomy to remove collar may increase risk of gastric dilation secondary to gastrointestinal hypomotility.

## Expected Course and Prognosis

■ Most patients receiving prompt, appropriate treatment will recover within 24–72 hours.
■ Patients experiencing severe CNS dysfunction, ileus, or complications from tremors/seizures have a more guarded prognosis.

## Abbreviations

- MAOI = monoamine oxidase inhibitor
- SSRI = selective serotonin reuptake inhibitor
- TCA = tricyclic antidepressant

## Suggested Reading

Andrade SF, Sakate M. The comparative efficacy of yohimbine and atipamezole to treat amitraz intoxication in dogs. *Vet Hum Toxicol* 2003;45(3):124–127.

Epstein SE, Poppenga R, Stump S. Amitraz toxicosis in 3 dogs after being in a rice field. *J Vet Emerg Crit Care* 2021;31(4):516–520.

Richardson JA. Amitraz. In: Peterson ME, Talcott PA (eds) *Small Animal Toxicology*, 3rd edn. St Louis: Elsevier, 2013; pp. 431–435.

Valtolina C, Adamantos S. Amitraz toxicity. *Stand Care* 2009;11(5):8–12.

**Author**: Sharon Gwaltney-Brant, DVM, PhD, DABT, DABVT
**Consulting Editor**: Robert H. Poppenga, DVM, PhD, DABVT

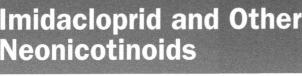

# Chapter 98

# Imidacloprid and Other Neonicotinoids

## DEFINITION/OVERVIEW

- Neonicotinoids are a relatively newer class of insecticides found in a variety of commercial preparations as well as topical spot-on veterinary products. They have rapidly become the most commonly used insecticides worldwide, replacing many older products over recent decades. Studies have shown them to be persistent and ubiquitous in the environment.
- Imidacloprid is one of the most widely used of these compounds and was the first commercially successful neonicotinoid insecticide. However, the neonicotinoid class also includes acetamiprid, clothianidin, dinotefuran, nitenpyram, thiacloprid, and thiamethoxam.
- Imidacloprid is used in topical flea products for dogs and cats and has a wide margin of safety given its high specificity for nicotinic receptors in insects.
- Neonicotinoids generally pose little risk of toxicity to pets, though reports of potential poisonings have increased, likely given the widespread utilization of these insecticides in recent years. Confirmed clinical cases of intoxication, however, remain rare.
- Neonicotinoids have been implicated in colony collapse disorder of bees, which has led to restrictions on product use in some countries and regions.

## ETIOLOGY/PATHOPHYSIOLOGY

### Mechanism of Action

- Neonicotinoids act on several types of postsynaptic nicotinic acetylcholine receptors in the CNS of insects, and these compounds likely have both agonistic and antagonistic effects.
- Binding to nicotinic acetylcholine receptors results in initial spontaneous discharge of nerve impulses with subsequent failure of nerve impulse transmission.
- While mammalian tissues contain multiple subtypes of nicotinic receptors, imidacloprid and other neonicotinoids are highly specific to insect nicotinic receptors and do not cross the blood–brain barrier in vertebrates, thus reducing potential toxicity to mammals.

### Pharmacokinetics – Absorption, Distribution, Metabolism, Excretion

- Absorption.
  - Topical imidacloprid spreads quickly over the skin via translocation. The drug is sequestered in hair follicles and glands but exhibits minimal to no systemic absorption.
  - Ingested imidacloprid is rapidly and almost completely absorbed from the gastrointestinal tract. The same has been shown for multiple neonicotinoids.

*Blackwell's Five-Minute Veterinary Consult Clinical Companion: Small Animal Toxicology*, Third Edition. Edited by Lynn R. Hovda, Ahna G. Brutlag, Robert H. Poppenga, and Steven E. Epstein. © 2024 John Wiley & Sons, Inc. Published 2024 by John Wiley & Sons, Inc.

- Distribution.
  - Distribution following oral administration occurs quickly, with peak levels generally noted within an hour to several hours, depending on the specific neonicotinoid.
  - With oral administration, imidacloprid and other neonicotinoids distribute widely to tissues but are not distributed to the CNS, fatty tissues, or bone.
  - Imidacloprid, nitenpyram, and other neonicotinoids do not accumulate in tissues.
  - With topical application, imidacloprid is distributed in the fatty layer of the skin.
- Metabolism.
  - Metabolism occurs primarily in the liver, with the rate of formation of most neonicotinoid metabolites demonstrated to be highest in rats, followed by humans, dogs, and cats.
  - Imidacloprid is oxidatively cleaved to the active metabolite 6-chloronicotinic acid. This metabolite is either conjugated with glycine and eliminated or is reduced to guanidine.
- Excretion.
  - In rats, 90% of imidacloprid is eliminated within 24 hours and 96% eliminated within 48 hours.
  - Routes of elimination for imidacloprid metabolites include urine (70–80%) and feces (20–30%).
  - The other neonicotinoids and their derivatives are also primarily eliminated via the urine.

## Toxicity

- Imidacloprid.
  - Topical imidacloprid at 50 mg/kg resulted in no adverse effects in dogs and cats.
  - A one-year feeding study of imidacloprid in dogs showed a NOEL (no observed effect level) of 41 mg/kg. Higher doses did result in elevated cholesterol levels and increased concentrations of liver cytochrome P450.
  - Dermal $LD_{50}$ of imidacloprid is over 5000 mg/kg in rats.
  - Acute oral $LD_{50}$ of technical-grade imidacloprid has been estimated to be 450 mg/kg in rats and 130–170 mg/kg in mice. Clinical signs and transient mild liver damage have been observed in rats at doses of 300 mg/kg.
  - Imidacloprid is not considered to be carcinogenic, mutagenic, or teratogenic, which is similar across all neonicotinoids. Topical imidacloprid products have been labeled for use in pregnant animals, as well as puppies and kittens as young as seven weeks. However, reproductive toxicity and fetotoxicity have been noted in experimental studies with other neonicotinoids.
- Nitenpyram.
  - Adult dogs and cats administered up to 10 times the therapeutic dose daily of nitenpyram for a month showed no adverse effects.
  - The NOEL of nitenpyram in a one-year study in dogs was shown to be 60 mg/kg/day.
  - Cats given 125 times the therapeutic dose of nitenpyram (125 mg/kg) exhibited hypersalivation, lethargy, vomiting, and tachypnea.
  - The acute oral $LD_{50}$ of nitenpyram in rats is 1575–1680 mg/kg, and the acute dermal $LD_{50}$ is >2000 mg/kg.
- Other neonicotinoids.
  - The acute oral $LD_{50}$ of thiacloprid in rats is 396–836 mg/kg. It was not acutely toxic by a dermal route in rabbits.
  - Two studies have shown acetamiprid's acute oral $LD_{50}$ to be 140–417 mg/kg in rats. It was not acutely toxic by a dermal route.

- Thiamethoxam showed an $LD_{50}$ of 1563 mg/kg in rats and 871 mg/kg in mice. It was not acutely toxic by a dermal route in rats.
- Clothianidin and dinotefuran were not acutely toxic via dermal, oral, or inhalational routes in the rat.

## Systems Affected

- Nervous – neonicotinoids block nicotinergic pathways, thus causing a build-up of acetylcholine at the neuromuscular junction. This results in insect hyperactivity, convulsions, paralysis, and eventually death. Signs in dogs and cats may include tremors, muscle weakness, ataxia, and impaired pupillary function (miotic or mydriatic pupils).
- Gastrointestinal – oral contact can cause excessive salivation. Nicotinic signs include salivation, vomiting, and diarrhea.
- Skin – signs of hypersensitivity reactions may include erythema, pruritus, and alopecia.
- Hepatobiliary – mild biochemical changes, perturbations of liver function, and liver enlargement with chronic overdose.

# SIGNALMENT/HISTORY

- Dogs and cats with exposure to normal topical application of products containing imidacloprid are not at risk for toxicosis. Exposure to extremely high doses may put pets at risk, especially if ingested.
- Diagnosis is generally based on history and clinical signs.

# CLINICAL FEATURES

- There is little published data regarding adverse effects in dogs and cats, but clinical signs are generally expected to be mild.
- Signs have been shown to occur within 15 minutes to two hours and typically resolve within 24 hours.
- Imidacloprid is bitter, so acute oral contact may cause excessive salivation or vomiting.
- Nicotinic signs in dogs and cats may include lethargy, salivation, vomiting, diarrhea, tremors, muscle weakness, and ataxia.
- Hypersensitivity reactions can occur with any topical product and have been reported. Signs may include erythema, pruritus, and alopecia.

# DIFFERENTIAL DIAGNOSIS

- Other oral toxicants causing hypersalivation, e.g., corrosive products, insoluble calcium oxalate-containing plants.
- Any other nontoxicant cause of hypersalivation or nausea, e.g., dental disease, oral ulceration or inflammation, other gastrointestinal disease, kidney disease, liver disease, pancreatitis, etc.
- Other tremorgenic toxins/toxicants (e.g., pyrethrins/pyrethroids, organophosphate or carbamate insecticides, metaldehyde, mycotoxins, penitrem A, methylxanthines, xylitol, elicit drugs) or primary neurological disease resulting in tremors, ataxia, or weakness.

# DIAGNOSTICS

- Hair and skin samples – somewhat helpful in establishing diagnosis.
  - Some laboratories can test for imidacloprid in these samples. However, as toxic tissue levels have not been established, this can only confirm exposure.

- Techniques utilized to detect imidacloprid and 6-chloronicotinic acid residues include high-performance liquid chromatography with UV detection, liquid chromatograpy-mass spectrometry and enzyme-linked immunosorbent assay.
- Clinical chemistry and urinalysis – not helpful in establishing diagnosis.

 **THERAPEUTICS**

- The goal of therapy is to reduce absorption and provide symptomatic and supportive care.
- There is no specific antidote for treatment of overdoses.

### Detoxification

- If exposure is dermal, bathing with a mild dishwashing detergent or follicle-flushing shampoo is recommended for removal.
- Emetics, adsorbents, or cathartics could be used depending on clinical signs observed, but absorption and elimination are so rapid that this approach is rarely indicated.

### Appropriate Health Care

- If exposure is via ingestion, recommended treatment includes dilution with water or milk. Oral therapy is not recommended if there is vomiting.
- Antihistamines or steroids may be utilized for treatment of acute hypersensitivity reactions.

 **COMMENTS**

### Expected Course and Prognosis

- Prognosis is generally considered good. The neonicotinoids have a wide margin of safety in mammals and thus seldom pose a problem to companion animals.
- Published reports of intoxication in dogs and cats are rare, but most are expected to recover with appropriate veterinary care in 24–72 hours.

### Abbreviations

See Appendix 1 for a complete list.
- NOEL = no observed effect level

### Suggested Reading

Ensley SM. Neonicotinoids. In: Gupta RC (ed.) *Veterinary Toxicology: Basic and Clinical Principles*, 3rd edn. Boston: Academic Press/Elsevier, 2018; pp. 521–524.
Gwaltney-Brant SM. Atypical topical spot-on products. In: Peterson M, Talcott P (eds) *Small Animal Toxicology*, 3rd edn. St Louis: Elsevier, 2013; pp. 744–745.
Rose PH. Nicotine and the neonicotinoids. In: Marrs TC (ed.) *Mammalian Toxicology of Insecticides*. Cambridge: Royal Society of Chemistry, 2012; pp. 184–220.
Sheets LP. Imidacloprid: a neonicotinoid insecticide. In: Krieger R (ed.) *Handbook of Pesticide Toxicology*, 3rd edn. San Diego: Academic Press, 2010; pp. 2055–2064.
Wismer T. Novel insecticides. In: Plumlee KH (ed.) *Clinical Veterinary Toxicology*. St Louis: Mosby, 2004; pp. 184–185.

**Authors**: Kate S. Farrell, DVM, DACVECC and Karl E. Jandrey, DVM, MAS, DACVECC
**Consulting Editor**: Robert H. Poppenga, DVM, PhD, DABVT

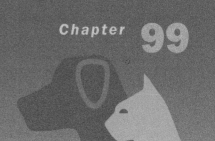

# Chapter 99

# Metaldehyde

## DEFINITION/OVERVIEW

- Metaldehyde is a polycyclic polymer of acetaldehyde.
- Primarily affects the CNS.
- Ingredient of slug and snail baits; also used as solid fuel for some camp stoves and is marketed as a color flame tablet for party goods.
- Snail and slug baits.
  - Purchased as liquids, granules, wettable powders, or pelleted baits.
  - May also contain other toxicants such as arsenate or insecticides.
  - Newer products containing iron phosphate (or iron EDTA) are now available and are considered less toxic (see Chapter 103 for a discussion of iron).

## ETIOLOGY/PATHOPHYSIOLOGY

### Mechanism of Action

- The exact mechanism is unknown.
  - It has been proposed that metaldehyde is converted to acetaldehyde after ingestion and that acetaldehyde is the primary toxic agent.
  - However, acetaldehyde was not found in the serum of rats during a dosing study and the authors recommended that this theory be reevaluated.
- Recent evidence suggests that metaldehyde may increase excitatory neurotransmitters or decrease inhibitory neurotransmitters; seizure threshold may be decreased.
  - Decreased levels of GABA, NE, and 5-HT are found in experimental mice.
  - MAO concentrations increased in treated mice.
- Metabolic acidosis and hyperthermia may be additional factors in clinical effects.

### Pharmacokinetics – Absorption, Distribution, Metabolism, Excretion

- Low water solubility.
- Lipid soluble.
- Hydrolyzed, in part, in acid environment of the stomach.
- Likely metabolized and detoxified by cytochrome P450.
- Acetaldehyde is metabolized to carbon dioxide and eliminated by the lungs.
- Urinary excretion as metaldehyde is less than 1% of dose.

*Blackwell's Five-Minute Veterinary Consult Clinical Companion: Small Animal Toxicology*, Third Edition.
Edited by Lynn R. Hovda, Ahna G. Brutlag, Robert H. Poppenga, and Steven E. Epstein.
© 2024 John Wiley & Sons, Inc. Published 2024 by John Wiley & Sons, Inc.

## Toxicity

- $LD_{50}$ values.
  - Canine $LD_{50}$: 210–600 mg/kg BW.
  - Feline $LD_{50}$: 207 mg/kg BW.
  - Rabbit $LD_{50}$: 290–1250 mg/kg BW.
  - Guinea pig $LD_{50}$: 175–700 mg/kg BW.
- Bait concentration ranges from 2.75% to 3.25%.
- At 210 mg/kg (lowest canine $LD_{50}$) and 3.25% bait, dosage for $LD_{50}$ is 6.5 grams bait/kg BW.

## Systems Affected

- Neuromuscular – seizures and muscle tremors.
- Hepatobiliary – delayed hepatotoxicosis has been reported but is not common.
- Multiple organ failure is possible secondary to convulsions and hyperthermia.

# SIGNALMENT/HISTORY

## Risk Factors

- Increased poisoning during predominant gardening and growing season.
- Increased risk when baits are overused or placed without protection from pets, or containers are left available or open.
- Dogs are much more likely to be poisoned than cats.
- Breed, age, or sex predilections are not known.

## Historical Findings

- Recent history of pets with access to treated garden areas.
- Recent purchase of slug baits.
- Baits not protected from access by pets.
- Occasionally, access to camp stove fuels or other metaldehyde sources.

## Location and Circumstances of Poisoning

- Prevalence is highest where slugs are a pest problem.
- Most common usage of baits is in coastal and low-lying areas with high prevalence of snails.
- Most consistent problems are also in warmer temperate to subtropical areas of United States.

## Interactions with Drugs, Nutrients, or Environment

- None reported.
- Conditions that inhibit cytochrome P450 might enhance toxicity.

# CLINICAL FEATURES

- Might occur immediately after ingestion or be delayed for up to three hours.
- Anxiety and panting are early signs.
- Muscle tremors.
- Seizures – may be intermittent early but progress to continuous; not necessarily evoked by external stimuli.
- Hyperthermia – temperature up to 108 °F (42.2 °C) common; probably caused by excessive muscle activity from convulsions; can lead to DIC or multiple organ failure if uncontrolled.
- Tachycardia and hyperpnea between convulsions – might note muscle tremors and anxiety; may be hyperesthetic to sounds, light, and/or touch.

- Nystagmus or mydriasis possible.
- Hypersalivation, vomiting, or diarrhea possible.
- Ataxia prior to or between seizures.

# DIFFERENTIAL DIAGNOSIS

- Strychnine toxicosis – causes intermittent seizures that can be evoked by external stimuli.
- Penitrem A or roquefortine toxicosis – mycotoxins usually found in moldy English walnuts or cream cheese; have been reported in other foodstuffs; cause a tremorgenic syndrome.
- Lead toxicosis – may cause seizures, behavior changes, blindness, vomiting, diarrhea.
- Zinc phosphide toxicosis – may cause seizures and hyperesthesia.
- Bromethalin toxicosis – may cause seizures.
- Organochlorine insecticide toxicosis – causes seizures in most mammals.
- Anticholinesterase insecticide (organophosphorus and carbamate insecticides) – may cause seizures; often accompanied by excessive salivation, miosis, lacrimation, dyspnea, urination, and defecation.
- Seizures – may be the result of a host of nontoxic conditions (e.g., neoplasia, trauma, infection, metabolic disorder, and congenital disorder).

# DIAGNOSTICS

- No specific or diagnostic features on CBC, chemistry, or UA.
- Increased serum muscle enzyme activities.
- Metabolic acidosis is typical.
- Changes in renal or hepatic values are possible but most likely secondary to uncontrolled hyperthermia.
- Radiographs may be indicated to evaluate for the presence of gastric material or severity of ingestion. Some metaldehyde bait pellets are radiopaque and may show up on radiographs.
- Metaldehyde testing can be performed on vomitus, stomach contents, serum, urine, or liver.
  - Keep samples frozen after collection.
  - Urine may yield low or negative values (see Pharmacokinetics).
  - Testing capabilities vary widely among laboratories, so check first to see what samples are recommended.

## Pathological Findings

- Lesions are not consistent or pathognomonic.
- Odor of acetaldehyde or formaldehyde in stomach contents.
- Hepatic, renal, or pulmonary congestion.
- Pulmonary edema and/or hemorrhage.
- Nonspecific agonal hemorrhages on heart and mucosal surfaces.
- Traumatic bruising or hemorrhage secondary to seizures.

# THERAPEUTICS

## Detoxification

- Recommend emesis at home if ingestion is reported less than two hours previous and animal is asymptomatic.
- Use hydrogen peroxide PO at 1–3 mL/kg BW; if no response, send patient to veterinary hospital.

- In hospital, recommend apomorphine 0.03 mg/kg IV (preferred) or 0.04 mg/kg IM or ropinirole topically 3.75 mg/m² in dogs.
  - Do not administer emetic to patients with seizures or that are comatose or hyperesthetic.
- In cats, xylazine at 0.44 mg/kg IM can be used as an emetic.
- Alternative to emetic is gastric lavage with water at 3–5 mL/kg, repeated until lavage fluid is clear.
- Follow gastric clearing with activated charcoal (1 g/kg BW) and sorbitol cathartic (4 g/kg BW PO).
- Symptomatic patients should have their symptoms controlled (e.g., muscle relaxant, anticonvulsant, thermoregulation, cooling measures, etc.) and once stabilized, they should be gastric lavaged under sedation or general anesthesia. The airway should be protected with an inflated ETT, and the stomach lavaged to remove any remaining product.

## Appropriate Health Care

- Emergency inpatient intensive care management until convulsions cease and hyperthermia is controlled.
- Acute care for metabolic acidosis may be essential to successful treatment.
  - Treat according to laboratory blood gas results.
  - If venous blood gas analysis reveals a severe metabolic acidosis (pH <7.0, BE ≤15, $HCO_3$ <11), sodium bicarbonate should be considered (0.5–1 mEq/kg slowly over 1–3 hours, IV).
- Control hyperthermia with cool water baths, ice packs, IV fluids, etc., until temperature reaches 103.5 °F; cooling measures should be discontinued at this temperature and regulated frequently.
- Antiemetic to prevent aspiration of vomitus.
- Aggressive IV fluid therapy is often necessary to aid in cooling measures, to treat the underlying metabolic acidosis, to correct dehydration, to correct electrolyte imbalances, and to aid in perfusion.
- Hepatoprotectants as needed.

## Antidote

- No antidote is available.

## Drug(s) of Choice

- Convulsions are controlled with diazepam, barbiturates, or general anesthesia and methocarbamol can be used to control muscle tremors. Seizures are frequently resistant to anticonvulsants and require general inhalant anesthesia for control.
  - Diazepam: 0.0.5–1 mg/kg IV or 0.5 mg/kg rectally; repeat in five minutes if needed.
  - Midazolam 0.05–0.3 mg/kg/h IV as CRI.
  - Barbiturates: phenobarbital 4–16 mg/kg IV.
  - Methocarbamol: 50–220 mg/kg IV to effect; do not exceed 330 mg/kg/day.
- SAMe 20 mg/kg PO q 24 hours for two weeks.
- Metaldehyde is lipid soluble; intravenous lipid emulsion administration can be considered in patients not responding to symptomatic and supportive care but efficacy is unknown.

## Precautions/Interactions

- Never induce vomiting in a convulsing patient.

## Patient Monitoring

- Periodically allow anticonvulsants to wear off to reevaluate seizure condition.
- Monitor for possible liver or renal damage during convalescence.

 **COMMENTS**

### Prevention/Avoidance

- Instruct owners on risks of metaldehyde.
- Advise clients on proper use, placement, and protection of metaldehyde from access by pets.
- Some manufacturers dye the product green or blue to assist with identification, which can result in confusion with other products (e.g., rodenticides).
- Some states require manufacturers to adjust the formulation to decrease palatability to pets.
- Use less toxic alternative products (e.g., iron phosphate or iron EDTA) for pest control.

### Possible Complications

- Liver or renal dysfunction is possible several days after recovery from the initial signs and is probably a sequela to the convulsions and hyperthermia.
- Aspiration pneumonia is a concern with any convulsing patient.
- Hyperthermia may lead to DIC or multiple organ failure.
- Temporary blindness or memory loss may occur.
- Concurrent toxicoses from additional ingredients (arsenate or insecticides) if they are present in the molluscicide.

### Expected Course and Prognosis

- Prognosis principally depends on the amount ingested and time to treatment.
- Delayed or nonaggressive treatment may result in death within hours of exposure.

### Abbreviations

See Appendix 1 for a complete list.

### Suggested Reading

Bergamini I, Mattavelli C, Grossi G, Magagnoli I, Giunti M. Conventional treatment of a metaldehyde-intoxicated cat with additional use of low-dose intravenous lipid emulsion. *JFMS Open Rep* 2020;6(2): 2055116920940177.

Brutlag AG, Puschner B. Metaldehyde. In: Peterson ME, Talcott PA (eds) *Small Animal Toxicology*, 3rd edn. St Louis: Elsevier, 2013; pp. 635–642.

Buhl KJ, Berman FW, Stone DL. Reports of metaldehyde and iron phosphate exposures in animals and characterization of suspected iron toxicosis in dogs. *J Am Vet Med Assoc* 2013;242:1244–1248.

Lelescu CA, Mureşan C, Muste A et al. Successful treatment of metaldehyde toxicosis with intravenous lipid emulsion in a dog. *Acta Vet Brno* 2017;86(4):379–383.

Yas-Natan E, Segev G, Aroch I. Clinical, neurological and clinicopathological signs, treatment and outcome of metaldehyde intoxication in 18 dogs. *J Small Anim Pract* 2007;48(8):438–443.

**Author**: Erica J. Howard, DVM
**Consulting Editor**: Robert H. Poppenga, DVM, PhD, DABVT

# Chapter 100

# Miscellaneous Insecticides (Fipronil and Spinosad)

## DEFINITION/OVERVIEW

- Fipronil and spinosad are two insecticides in current clinical use for small animals. While they have distinct structural differences, there are important similarities in their mechanisms of action.
- Both compounds owe their wide margin of safety to a relative selectivity for receptors in the insect nervous system. At therapeutic doses and mild to moderate overdoses, adverse effects in mammals are generally limited to gastrointestinal upset, lethargy, and dermal irritation.
- Exception: Fipronil is highly toxic to rabbits and is absolutely contraindicated in this species.

## ETIOLOGY/PATHOPHYSIOLOGY

### Mechanism of Action

- Fipronil is an antiparasitic agent of the phenylpyrazole class. Mechanistically, it interferes with the function of GABA-mediated chloride channels (by binding to $GABA_A$ receptors), preventing chloride uptake and leading to excessive neuronal stimulation. It has a substantially higher binding affinity (>500-fold) for the $GABA_A$ complexes of insects relative to those of mammals, accounting for its broad margin of safety in most mammalian species.
- Spinosad is a combination of two macrocyclic lactones, spinosyn A and D. It is a nicotinic acetylcholine receptor agonist with specific activity on the D-alpha receptors in the insect nervous system. Spinosad binding causes hyperexcitation of insect motor neurons, resulting in paralysis and death. Interference with GABA-mediated chloride channels appears to be a secondary mechanism of action.

### Pharmacokinetics – Absorption, Distribution, Metabolism and Excretion

- Fipronil products are labeled for topical use in dogs or cats. Dermally applied fipronil is quite lipophilic, concentrating in skin oils and hair follicles. It spreads across the body surface, via the skin oils, within 24 hours of dermal application. When applied topically, <5% of the drug is absorbed systemically. It may be ingested if an animal licks the product off itself or a housemate. Oral bioavailability is typically 50–85% of the total ingested dose.
- Spinosad products are labeled for oral use in dogs or cats. It is rapidly absorbed from the GI tract, with an oral bioavailability of approximately 70%. It is concentrated particularly in adipose tissues, and is eliminated over days to weeks, primarily in the feces.

*Blackwell's Five-Minute Veterinary Consult Clinical Companion: Small Animal Toxicology*, Third Edition.
Edited by Lynn R. Hovda, Ahna G. Brutlag, Robert H. Poppenga, and Steven E. Epstein.
© 2024 John Wiley & Sons, Inc. Published 2024 by John Wiley & Sons, Inc.

## Toxicity (End-use Products)

- Fipronil: oral LD$_{50}$ (rat): 5000 mg/kg.
- Spinosad: oral LD$_{50}$ (rat): >3600 mg/kg.

## Systems Affected

- Fipronil.
  - Skin/exocrine – erythema, dermatitis, pruritus, alopecia.
  - Gastrointestinal – transient hyporexia/anorexia; hypersalivation and vomiting with oral exposures.
  - Nervous – hiding, lethargy. Rabbits may experience ataxia, tremors, and seizures.
- Spinosad.
  - Skin/exocrine – pruritus.
  - Gastrointestinal – vomiting, hyporexia/anorexia, diarrhea, hypersalivation.
  - Nervous – depression/lethargy, ataxia, tremors, seizures.

 # SIGNALMENT/HISTORY

## Risk Factors

- Smaller animals are more likely to be accidentally or improperly overdosed with medications labeled for larger animals. The latter often occurs when a pet owner attempts to split a dose of a product labelled for a larger pet among several smaller pets.
- Spinosad should be used with caution in patients with a history of seizures, due to the theoretical potential that it may lower the seizure threshold in these animals.
- Rabbits are at severe risk from exposure to fipronil and it is absolutely contraindicated in this species.

## Location and Circumstances of Poisoning

- Fipronil is intended for topical application, sometimes in products containing other active ingredients. Overdoses may occur from inadvertent or intentional overapplication of the product, or from using a product labeled for a larger weight class of animal. Topical products are sometimes accidentally given by mouth, or may be licked off the fur/skin of a housemate. Canine and feline labeled products are sometimes inappropriately applied to rabbits.
- Spinosad is given orally, sometimes in products containing other active ingredients. Overdoses may occur by accidentally repeating a dose, or by giving a dose labeled for a larger weight class of animal.
- Toxic exposures are more common during warmer months when risk for ectoparasitism is highest and need for these products is the greatest. When these products are used year-round, incidence of intoxication shows less seasonal variation.

## Interactions with Drugs, Nutrients, or Environment

- Spinosad should not be used concurrently with high-dose ivermectin (as for conditions such as demodectic mange) as it may increase the risk for ivermectin intoxication. This interaction is not observed when spinosad is used with low-dose ivermectin (as for monthly heartworm prevention).

 # CLINICAL FEATURES

- Dermatological signs in dogs and cats may be seen within minutes to several days of topical application of fipronil.
- Gastrointestinal signs in dogs and cats may be seen within minutes to 2–3 days after ingestion of fipronil or spinosad.

- Rabbits will typically develop signs within a week of exposure to fipronil. Initial signs can be mild and nonspecific, and often include hyporexia/anorexia and lethargy/depression. These can be followed as long as 2–3 weeks later by ataxia, tremors, and seizures.
- Because initial signs in rabbits might be mild and nonspecific, these animals are sometimes not presented for care until more dramatic neurological signs have developed. The owner may be unaware of a link between the fipronil exposure and clinical signs, so a thorough history is essential in order to correctly identify the cause.

 ## DIFFERENTIAL DIAGNOSIS

- Animals having GI signs: primary gastrointestinal disease of any origin.
- Animals having dermal signs: primary dermatological disease of any origin. Hypersensitivity reaction to other drugs, vaccines, insect or arachnid envenomation.
- Animals experiencing ataxia, seizures, or tremors: other intoxications, including bromethalin, metaldehyde, baclofen, tremorgenic mycotoxins, ethanol, ethylene glycol, marijuana, ivermectin. Epilepsy, either idiopathic or secondary to metabolic disease, intracranial neoplasia, or cerebrovascular disease. Hypoglycemia, particularly in young and/or very small patients.

 ## DIAGNOSTICS

- History of use or inadvertent exposure.
- Routine laboratory workup is typically unrewarding in diagnosing intoxication caused by these compounds, but may be helpful in ruling out alternative differentials.
- Plasma or serum can be tested for the presence of fipronil, although this service is offered by only a handful of laboratories

 ## THERAPEUTICS

### Detoxification

- Topical fipronil products can be removed from the skin and coat by bathing the patient using a liquid dish detergent and rinsing thoroughly. These detergents contain degreasing agents, which remove the lipophilic products from skin and coat more effectively than shampoos labeled for humans or pets. Bathing is most effective if performed within 24–48 hours of product application. In some cases, 1–2 repeat baths may be necessary for full removal.
- Patients that are hypersalivating after grooming a topical product off the coat may benefit from gentle oral irrigation with clean water or isotonic saline solution. Encouraging the animal to drink water or eat food may also help remove the adverse taste from the mouth.
- In case of ophthalmic exposure to a topical product, the eyes should be gently irrigated with room-temperature water or an eyewash solution for 10–15 minutes.
- For ingested products, emesis induction may be considered. Chewable tablets are rapidly absorbed, so emesis longer than 60 minutes post ingestion is generally of minimal benefit. Emesis induction is not indicated in rabbits due to their inability to vomit. Emesis should not be induced in any patient showing signs of intoxication, with decreased level of consciousness, or impaired ability to protect the airway.
- A dose of activated charcoal with a cathartic may be considered in patients with large ingestions. The same contraindications apply as with emesis induction.

## Appropriate Health Care

- Patients experiencing mild dermatological or gastrointestinal signs can usually be managed on an outpatient basis.
- Patients experiencing neurological signs, including rabbits exposed to fipronil, should be hospitalized.
- Patients that have received spinosad and ivermectin, and are subsequently exhibiting signs consistent with ivermectin intoxication, should be managed as with other ivermectin cases.

## Antidotes

- No specific antidotes exist to fipronil or spinosad. Treatment of affected patients is symptomatic and supportive.

## Drug(s) of Choice

Note: Dosages that follow are for dogs, unless otherwise specified. Appropriate drugs and dosages should be confirmed for other species.

- For dermal irritation or pruritus.
    - Steroids: prednisone 0.5–1.1 mg/kg PO divided q 12 hours, tapering dose as needed.
    - Antihistamines: diphenhydramine 2.2 mg/kg PO q 8–12 hours, not to exceed 50 mg per dose.
- For evidence of secondary bacterial infection with open or ulcerated skin: cefpodoxime 5–10 mg/kg PO q 24 hours.
- For severe or persistent vomiting secondary to ingestion of products: maropitant 1 mg/kg SQ q 24 hours.
- For rabbits experiencing seizures after fipronil exposure.
    - Diazepam 0.5–1 mg/kg IV or per rectum.
    - Midazolam 1–2 mg/kg IM or IV.

## Precautions/Interactions

- High-dose ivermectin therapy should not be used concurrently in an animal receiving spinosad.

 **COMMENTS**

### Prevention/Avoidance

- Rabbit owners should be informed that fipronil is very toxic to this species and should never be used.
- In homes shared between rabbits and dogs or cats, the safest option is to keep rabbits separated from the other species for 48 hours after a fipronil product is applied to the dogs or cats.
- All small animal owners should be cautioned that antiparasitic products should never be used in a manner that deviates from the product label, unless such use is at the specific direction of their veterinarian.

### Expected Course and Prognosis

- Prognosis is generally excellent for dogs and cats experiencing gastrointestinal or dermal effects from exposure to fipronil or spinosad.
- A rabbit with exposure to fipronil has a guarded prognosis and requires careful monitoring for 3–4 weeks post exposure. If clinical signs develop, hospitalization is strongly recommended.
- Prognosis for rabbits developing neurological signs after exposure to fipronil is guarded to poor, particularly if they are not managed as an inpatient.

## Suggested Reading

Anadon A, Gupta RC. Fipronil. In: Gupta RC (ed.) *Veterinary Toxicology: Basic and Clinical Principles*, 3rd edn. New York: Elsevier, 2018; pp. 533–537.

Cooper PE, Penaliggon J. Use of Frontline spray on rabbits. *Vet Rec* 1997;140(20):535–536.

d'Ovidio D, Cortellini S. Successful management of fipronil toxicosis in two pet rabbits. *Open Vet J* 2022;12(4):508–510.

Dunn ST, Hedges L, Sampson KE et al. Pharmacokinetic interaction of the antiparasitic agents ivermectin and spinosad in dogs. *Drug Metab Dispos* 2011;39(5):789–795.

Plumb DC. Spinosad. In: Plumb DC (ed.) *Plumb's Veterinary Drug Handbook*, 9th edn. Ames: Wiley-Blackwell, 2018; pp. 367–378.

**Author:** James Eucher, DVM, DHSc, MS, MPH, DABT
**Consulting Editor:** Robert H. Poppenga, DVM, PhD, DABVT

# Chapter 101

# Organophosphorus and Carbamate Anticholinesterase Pesticides

## DEFINITION/OVERVIEW

- Organophosphate (OP) and carbamate cholinesterase-inhibiting pesticides are still common causes of toxicosis in dogs and cats, although the incidence appears to be steadily decreasing nationwide. This is likely due to the removal of several products from the home market and the introduction and increasing popularity of several other less toxic insecticides.
- Chlorpyrifos, once found in flea collars and other pesticide products, was withdrawn in 2000 and diazinon followed in 2004. Older products are still found (and used) in homes, garages, barns, and other storage facilities and remain a source of poisoning.
- Products currently licensed for use on animals, in the house, on the lawn and garden, or for farm or agricultural use are all potential sources of poisoning.
- Carbamate *fungicides* that do not inhibit cholinesterase activity are in a different category and not discussed in this chapter.

## ETIOLOGY/PATHOPHYSIOLOGY

- In addition to systemic oral exposure, dogs and cats can be poisoned through ophthalmic, respiratory, and dermal routes. Onset and duration of clinical signs and toxicity vary depending on the particular OP or carbamate, the form of the pesticide (e.g., liquid, powder, sustained-release plastic), as well as the route of exposure.

### Mechanism of Action

- Competitive inhibitors of cholinesterase enzymes. Enzyme inhibition allows acetylcholine, a neurotransmitter, to accumulate at nerve junctions in the parasympathetic/sympathetic nervous systems, peripheral nervous system, and central nervous system (CNS). This results in initial and excessive stimulation of muscarinic, nicotinic, and CNS cholinergic receptors.
- There are two main enzymes with cholinesterase activity.
  - Acetylcholinesterase ("true" cholinesterase) – present in the red blood cell membrane and in the cholinergic synapses in the central and peripheral nervous systems.
  - Pseudocholinesterase (plasma cholinesterase) – found in the plasma, liver, pancreas, and CNS.

### Pharmacokinetics – Absorption, Distribution, Metabolism, Excretion

- Precise pharmacokinetics vary with each compound.
- Well absorbed across intact skin, lungs, cornea, and gastrointestinal tract.

---

*Blackwell's Five-Minute Veterinary Consult Clinical Companion: Small Animal Toxicology*, Third Edition. Edited by Lynn R. Hovda, Ahna G. Brutlag, Robert H. Poppenga, and Steven E. Epstein. © 2024 John Wiley & Sons, Inc. Published 2024 by John Wiley & Sons, Inc.

- Widely distributed and many accumulate in fat.
- Metabolized in liver.
- Excreted in urine as metabolites.
- Organophosphates.
  - Liver microsomal enzymes convert some OPs to a more toxic "oxon" compound. OPs irreversibly bind to cholinesterase enzymes, increasing the toxicity and duration of action.
  - Different OPs bind to cholinesterase with different affinity. Some "age" or become more strongly bound with the passage of time.
- Carbamates.
  - Inhibition of cholinesterase enzymes is due to carbamylation of the enzyme esters. Binding is labile, reversible, and not as long lasting as seen with OPs.

## Toxicity

- Varies widely depending on the compound.
- Organophosphorus compounds.
  - Very highly toxic compounds include disulfoton, fensulfothion, parathion, terbufos, TEPP (tetraethyl pyrophosphate), and others.
  - Compounds with intermediate toxicity include coumaphos, famphur, trichlorfon, and others.
  - Intermediate to low toxicity compounds include chlorpyrifos, diazinon, dichlorvos, fenthion, malathion, and others.
  - Oral $LD_{50}$ of chlorpyrifos in cats is very low (10–40 mg/kg).
- Carbamate compounds.
  - Extremely toxic compounds include aldicarb, carbofuran, methomyl, carbofuran, and others.
  - Aminocarb, bendiocarb, and propuxur are among the highly toxic compounds.
  - Moderately toxic compounds include carbaryl and others.

## Systems Affected

- Virtually all systems in the body are affected to some extent by OPs or carbamates, with effects dependent on the specific neuroeffector junction involved.
- Accumulation of acetylcholine at autonomic junctions results in stimulation of end-organs, with excessive secretions and smooth muscle contractions the expected outcome.
- Variable effects are observed at skeletal muscle junctions where both stimulatory and, to a lesser extent, inhibitory effects occur.
- Gastrointestinal – stimulation of muscarinic synapses results in the acute onset of salivation (S), lacrimation (L), urination (U), defecation (D), and gastroenteritis (GE) (this is where the mnemonic SLUDGE comes from).
- Nervous – stimulation results in variable and diverse signs, ranging from CNS excitation (e.g., hyperexcitability, seizures) to lethargy (e.g., chlorpyrifos in cats).
- Neuromuscular – tremors and muscle weakness as part of nicotinic stimulation; paresis or frank paralysis following the acute cholinergic crisis (intermediate syndrome).
- Cardiovascular – inhibitory effect on sinoatrial node results in bradycardia.
- Ophthalmic – miosis or mydriasis from either muscarinic or nicotinic stimulation.
- Respiratory – vapors produce irritation to mucous membranes and bronchospasm. Dyspnea can result from bronchoconstriction and fluid accumulations.

# SIGNALMENT/HISTORY

## Risk Factors

- Cats are more sensitive than dogs, especially to chlorpyrifos; however, poisonings are more frequently reported in dogs.
- Younger animals may be at greater risk.
- Thin animals or those with a naturally lean body mass may be more susceptible to intoxication from lipophilic OPs.

## Historical Findings

- Chewed-up containers or disturbed earth around recently treated rose bushes, shrubs, and flower/vegetable gardens.
- Intoxications have been reported following ingestion of livestock insecticide ear tags.
- Outdoor inhalation exposures as a result of aerial application is uncommon.
- Rapid onset of SLUDGE syndrome (the author has also been using the mnemonic DUMBSLED to describe diarrhea, urination, miosis/mydriasis, bradycardia, salivation, lacrimation, emesis, and dyspnea).
- Products are often used to intentionally poison pets, disguised in food products.

# CLINICAL FEATURES

- Local effects from direct contact with the product. Signs may be seen in just a few moments or delayed for days with dermal exposure or following ingestion of delayed-release products (e.g., embedded livestock ear tags).
- Ophthalmic – irritation, lacrimation, photophobia, and miosis or mydriasis. Pupil size generally returns to normal in 12–36 hours.
- Respiratory – respiratory irritation with bronchospasm; absorption across mucous membranes.
- Dermal – irritation; absorption can occur across intact skin with systemic toxicity if concentration and duration of exposure are high enough.
- Systemic effects may occur as early as 5–60 minutes, usually occur by six hours, and rarely after 12 hours unless exposure was dermal or compound was in a delayed-release form.
- CNS – agitation or depression, aggression, seizures, respiratory depression and failure (centrally mediated), death.
- Muscarinic signs – most commonly observed and generally associated with the SLUDGE syndrome. Other signs include bradycardia, dyspnea, and miosis. Not all signs are typically observed and one must look for a preponderance of evidence.
- Nicotinic signs – facial twitching (especially in cats), weakness, ataxia, muscle tremors, tachycardia, paralysis, and mydriasis.
- Intermediate syndrome: signs generally occur 24–72 hours after the onset of acute signs and may last from several days to weeks.
  - Occurs most commonly with lipophilic OPs.
  - Acute or chronic; can be seen following prolonged dermal exposure.
  - Due to downregulation of the cholinergic receptors, particularly muscarinic, and eventual fatigue of the nicotinic receptors.
  - Neuromuscular weakness predominantly affects the thoracic limb, neck, and respiratory muscles. Cervical ventroflexion is common.

- Other signs include cranial nerve deficits, anorexia, muscle tremors, abnormal postures or behaviors, lethargy, and seizures.
- Death from hypoventilation and respiratory depression.

# DIFFERENTIAL DIAGNOSIS

- Amphetamine, methylphenidate, methamphetamine, cocaine, and other human CNS stimulant compounds.
- Concentrated pyrethrin/permethrin/pyrethroid topical products.
- Metaldehyde.
- Strychnine.
- Neurotoxic cyanobacteria or blue-green algae.
- Lead.
- Nicotine.
- Methylxanthines (e.g., theobromine, theophylline, caffeine).
- Toxic mushrooms.
- Chlorinated hydrocarbon pesticides.
- Tremorgenic mycotoxins found in moldy food and compost (penitrem A, roquefortine).
- Zinc phosphide-containing rodenticides.
- Convulsant form of bromethalin intoxication.
- Severe gastroenteritis or pancreatitis from infectious, environmental, or other causes.

# DIAGNOSTICS

- Analysis of stomach contents or vomitus for the parent compound.
- Modern analytical methods can detect OP and carbamate residues and metabolites in blood/serum and body organs such as liver, kidney, and fat.
- Positive response to a test dose of atropine (0.02 mg/kg IV).
- Blood cholinesterase activity antemortem and brain cholinesterase activity postmortem. Levels less than 50% of normal are considered suspicious and less than 25% of normal are diagnostic.
- Cholinesterase testing: cautious interpretation of measured activity, considering onset of signs and when sample was taken. Reversal of cholinesterase inhibition can occur over time, particularly with carbamate exposures. Anemia can lead to low cholinesterase values.
- Plasma cholinesterase – may be more appropriate for cats and avian species; can be used for other species.
- Whole blood cholinesterase – measures cholinesterase in plasma and RBC membranes; can be used for all species, including cats.
- Brain cholinesterase – some inhibitors do not cross the blood–brain barrier well; it has been difficult for laboratories to establish reference ranges for many species, depending on which part of the brain is collected and tested.

### Pathological Findings

- Nonspecific lesions; endocardial and epicardial petechial hemorrhages; pulmonary edema; pancreatitis in dogs can occur.

# THERAPEUTICS

## Detoxification

- Oral exposure.
    - Early induction of emesis depending on the carrier. Many liquid products have petroleum-based carriers, and emesis is NOT indicated for these due to aspiration risk.
    - If significant emesis occurs spontaneously, further induction is unnecessary.
    - Gastric lavage may be an option.
    - Activated charcoal, single or multiple doses 4–6 hours apart (first dose with sorbitol, later doses without) – depends if diarrhea is already present.
    - Flea collars or pesticide-embedded ear tags that are ingested might need to be removed by emesis, whole-bowel irrigation, endoscopy, or surgery if deemed appropriate.
- Dermal exposure.
    - Clip hair if possible.
    - Bathe thoroughly in warm water and soap. Rinse and repeat several times.
    - Personal protection important when bathing.
- Ophthalmic exposure.
    - Lavage with tepid water for 10–15 minutes while patient is sedated.
    - Ophthalmic ointment for irritation.
- Respiratory exposure.
    - Move to fresh air.
    - Humidified oxygen as needed for severe dyspnea.

## Appropriate Health Care

- Close monitoring of heart rate. Bradycardia is most common; tachycardia can occur.
- Blood pressure and cardiovascular support as needed.
- Oxygen as needed for dyspnea or hypoxemia.
- Thermoregulation and maintain hydration status.
- Severe respiratory depression or secondary aspiration pneumonia can occur; be prepared to provide ventilatory support as needed.
- Venous blood gas monitoring to detect metabolic acidosis; bicarbonate only if severe.
- Monitor closely for pancreatitis (dogs) and hemorrhagic gastroenteritis (dogs and cats).

## Antidotes

- Atropine – effective *only* for SLUDGE or DUMBSLED signs. Primarily used to control bronchial secretions and bradycardia. Dosage range for this is very wide.
    - Mild-to-moderate toxicity.
        - Dosage range of 0.1–0.5 mg/kg BW.
        - Give ¼ of dose IV and remainder IM or SQ.
        - Repeat every 1–2 hours as needed until the animal is stable and secretions are controlled.
    - Serious and life-threatening toxicity.
        - Use the high end of the dosage range (1–2 mg/kg BW).
        - Give ¼ of the dose IV, wait 15 minutes and give the remainder SQ or IM.
        - Repeat every 1–2 hours until animal is stable and secretions are controlled.

- Secretions and then heart rate should be the guide to redosing.
- Pay particular attention to respiratory secretions as animals can die from hypoxia if not enough atropine is administered.
- Pralidoxime chloride (2-PAM) – used for OP toxicosis to reverse the initial binding of OP with acetylcholinesterase. Questionable efficacy in carbamate toxicoses.
  - 20 mg/kg BW IM or IV q 8–12 hours slowly over 15–30 minutes; stop if signs get worse.
  - Rapid IV administration of 2-PAM has been associated with tachycardia, laryngospasm, neuromuscular blockade, muscle rigidity, and death.
  - Greatest efficacy when given within the first 24 hours after exposure.
  - Generally see effects after 1–2 doses; if no response after 3–4 doses, discontinue use.
  - Has been suggested to be beneficial in treatment of intermediate syndrome, even when signs occur later than 24 hours post exposure. It appears to work well on the most commonly affected muscles, such as the diaphragm and cervical muscles.

## Drug(s) of Choice

- Fluid therapy: IV fluids to maintain hydration. Use PCV/TPP to monitor, but generally run fluids at 2–3× maintenance or greater as significant amounts of fluid are lost with secretions and decontamination procedures.
- Seizures.
  - Diazepam: 0.25–0.5 mg/kg IV, to effect.
  - Phenobarbital: 10–20 mg/kg IV, to effect.
- Antiemetics if vomiting is severe or persistent, and prior to or after the use of activated charcoal.
  - Maropitant: 1 mg/kg SQ q 24 hours.
  - Ondansetron: 0.1–0.2 mg/kg IV q 6–12 hours (dogs and cats).
- GI protectants, as needed.
  - H$_2$-blockers (not as commonly used).
    - Famotidine 0.1–0.2 mg/kg PO, SQ, IM, IV q 12 hours for dogs; 0.2 mg/kg q 12–24 hours IM, SQ, PO, IV (slowly) for cats.
    - Ranitidine 2 mg/kg q 8 hours IV, PO for dogs; 2.5 mg/kg q 12 hours IV or 3.5 mg/kg q 12 hours PO for cats.
    - Cimetidine 10 mg/kg PO, IM, IV q 6–8 hours.
  - Omeprazole: 1–2 mg/kg daily PO for dogs; 1 mg/kg daily PO for cats.
  - Sucralfate: 0.5–1 g q 8–12 hours PO for dogs; 0.25 g q 8–12 hours PO for cats.

## Precautions/Interactions

- Do NOT use 2-PAM in combination with phenothiazines, morphine, or succinylcholine.
- Use atropine judiciously. Use enough to keep the animal from drowning in secretions. Initial tachycardia should not preclude the use of atropine, but close monitoring is necessary.

## Surgical Considerations

- Endoscopic or surgical removal may be necessary if the animal has swallowed a flea collar or pesticide-embedded livestock ear tag.

## Environmental Issues

- Properly store and dispose of these pesticides to avoid environmental/groundwater contamination.

## Patient Monitoring

- Pay close attention to secretions. Use an appropriate amount of atropine to control secretions. Replace IV fluids to correct fluid losses from secretions and decontamination procedures.
- Monitor cardiovascular and respiratory system, body temperature, and hydration status (discussed above).

 ## COMMENTS

### Prevention/Avoidance

- Keep pesticides away from pets, follow label directions, and properly store and dispose of old or unused products.
- Fence or otherwise keep pets out of rose gardens, vegetable gardens, and any other areas where pesticides are applied.

### Expected Course and Prognosis

- Good with early and aggressive care. Animals developing the intermediate syndrome may need care for several days to weeks. Pancreatitis and hemorrhagic gastroenteritis complicate the recovery.

### Abbreviations

See Appendix 1 for a complete list.
- DUMBSLED = diarrhea, urination, miosis/mydriasis, bradycardia, salivation, lacrimation, emesis, dyspnea
- SLUDGE = salivation, lacrimation, urination, diarrhea, gastroenteritis
- TEPP = tetraethyl pyrophosphate

### Suggested Reading

Asokan VR, Kerl ME, Evans T, Harmon H. Organophosphate intoxication in 2 dogs from ingestion of cattle ear tags. *J Vet Emerg Crit Care* 2019;29(4): 424–430.
Bahri L. Pralidoxime. *Compend Contin Educ Vet* 2002;24(11):884–886.
Hopper K, Aldrich J, Haskins C. The recognition and treatment of the intermediate syndrome of organophosphate poisoning in a dog. *J Vet Emerg Crit Care* 2002;12(2): 99–102.
Means C. Organophosphate and carbamate insecticides. In: Peterson ME, Talcott PA (eds) *Small Animal Toxicology*, 3rd edn. St Louis: Elsevier, 2013; pp. 715–724.
Tecles F, Panizo C, Subiela SM et al. Effects of different variables on whole blood cholinesterase analysis in dogs. *J Vet Diagn Invest* 2002;14:132–139.

**Author:** Patricia A. Talcott, DVM, PhD, DABVT
**Consulting Editor:** Robert H. Poppenga, DVM, PhD, DABVT

# Chapter 102

# Pyrethrins and Pyrethroids

## DEFINITION/OVERVIEW

- Pyrethrins are derived from *Chrysanthemum* flowers; pyrethroids are synthetic or semisynthetic derivatives of pyrethrins.
- Used as topical and environmental insecticides in a variety of formulations including sprays, shampoos, dips, collars, ear tags, dusts, spot-on/pour-on liquids, and granules.
- Signs of toxicosis include hypersalivation, hyper- or hypothermia, dyspnea, paresthesia, vomiting, hyperexcitability, tremors, ataxia, weakness, seizures, and death.

## ETIOLOGY/PATHOPHYSIOLOGY

- Pyrethrins and pyrethroids are frequently formulated with other ingredients to enhance insecticidal activity. Methoprene and pyriproxyfen are insect growth regulators that prevent immature insect stages from maturing by interfering with insect-specific growth hormones. Piperonyl butoxide inhibits insect metabolism of pyrethroids.

### Mechanism of Action

- Pyrethrins and pyrethroids cause hyperexcitability of cells by slowing the closing of neuronal sodium channels. Some pyrethroids can also exhibit activity on GABA-gated chloride channels.
- Sodium channels are found in large numbers in peripheral muscle, salivary glands, and CNS, which explains the manifestation of signs seen with overdoses.
- The effect on sodium influx is temperature dependent, with increased activity at cooler body temperatures.
- Paresthesia (tingling, burning, numbing, itching) following topical application of some pyrethroids (e.g., permethrin) is caused by direct action on cutaneous sensory nerves.

### Pharmacokinetics – Absorption, Distribution, Metabolism, Excretion

- Rapidly absorbed following ingestion; oral bioavailability in dogs is ~50%.
- Transdermal absorption varies but generally is quite low.
- Highly lipophilic and distributes to tissues with high lipid concentrations such as CNS, adipose tissue, liver, kidneys, and milk; pyrethrins and pyrethroids do not cross the placenta.
- Metabolism occurs in small intestine, liver, and blood, primarily via hydrolysis to inactive metabolites. Some metabolites are further conjugated with amino acids, glucuronide, or sulfate.
- Metabolites are eliminated primarily through urine, although some pyrethroids (e.g., permethrin) have significant biliary excretion.

*Blackwell's Five-Minute Veterinary Consult Clinical Companion: Small Animal Toxicology*, Third Edition. Edited by Lynn R. Hovda, Ahna G. Brutlag, Robert H. Poppenga, and Steven E. Epstein. © 2024 John Wiley & Sons, Inc. Published 2024 by John Wiley & Sons, Inc.

## Toxicity

■ Toxicity varies with animal species and the specific pyrethrin/pyrethroid product, concentration, and formulation.
■ Generally, products containing <1% pyrethrin/pyrethroid are well tolerated by mammals, including cats.
■ Cats are particularly sensitive to many concentrated (>5%) pyrethroids. Most cats tolerate concentrated (40–60%) etofenprox products when applied per label.
■ Dermal paresthesia at concentrated pyrethroid application site can result in signs of agitation, scratching, panting, hyperactivity, depression, and reluctance to move.
■ Oral exposure can result in hypersalivation and/or vomiting without neurological involvement.
■ Pyrethroids have no anticholinesterase activity, so potentiation of organophosphorus or carbamate insecticides is not expected if used together.

## Systems Affected

■ Gastrointestinal – hypersalivation, vomiting, diarrhea, gastritis.
■ Skin/exocrine – paresthesia, localized dermal hypersensitivity reaction.
■ Nervous – hyperesthesia, hyperexcitability, ataxia, paw/facial twitching, muscle fasciculation, tremor, seizure.
■ Endocrine/metabolic – hyperthermia due to prolonged muscle activity; adrenal stimulation resulting in hyperglycemia.
■ Ophthalmic – mydriasis, transient blindness, significant contact irritation due to carrier agents in the product.
■ Respiratory – respiratory distress secondary to unmanaged neurological symptoms.
■ Renal/urological – myoglobinuria secondary to uncontrolled/prolonged tremors or seizures; potential for AKI.

 # SIGNALMENT/HISTORY

### Risk Factors

■ Felines are especially sensitive to some concentrated pyrethroids (e.g., 45% permethrin), but tolerate concentrated forms of others (e.g., 40% etofenprox).
■ Very young, very old, anemic, sick, debilitated, or stressed animals are at increased risk of toxicosis.
■ Heavy flea, tick, or other parasite infestations can increase risk of toxicosis.
■ Use of more than one pyrethroid product can result in additive effects and increase risk of toxicosis; this is primarily a concern with concentrated (>5%) pyrethroids.

### Historical Findings

■ Patients can present with a history of product application or misuse within the previous 12–24 hours.
■ Cats can present after a canine pyrethroid spot-on product was applied to another pet with which they had physical contact.
■ Patients (commonly dogs) can present after ingesting large quantities of pyrethroid-based granular yard insecticides, pyrethroid flea collars, or contents of tubes of topical spot-on products.

### Location and Circumstances of Poisoning

■ Most exposures occur in or around the home.
■ Exposure to pyrethroid-containing livestock or agricultural products can occur in farming environments.

CLINICAL FEATURES

- Onset of signs of toxicosis can occur within minutes to several hours following exposure depending on species involved, route of exposure, pyrethrin/pyrethroid, formulation, and dosage.
- Signs include hypersalivation, hyper- or hypothermia, paresthesia, "paw flicking," vomiting, hyperexcitability, tremors, ataxia, weakness, dyspnea, seizures, and death.
- Paresthesia effects can result in reluctance to move, hiding, hyperactivity, agitation, panting, and attempts to scratch the site of application.

 DIFFERENTIAL DIAGNOSIS

- Intoxications: organophosphate or carbamate insecticides, organochlorine insecticides, strychnine, metaldehyde, 4-aminopyridine, methylxanthines, tremorgenic mycotoxins, CNS stimulant drugs (amphetamine, cocaine, etc.), nicotine, xylitol.
- Hepatic encephalopathy, uremic encephalopathy, hypoglycemia, hypocalcemia.
- CNS trauma, CNS neoplasia, CNS inflammation/infection.

 DIAGNOSTICS

### Clinical Pathological Findings

- Baseline PCV/TS and blood glucose.
- CBC, serum chemistry, UA, particularly in geriatric patients or those with metabolic disease.
- In cases with severe tremors or seizures, a CK and coagulation panel can be helpful in determining other underlying etiologies or secondary complications (e.g., DIC).

### Other Diagnostics

- Gas chromatographic analysis of hair samples or tissues (fat, brain, liver) can confirm exposure to pyrethroids; turn-around times make this impractical for diagnosing emergent cases.
- Tissue pyrethroid concentrations do not correlate with degree of clinical illness.

### Pathological Findings

No specific gross or microscopic pathological findings are expected.

 THERAPEUTICS

- Treatment goals are to manage clinical signs, provide supportive care, remove the source of the intoxication when feasible, and monitor for development of complications due to prolonged tremors or seizures.
- Minor signs such as hypersalivation, facial/ear twitching, paw flicking, or single episodes of vomiting or diarrhea can occur as adverse effects following the appropriate use of pyrethroid products in dogs and cats. These signs are generally transient and do not usually require specific treatment.

### Detoxification

- Manage severe clinical signs (tremors, seizures) first before attempting decontamination.
- Cats can hypersalivate due to the unpleasant taste of a topically applied product as they attempt to groom themselves. These reactions can be managed by offering milk or liquid from canned, water-packed tuna to dilute the product taste.

- Patients with exposure due to grooming product off themselves or other animals will not have sufficient product in the GI tract to warrant gastrointestinal decontamination.
- Do not induce emesis in symptomatic patients due to risk of aspiration pneumonia. Do not administer activated charcoal to patients showing more than mild signs due to risk of aspiration.
- Patients that have ingested large quantities of pyrethroid solids (e.g., collars, granules) and are not showing signs can have emesis induced.
  - Dogs.
    - 3% hydrogen peroxide 2 mL/kg PO up to maximum of 45 mL; feeding a small, moist meal can improve efficacy.
    - Apomorphine: 0.02–0.04 mg/kg IV, SQ, IM; can cause CNS depression.
    - Ropinirole (dogs only): 3.75 mg/m$^2$ topically into conjunctival sac; follow product dosing chart for appropriate number of drops.
  - Cats: alpha-2-adrenergic agents (reverse sedative effects with atipamezole or yohimbine).
    - Dexmedetomidine 0.001–0.002 mg/kg IV or 0.04 mg/kg IM.
    - Xylazine 0.44 mg/kg IM, SQ.
- Activated charcoal (1–3 g/kg) with cathartic for asymptomatic patients that have ingested large amounts of solid pyrethroids.
- For dermal exposures, medically manage any severe signs, then bathe with liquid dish detergent using warm water; several applications of detergent might be necessary. Keep patient warm following bathing.

## Appropriate Health Care

- Manage severe tremors and/or seizures. Do not overmedicate in attempts to eliminate minor tremors or twitching. Aim to manage tremors to the point that the patient can maintain a normal body temperature, ambulate normally, and eat/drink without problems.
- Intravenous fluids can aid in providing cardiovascular support, maintaining hydration, and cooling hyperthermic patients; fluids will not enhance elimination of pyrethroids, so diuresis is not warranted.
- Thermoregulation is vital. Tremoring/seizing patients frequently present hyperthermic due to muscle activity. Managing tremors/seizures followed by bathing often results in resolution of hyperthermia without need for aggressive cooling measures. Patients that develop hypothermia following sedation and bathing can experience exacerbation of muscle tremors as pyrethroids are more potent at lower body temperatures.
- Patients experiencing local paresthesia reactions can respond to vitamin E oil or cool packs applied directly to product application site.

## Antidote

There is no specific antidote.

## Drug(s) of Choice

Methocarbamol: 50–220 mg/kg IV; administer ½ of dose at ~2 mL/min, wait for patient to relax, then continue slowly to effect. Can follow bolus with CRI of 8.8–12.2 mg/kg/h; dosages exceeding 330 mg/kg/day might be required in severe cases but monitor carefully for methocarbamol-induced respiratory depression.

## Precautions/Interactions

Atropine is not indicated in treating pyrethroid toxicosis.

### Alternative Drugs

- Midazolam: 0.05–0.31 mg/kg/h IV CRI +/– propofol; monitor respiration and body temperature closely in anesthetized patients.
- Propofol: 1.5–19 mg/kg/h IV CRI; monitor respiration and body temperature closely in anesthetized patients.
- Phenobarbital: 2–8 mg/kg IV to effect; monitor respiration and body temperature closely in anesthetized patients.
- Pentobarbital: 4–16 mg/kg IV to effect; monitor respiration and body temperature closely in anesthetized patients.
- Diazepam: 0.13–1.5 mg/kg IV, 0.47–1.7 mg/kg per rectum; rarely effective as sole agent for tremors or seizures, but can reduce hyperesthesia when used in combination with methocarbamol.
- Intravenous lipid emulsions (ILE): 20% solution, 1.5 mL/kg bolus followed by 0.5 mL/kg/min for 30–60 minutes; repeat in 4–6 hours if still symptomatic and serum is not lipemic; discontinue if no effect after two doses; use should be restricted to patients unresponsive to other treatment or where euthanasia is being considered due to cost/duration of treatment; adverse events with ILE therapy include hemolysis and pancreatitis.

### Patient Monitoring

- Monitor for return of tremors.
- Reassess thermoregulation measures and decontamination effectiveness if tremors continue to recur.
- Monitor for development of complications from tremors/seizures (e.g., rhabdomyolysis, DIC, renal injury, etc.).

 **COMMENTS**

### Prevention/Avoidance

- Secure pesticides where they cannot be accessed by pets.
- Always use pesticide products per label directions.
- Never apply a product labeled only for dogs to other species.

### Possible Complications

- Rhabdomyolysis +/- myoglobinuric ARF due to prolonged muscular exertion from tremors or seizures.
- Prolonged hyperthermia can result in development of DIC.

### Expected Course and Prognosis

- Most cases that are treated promptly and aggressively have good outcomes.
- Failure to obtain prompt treatment can result in complications (e.g., rhabdomyolysis, DIC) that can worsen prognosis.

### Suggested Reading

Boland LA, Angles JM. Feline permethrin toxicity: retrospective study of 42 cases. *J Feline Med Surg* 2010;12(2):61–71.

Draper WE, Boldfer L, Cottam E, McMichael M, Schubert T. Methocarbamol CRI for symptomatic treatment of pyrethroid intoxication: a report of three cases. *J Am Anim Hosp Assoc* 2013;49(5):325–328.

Kelmer E, Oved S, Abu Ahmad W et al. Retrospective evaluation of factors associated with the morbidity and outcome of permethrin toxicosis in cats. *Israel J Vet Med* 2020;75(3):142–147.

Kuo K, Odunayo A. Adjunctive therapy with intravenous lipid emulsion and methocarbamol for permethrin toxicity in 2 cats. *J Vet Emerg Crit Care* 2013;23(4):436–441.

Pelizzola M, Mattavelli C, Trola R et al. Low-dose intravenous lipid emulsion as a safe treatment for lipophilic intoxications in five cats. *Vet Rec Case Rep* 2018;6(4):e000663.

**Author**: Sharon Gwaltney-Brant DVM, PhD, DABVT, DABT
**Consulting Editor**: Robert H. Poppenga, DVM, PhD, DABVT

# Metals and Metalloids

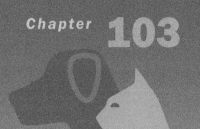

# Chapter 103

# Iron

## DEFINITION/OVERVIEW

- Iron is an essential element for living organisms, as it is needed for the transport and binding of oxygen, as well as for many oxidation-reduction reactions.
- In companion animals, oral toxicosis is predominant but iron can be toxic by injectable routes as well.
- Iron may be lethal when ingested in large quantities of readily ionized and soluble iron due to its oxidation-reduction properties.
- Sources of large concentrations of readily ionizable iron include multivitamins, dietary mineral supplements, human prenatal supplements, fertilizers, molluscicides, oxygen absorber packets, and some types of hand warmers.
- Circulating iron in excess of the total iron-binding capacity (TIBC), or free iron, is very reactive. It can cause direct oxidative damage to any cell type, as well as secondary damage through processes such as lipid peroxidation.
- Damage to mitochondria results in compromise to cellular respiration.
- Primary systems affected are GI, hepatic, cardiovascular, and CNS

## ETIOLOGY/PATHOPHYSIOLOGY

- Iron toxicosis is generally associated with ingestion of iron-fortified pills (e.g., vitamins/minerals or prenatal supplements), but other sources include iron-fortified fertilizers, newer molluscicide products, oxygen absorber packets, and some types of hand warmers.
- In order for iron to be absorbed and toxic, it must be in a readily ionized and soluble form.
- Metallic iron, iron-containing alloys, and iron oxide (rust) are not readily ionizable. Thus they are not associated with iron toxicosis.
- Take care when calculating iron ingestion; iron salts in supplements and medications vary in elemental iron content (between 12% and 63%; see Table 103.1).

### Mechanism of Action

- Large oral doses of ionizable iron can damage the GI mucosal integrity, allowing increased iron absorption.
- Free circulating iron (in excess of TIBC) is very reactive and causes oxidative damage to membranes. These interactions produce highly reactive hydroxyl ions and hydroxyl radicals which cause further membrane damage.
- Reduction-oxidation cycling of iron from ferric to ferrous states and back can result in highly reactive free radicals.
- Damage is primarily focused on tissues of highest exposure to free iron: GIT, cardiovascular, and hepatic.

---

*Blackwell's Five-Minute Veterinary Consult Clinical Companion: Small Animal Toxicology*, Third Edition.
Edited by Lynn R. Hovda, Ahna G. Brutlag, Robert H. Poppenga, and Steven E. Epstein.
© 2024 John Wiley & Sons, Inc. Published 2024 by John Wiley & Sons, Inc.

**TABLE 103.1 Percentage of elemental iron in common soluble iron salts.**

| Salt | Percentage of elemental iron |
| --- | --- |
| Iron (as ferric salt) | 100 |
| Iron (as ferrous salt) | 100 |
| Ferric ammonium citrate | 15 |
| Ferric chloride | 34 |
| Ferric hydroxide | 63 |
| Ferric phosphate | 37 |
| Ferric pyrophosphate | 30 |
| Ferrocholinate | 12 |
| Ferroglycine sulfate | 16 |
| Ferrous fumarate | 33 |
| Ferrous carbonate | 48 |
| Ferrous gluconate | 12 |
| Ferrous lactate | 24 |
| Ferrous sulfate (anhydrous) | 37 |
| Ferrous sulfate (hydrate) | 20 |
| Peptonized iron | 17 |

- Vasodilation and vascular damage result in systemic shock, leading to a metabolic acidosis.
- Vascular damage can result in hemorrhage.
- Mitochondrial damage results in compromise of cellular respiration, further contributing to systemic metabolic acidosis.

### Pharmacokinetics – Absorption, Distribution, Metabolism, Excretion

- Iron absorption is titrated at the GI mucosa depending on the body's requirements.
- Iron must be ionized in order to be absorbed.
- Ferrous iron is more bioavailable than ferric; both are absorbable if ionized.
- Once absorbed, iron is distributed to tissues, transported by iron-binding proteins.
- Saturation of these iron-binding proteins results in "free iron" being circulated in the serum to tissues.
- Unused iron is sequestered in tissues as ferritin molecules.
- Unlike most metals, animals are unable to excrete excess iron. Even in overdose situations, excess iron is incorporated into ferritin in cells in order to sequester it.
- Minimal amounts of iron are lost from the body, primarily via exfoliation of GIT cells or via blood loss.

### Toxicity

- Oral toxic dose (dogs).
  - <20 mg/kg of ionizable iron is nontoxic.
  - 20–60 mg/kg of ionizable iron can result in clinical signs.
  - >60 mg/kg of ionizable iron can result in serious clinical disease.
- Injectable iron is more toxic due to much greater bioavailability.

## Systems Affected

- Gastrointestinal – GI erosions, ulcerations, and hemorrhage result from direct oxidative damage and adherence of pills to GI mucosal surfaces, increasing iron permeability.
  - Potential for stricture formation in esophagus or GIT after recovery.
- Cardiovascular – oxidative damage results in vasodilation, vascular leakage, and hemorrhage.
- Metabolic – compromised cellular respiration and lactic acidosis secondary to hypovolemia and hypotension contribute to acid–base imbalances (e.g., metabolic acidosis).
- Hepatobiliary – free iron damages hepatocellular membranes and subcellular organelles, which can lead to coagulation deficits.
- Nervous – typically secondary to effects on other systems, such as CNS edema following vascular injury and hepatic encephalopathy following hepatic injury.

 # SIGNALMENT/HISTORY

### Risk Factors

- All species and ages are potentially susceptible.
- Dogs are more likely to ingest large amounts of the described iron-containing agents, due to indiscriminate eating behavior.

### Historical Findings

- Owners frequently report ingestion of large numbers of vitamin/mineral pills.

### Location and Circumstances of Poisoning

- Most frequent ingestion occurs inside households when dogs gain access to bottles of vitamins/mineral pills.
- Much less common toxic exposures include ingestions of iron-fortified fertilizers, some types of iron-containing hand warmers, or oxygen absorber packets in food packaging.
- Exposure of dogs to iron-containing molluscicides has increased due to wider availability of products designed to replace metaldehyde formulations.

 # CLINICAL FEATURES

- Toxicosis is unlikely to develop in animals that remain asymptomatic for 6–8 hours.
- Gastrointestinal signs are often the first to be noted after oral exposures.
- Iron toxicosis occurs in four phases, the severity and timing of each phase depends on the dose and amount of damage to tissues.
  - Stage I (0–6 hours).
    - Vomiting.
    - Diarrhea.
    - Lethargy.
    - GI hemorrhage.
    - Abdominal pain.
  - Stage II (6–24 hours): apparent recovery.
  - Stage III (12–96 hours).
    - Vomiting/diarrhea/GI hemorrhage/abdominal pain.
    - Lethargy.
    - Shock.

   - ○ Tremors.
   - ○ Metabolic acidosis.
- Stage IV (2–6 weeks): GIT stricture formation secondary to initial mucosal damage resulting in GI obstruction.

# DIFFERENTIAL DIAGNOSIS

- Primary gastrointestinal disease – mesenteric torsion, GDV, obstruction, pancreatitis, septic peritonitis, acute hemorrhagic diarrhea syndrome, gastroenteritis, infectious, parasitic.
- Secondary gastrointestinal disease – hypoadrenocorticism, endotoxin ingestion from garbage, caustic/corrosive ingestion, heat stroke, "shock gut", snake bite.
- Primary metabolic disease – renal, hepatic, etc.

# DIAGNOSTICS

Serum analysis for total iron and TIBC.
- Normal serum iron binding capacity is 3–4 times the serum iron concentration.
- Serum iron > TIBC indicates treatment for iron toxicosis is required.
- For chewable tablets or liquid solution ingestions, check serum iron levels 2–3 hours post ingestion.
- For capsules or nonchewable tablets, check serum iron levels 4–6 hours post ingestion.
    - ○ Expected range in dogs: 94–122 mcg/dL.
    - ○ Chelation indicated: >250–500 mcg/dL.
    - ○ Avoid hemolyzed serum samples; hemolysis increases iron content.
- Absorption rates can vary and serum iron concentrations may change rapidly.
- Monitor every 2–4 hours until levels peak, then every 6–8 hours in patients on chelation therapy.
- Check serum iron 5–6 hours post ingestion in asymptomatic patients.

### Clinical Pathological Findings

- CBC, chemistry, UA, venous blood gas analysis – leukocytosis, hypoglycemia, hyperglycemia, metabolic acidosis, normal to high AST, ALT, ALP, and serum bilirubin.
- Blood pressure for hypotension.
- Coagulation profile for DIC.

### Other Diagnostics

- Radiographs may aid in visualizing pill bezoars or pills adhered to esophageal/gastric mucosa.

### Pathological Findings

- Primary gross lesions are of damage to the GIT, liver, and vascular systems.
- Damage to the GIT can range from erythema to complete epithelial necrosis.
- Hemorrhage in the GIT and liver is often observed, and can be seen in any organ system. Hepatomegaly may also be evident.
- Pathological lesions of edema and hemorrhage in any organ system can occur due to damage to vasculature.
- Cellular damage to vascular endothelium, hepatocytes, and myocardial cells may be seen histologically.

# THERAPEUTICS

- General therapy aims to minimize further iron absorption, correct hypovolemic shock, correct metabolic acidosis, treat GI signs, and eliminate free iron.

## Detoxification

- Activated charcoal does not bind to iron and should not be used.
- Oral milk of magnesia or aluminum hydroxide will precipitate iron in the GIT as insoluble iron hydroxide. Dose at 5–30 mL PO q 8–12 hours (may cause diarrhea).
- Remove unabsorbed iron from stomach to reduce duration and severity of clinical signs.
- Induce emesis in asymptomatic patient, early post ingestion. Caution is advised if there is evidence of gastric damage.
- Gastric lavage should be performed when emesis is contraindicated or pill bezoars are identified (e.g., radiographically). Also consider whole-bowel irrigation or enema.
- Emergency gastrotomy may be indicated if lavage fails to remove pills or bezoars, and a toxic amount of iron has been ingested.

## Appropriate Health Care

- Inpatient monitoring with toxic doses and hospitalization if symptomatic.
- Home monitoring optional for patients that remain asymptomatic for eight hours post ingestion.
- Treat shock and metabolic acidosis appropriately.
- IV fluids as needed for dehydration and hypovolemia for 24–72 hours or PRN until clinical signs resolve; this will also enhance urinary elimination of chelated iron.

## Antidote

- Chelation recommended when serum iron >250–500 mcg/dL or serum iron >TIBC.
    - Deferoxamine mesylate is an effective iron chelator and is given at 15 mg/kg/h, slow IV infusion, or 40 mg/kg IM q 4–6 hours or slow IV q 4–6 hours.
    - Duration of chelation therapy is until TIBC is greater than serum iron or serum iron <300 mcg/dL.
    - Ascorbic acid 10–15 mg/kg PO, SQ, IM, q 4–6 hours.
        - Only give with deferoxamine chelation to enhance iron excretion.
        - Start after iron fully removed from GI tract.

## Drug(s) of Choice

- Antiemetics.
    - Maropitant 1 mg/kg, SQ q 24 hours.
    - Ondansetron 0.1–0.2 mg/kg, SQ, IV q 8–12 hours.
    - Metoclopramide 0.2–0.5 mg/kg, PO, IM, SQ q 8 hours or 1–2 mg/kg/day, CRI IV.
- Proton pump inhibitors.
    - Omeprazole 0.5–1.0 mg/kg, PO q2 4 hours in dogs; 0.7 mg/kg, PO q 24 hours in cats.
    - Pantoprazole 1 mg/kg, IV q 24 hours in dogs.
- $H_2$ antagonist: famotidine 0.5–1.0 mg/kg, PO, SQ, IM, or IV q 12–24 hours.
- Sucralfate 0.25–1 g, PO q 8–12 hours.

## Precautions/Interactions

- Gastric lavage is contraindicated when hematemesis is present due to increased risk of perforation.

- IV deferoxamine must be given slowly or it may precipitate cardiac arrhythmias.
- Deferoxamine is teratogenic. Use in pregnant patients only if the benefits outweigh the risks.
- Deferoxamine-iron chelates are eliminated in the urine. Caution is advised for patients with poor renal function.

## Surgical Considerations

- Emergency gastrotomy is indicated in cases where a toxic dose has been ingested and gastric lavage has failed to remove radiographically visible pills/bezoars.

## Patient Monitoring

- Monitor serum iron and TIBC every 6–8 hours while on chelation therapy. Patient should remain in hospital until they can maintain expected serum iron and TIBC for 24 hours post chelation therapy.
- Monitor hydration status, serum hepatic enzymes, acid–base status, and GIT effects.
- In severely symptomatic animals, advise clients to monitor their pet for normal dietary intake and fecal production for 6–8 weeks to evaluate for stricture development.

## Diet

- Limit oral intake during the first 24 hours in severely symptomatic animals.
- Following evaluation of GI damage, either start patient on a bland, easily digestible, soft food diet to allow mucosal repair or allow patient to return to a normal diet.

 # COMMENTS

- Caution with inducing emesis or gastric lavage as GI damage can increase risks of perforations.
- It is critical to remove any remaining iron material or pills to prevent further absorption or GI damage.

## Prevention/Avoidance

- Prevention is only achieved by limiting the potential animal exposure.

## Possible Complications

- Stricture formation is a possible sequela to GI mucosal damage.

## Expected Course and Prognosis

- In patients asymptomatic by eight hours, the prognosis is very good. These animals are unlikely to develop clinical signs.
- In patients adequately decontaminated prior to development of clinical signs, the prognosis is fair to guarded until they are asymptomatic for eight hours or until the serum iron < TIBC at 6–8 hours post ingestion.
- In symptomatic patients, the prognosis is guarded until chelation therapy results in serum iron < TIBC. The prognosis is based on the severity of clinical signs and the amount of damage already done.

## See Also

Chapter 2 Emergency Management of the Poisoned Patient

## Abbreviations

See Appendix 1 for a complete list.
- TIBC = total iron-binding capacity

## Suggested Reading

Albretsen JC. Iron. In: Plumlee H (ed.) *Clinical Veterinary Toxicology*. St Louis: Mosby, 2004; pp. 202–204.

Brutlag AG, Flint CTC, Puschner B. Iron intoxication in a dog consequent to the ingestion of oxygen absorber sachets in pet treat packaging. *J Med Toxicol* 2012;8:76–79.

Hall JO. Iron. In: Peterson ME, Talcott PA (eds) *Small Animal Toxicology*, 3rd edn. St Louis: Elsevier, 2013; pp. 595–600.

Hooser SB. Iron. In: Gupta RC (ed.) *Veterinary Toxicology Basic and Clinical Principles*, 2nd edn. San Diego: Elsevier, 2012; pp. 517–521.

## Acknowledgments

The author and book editors acknowledge the prior contribution of Jeffery O. Hall.

**Author:** Chelsea Sykes, DVM
**Consulting Editor:** Robert H. Poppenga, DVM, PhD, DABVT

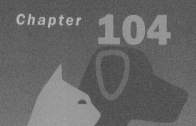
# Lead

## DEFINITION/OVERVIEW

- Historically, lead has been used for many purposes, but its use in products such as paint and gasoline has declined due to its acute and chronic toxicity to humans, especially children; incidences of poisoning in dogs and cats have declined as a consequence.
- Ingestion of some form of lead – paint and paint residues or dust from sanding; car batteries; linoleum; solder; plumbing materials and supplies; lubricating compounds; putty; tar paper; lead foil; golf balls; lead object (e.g., shot, fishing sinkers, drapery weights), leaded glass.
- Use of improperly glazed ceramic food or water bowl.
- Lead paint or lead-contaminated dust or soil are common sources for exposure; cats ingest lead as a result of self-grooming.
- Intoxication (blood lead >0.35 ppm, although somewhat variable) owing to acute or chronic exposure to some form of lead.

## ETIOLOGY/PATHOPHYSIOLOGY

### Mechanism of Action

- Cell damage is due in part to the ability of lead to substitute for other polyvalent cations (especially divalent cations such as Ca and Zn) important for cell homeostasis.
- Lead binds to sulfhydryl and other nucleophilic functional groups, causing inhibition of several enzymes and changes in calcium and vitamin D metabolism.
- Lead causes increased production of reactive oxygen species, resulting in oxidative damage.
- Diverse biological processes are affected, including metal transport, energy metabolism, apoptosis, ion conduction, cell adhesion, inter- and intracellular signaling, enzymatic processes, protein maturation, and genetic regulation.
- Lead inhibits hemoglobin production by interfering with several enzymatic steps in the heme pathway; this contributes to anemia associated with chronic lead intoxication.

### Pharmacokinetics – Absorption, Distribution, Metabolism, Excretion

- Ingestion of lead is the most common route of exposure.
- Bioavailability is dependent on the form of lead ingested, the physiological state and age of the animal, and diet.
- Lead bioavailability is greater in young animals, animals that are deficient in calcium, iron, zinc or vitamin D, and pregnant or lactating animals.
- It is widely distributed in the body and can cross the blood–brain barrier.
- It accumulates in active bone matrix; bone serves as a relatively inert long-term storage site.
- After absorption, a large proportion of lead is carried on erythrocyte membranes.

*Blackwell's Five-Minute Veterinary Consult Clinical Companion: Small Animal Toxicology*, Third Edition.
Edited by Lynn R. Hovda, Ahna G. Brutlag, Robert H. Poppenga, and Steven E. Epstein.
© 2024 John Wiley & Sons, Inc. Published 2024 by John Wiley & Sons, Inc.

- Excretion is primarily via the bile with relatively little naturally excreted in the urine; chelation therapy greatly increases urinary excretion of the metal.
- The half-life of lead is multiphasic: 1.2 days in blood, 184 days in soft tissues, and >4500 days in bone.

## Toxicity

- Variable depending on form of lead, species, and age of animal.
- Not well defined in cats.
- Dogs: acutely toxic dosages range from 190 to 1000 mg/kg body weight, whereas a chronic cumulative dosage is approximately 1.8–2.6 mg/kg body weight.

## Systems Affected

- Gastrointestinal – unknown mechanism, likely damage to peripheral nerves.
- Nervous – capillary damage; alteration of membrane ionic channels and signaling molecules.
- Renal/urological – damage to proximal tubule cells due to enzyme disruption and oxidative damage.
- Hemic/lymph/immune – interference with hemoglobin synthesis, increased fragility and decreased survival of RBCs, release of reticulocytes and nucleated RBCs from bone marrow, inhibition of 5'-pyrimidine nucleotidase causing retention of RNA degradation products, aggregation of ribosomes resulting in basophilic stippling.

# SIGNALMENT/HISTORY

## Risk Factors

- Housing in older, nonrenovated buildings where lead-based paint was used.
- Housing in older buildings undergoing renovation where environmental lead contamination is more likely to occur.
- Low socioeconomic status of the pet owner.
- Younger animals (<1 year) due to increased bioavailability.
- Dogs more commonly intoxicated than cats.
- Dietary deficiencies of calcium, iron, zinc, and vitamin D.

## Historical Findings

- History of renovation of older house or building or ingestion of lead objects.

## Location and Circumstances of Poisoning

- Dogs are more likely to ingest lead-containing paint or lead objects; cats are exposed to lead-containing dusts as a result of grooming.

# CLINICAL FEATURES

- Primarily gastrointestinal and neurological signs.
- Gastrointestinal – often precede CNS signs; predominant with chronic, low-level exposure.
- CNS – occur more often with acute exposure; more common in younger animals.
- Renal – proximal tubular nephropathy has been reported.

- Common clinical signs include emesis, diarrhea, anorexia, abdominal pain, regurgitation due to megaesophagus, lethargy, hysteria, seizures, and blindness. In cats, central vestibular abnormalities such as vertical nystagmus and ataxia reported.

# DIFFERENTIAL DIAGNOSIS

## Dogs

- Infectious encephalitides.
- Epilepsy.
- Bromethalin, methylxanthine, organophosphorus/carbamate insecticide, tremorgenic myco-toxin or NSAID toxicoses.
- Heat stroke.
- Intestinal parasitism.
- Intussusception.
- Foreign body.
- Pancreatitis.
- Infectious canine hepatitis.

## Cats

- Degenerative or storage diseases.
- Hepatic encephalopathy.
- Infectious encephalitides.
- Organophosphorus/carbamabe insecticide, bromethalin, or methylxanthine toxicosis.

# DIAGNOSTICS

## Clinical Pathological Findings

- Between 5 and 40 nucleated RBCs/100 WBCs without anemia; absence of nucleated RBC does not rule out the diagnosis.
- Anisocytosis, polychromasia, poikilocytosis, target cells, hypochromasia.
- Basophilic stippling of RBCs; often difficult to detect.
- Neutrophilic leukocytosis.
- Cats – elevated AST and ALP reported.
- Urinalysis – mild nonspecific renal damage; glucosuria; proteinuria; hemoglobinuria.

## Other Diagnostics

- Imaging: presence of radiopaque material in the gastrointestinal tract (presence or absence is not diagnostic); radiographic lead lines (precipitation of lead salts) within the epiphyseal plate of long bones is uncommon.
- Lead detection.
    - Antemortem whole-blood lead concentration: >0.35 ppm (35 mcg/dL); postmortem liver and/or kidney lead concentration: >5 ppm (wet weight).
    - Blood lead concentrations fluctuate and do not necessarily correlate with total body burden.
    - Lower values – must be interpreted in conjunction with history and clinical signs.
    - No normal "background" blood lead concentrations; typically less than 0.05 ppm.
    - Blood concentrations – do not correlate with occurrence or severity of clinical signs.

- CaNa₂EDTA mobilization test – collect one 24-hour urine sample; administer CaNa₂EDTA (75 mg/kg IM); collect a second 24-hour urine sample; with toxicosis, urine lead increases 10–60-fold post EDTA (succimer could conceivably be substituted for CaNa₂EDTA but this has not been evaluated).
- Point-of-care testing is available but results might underestimate true blood lead concentrations; confirmation of results using other techniques such as GFAAS or ICP-MS is recommended.

## Pathological Findings

- Gross: may note paint chips or lead objects in gastrointestinal tract.
- Intranuclear inclusion bodies: may note in hepatocytes or renal tubular epithelial cells; intracellular storage form of lead; considered pathognomonic.
- Cerebrocortical lesions: spongiosis, vascular hypertrophy, gliosis, neuronal necrosis, demyelination.

 # THERAPEUTICS

## Detoxification

- Evacuation of gastrointestinal tract – saline cathartics; sodium or magnesium sulfate (dogs, 2–25 g and cats 2–5 g PO as 20% solution or less).
- Sulfate-containing cathartics potentially precipitate lead in the gastrointestinal tract to the less bioavailable lead sulfate salt.
- Endoscopic or surgical removal of lead objects in the gastrointestinal tract might be warranted in some cases.

## Drug(s) and Antidotes of Choice

- Reduction of lead body burden with chelation therapy – CaNa₂EDTA (dogs and cats, 25 mg/kg SQ, IM, IV q 6 hours for 2–5 days); dilute to a 1% solution with D₅W before administration; may need multiple treatment courses if blood lead concentration is high; allow five-day rest period between treatment courses.
- Succimer – alternative to CaNa₂ EDTA; orally administered chelating agent; 10 mg/kg PO q 8 hours for five days followed by 10 mg PO q 12 hours for two weeks; allow two-week rest period between treatments; may administer per rectum if clinical signs such as emesis preclude oral administration; cats successfully treated with 10 mg/kg PO q 8 hours for 17 days. Advantages over other chelators: can be given PO, allowing for outpatient treatment; does not increase lead absorption from the gastrointestinal tract; not reported to be nephrotoxic; chelation of essential elements such as zinc and copper is not clinically significant.
- CaNa₂EDTA more effective at removing lead from bone; succimer more effective at removing lead from soft tissues.
- Control seizures – diazepam (given to effect; dogs and cats, 0.5 mg/kg IV) or phenobarbital sodium (administer in increments of 10–20 mg/kg IV to effect).
- Alleviation of cerebral edema – mannitol (0.25–2 g/kg of 15–25% IV, slow infusion over 30–60 minutes) and dexamethasone (2.2–4.4 mg/kg IV).
- Some evidence that antioxidants or thiol-containing drugs may be useful – vitamins C and E, alpha-lipoic acid, N-acetylcysteine; optimal doses not determined.
- B-vitamins, especially thiamine, may also be useful; optimal doses not determined.
- Balanced electrolyte fluids – Ringer's solution; correction of hydration deficit.

## Appropriate Health Care

- Inpatient – first course of chelation, depending on severity of clinical signs.
- Outpatient – orally administered chelators.

## Precautions/Interactions

- $CaNa_2EDTA$ – safety in pregnancy not established; teratogenic at therapeutic doses although in human medicine it is recommended over succimer for pregnant patients; do not administer to patients with renal impairment or anuria; establish urine flow before administration; do not administer orally; depletion of zinc, iron, and manganese with long-term therapy.
- Succimer – safety in pregnancy not established; fetotoxic at doses much higher (100–1000 mg/kg) than recommended therapeutic dose; depletion of essential metals is not clinically significant.

## Patient Monitoring

- Assess blood lead concentrations before additional courses of chelation therapy or 10–14 days after cessation of chelation therapy.

## Diet

- Provide a good-quality, nutritionally complete diet.

 **COMMENTS**

## Prevention/Avoidance

- Client awareness of potential sources of exposure and avoidance of contact with those sources.
- Test paint, soil, or dust prior to allowing animal access if likelihood of lead contamination.
- Depending on the circumstances of exposure, environmental clean-up might be warranted to avoid continued exposure.
- Inform client of the potential of adverse human health effects of lead.
- Notify public health officials and consult with family physician for possible blood lead testing.
- Given the ubiquitous nature of lead in the environment, its detection at low concentrations in pet foods is possible; the low concentrations have not been shown to be of concern.

## Possible Complications

- Uncontrolled seizures can result in permanent neurological deficits.
- Blindness.

## Expected Course and Prognosis

- Signs should dramatically improve within 24–48 hours after initiating chelation therapy.
- Prognosis – favorable with treatment.
- Uncontrolled seizures – guarded prognosis.

## Abbreviations

See Appendix 1 for a complete list.
- $CaNa_2$ EDTA = calcium disodium ethylene diamine tetraacetate
- GFAAS = graphite furnace atomic absorption spectrometry
- ICP-MS = inductively coupled plasma-mass spectrometry

## Suggested Reading

Knight TE, Kumar MSA. Lead toxicosis in cats – a review. *J Feline Med Surg* 2003;5:249–255.

Knight TE, Kent, M, Junk JE. Succimer for treatment of lead toxicosis in two cats. *J Am Vet Med Assoc* 2001;218:1946–1948.

Langlois DK, Kaneene JB, Yuzbasiyan-Gurkan V et al. Investigation of blood lead concentrations in dogs living in Flint, Michigan. *J Am Vet Med Assoc* 2017;251(8):912–921.

Morgan RV, Moore FM, Pearce LK et al. Clinical and laboratory findings in small companion animals with lead poisoning: 347 cases (1977–1986). *J Am Vet Med Assoc* 1991;199:93–97.

Morgan RV, Pearce LK, Moore FM et al. Demographic data and treatment of small companion animals with lead poisoning: 347 cases (1977–1986). *J Am Vet Med Assoc* 1991;199:98–102.

Ramsey DT, Casteel SW, Fagella AM et al. Use of orally administered succimer (meso-2,3-dimercaptosuccinic acid) for treatment of lead poisoning in dogs. *J Am Vet Med Assoc* 1996;208:371–375.

**Author**: Robert H. Poppenga, DVM, PhD, DABVT
**Consulting Editor**: Lynn Hovda, RPh, DVM, MS, DACVIM

# Chapter 105

# Zinc

## DEFINITION/OVERVIEW

- Zinc (Zn) toxicosis results from the ingestion of zinc-containing objects such as pennies (see later in this chapter), metallic nuts, bolts, staples, galvanized metal (e.g., nails), pieces from board games, zippers, toys, and jewelry or from products containing zinc salts such as zinc oxide.
- Zinc-containing products include the following.
  - Zinc carbonate and gluconate (dietary supplements), Zn acetate (throat lozenges).
  - Zinc chloride (deodorants), Zn pyrithione (shampoo), Zn oxide (sunblock, diaper creams, calamine lotion).
  - Zn sulfide (paint).
  - Metallic zinc (coins, nut, bolts), brass (alloy of zinc and copper).
- The most common cause of Zn toxicosis is penny ingestion.
  - US pennies minted after 1982 contain 97.5% Zn.
  - Canadian pennies minted from 1997 through 2001 contain 96% Zn.
- Toxicosis initially presents as gastrointestinal upset with vomiting and anorexia but can progress to intravascular hemolytic anemia. Secondary multiorgan failure (renal, hepatic, pancreatic, cardiac), DIC, and cardiopulmonary arrest can occur in severe toxicosis.
- Zinc salt-containing products such as zinc oxide in skin protectants (i.e., diaper rash cream and sunblock) and zinc acetate in throat lozenges can cause gastroenteritis but are not expected to cause Zn toxicosis with acute ingestion.

## ETIOLOGY/PATHOPHYSIOLOGY

### Mechanism of Action

- Unknown: mechanisms have been proposed but none confirmed.
- Intravascular hemolysis is common.
- High concentrations of zinc may be found in serum, red blood cells, liver, kidneys, and pancreas following toxicosis.

### Pharmacokinetics – Absorption, Distribution, Metabolism, Excretion

- Zinc absorption primarily occurs in the small intestine after oral exposure. The acidic environment of the stomach promotes leaching of zinc from ingested objects, allowing for absorption.
- Metabolism occurs in the liver, with metallothionein playing a significant role.
- Excretion occurs primarily via the feces, with a small amount excreted in the urine. Urinary excretion plays a bigger role in toxicosis, especially with chelation therapy.

*Blackwell's Five-Minute Veterinary Consult Clinical Companion: Small Animal Toxicology*, Third Edition.
Edited by Lynn R. Hovda, Ahna G. Brutlag, Robert H. Poppenga, and Steven E. Epstein.
© 2024 John Wiley & Sons, Inc. Published 2024 by John Wiley & Sons, Inc.

## Toxicity

- Although an $LD_{50}$ of 100 mg/kg acute Zn salt ingestion in dogs has been reported, source or study supporting this $LD_{50}$ is unknown.
- Ingestion of one penny (2.5 g) can cause toxicosis in most dogs.
- Acute ingestion of topical Zn salt-containing products generally causes gastrointestinal upset; subacute and chronic exposure has been documented to cause systemic zinc toxicosis.

## Systems Affected

- Hemic – intravascular hemolysis, Heinz body anemia, coagulopathy, DIC, leukocytosis with neutrophilia, left shift, monocytosis, lymphopenia.
- Gastrointestinal – anorexia, vomiting, diarrhea.
- Endocrine – pancreatitis.
- Renal – pigmenturia (hemoglobinuria, bilirubinuria), azotemia, oliguria/anuria.
- Nervous – depression, ataxia, seizures.
- Hepatic – hyperbilirubinemia, elevated liver enzymes, hepatic necrosis.

# SIGNALMENT/HISTORY

- Toxicosis can occur in any species but is frequently reported in young, small-breed dogs (<25 pounds) that are often unable to pass the metallic object out of the stomach.

## Risk Factors

- Young animals may ingest more foreign objects due to indiscriminate eating.

## Historical Findings

- Ingestion of topical cream or metallic object.
- History of vomiting, lethargy, anorexia, jaundice, abnormal or red-colored urine.

## Location and Circumstance of Poisoning

- Most exposures to coins or zinc salts occur in the home.
- Kennels or workplaces may pose added risks for other Zn metal or salt ingestion.

## Interaction with Drugs, Nutrients, or Environment

- Zinc may interfere with copper or iron absorption, although this is unlikely to be a concern with acute exposures.
- Zinc absorption may be decreased with high dietary levels of phytates, calcium, or phosphorus and increased with certain amino acids and EDTA.

# CLINICAL FEATURES

- The most common signs are anorexia, vomiting, diarrhea, lethargy, depression, pale or icteric mucous membranes, and icteric sclera and skin. Orange-tinged feces and pigmenturia may be noted.
- GI signs may begin minutes after ingestion. The onset of hemolysis is dependent upon the rate at which a zinc-containing object breaks down in the stomach, which might take hours to days.
- Animals with hemolytic anemia will often be tachycardic with weak or bounding pulses. A heart murmur may be noted on auscultation.

- Severe depression and seizures can develop at later stages.
- Death is often due to cardiovascular collapse and multiorgan failure.

 # DIFFERENTIAL DIAGNOSIS

- Hemolysis: IMHA, babesiosis, onions, garlic, chives, naphthalene mothballs, acetaminophen, snake and spider envenomation, propylene glycol, and caval syndrome.
- Gastrointestinal signs: primary gastrointestinal infectious and inflammatory diseases, foreign body ingestion, dietary indiscretion, and secondary to metabolic disease.

 # DIAGNOSTICS

## Clinical Pathological Findings

- CBC.
  - Hemolytic anemia, Heinz body formation, regenerative anemia. Spherocytosis and target cells are inconsistently noted.
  - Leukocytosis with neutrophilia, left shift, monocytosis, lymphopenia.
  - Thrombocytopenia in animals with DIC.
- Serum chemistry.
  - Hyperbilirubinemia, elevated AST, ALP, and less commonly GGT and ALT.
  - Azotemia.
  - Elevated amylase and lipase.
- Urinalysis: bilirubinuria, hemoglobinuria, isosthenuria, tubular casts.
- Coagulation panel: prolonged PT/PTT, hypofibrinogenemia, thrombocytopenia, high FDPs suggestive of DIC.

## Other Diagnostics

- Abdominal radiographs to evaluate for metallic object in GI tract. Repeat after object removal to ensure all metal is removed.
- Serum Zn levels often exceed 5 ppm (normal range 0.7–2 ppm for dogs and cats). Contact reference lab for instruction prior to submission as specific tubes are required.

## Pathological Findings

- Gross lesions include icterus, splenomegaly, hepatomegaly, and pigmenturia.
- Histological lesions include evidence of pigmentary nephropathy, hepatic necrosis, pancreatic acinar cell necrosis. Macrophages may contain hemosiderin.
- Tissue Zn levels can be measured in liver, kidney, and pancreas samples collected postmortem.

 # THERAPEUTICS

Main goal of treatment is stabilization and rapid removal of zinc objects if present.

## Detoxification

- Induce emesis in asymptomatic animals with evidence of a metallic foreign object in the stomach. Not always efficacious.
- Removal of the metallic object via endoscopy or laparotomy/gastrotomy after initial stabilization. Zinc levels decrease rapidly after removal of the object.
- Activated charcoal does not bind to zinc and is not indicated.

## Drug(s) and Antidotes of Choice

- $H_2$ receptor antagonists, such as famotidine 0.5–1 mg/kg IV, SQ, IM, PO q 12–24 hours, can be given to help reduce stomach acidity and decrease the rate of Zn release from ingested metal.
- Antiemetics such as maropitant 1 mg/kg SQ q 24 hours for vomiting.

## Alternative Drugs

- For stomach acid reduction.
  - Proton pump inhibitors such as omeprazole 0.5–1 mg/kg PO q 12–24 hours or pantoprazole 0.7–1 mg/kg IV q 24 hours.
  - Oral antacid such as calcium carbonate 25–50 mg/kg PO q 2–4 hours can be used in nonvomiting animals.

## Appropriate Health Care

- IV fluids to maintain hydration and perfusion.
- Red blood cell transfusion(s) may be needed for patients with clinical signs associated with anemia; plasma transfusion(s) may be needed for coagulopathy.

## Precautions/Interactions

- Chelation using $CaNa_2EDTA$ is controversial and should not be necessary once the object or source has been removed. Zinc concentrations will rapidly decrease once the source is removed. Chelation therapy may increase absorption of Zn if initiated before the metal is removed and $CaNa_2EDTA$ can also exacerbate GI signs and cause nephrotoxicity.
- Avoid other nephrotoxic drugs such as NSAIDs and aminoglycosides because of the risk of renal failure.
- The use of blood products from a universal donor in dogs (DEA 1.1 negative) may decrease transfusion reactions if blood type or cross-match cannot be performed prior to blood product administration.

## Patient Monitoring

- Hospitalization and monitoring for 24–72 hours following object removal.
- Minimize patient stress prior to stabilization.
- Recumbent animals will need soft bedding and positional rotation every four hours.
- During hospitalization: PCV q 6–12 hours, serum chemistry q 12–24 hours. If persistent chemistry abnormalities at discharge, recheck blood work 1–2 weeks post discharge to assess response to therapy.
- Urinary catheterization can be done for recumbent patient comfort and to monitor urine output if concerned about acute renal failure.
- It should be unnecessary to recheck blood and urine Zn levels as they should decrease rapidly following Zn object removal. If clinical improvement is not noted, recheck blood levels, reassess patient for additional Zn exposure, and rule out other causes for clinical signs noted.

 # COMMENTS

### Prevention/Avoidance

- Inform clients of the hazard of ingesting zinc-containing objects or products and ensure that pets do not have access to areas where exposure may occur.
- Advise owners to avoid use of topical zinc-containing preparations without veterinary supervision.

## Possible Complications

- Multiple organ failure (especially liver and kidney), DIC, pancreatic disease, seizures, and cardiopulmonary arrest can occur even with aggressive therapy.

## Expected Course and Prognosis

- Animals may show improvement within 24–72 hours after object removal.
- Complete recovery is possible.
- Prognosis is guarded to good depending on degree of morbidity prior to object removal.
- Development of multiorgan failure (especially kidney and liver), DIC, seizures, or cardiopulmonary arrest indicates a need for more aggressive care and worsening prognosis.

## See Also

## Abbreviations

See Appendix 1 for a complete list.

## Suggested Reading

Ambar N, Tovar T. Suspcted hemolytic anemia secondary to acute zine toxicity after ingestion of "max strength" (zinc oxide) diaper rash cream. *J Vet Emerg Crit Care* 2022;32:125–128.

Cummings JE, Kovacic JP. The ubiquitous role of zinc in health and disease. *J Vet Emerg Crit Care* 2009;19:215–240.

Gurnee CM, Drobatz KJ. Zinc intoxication in dogs: 19 cases (1991–2003). *J Am Vet Med Assoc* 2007;230:1174–1179.

Talcott PA. Zinc poisoning. In: Peterson ME, Talcott PA (eds) *Small Animal Toxicology*, 3rd edn. St Louis: Elsevier, 2013; pp. 847–852.

Van der Merwe D, Tawde S. Antacids in the initial management of metallic zinc ingestion in dogs. *J Vet Pharmacol Ther* 2008;32:2003–2006.

## Acknowledgment

The authors and editors acknowledge the prior contributions of Dr Kathryn M. Meurs, DVM, PhD, and Patricia A. Talcott, DVM, PhD, DABVT, who authored this topic in a previous edition.

**Author**: Katherine L. Peterson, DVM, DACVECC, DABT
**Consulting Editor**: Robert H. Poppenga, DVM, PhD, DABVT

# Nondrug Consumer Products

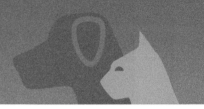

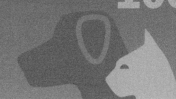

# Chapter 106

# Glow Jewelry and Toys (Dibutyl Phthalate)

## DEFINITION/OVERVIEW

- Many types of recreational and consumer glow jewelry or glow-in-the-dark jewelry contain an oily, chemiluminescent substance known as dibutyl phthalate.
- Common types of glow jewelry include rings, necklaces, bracelets, and earrings. Other glow products include wands, swords, insects, empty eggs, and many other colorful products. (Figures 106.1 and 106.2).
- Toxicosis occurs more often in cats than other small animals.
- A few glow stick-type products contain hydrogen peroxide in phthalic ester and phenyl oxalate ester or contain batteries; these products are not covered in this chapter.
- Dibutyl phthalate is also widely used in the manufacturing of products including plastics, glues, dyes, printing ink, solvents for perfume, safety glass, and as insect repellants for use in clothing.

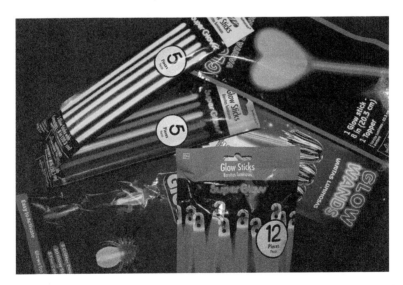

■ **Figure 106.1** Colorful packaging can be very attractive to dogs. Source: Courtesy of Tyne K. Hovda.

*Blackwell's Five-Minute Veterinary Consult Clinical Companion: Small Animal Toxicology*, Third Edition.
Edited by Lynn R. Hovda, Ahna G. Brutlag, Robert H. Poppenga, and Steven E. Epstein.
© 2024 John Wiley & Sons, Inc. Published 2024 by John Wiley & Sons, Inc.

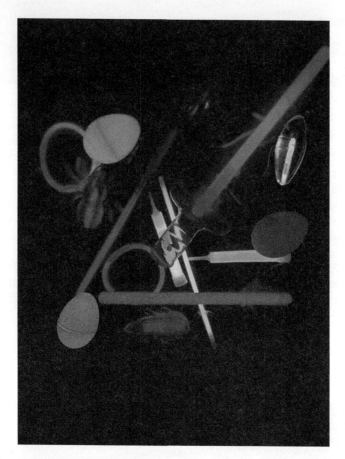

■ Figure 106.2 Several different glow products. Source: Courtesy of Tyne K. Hovda.

 **ETIOLOGY/PATHOPHYSIOLOGY**

### Mechanism of Action

- Dibutyl phthalate is an irritant to the eyes, skin, and mucous membranes.
- The unpleasant, bitter taste tends to limit oral exposure.

### Toxicity

- Dibutyl phthalate has a low order of acute toxicity with a wide margin.
- Oral $LD_{50}$ (rats) >8 g/kg; lethal exposure for other species is unknown.
- Rats receiving an oral dose of 1 mg/kg twice a week for 1.5 years had no adverse effects; rats and other laboratory animals tolerated 2 g/kg orally once daily for 10 days.
- Glow jewelry contains small amounts of dibutyl phthalate, with most pieces containing less than 5 mL of liquid. Most packages do not show the amount of dibutyl phthalate present. Approximate values are as follow.
  - Earrings and bracelets 0.3–0.5 mL.
  - Necklaces 1–2 mL.
  - Large wands 3–5 mL.

### Systems Affected

- Gastrointestinal – oral irritation, profuse hypersalivation, agitation secondary to oropharyngeal discomfort, vomiting.

- Skin/exocrine – irritation, burning, redness, contact dermatitis.
- Ophthalmic – stinging and burning sensation, profuse lacrimation, photophobia, conjunctival edema, conjunctivitis.
- Respiratory – labored breathing and respiratory paralysis have been noted in experimentally fatally poisoned animals (rare and not reported with glow jewelry).

 # SIGNALMENT/HISTORY

- Any age or breed of dog or cat may be affected.
- History of biting or chewing product.
- Reported to occur more often in cats; self-grooming in cats increases potential for oral and ocular exposure.

## Location and Circumstances of Poisoning

- The presence of children in the household may increase exposure as they are more likely to own and play with glow jewelry, leaving it in places where dogs and cats can find it.

 # CLINICAL FEATURES

- Clinical signs are typically due to the unpleasant and bitter chemical taste of the product, resulting in an acute onset of profuse hypersalivation or emesis.
- Other clinical signs include agitation, aggressiveness, or abnormal behaviors such as hiding or running away.
- Pets biting into the sticks or ingesting the liquid should be evaluated in a dark room for evidence of product on their haircoat. If present, bathe with a mild soap.
- Contact with thin haircoat or hairless areas results in a mild burning and stinging sensation.
- Cats may develop pruritus and can self-traumatize with itching and scratching.
- Ocular exposure may result in conjunctivitis or corneal abrasion. The presence of corneal ulceration should be ruled out with fluorescein staining.

 # DIFFERENTIAL DIAGNOSIS

- Other irritant products such as perfumes and alcohols.
- Oxalate-containing plants.
- Oral ingestion of topical flea and tick products.

 # DIAGNOSTICS

- In general, laboratory diagnostics are not necessary.
- Consider blood work in significantly symptomatic animals, pediatric, and geriatric patients, or patients with underlying disorders.

 # THERAPEUTICS

- Goals of treatment include decontamination, oropharyngeal lavage, antiemetics, fluids, and bathing.

## Detoxification

- Emesis and gastric lavage are not indicated.
- Activated charcoal is unnecessary.

- Gently wipe mouth and surrounding area and rinse with cool water or offer a small amount of palatable liquid (e.g., chicken broth, milk, canned tuna water, or canned cat food) to dilute the product and help remove the taste.
- The signs are generally self-limiting and related to the taste of dibutyl phthalate; signs quickly resolve with decontamination.
- Bathe with a mild, noninsecticidal pet shampoo or dish soap and rinse well with tepid water. Examine pet in a darkened room to ensure that all the glow product has been completely removed from the haircoat.

### Appropriate Health Care

- A thorough ocular exam is necessary if ophthalmic signs are present.
- When an ocular exposure to dibutyl phthalate has occurred, the eyes should be lavaged thoroughly with eye wash for 10–15 minutes.
- Slit lamp or fluorescein testing may be necessary to evaluate for corneal ulceration. Ulceration should be treated with ophthalmic medication as deemed medically appropriate.
- Fluids (SQ or IV) may be needed in symptomatic patients.

### Antidotes and Drug(s) of Choice

- No antidote.
- Antiemetic.
  - Maropitant 1 mg/kg SQ or IV (in dogs over 4 months) q 24 hours.
  - Ondansetron 0.5–1 mg/kg IV q 12 hours for dogs; 0.1–1 mg/kg IV, SQ, IM q 6–12 hours for cats.

# COMMENTS

### Prevention/Avoidance

- Pet parents should be informed about the exposure to glow jewelry, particularly during holidays like Halloween or Fourth of July.

### Expected Course and Prognosis

- Most reactions are self-limiting and can be treated at home without veterinary intervention.
- For symptomatic animals, little treatment is required.
- Many of the signs are associated with the bitter taste of the product and resolve quickly once the product is gone.
- Animals with an ocular exposure should be evaluated by a veterinarian.
- Prognosis for complete recovery is excellent.

### Abbreviations

See Appendix 1 for a complete list.

### Suggested Reading

Hoffman RJ, Nelson LS, Hoffman RS. Pediatric and young adult exposure to chemiluminescent glow sticks. *Arch Ped Adol Med* 2002;156(9):901–904.

Kamrin MA. Phthalate risks, phthalate regulation, and public health: a review. *J Toxicol Environ Health B Crit Rev* 2009;12(2):157–174.

Rosendale ME. Glow jewelry (dibutyl phthalate) ingestion in cats. *Vet Med* 1999;94(8):703.

**Author**: Tyne K. Hovda, DVM
**Consulting Editor**: Lynn R. Hovda, RPH, DVM, MS, DACVIM

# Chapter 107

# Fluoride

## DEFINITION/OVERVIEW

- Fluoride toxicosis can develop from exposure to highly corrosive hydrofluoric acid as well as other corrosive and noncorrosive products containing fluoride salts such as sodium fluoride.
- This chapter will focus on fluoride ingestion of products that do not contain hydrofluoric acid. See Chapter 13 for more information on this toxicant.
- Noncorrosive fluoride products include a variety of fluoride salts, with sodium fluoride commonly present in over-the-counter items used for prophylactic dental care, multivitamins, osteoporosis treatment, and insecticides. Noncorrosive fluoride is also found in most municipal drinking water supplies.
- Corrosive fluoride products may be found in oven cleaners, toilet cleaners, and other cleaning solutions.
- Fluoride is released in the environment through volcanic eruptions, sea water, emissions from mining activities, and manufacturing of various products including glass, steel, brick, copper, nickel, and glues.
- Common signs of mild fluoride ingestion include vomiting and diarrhea, which typically require minimal supportive care. Larger ingestions may result in electrolyte abnormalities requiring more aggressive care.
- Concentrated fluoride salts can be caustic to the GIT and in severe toxicosis lead to metabolic disturbances that result in arrhythmias and respiratory muscle paralysis.
- Long-term chronic overdoses without calcium supplementation may cause skeletal and dental fluorosis, leading to abnormal tooth structure, fractures, and malformations.

## ETIOLOGY/PATHOPHYSIOLOGY

### Mechanism of Action

- When fluoride salts are ingested, they react with the acidic environment of the stomach to create hydrofluoric acid, which is highly corrosive.
- Once absorbed, hydrofluoric acid interferes with calcium metabolism and may cause hypocalcemia. It also interferes with Na/K ATPase, leading to an efflux of K from the cell, resulting in hyperkalemia.
- In the hydroxyapatite of the bone, fluoride substitutes for hydroxyl groups which causes changes to the mineralization and structure of the bone.
- In severe toxicosis, hypocalcemia and hyperkalemia can be severe enough to cause ECG changes and secondary cardiac arrhythmias may result.

*Blackwell's Five-Minute Veterinary Consult Clinical Companion: Small Animal Toxicology*, Third Edition. Edited by Lynn R. Hovda, Ahna G. Brutlag, Robert H. Poppenga, and Steven E. Epstein. © 2024 John Wiley & Sons, Inc. Published 2024 by John Wiley & Sons, Inc.

- Respiratory muscle paralysis from hypocalcemia and cardiac arrest from hyperkalemia are the most common causes of death.

## Toxicokinetics

- Sodium fluoride and other soluble fluoride salts are rapidly absorbed from the GIT and reach peak plasma levels 30 minutes after ingestion. The primary site of absorption is the stomach with a lesser amount in the small intestine.
- Uptake of fluoride by older animals is less than that of young animals.
- Carbohydrates and fat can reduce or delay fluoride absorption.
- Absorption and distribution occur in a pH-dependent manner.
- Fluoride is distributed to soft and bony tissues before accumulating in the bone, causing a rapid decline in fluoride plasma concentrations.
- Fluoride is not protein bound and circulates as a free ion until it binds to the bone over several hours after ingestion.
- Accumulation of fluoride in bony tissues is a reversible process.
- Fluoride is 50% excreted by the kidneys with the remainder excreted in feces, sweat, saliva, and milk or retained by the bone.
- Urinary excretion of fluoride is lower with acidic urine and enhanced with alkaline urine.
- Elimination half-life is 2–9 hours in people with normal kidney function but can be prolonged with kidney disease; unknown half-life in small animals.

## Toxicity

- Very little information exists in the veterinary literature regarding acute fluoride toxicosis in small animals.
- Anecdotally, fluoride ion <5 mg/kg results in mild clinical signs; higher doses may require more aggressive care.
- Sodium fluoride is 45% fluoride ion by weight (1 mg sodium fluoride = 0.45 mg fluoride ion).
- Fluoride toothpaste typically contains up to 1.1 mg fluoride ion per gram of toothpaste. Mouthwashes or rinses typically contain 0.05–0.2% sodium fluoride and have approximately 0.02–0.9 mg of fluoride ion/mL of rinse. Verify amounts for each brand.
- Fluoride salts induce oxidative stress by generating free oxygen radicals causing lipid peroxidation which results in cell membrane damage, with liver and kidney most significantly affected.

## Systems Affected

- Cardiovascular – cardiac arrhythmias secondary to profound hyperkalemia and hypocalcemia (severe toxicosis).
- Gastrointestinal – GI irritation, nausea, vomiting, anorexia, abdominal pain, HGE, ulceration, oral irritation. Tooth discoloration and enamel defects can occur in young animals or with chronic exposure.
- Hemic/lymphatic/immune – hypocalcemia, hyperkalemia.
- Hepatobiliary – increased hepatic enzymes.
- Respiratory – coughing, respiratory irritation, respiratory muscle paralysis (severe toxicosis).
- Musculoskeletal – painful muscle spasms/tremors, weakness, skeletal fluorosis (chronic).
- Nervous – hyperactive reflexes.
- Skin/exocrine – dermal irritation.
- Renal – increased BUN and creatinine with chronic exposure.

# SIGNALMENT/HISTORY

### Risk Factors

- Any age, sex, and breed of pet can be affected.
- Animals drinking water from a source with high fluoride content chronically.
- Young animals may be predisposed to tooth and bone damage with chronic exposure.

### Historical Findings

- Witnessed ingestion or discovery of chewed-up packaging.
- Owners may report drooling, vomiting, and anorexia.
- Owners may report neurological abnormalities in extreme ingestions due to hypocalcemia.
- Chronic lameness, frequent fractures, and bony injury with minimal trauma may be indicative of chronic fluoride toxicosis.

### Location and Circumstances of Poisoning

- Exposure typically occurs within the home, specifically in the bathroom, where the pet has access to toothpaste, mouthwash, fluoride supplements or vitamins containing fluoride.
- In areas with municipal drinking water sources containing fluoride, chronic overexposure may occur if excessive fluoride has been inadvertently added to the water source.

# CLINICAL FEATURES

- Clinical signs may be present within a few hours after exposure.
- Mucous membrane erythema, oral irritation, vomiting, hypersalivation, nausea, abdominal pain, or dysphagia may be present.
- Cardiac arrhythmias, muscle tremors, or muscle weakness may be noted with severe toxicosis.
- Clinical signs with chronic exposure include dry skin and hair coat, lameness, and periosteal overgrowth near joints, and discoloration and enamel defects to the teeth.

# DIFFERENTIAL DIAGNOSIS

- Gastrointestinal – GI irritants or other corrosives, plants such as azalea or rhododendron, calcium oxalate-containing plants, saponin-containing plants, dietary indiscretion.
- Hypocalcemia – nursing, hypoparathyroidism, calcium channel blocker toxicosis.
- Hyperkalemia – iatrogenic supplementation, acute kidney failure, urinary obstruction, uroabdomen, hypoadrenocorticism.
- Cardiac arrhythmias – primary cardiac disease, electrolyte derangements, stimulant toxicosis (methylxanthines, SSRI, methylphenidate).

# DIAGNOSTICS

### Clinical Pathological Findings

- Serum chemistry – hyperkalemia, hypocalcemia, hypomagnesemia, elevated hepatic enzymes, particularly ALT, AST, total bilirubin and ALP. Elevated BUN and creatinine in chronic exposures.

## Other Diagnostics

- ECG – QT prolongation, arrhythmias secondary to potassium, magnesium, and calcium abnormalities.

## Pathological Findings

- Primarily limited to irritant or corrosive damage in the GIT.
- Chronic fluorosis causes exostosis of long bones as well as mottled, pitted, or excessively worn teeth/enamel.
- Chronic exposure has been shown to cause renal cell apoptosis, atrophic glomeruli, glomerular capsule and tubule dilation, severe tubule leakage and necrosis of glomeruli and tubules in young pigs. It is reasonable to assume this would be a concern in small animals as well, though not documented.
- Chronic exposure has been shown to cause hepatocellular necrosis, degenerative changes, hepatic hyperplasia, extensive vacuolization in hepatocytes, centrilobular necrosis, congested and dilated central vein and blood sinusoids in albino rats. It is reasonable to assume this would be a concern in small animals as well, though not documented.

 ## THERAPEUTICS

- Treatment for most fluoride ingestions is supportive care for GI signs.
- Larger exposures may require decontamination, neutralization of the fluoride with antacids or calcium, fluid therapy, correction of electrolyte abnormalities, and GI supportive care.
- Quinidine, a potassium channel blocker, has been shown to be protective in cases of arrhythmias secondary to severe hyperkalemia in dogs.

## Detoxification

- Before decontamination is initiated, determine which type of fluoride was ingested (e.g., corrosive vs noncorrosive), if possible.
- Noncorrosive.
  - Emesis should be induced if ingestion was within two hours for a tablet-based product or 30 minutes for a gel or powder.
  - With large recent tablet exposures, if emesis return is low yield, consider gastric lavage with a large-bore stomach tube and an inflated endotracheal tube to protect the airway.
- Corrosive.
  - Emesis is contraindicated.
  - With large exposures, calcium gluconate solution can be administered orally or via stomach tube to bind fluoride ions.

## Appropriate Health Care

- Maintain hydration and perfusion with IV fluid therapy until clinical signs resolve.
- Correct electrolyte abnormalities.
  - Calcium gluconate for hypocalcemia.
  - Regular insulin administration and dextrose supplementation can be considered for severe hyperkalemia.
- If indicated, monitor cardiac function with a continuous ECG to evaluate for the presence of arrhythmias.

## Antidote

- No antidote is available.

## Drug(s) of Choice

- GI supportive therapy.
  - Antiemetics as needed for vomiting.
    - o Dolasetron mesylate 0.6 mg/kg IV, SQ, PO q 24 hours.
    - o Maropitant 1 mg/kg SQ q 24 hours.
    - o Metoclopramide 0.2–0.5 mg/kg SQ, IV, PO q 8 hours.
    - o Ondansetron 0.1–0.2 mg/kg IV q 8–12 hours.
  - Famotidine 0.5–1 mg/kg IV, SQ, PO q 12–24 hours, extending longer if GI ulceration is present.
  - Sucralfate 0.25–1 g/kg PO q 8 hours × 3–5 days, extending longer if GI ulceration is present.
- Neutralize fluoride.
  - Calcium carbonate. No established dose available.
  - Magnesium hydroxide 5–15 mL q 24 hours.
- Electrolyte correction.
  - Calcium gluconate 10% 50–150 mg/kg IV over 20–30 minutes to effect for hypocalcemia; monitor heart rate and an ECG during administration.
  - Regular insulin 0.5 U/kg IV and dextrose 1–2 g/kg (2–4 mL/kg 50% dextrose) IV for severe hyperkalemia.
- Ventricular arrhythmia: quinidine 200 mg TOTAL dose in dogs.

## Precautions/Interactions

- Electrolyte supplementation needs to be performed with cardiac monitoring and regular rechecks of serum levels to determine if further supplementation is necessary.
- Aluminum hydroxide can alter the absorption of other drugs and should be administered one hour apart from other oral medications.

## Alternative Drugs

- Use of tamarind (*Tamarandus indica* L.) has been shown to decrease bone retention and facilitate urinary excretion of fluoride in experimental dogs receiving 10 grams of commercially available tamarind paste daily for three months when fed along with 10 mg sodium fluoride per day.

## Extracorporeal Therapy

- While there are currently no reports of success in small animal patients, due to the renal clearance of fluoride, it is a reasonable treatment to consider in patients with severe poisoning and acute kidney injury.

## Surgical Considerations

- Ulcerations of the GIT could potentially cause perforation, necessitating surgical intervention (rare).

## Patient Monitoring

- Serum electrolytes should be monitored every 2–4 hours during initial management of severely symptomatic cases to guide supplementation.

## Diet

- The additional use of dairy products (e.g., milk, yogurt, etc.) to neutralize fluoride may be beneficial, provided the patient is not vomiting, particularly if decontamination and veterinary care are not available.
- Calcium supplementation may be needed initially, but no long-term diet changes are recommended.
- Bland diet can be considered in patients with GI signs.

 COMMENTS

### Prevention/Avoidance

- Store fluoride-containing products away from pets.
- Be aware of local warnings regarding high levels of fluoride in municipal drinking water and avoid its use in animals.

### Possible Complications

- In severe cases, if electrolyte abnormalities cannot be corrected, death from cardiac arrest or respiratory muscle paralysis is possible. Mechanical ventilation may be necessary until respiratory muscle paralysis resolves.

### Expected Course and Prognosis

- Most OTC noncorrosive fluoride exposures result in mild clinical signs and should resolve with supportive care within 24 hours.
- Prognosis is good with small ingestions or with early intervention and appropriate management. Large ingestions with late intervention have a guarded prognosis.

### Synonyms

Skeletal fluorosis, sodium fluoride toxicosis, fluoride silicate toxicosis, fluoridosis.

### See Also

Chapter 13, Hydrofluoric Acid

### Abbreviations

See Appendix 1 for a full list.

### Suggested Reading

Azab AE, Albasha MO, Jbireal JM et al. Sodium fluoride induces hepato-renal oxidative stress and pathophysiological changes in experimental animals. *Open J Apoptosis* 2018;7:1–23.

Boink AB, Wemer J, Meulenbelt J et al. The mechanism of fluoride-induced hypocalcaemia. *Hum Exp Toxicol* 1994;13:149–155.

Mishra R, Jain S, Bhatnger, M, Shukla SD. Fluoride toxicity myth or fact? A review. *Cell Tissue Res* 2020;20(1):6869–6882.

Su MK. Hydrofluoric acid and fluorides. In: Nelson LS et al. (eds) *Goldfrank's Toxicologic Emergencies*, 11th edn. New York: McGraw-Hill, 2019; pp. 1397–1402.

Ullah R, Zafar MS, Shahani N. Potential fluoride toxicity from oral medicaments: a review. *Iran J Basic Med Sci* 2017;20(8):841–848.

**Author:** Renee D. Schmid, DVM, DABT, DABVT
**Consulting Editor:** Lynn R. Hovda, RPh, DVM, MS, DACVIM

# Plants and Biotoxins

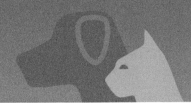

# Azaleas and Rhododendrons

## DEFINITION/OVERVIEW

- There are over 1000 species of azaleas/rhododendrons in the Ericaceae family. Typically, the smaller, deciduous forms are referred to as azaleas (Figure 108.1), and the larger, evergreen forms are called rhododendrons (Figures 108.2 and 108.3), but there may be some exceptions. Both forms have showy flowers.
  - Included in the Ericaceae family are mountain laurel (*Kalmia latifolia*) and Japanese pieris (*Pieris japonicus*) and both have similar toxic effects.
- Azaleas/rhododendrons are found on all continents. They occur naturally in nature, cultivated as shrubs or small trees, and as indoor ornamentals.

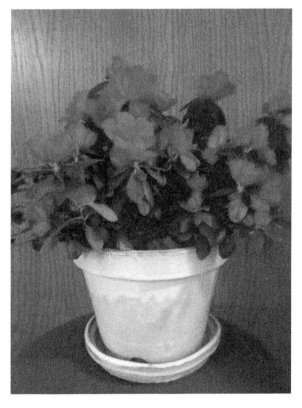

■ Figure 108.1 Smaller azalea as an indoor potted plant. Source: Courtesy of Lynn R. Hovda.

*Blackwell's Five-Minute Veterinary Consult Clinical Companion: Small Animal Toxicology*, Third Edition.
Edited by Lynn R. Hovda, Ahna G. Brutlag, Robert H. Poppenga, and Steven E. Epstein.
© 2024 John Wiley & Sons, Inc. Published 2024 by John Wiley & Sons, Inc.

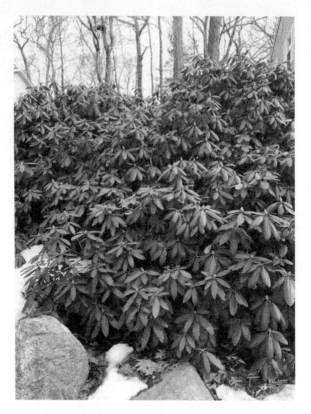

■ **Figure 108.2** Larger, more robust rhododendron shrub. Source: Courtesy of Lynn R. Hovda.

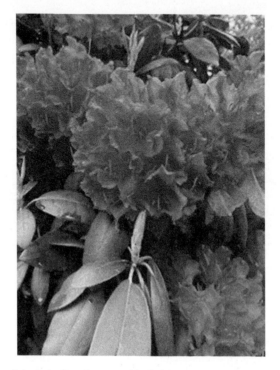

■ **Figure 108.3** Close-up of rhododendron flower and leaf with bud. Source: Courtesy of Lynn R. Hovda.

- Diterpenoid grayanotoxins (previously known as andromedotoxins or rhodotoxins) are found to some extent in all plants in the Ericaceae family.
- All parts of the plant are toxic, but concentrations of toxin may vary between plants.
- Gastrointestinal signs predominate, with CV and neurological signs occurring much less often.
- Clinical signs usually occur quickly (within a few hours of ingestion) but may be delayed up to 12 hours. Most are gone by 24 hours; longer if neuro signs occur.

 # ETIOLOGY/PATHOPHYSIOLOGY

## Mechanism of Action

- Grayanotoxins bind to group II receptor sites in voltage-gated sodium channels within cells in the heart, nerve, and skeletal muscle, thus increasing permeability of sodium ions, and resulting in prolonged depolarization/excitability of the affected cell membranes.

## Toxicokinetics

- Absorption is thought to be rapid with clinical signs within 1–6 hours; may be delayed up to 12 hours.
- Metabolism and excretion are also thought to be rapid.

## Toxicity

- Grayanotoxins I and III are currently considered the principal toxic isomers; I is most common. Concentrations of various grayanotoxins (I through XXV) vary among plants.
- All parts of the plant, including nectar and flowers, and especially leaves, are toxic.
- Secondary products such as Labrador tea, alternative medicine concoctions, and honey ("mad honey") may also be toxic.
- Ingestion of 0.2% of animal's body weight (documented in cattle) may cause clinical signs.

## Systems Affected

- Gastrointestinal – early onset of hypersalivation and gastroenteritis (with repeated swallowing, anorexia, persistent vomiting, abdominal pain, bloat, diarrhea).
- Cardiovascular – changes in heart rate and rhythm (bradycardia, tachycardia, AV block, hypotension, arrhythmias).
- CNS – ranges from depression or weakness (lasting 2–3 days in some cases) to coma.

 # SIGNALMENT/HISTORY

## Risk Factors

- There is no breed or species predilection.
- Animals with underlying cardiac disease are at increased risk.

## Historical Findings

- Diagnosis is typically made through history of ingestion and identification of plant material.

## Location and Circumstances of Poisoning

- Access and ingestion of wild or ornamental plants and/or trimmings.

 # CLINICAL FEATURES

- Onset of clinical signs is usually rapid, within 1–6 hours, but signs may be delayed for up to 12 hours. Most clinical signs resolve within 24 hours, but CNS signs can persist for 2–3 days.

- Gastrointestinal signs typically predominate and occur early in toxicity – hypersalivation, retching, vomiting, diarrhea (rare), abdominal pain, anorexia, possible hemorrhagic enteritis, bloat.
- Cardiovascular signs – bradycardia or tachycardia (less common, possibly a reflex secondary to hypotension), arrhythmias, hypotension, CV block, cardiopulmonary arrest.
- Neurological signs – depression, weakness, reluctance to stand (may be related to CV events), tremors, seizures, paralysis, coma.
- Other reported clinical signs may include transient blindness, dyspnea, vocalization.

# DIFFERENTIAL DIAGNOSIS

- Infectious or metabolic disease (viral, bacterial, HE).
- Other toxicants.
  - *Taxus* spp. and cardiac glycoside-containing plants (foxglove, oleander, etc.).
  - Prescription medications used in veterinary or human medicine for cardiac disease (particularly digitalis).
  - Prescription medications used in veterinary or human medicine that have cardiac effects without being specifically prescribed for cardiac disease.
  - Organophosphorus- and carbamate-containing pesticides.
- Underlying cardiac disease.

# DIAGNOSTICS

## Clinical Pathological Findings

- Clinical laboratory tests (serum chemistry and CBC) typically do not show primary abnormalities, but there may be secondary metabolic acidosis (from seizures) or dehydration and electrolyte imbalance secondary to prolonged vomiting.

## Other Diagnostics

- LC/MS is available to determine presence of grayanotoxins in stomach contents, serum, or urine.

## Pathological Findings

- Nonspecific – plant material in the GIT, mild hemorrhagic enteritis, renal tubular damage, possible aspiration pneumonia.

# THERAPEUTICS

## Detoxification

- Bathe animal to remove nectar if present.
- Early emesis if asymptomatic.
- Gastric lavage to remove large amounts of plant material (retain for toxin identification).
- Activated charcoal with cathartic (1 g/kg) single dose if no risk of aspiration and if GIT motility is normal. Monitor serum sodium as needed.

## Appropriate Health Care

- Pay close attention to hydration (vomiting may be severe).
- Monitor vitals including blood pressure frequently.
- Consider continuous ECG and BP monitoring.

- SX – hospitalize in a darkened area without excess stimulation (seizures may occur and neurological signs may persist for a few days).
- ASX – can be discharged after 8–12 hours.

### Antidote

- There is no specific antidote.

### Drug(s) of Choice

- Early, cautious use of IV fluids to maintain blood pressure and hydration, with care to avoid overloading.
- GI signs.
  - Antiemetics.
    - ○ Maropitant 1 mg/kg SQ or IV q 24 hours.
    - ○ Ondansetron 0.5 mg/kg IV q 8–12 hours.
  - GI protectants as needed.
    - ○ $H_2$-blockers: famotidine 0.5–1 mg/kg PO, SQ, IM, IV q 12–24 hours.
    - ○ Proton pump inhibitor.
      - ◇ Omeprazole 0.5–1 mg/kg PO q 12–24 hours.
      - ◇ Pantoprazole 0.7–1 mg/kg IV q12 hours.
    - ○ Sucralfate 0.25–1 g PO q 8 hours × 5–7 days if evidence of active ulcer disease.
- CV signs.
  - Bradycardia.
    - ○ Atropine 0.02–0.04 mg/kg IV, IM, or SQ.
    - ○ Glycopyrrolate.
      - ◇ Dog: 0.011 mg/kg IV or IM.
      - ◇ Cat: 0.005–0.01 mg/kg IV or IM, 0.01–0.02 mg/kg SQ.
    - ○ Temporary pacemaker for severe cases of unresponsive bradycardia.
  - Ventricular dysrhythmias or sustained tachycardia unresponsive to fluid therapy.
    - ○ Lidocaine.
      - ◇ Dogs: 2–4 mg/kg IV while monitoring ECG. If effective, follow with CRI of 50–100 mcg/kg/min.
      - ◇ Cats (for severe ventricular dysrhythmias): 0.25–0.5 mg/kg slow IV while monitoring ECG. Use with caution in cats.
  - Hypotension.
    - ○ If persistent and refractory to fluid therapy – vasopressors.
      - ◇ Norepinephrine 0.1 2.0 mcg/kg/min IV CRI.
      - ◇ Dopamine 10–20 mcg/kg/min IV CRI.
- CNS signs.
  - Seizures.
    - ○ Benzodiazepines.
      - ◇ Diazepam 0.25–0.5 mg/kg IV.
      - ◇ Midazolam 0.1–0.5 mg/kg IV.
    - ○ Long-acting anticonvulsant for seizures if benzodiazepine unsuccessful.
      - ◇ Phenobarbital 2–5 mg/kg IV.
      - ◇ Levetiracetam 30–60 mg/kg IV q 8 hours PRN.
  - Tremors.
    - ○ Methocarbamol 55–220 mg/kg IV q 4–6 hours PRN, start low and titrate to effect. Monitor for excessive sedation and respiratory depression if exceeding 330 mg/kg/day.

## Alternative Drugs

- Intralipid therapy has been used successfully in goats, but this treatment is experimental and not routinely recommended for this toxin.

 **COMMENTS**

### Prevention/Avoidance

- Clippings should be kept out of pet's environment.
- Flowering plants are tempting to cats and should be kept out of reach.

### Possible Complications

- Acute kidney injury due to prolonged hypotension.
- Aspiration pneumonia.

### Expected Course/Prognosis

- Prognosis is good with early and appropriate therapy.
- Development of cardiac compromise complicates therapy and lowers prognosis.
- Neurological signs may persist for days.

### See Also

Chapter 112 Cardiac Glycosides
Chapter 121 Yew

### Abbreviations

See Appendix 1 for a complete list.

### Suggested Reading

Bischoff K, Smith MC, Stump S. Treatment of *Pieris* ingestion in goats with intravenous lipid emulsion. *J Med Toxicol* 2014;10(4):411–414.
Burrows GE, Tyri RJ. *Toxic Plants of North America*. Ames: ISU Press, 2006.
Jansen SA, Kleerekooper I, Hofmam Z et al. Grayanotoxin poisoning: 'Mad honey disease' and beyond. *Cardiovasc Toxicol* 2012;12(3):208–215.
Knight AP. *A Guide to Poisonous House and Garden Plants*. Jackson: Teton NewMedia, 2006.
Milewski LM, Khan SA. An overview of potentially life-threatening poisonous plants in dogs and cats. *J Vet Emerg Crit Care* 2006;16(1):25–33.

**Author:** Tiffany Hughes, DVM
**Consulting Editor:** Lynn R. Hovda, RPh, DVM, MS, DACVIM

# Chapter 109

# Blue-green Algae (Cyanobacteria): Anatoxin-A

## DEFINITION/OVERVIEW

- Harmful algal blooms resulting in cyanobacterial proliferations and poisonings are becoming more common due to eutrophication of freshwater and brackish ecosystems.
- Most cyanobacteria blooms do not produce toxins. However, determining toxin production and severity is not possible with the naked eye. All blooms are potentially toxic.
- Cyanotoxin exposure can lead to an acute intoxication affecting the liver, skin, or CNS.
- Anatoxins are neurotoxic cyanotoxins produced mainly by *Anabaena* but other genera such as *Planktothrix, Oscillatoria, Microcystis, Aphanizomenon,* and others are capable of producing anatoxins.
- Three anatoxins have been identified; anatoxin-a, its homologue, homoanatoxin-a, and anatoxin-a$_s$.
- Overall prognosis is poor, with death occurring minutes to hours after neurotoxin exposure.

## ETIOLOGY/PATHOPHYSIOLOGY

### Mechanism of Action

- Anatoxin-a and homoanatoxin-a are potent cholinergic agonists at nicotinic acetylcholine receptors, resulting in continuous electrical stimulation at the neuromuscular junction.
- Anatoxin-a$_s$ is a naturally occurring irreversible acetylcholinesterase inhibitor leading to increased acetylcholine concentrations in the synapse. Anatoxin-a$_s$ is incapable of crossing the blood–brain barrier so effects and clinical signs are peripheral.

### Toxicokinetics

- Data on the toxicokinetics of anatoxin-a, homoanatoxin-a, and anatoxin-a$_s$ have not been established.
- For anatoxin-a, rapid absorption is suspected based on rapid onset of clinical signs after oral exposure.
- Excretion of anatoxin-a is thought to occur via feces and urine based on detection of unchanged toxin in urine and bile.

### Toxicity

- The reported IP $LD_{50}$ of anatoxin-a in mice is 200 mcg/kg while the IV $LD_{50}$ is estimated at less than 100 mcg/kg. The oral toxicity of anatoxin-a is much higher, with an oral $LD_{50}$ in mice reported as greater than 5000 mcg/kg.

*Blackwell's Five-Minute Veterinary Consult Clinical Companion: Small Animal Toxicology*, Third Edition. Edited by Lynn R. Hovda, Ahna G. Brutlag, Robert H. Poppenga, and Steven E. Epstein. © 2024 John Wiley & Sons, Inc. Published 2024 by John Wiley & Sons, Inc.

- The reported IP $LD_{50}$ of homoanatoxin-a in mice is 250 mcg/kg.
- Anatoxin-a$_s$ is much more toxic than anatoxin-a or homoanatoxin-a. The reported IP $LD_{50}$ in mice is 20 mcg/kg.

## Systems Affected

- Anatoxin-a and homoanatoxin-a.
  - Nervous – muscle tremors, muscle rigidity, paralysis (including respiratory), and cyanosis.
- Anatoxin-a$_s$
  - Nervous – salivation, lacrimation, defecation, urination, muscle tremors.

# SIGNALMENT/HISTORY

- Dogs are more commonly affected by anatoxin-a, but other species may develop toxicosis if a sufficient dose is ingested.
- Backyard ponds that are poorly maintained and allow for cyanobacterial proliferation may pose a risk to dogs.

## Risk Factors

- Dogs that enjoy swimming are more likely to consume toxic amounts of an algal bloom than dogs that refrain from water.
- Algal bloom prevalence is higher during increased water temperature and elevated nutrient concentrations in the water.
- Use of a dietary supplement containing naturally harvested blue-green algae.

## Historical Findings

- Witnessed exposure to water with or without visible algal bloom. Toxins may persist in the water post bloom.
- Algal material on coat or present in vomit.
- Owners frequently report rapid onset of clinical presentation, usually within 30 minutes of access to water.
- Other animals (especially livestock) may be found dead near the water source.

## Location and Circumstances of Poisoning

- Lakes, streams, ponds, removed algal material (bucket).
- Algal bloom prevalence is highest during increased water temperature and elevated nutrient concentrations in the water.
- Steady winds that propel toxic blooms to shore allow for ingestion by thirsty animals.
- Different cyanobacteria reside in the benthic zone (i.e., on the sediment) and in the pelagic zone (water column). Blooms of pelagic species are usually easily detected at the water surface of ponds, rivers, or lakes. Blooms of benthic species are difficult to detect since algae reside on the surface of sediment and stones in rivers or lakes.

# CLINICAL FEATURES

- Anatoxin-a and homoanatoxin-a – clinical signs include rapid onset of rigidity and muscle tremors, followed by paralysis, cyanosis, and death as a result of potent cholinergic stimulation. Progression is very rapid, and death usually occurs within minutes to a few hours of exposure.

■ Anatoxin-a$_s$ – rapid onset of excessive salivation (the "s" stands for salivation), lacrimation, diarrhea, and urination associated with muscarinic overstimulation. Clinical signs of nicotinic overstimulation include tremors, incoordination, and convulsions. Respiratory arrest and recumbency may be seen prior to death. Progression is very rapid, and animals may die within 30 minutes of exposure.

 DIFFERENTIAL DIAGNOSIS

■ Anatoxin-a and homoanatoxin-a – strychnine, metaldehyde, avitrol, penitrem A/roquefortine mycotoxins, methylxanthines, pyrethrin/pyrethroid insecticides, organochlorine insecticides, poisonous plants (cyanide, oleander, poison hemlock), illicit substances (amphetamine derivatives), ephedra-containing compounds.
■ Anatoxin-a$_s$ – organophosphorus and carbamate insecticides, slaframine.

 DIAGNOSTICS

### Clinical Pathological Findings

■ No significant findings.

### Other Diagnostics

■ Save gastric contents and water source samples for diagnostic testing.
■ Toxicology testing.
  • Toxicity is strain specific and identification of a potential toxin-producing strain should be followed up by toxicant detection to predict toxicity level.
  • Anatoxin-a$_s$ – depressed blood cholinesterase activity.
  • Identification of the cyanobacteria in the suspect water source or stomach contents; however, positive identification does not confirm intoxication because the toxicity of cyanobacteria is strain specific, and morphological observations alone cannot predict the hazard level.
  • Detection of anatoxin-a or homoanatoxin-a in gastric contents, urine, bile, and suspect source material.
  • Mouse bioassay (IP injection of algal bloom extract) was used in the past to determine the toxicity of crude algal biomass in suspicious blue-green algae poisonings.

### Pathological Findings

■ Detection of algal bloom material in GI tract and/or on legs. No lesions are usually present.

 THERAPEUTICS

■ The treatment goals are to prevent further exposure and absorption, control CNS signs, and provide supportive care.
■ Treatment is often unsuccessful due to the rapid onset of clinical signs and death.
■ Anatoxin-a and homoanatoxin-a toxicosis – general supportive care and specific measures to control seizures should be performed.
■ Anatoxin-a$_s$ toxicosis – atropine should be given at a test dose to determine its efficacy in animals with life-threatening clinical signs. After the test dose, atropine can be given repeatedly until cessation of salivation.

## Detoxification

- Emesis may be induced in asymptomatic animals with recent exposures.
- Activated charcoal can be attempted, but efficacy is questionable.
- Bathe all animals with dermal exposure very thoroughly. Protective clothing must be worn by staff members during bathing (risk of dermatitis).

## Appropriate Health Care

- All intoxicated animals will need intensive care.
- Ventilation should be closely monitored in patients with severe neurological impairment using venous or arterial (preferred) $pCO_2$ or end-tidal capnography. Mechanical ventilation is indicated for patients with hypoventilation.

## Antidote

- No antidote available.

## Drug(s) of Choice

- Seizures.
  - Diazepam 2–5 mg/kg IV. These doses are much higher than normally used for seizure control. In general, if a 2 mg/kg IV dose does not control seizures, switch to phenobarbital.
  - Phenobarbital 2–20 mg/kg IV q 6–12 hours (may have to use very high doses).
  - Propofol 3–6 mg/kg IV to effect. CRI may be useful, 0.1–0.6 mg/kg/min.
  - Levetiracetam 20–60 mg/kg IV slowly. Repeat 10–20 mg/kg IV q 6–8 hours as needed.
- Tremors: methocarbamol 55–220 mg/kg IV.
- Atropine 0.02–0.04 mg/kg IV to effect in anatoxin-a$_s$ intoxication.

## Precautions/Interactions

- Wear protective clothing while handling/bathing affected animals. Significant contact dermatitis may occur.
- Carefully monitor for anticholinergic effects and reduce or discontinue atropine if adverse effects occur.

## Patient Monitoring

- Monitor biochemical profile, blood gases, and respiratory function.

    **COMMENTS**

### Prevention/Avoidance

- Deny dogs access to water with visible algal blooms.
- Reduce fertilizer runoff and applications in fields surrounding ponds used for drinking water.
- Remove algal blooms from ponds immediately and discard material safely.

### Possible Complications

- DIC, rhabdomyolysis, and myoglobinuria with subsequent renal failure are possible if prolonged, untreated tremors/seizures or hyperthermia present.

## Expected Course and Prognosis

- Animals poisoned with blue-green algae toxins are often found dead.
- Blue-green algae intoxications progress so rapidly that treatment is often too late.
- Prognosis is poor.

## Synonyms

Anatoxin toxicosis, anatoxin poisoning, neurotoxic algae poisoning.

## Abbreviations

See Appendix 1 for a complete list.

## Suggested Reading

Puschner B. Cyanobacterial (blue-green algae) toxins. In: Gupta RC (ed.) *Veterinary Toxicology: Basic and Clinical Principles*, 3rd edn. San Diego: Elsevier, 2018; pp. 763–777.

Puschner B, Hoff B, Tor ER. Diagnosis of anatoxin-a poisoning in dogs from North America. *J Vet Diagn Invest* 2008;20:89–92.

Puschner B, Pratt C, Tor ER. Treatment and diagnosis of a dog with fulminant neurological deterioration due to anatoxin-a intoxication. *J Vet Emerg Crit Care* 2010;20(5):518–522.

Wood SA, Selwood AI, Rueckert A et al. First report of homoanatoxin-a and associated dog neurotoxicosis in New Zealand. *Toxicon* 2007;50(2):292–301.

**Authors**: Adrienne Bautista, DVM, PhD, DABVT and Birgit Puschner, DVM, PhD, DABVT
**Consulting Editor**: Lynn R. Hovda, RPh, DVM, MS, DACVIM

# Blue-green Algae (Cyanobacteria): Microcystins

## DEFINITION/OVERVIEW

- Blue-green algal (cyanobacterial) proliferations occur in freshwater and brackish ecosystems under certain environmental conditions, potentially resulting in toxin production and leading to harmful algal blooms (Figure 110.1).
- Dietary supplements containing blue-green algae are potential sources for exposure as well as toxin-contaminated water sources.
- Most cyanobacteria blooms do not produce toxins. However, determining toxin production and severity is not possible with the naked eye. All blooms are potentially toxic.
- Cyanotoxin exposure can lead to an acute intoxication affecting the liver, skin, or CNS. Hepatotoxic blue-green algae poisonings are more frequently reported than dermal and neurotoxic algal intoxications.
- Microcystins (MCs) are hepatotoxic cyanotoxins that have been found worldwide and are produced by *Microcystis, Anabaena, Planktothrix, Nostoc*, and other genera.
- MCs are the most common cyanotoxins present in inland lakes of the United States.
- Mammals, reptiles, amphibians, aquatic species, invertebrates, and even some plant species are susceptible to the toxic effects of microcystins.

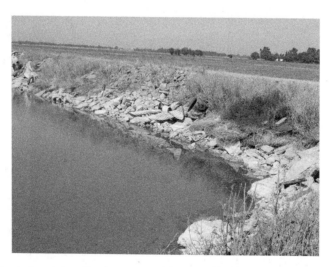

■ Figure 110.1 *Microcystis* sp. algal bloom; pond in northern California, August 2008. Bloom resulted in illness and death of cattle. Outbreak occurred during a period of high ambient temperature (above 100 °F for days) after strong winds had concentrated the algal material at one side of the pond, which was the only water access these cattle had. Source: Courtesy of Birgit Puschner.

*Blackwell's Five-Minute Veterinary Consult Clinical Companion: Small Animal Toxicology*, Third Edition. Edited by Lynn R. Hovda, Ahna G. Brutlag, Robert H. Poppenga, and Steven E. Epstein.
© 2024 John Wiley & Sons, Inc. Published 2024 by John Wiley & Sons, Inc.

- More than 100 different structural variants of microcystins have been identified, with the microcystin-LR congener being the most extensively studied.

 # ETIOLOGY/PATHOPHYSIOLOGY

## Mechanism of Action

- Microcystins target the liver by inhibiting protein phosphatases 1 and 2A. The resulting disruption of cytoskeletal components and associated rearrangement of filamentous actin within hepatocytes cause severe liver damage. Free radical formation and mitochondrial alterations may also contribute to the pathological changes, most notably acute centrilobular necrosis.

## Toxicokinetics

- There are very limited data on the kinetics of microcystins, especially in relation to species variations.
- Absorption occurs in the small intestine with rapid distribution to liver hepatocytes via organic anion transporters (OATs). Microcystins can also reach lung, heart, and capillaries.
- Some data suggest conjugation with glutathione and cystine as major detoxification pathways, although the exact route of metabolism has yet to be defined.
- The kidney appears to be important for excretion based on radiolabeled experiments in rodents.

## Toxicity

- The $LD_{50}$ for microcystins varies between 50 and 11 000 mcg/kg, depending on the exact microcystin structure, the species affected, and the route of administration.
- In mice, the oral $LD_{50}$ value for microcystin-LR is 10.9 mg/kg, while the IP $LD_{50}$ is 50 mcg/kg. Most algal blooms contain a number of structural variants of microcystins, and thus it is difficult to estimate the potential toxicity of a bloom (Figure 110.2).
- Chronic and subchronic toxicity data do exist for domestic animals.

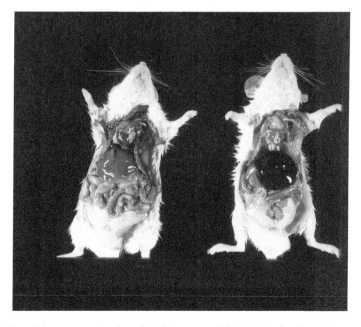

■ **Figure 110.2** Mouse bioassay: massive hepatic enlargement with dark discoloration subsequent to intraperitoneal injection with 0.5 mL of algal extract (R mouse). Control mouse (L) was given 0.5 mL of deionized water IP. Algal bloom had resulted in illness and death of cattle in northern California and was identified morphologically as a *Microcystis* sp. Source: Courtesy of Birgit Puschner.

## Systems Affected

- Hepatobiliary – diarrhea, weakness, pale mucous membranes, icterus, shock, liver failure.
- Hemic – coagulopathy can develop as a result of liver failure.
- Nervous – encephalopathy can develop as a result of liver failure.

 # SIGNALMENT/HISTORY

- Dogs are the most common species affected by microcystins, although many species may develop toxicosis if a sufficient dose is ingested.
- Backyard ponds that are poorly maintained and allow for cyanobacterial proliferation may pose a risk to dogs.

### Risk Factors

- Dogs that enjoy swimming are more likely to consume toxic amounts of an algal bloom than dogs that refrain from water.
- Algal bloom prevalence is higher during increased water temperature and elevated nutrient concentrations in the water.
- Use of a dietary supplement containing naturally harvested blue-green algae.

### Historical Findings

- Witnessed exposure to water with or without surface algal bloom. Toxins may persist in the water post bloom.
- Algal material on coat or present in vomit.
- Owners frequently report rapid onset of clinical presentation, usually within 30 minutes of access to water.
- Other animals (especially livestock) may be found dead near the water source.

### Location and Circumstances of Poisoning

- Lakes, streams, ponds, removed algal material (bucket).
- Most microcystin-producing algal blooms are found in fresh water, but they have also occurred in saline environments.
- Algal bloom prevalence is highest during increased water temperature and elevated nutrient concentrations in the water.
- Steady winds that propel toxic blooms to shore allow for ingestion by thirsty animals.
- Different algal species reside in the benthic zone (i.e., on the sediment) or in the pelagic zone (water column). Blooms of pelagic species are usually easily detected at the water surface of ponds, rivers, or lakes. Blooms of benthic species are difficult to detect since algae reside on the surface of sediment and stones in rivers or lakes.

 # CLINICAL FEATURES

- Acute hepatotoxicosis with clinical signs of diarrhea, weakness, pale mucous membranes, and shock.
- Progression of disease is rapid, and death generally occurs within several hours of exposure.

# DIFFERENTIAL DIAGNOSIS

- Other causes of acute liver failure such as amanitins, aflatoxins, cocklebur, xylitol, cycad palms, acetaminophen.

# DIAGNOSTICS

## Clinical Pathological Findings

- Increase in serum ALP, AST, ALT, and in bilirubin, hyperkalemia, and hypoglycemia.

## Other Diagnostics

- Save gastric contents and water source samples for diagnostic testing.
- Toxicology testing.
  - Identification of the cyanobacteria in the suspect water source or stomach contents; however, positive identification does not confirm intoxication because the toxicity of the cyanobacteria is strain specific, and morphological observations alone cannot predict the hazard level.
  - Detection of microcystins in gastric contents and suspect source material (e.g., water, dietary supplement).
  - Enzyme-linked immunosorbent assay to screen for microcystins in water. Confirmation required with an alternate method such as LC-MS/MS at a diagnostic laboratory.
  - Mouse bioassay (IP injection of algal bloom extract) was used in the past to determine the toxicity of crude algal biomass in suspicious blue-green algae poisonings (see Figure 110.2).

## Pathological Findings

- Detection of algal bloom material in GI tract and/or on legs. Grossly evident liver enlargement.
- Histological lesions include progressive centrilobular hepatocyte rounding, dissociation, necrosis, breakdown of the sinusoidal endothelium, and intrahepatic hemorrhage.

# THERAPEUTICS

- The treatment goals are to prevent further exposure and absorption, control any CNS signs, and provide supportive care to treat hypovolemia and electrolyte imbalances.
- Treatment is often unsuccessful due to the rapid onset of clinical signs and death.

## Detoxification

- Emesis may be induced in asymptomatic animals with recent exposures.
- Activated charcoal can be attempted, but efficacy is questionable.
- Bathe all animals with dermal exposure very thoroughly. Protective clothing must be worn by staff members during bathing.

## Appropriate Health Care

- All intoxicated animals will need prompt emergency and intensive care.

## Antidote

- No antidote available.

## Drug(s) of Choice

- Manage acute signs of hepatic hemorrhagic shock with IV crystalloids, colloids, and blood products as needed. Initial shock boluses of 20 mL/kg of crystalloids can be given over 10–20 minutes during initial stabilization.

- The use of blood products (pRBC, WB, FFP, or FP) may be necessary to increase oxygen-carrying capacity and replace coagulation factors. Patients should be blood typed prior to transfusion.
  - Blood products (whole blood, pRBC, etc.) 10–20 mL/kg IV to effect.
  - FFP or FP 10–20 mL/kg IV over 1–4 hours.
- Vitamin $K_1$ (phytonadione) 1–5 mg/kg q 24 hours PO, SQ to address clotting issues.
- Hepatoprotectants.
  - SAMe 18–20 mg/kg PO q 24 hours.
  - Silymarin 20–50 mg/kg PO q 24 hours.

### Alternative Drugs

- Cholestyramine – bile acid sequestrant; no data on efficacy in microcystin toxicosis is available. 172 mg/kg (78.4 mg/lb) PO q 24 hours.

### Precautions/Interactions

- Wear protective clothing while handling/bathing affected animals.

### Patient Monitoring

- Intensive care and monitoring will be needed, including blood glucose, electrolytes, CBC, serum biochemistry, and coagulation parameters.

 **COMMENTS**

### Prevention/Avoidance

- Deny dogs access to water with visible algal blooms.
- Reduce fertilizer runoff and applications in fields surrounding ponds used for drinking water.
- Remove algal blooms from ponds immediately and discard material safely.
- Evaluate the source of blue-green algae dietary supplements.

### Possible Complications

- DIC, hepatic encephalopathy, and renal failure.

### Expected Course and Prognosis

- Animals poisoned with cyanotoxins are often found dead.
- Blue-green algae intoxications progress so rapidly that treatment is often too late.
- Prognosis is poor.

### Public Health

- Toxin-producing algal blooms also pose a significant human health risk. Cases of human contact dermatitis, upper respiratory irritation, and death have occurred. Microcystins are considered possible carcinogens as tumor promoters.
- Suspect blooms should be reported to local environmental regulatory authorities.
- A guideline value of no more than 1 mcg/l of microcystins in lifetime drinking water has been set by the World Health Organization.

## Synonyms

Blue-green algae toxicosis, blue-green algae poisoning, microcystin poisoning.

## Abbreviations

See Appendix 1 for a complete list.

## Suggested Reading

Bautista AC, Moore CE, Lin Y et al. Hepatopathy following consumption of a commercially available blue-green algae dietary supplement in a dog. *BMC Vet Res* 2015;11:136.

DeVries SE, Galey FD, Namikoshi M et al. Clinical and pathologic findings of blue-green algae (*Microcystis aeruginosa*) intoxication in a dog. *J Vet Diagn Invest* 1993;5(3):403–408.

Foss AJ, Aubel MT, Gallagher B, Mettee N et al. Diagnosing microcystin intoxication of canines: clinico-pathological indications, pathological characteristics, and analytical detection in postmortem and antemortem samples. *Toxins* 2019;11(8):456.

Loftin KA, Graham JL, Hilborn ED et al. Cyanotoxins in inland lakes of the United States: occurrence and potential recreational health risks in the EPA National Lakes Assessment 2007. *Harmful Algae* 2016;56:77–90.

Puschner B. Cyanobacterial (blue-green algae) toxins. In: Gupta RC (ed.) *Veterinary Toxicology: Basic and Clinical Principles*, 3rd edn. San Diego: Elsevier, 2018: pp. 763–777.

Rankin KA, Alroy KA, Kudela RM et al. Treatment of cyanobacterial (microcystin) toxicosis using oral cholestyramine: case report of a dog from Montana. *Toxins* 2013;5(6):1051–1063.

**Authors**: Adrienne Bautista, DVM, PhD, DABVT and Birgit Puschner, DVM, PhD, DABVT
**Consulting Editor**: Lynn R. Hovda, RPh, DVM, MS, DACVIM

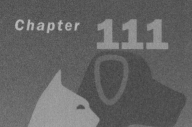
# Blue-green Algae (Cyanobacteria): Others

## DEFINITION/OVERVIEW

- Although microcystins and anatoxins make up a majority of the documented animal poisonings from blue-green algal (cyanobacterial) proliferations, other cyanotoxins exist and may pose an increased risk under certain environmental conditions.
- Most cyanobacteria blooms do not produce toxins. However, determining toxin production and severity is not possible with the naked eye. All blooms are potentially toxic.
- Cyanotoxin exposure can lead to an acute intoxication affecting the liver, skin, or CNS.
- Dermatotoxins include lyngbya-, aplysia-, and debromoaplysiatoxin produced by *Lyngbya*, *Schizothrix*, and *Planktothrix* (Figure 111.1).
- Nodularins are hepatotoxic cyanotoxins, similar to microcystins, that are only produced by *Nodularia*.
- Cylindrospermopsins are produced by *Cylindrospermopsis*, *Aphanizomenon*, *Anabena*, and *Lyngbya* and have caused acute deaths in cattle.
- Beta-N-methylamino-l-alanine (BMAA), neurotoxic amino acid, is thought to be produced by all types of blue-green algae and has been implicated in avian vacuolar myelopathy (not further discussed).

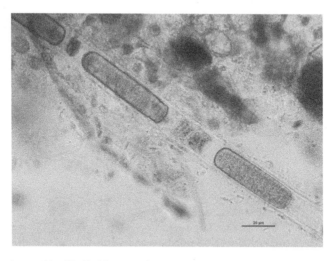

■ **Figure 111.1** *Lyngbya* sp. identified in lake water from northern California, June 2013. Dog with access to water had an outbreak of dermatitis after swimming. Debromoaplysiatoxin was detected in the water sample. Source: Courtesy of Birgit Puschner.

*Blackwell's Five-Minute Veterinary Consult Clinical Companion: Small Animal Toxicology*, Third Edition.
Edited by Lynn R. Hovda, Ahna G. Brutlag, Robert H. Poppenga, and Steven E. Epstein.
© 2024 John Wiley & Sons, Inc. Published 2024 by John Wiley & Sons, Inc.

- Saxitoxins, although commonly associated with paralytic shellfish poisoning, are produced by a number of freshwater blue-green algae, including certain species of *Aphanizomenon*, *Cylindrospermopsis*, *Anabena*, *Lyngbya*, and *Planktothrix*.

 ## ETIOLOGY/PATHOPHYSIOLOGY

### Mechanism of Action

- Lyngbya-, aplysia-, and debromoaplysiatoxins are all activators of protein kinase C, an enzyme important in controlling the function of other proteins.
- Nodularins are cyclic pentapeptide cyanotoxins similar in chemical structure, toxicity, and mode of action to microcystins leading to severe liver damage.
- Cylindrospermopsins are potent inhibitors of protein synthesis which can lead to injury in a multitude of organs, including liver, kidney, heart, and gastrointestinal tract.
- Saxitoxins block voltage-gated sodium channels leading to neuromuscular, respiratory, and cardiovascular effects.

### Toxicokinetics

- Lyngbyatoxin A is slightly lipophilic and has been found to penetrate the skin within hours. Other data on the toxicokinetics of lyngbya-, aplysia-, and debromoaplysiatoxins are lacking.
- There are limited data on the kinetics of nodularins and it is assumed they behave similar to microcystins, targeting the liver and kidneys after absorption by the small intestines. Lymphoid organs can also be affected.
- Data on the toxicokinetics of cylindrospermopsin in small animals are very limited. Studies in other species have shown effects on various organs including the liver, kidneys, adrenal glands, intestine, lung, thymus, and heart.
- From the limited data on the toxicokinetics of saxitoxins in cats, they can reach the CNS and are also distributed to the liver, kidney, and spleen. Excretion is mainly via urine.

### Toxicity

- Reported IP $LD_{50}$ of lyngbyatoxin A in mice is 0.25 mg/kg.
- The $LD_{50}$ for nodularins in small animals is unknown. A reported IP $LD_{50}$ of nodularins in rats is 30–50 mcg/kg.
- An oral $LD_{50}$ of pure cylindrospermopsin is not available in animals.
- The IP $LD_{50}$ of the most potent saxitoxin in mice is 10 mcg/kg.
- Chronic and subchronic toxicity data do exist for domestic animals.

### Systems Affected

- Lyngbya-, aplysia-, and debromoaplysiatoxins.
  - Skin/exocrine – pruritus, erythema, blister formation, dermatitis.
- Nodularins.
  - Hepatobiliary – vomiting, diarrhea, weakness, pale mucous membranes, icterus, shock.
- Cylindrospermopsin.
  - Hepatobiliary – vomiting, diarrhea, weakness, pale mucous membranes, icterus, shock.
- Saxitoxins.
  - Cardiovascular – hypotension, shock.
  - Nervous – weakness, muscle tremors, respiratory arrest.

**SIGNALMENT/HISTORY**

- Dogs are more likely to be affected by these other cyanobacterial toxins although many species may develop toxicosis if a sufficient dose is ingested.
- Backyard ponds that are poorly maintained and allow for cyanobacterial proliferation may pose a risk to dogs.

### Risk Factors

- Dogs that enjoy swimming are more likely to consume or come in contact with toxic amounts of an algal bloom than dogs that refrain from water.
- Algal bloom prevalence is higher during increased water temperature and elevated nutrient concentrations in the water.

### Historical Findings

- Witnessed exposure to water with or without visible algal bloom. Toxins may persist in the water post bloom.
- Algal material on coat or present in vomit.
- Owners frequently report rapid onset of clinical presentation after access to water.
- Other animals (especially livestock) may be found dead near the water source.

### Location and Circumstances of Poisoning

- Lakes, streams, ponds, removed algal material (bucket).
- Algal bloom prevalence is highest during increased water temperature and elevated nutrient concentrations in the water.
- Steady winds that propel toxic blooms to shore allow for ingestion by thirsty animals.

 **CLINICAL FEATURES**

- Lyngbya-, aplysia-, and debromoaplysiatoxins – acute onset of pruritus and erythema followed by dermatitis with or without blister formation. Prognosis is good.
- Nodularins – acute hepatotoxicosis with clinical signs of vomiting, diarrhea, weakness, pale mucous membranes developing a few hours after exposure. Death may occur 1–5 days following exposure.
- Cylindrospermopsin – hepatoxicities.
- Saxitoxins – neuromuscular weakness, respiratory arrest, and cardiovascular shock that may be responsive to adrenergic agonists.

 **DIFFERENTIAL DIAGNOSIS**

- Lyngbya-, aplysia-, and debromoaplysiatoxins – other causes of dermatitis such as insect bites, bacterial infections, parasites, and allergic reactions.
- Nodularins – other causes of acute liver failure such as microcystins, amanitins, aflatoxins, cocklebur, xylitol, cycad palms, acetaminophen.
- Cylindrospermopsin – other causes of acute liver failure such as microcystins, amanitins, aflatoxins, cocklebur, xylitol, cycad palms, acetaminophen.
- Saxitoxins – anatoxins, organophosphorus and carbamate insecticides, strychnine, zinc phosphide, metaldehyde, amphetamines, certain drugs of abuse, and neurotoxic plants.

# DIAGNOSTICS

## Clinical Pathological Findings

- Nodularins and cylindrospermopsin – increase in serum ALP, AST, ALT, and in bilirubin, hyperkalemia, hypoglycemia.

## Other Diagnostics

- Save gastric contents and water source samples for diagnostic testing.
- Toxicology testing.
  - Toxicity is strain specific and identification of a potential toxin-producing strain should be followed up by toxicant detection to predict toxicity level.
  - Identification of the algae in the suspect water source or stomach contents; however, positive identification does not confirm intoxication because the toxicity of the cyanobacteria is strain specific, and morphological observations alone cannot predict the hazard level.
  - Detection of specific cyanotoxin in gastric contents, urine, bile, postmortem tissues, and suspect source material.
  - Mouse bioassay (IP injection of algal bloom extract) was used in the past to determine the toxicity of crude algal biomass in suspicious blue-green algae poisonings.

## Pathological Findings

- Detection of algal bloom material in GI tract and/or on legs.
- Nodularins – gross liver enlargement; histological lesions include hepatic and renal necrosis, along with possible lymphoid depletion.
- Cylindrospermopsin – gross liver enlargement, epicardial hemorrhage, subserosal gastrointestinal hemorrhage; histologically there is hepatic necrosis.

 # THERAPEUTICS

- The treatment goals are to prevent further exposure and absorption, control any CNS signs, and provide supportive care.
- Lyngbya-, aplysia-, and debromoaplysiatoxins – provide supportive therapy to treat pruritus, dermatitis, and potentially secondary bacterial infections.
- Nodularins and cylindrospermopsin – provide supportive therapy to treat hypovolemia and electrolyte imbalances.
- Saxitoxins – general supportive care and specific measures to control shock should be performed.

## Detoxification

- Emesis may be induced in asymptomatic animals with recent exposures.
- Activated charcoal can be attempted, but efficacy is questionable.
- Bathe all animals with dermal exposure very thoroughly. Protective clothing must be worn by staff members during bathing (risk of dermatitis).

## Appropriate Health Care

- All intoxicated animals will need prompt emergency and intensive care.
- Ventilation should be closely monitored in patients with severe neurological impairment using venous or arterial (preferred) $pCO_2$ or end-tidal capnography. Mechanical ventilation is indicated for patients with hypoventilation.

## Antidote

- No antidote available.

## Drug(s) of Choice

- Manage acute signs of hepatic hemorrhagic shock with IV crystalloids, colloids, and blood products as needed. Initial shock boluses of 20 mL/kg of crystalloids can be given over 10–20 minutes during initial stabilization.
- The use of blood products (pRBC, WB, FFP, or FP) may be necessary to increase oxygen-carrying capacity and replace coagulation factors. Patients should be blood typed prior to transfusion.
  - Blood products (whole blood, pRBC, etc.) 10–20 mL/kg IV to effect.
  - FFP or FP 10–20 mL/kg IV over 1–4 hours.
- Seizures.
  - Diazepam 2–5 mg/kg IV. These doses are much higher than normally used for seizure control. In general, if a 2 mg/kg IV dose does not control seizures, switch to phenobarbital.
  - Phenobarbital 2–20 mg/kg IV q 6–12 hours (may have to use very high doses).
  - Propofol 3–6 mg/kg IV to effect. CRI may be useful, 0.1–0.6 mg/kg/min.
  - Levetiracetam 20–60 mg/kg IV slowly. Repeat 10–20 mg/kg IV q 6–8 hours as needed.
- Tremors: methocarbamol 55–220 mg/kg IV.
- Atropine 0.02–0.04 mg/kg IV to effect in anatoxin-a$_s$ intoxication.
- Vitamin K$_1$ (phytonadione) 1–5 mg/kg q 24 hours PO, SQ to address clotting issues.
- Hepatoprotectants.
  - SAMe 18–20 mg/kg PO q 24 hours.
  - Silymarin 20–50 mg/kg PO q 24 hours.
- Antipruritic: prednisone/prednisolone 1–2 mg/kg PO q 24 hours.
- Diphenhydramine 2.2 mg/kg PO q 8–12 hours in dermatoxin intoxication.

## Alternative Drugs

- Cholestyramine – bile acid sequestrant; no data on efficacy in nodularin or cylindrospermopsin toxicosis are available. 172 mg/kg (78.4 mg/lb) PO q 24 hours.

## Precautions/Interactions

- Wear protective clothing while handling/bathing affected animals. Significant contact dermatitis may occur.

## Patient Monitoring

- Nodularin and cylindrospermopsin toxicosis – monitor liver function, coagulation status.
- Saxitoxin toxicosis – monitor biochemical profile, blood gases, respiratory and cardiovascular function.

 **COMMENTS**

### Prevention/Avoidance

- Deny dogs access to water with visible algal blooms.
- Reduce fertilizer runoff and applications in fields surrounding ponds used for drinking water.
- Remove algal blooms from ponds immediately and discard material safely.

## Possible Complications

- DIC, rhabdomyolysis, and myoglobinuria with subsequent renal failure are possible if prolonged, untreated tremors/seizures or hyperthermia present.

## Expected Course and Prognosis

- Animals poisoned with blue-green algae toxins are often found dead.
- Blue-green algae intoxications often progress rapidly such that treatment is often too late.
- Prognosis depends on amount and type of blue-green algae toxin animal is exposed to.
- Prognosis is good to fair for animals solely exposed to dermatotoxins.

## Public Health

- Toxin-producing algal blooms also pose a significant human health risk. Cases of human contact dermatitis, upper respiratory irritation, and death have occurred.
- Suspect blooms should be reported to local environmental regulatory authorities.

## Synonyms

Blue-green algae toxicosis, blue-green algae poisoning, paralytic shellfish poisoning.

## Abbreviations

See Appendix 1 for a complete list.

## Suggested Reading

Andrinolo D, Michea LF, Lagos N. Toxic effects, pharmacokinetics and clearance of saxitoxin, a component of paralytic shellfish poison (PSP), in cats. *Toxicon* 1999;37(3):447–464.

Griffiths DJ, Saker ML. The Palm Island mystery disease 20 years on: a review of research on the cyanotoxin cylindrospermopsin. *Environ Toxicol* 2003;18(2):78–93.

Puschner B. Cyanobacterial (blue-green algae) toxins. In: Gupta RC (ed.) *Veterinary Toxicology: Basic and Clinical Principles*, 3rd edn. San Diego: Elsevier, 2018; pp. 763–777.

Puschner B, Bautista AC, Wong C. Debromoaplysiatoxin as the causative agent of dermatitis in a dog after exposure to freshwater in California. *Front Vet Sci* 2017;4:50.

Simola O, Wiberg M, Jokela J et al. Pathologic findings and toxin identification in cyanobacterial (*Nodularia spumigena*) intoxication in a dog. *Vet Pathol* 2012;49(5):755–759.

**Authors:** Adrienne Bautista, DVM, PhD, DABVT and Birgit Puschner, DVM, PhD, DABVT
**Consulting Editor:** Lynn R. Hovda, RPh, DVM, MS, DACVIM

# Chapter 112

# Cardiac Glycosides

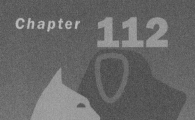

## DEFINITION/OVERVIEW

- A significant number of plants (and smaller number of animals) contain naturally occurring cardiotoxic cardenolides or bufadienolides that cause GI disturbances as well as severe cardiac arrhythmias. Approximately 400 cardiac cardenolides have been described. Digoxin and digitoxin, the most widely known of these toxins, were first used to treat congestive heart failure in human beings and are still occasionally used in human and veterinary medicine. Ingestion of pharmaceutical products containing these compounds is generally associated with more severe toxicity than ingestion of plants.
- Common plants containing cardiac glycoside toxins include the following.
  - Desert rose (*Adenium obesum;* Figure 112.1).
  - Dogbane (*Apocynum* spp.).
  - Purple or common foxglove (*Digitalis purpurea;* Figures 112.2 and 112.3).
  - Giant milkweed (*Calatropis* spp.).
  - Kalanchoe (*Kalanchoe* spp.; Figure 112.4).
  - Lily of the valley (*Convallaria majalis;* Figure 112.5).
  - Milkweed (*Asclepias* spp.; Figures 112.6 and 112.7).
  - Oleander (*Nerium oleander;* Figures 112.8 and 112.9).
  - Oubain (*Strophanthus gratus*).
  - Spring pheasant's eye (*Adonis vernalis*).
  - Squill (*Urginea indica* and *U. maritima*).
  - Star of Bethlehem (*Ornithogalum umbellatum*).
  - Wormseed wallflower (*Erysimum cheiranthoides*).
  - Wooly foxglove (*Digitalis lantana*).
  - Yellow oleander (*Cascabela thevetia* [*Thevetia peruviana*]; Figure 112.10).
- Common names are often used interchangeably to describe any of several different plants. Confirming the scientific name is essential for accurate identification.
- Different plants may have varying levels of toxicity, and concentrations of these glycosides may differ in separate parts of the plant (i.e., stem, leaves, seeds, or fruit).
- Many of these are cultivated for indoor and outdoor uses and sold at grocery and garden stores (see Figure 112.2). Several may also be found growing in the wild.

*Blackwell's Five-Minute Veterinary Consult Clinical Companion: Small Animal Toxicology*, Third Edition.
Edited by Lynn R. Hovda, Ahna G. Brutlag, Robert H. Poppenga, and Steven E. Epstein.
© 2024 John Wiley & Sons, Inc. Published 2024 by John Wiley & Sons, Inc.

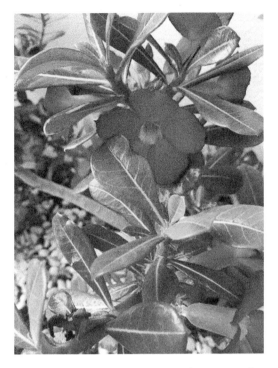

■ **Figure 112.1** Desert rose (*Adenium obesum*). Source: Courtesy of Lynn R. Hovda.

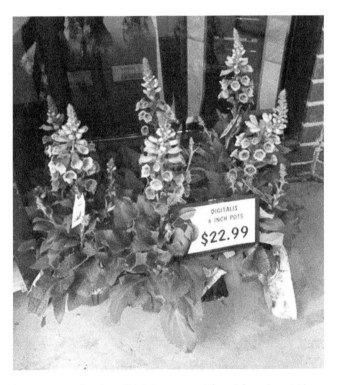

■ **Figure 112.2** Purple or common foxglove (*Digitalis purpurea*) found for sale outside a grocery store. Source: Courtesy of David Brown, University of Minnesota, St Paul, MN.

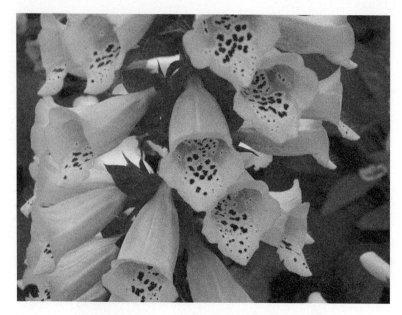

■ **Figure 112.3** Close-up of common foxglove (*Digitalis purpurea*). Source: Courtesy of Lynn R. Hovda.

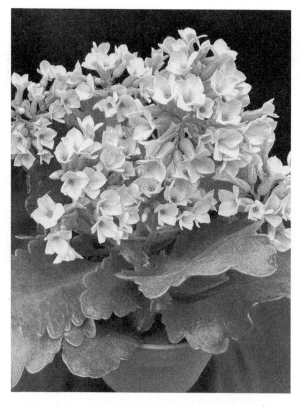

■ **Figure 112.4** Kalanchoe (*Kalanchoe* spp.). Source: Courtesy of Tyne K. Hovda.

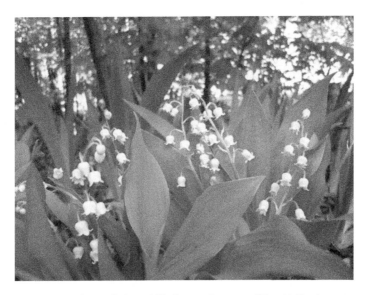

■ **Figure 112.5** Lily of the valley (*Convallaria majalis*). Source: Courtesy of Tyne K. Hovda.

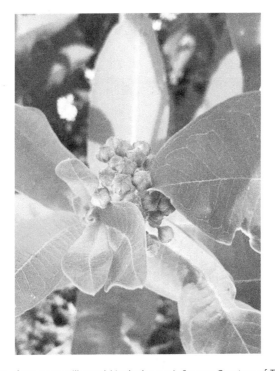

■ **Figure 112.6** Early buds of common milkweed (*Asclepias* spp.). Source: Courtesy of Tyne K. Hovda.

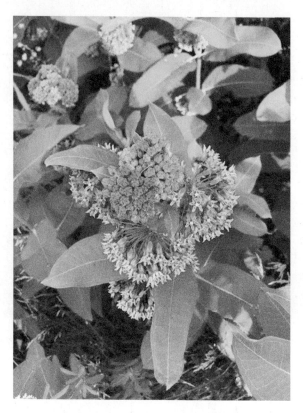

■ **Figure 112.7** Closeup of common milkweed flower (*Asclepias* spp.). Source: Courtesy of Tyne K. Hovda.

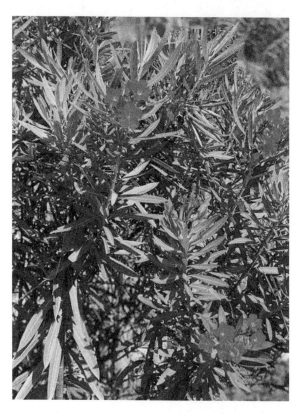

■ **Figure 112.8** Oleander (*Nerium oleander*) shrub found growing along the highway in Puerto Vallarta, Mexico. Source: Courtesy of Lynn R. Hovda.

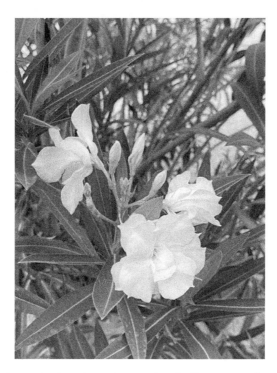

■ **Figure 112.9** Oleander flower (*Nerium oleander*). Most oleander flowers are red or pink, but other colors such as white, very pale yellow, salmon, and peach may also be found. Source: Courtesy of Tyne K. Hovda.

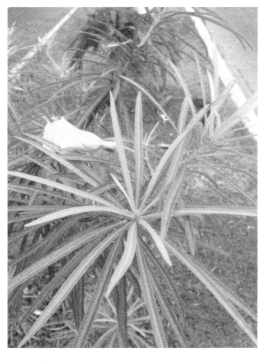

■ **Figure 112.10** Yellow oleander (*Cascabela thevetia* [*Thevetia peruviana*]). Source: Courtesy of Lynn R. Hovda.

# ETIOLOGY/PATHOPHYSIOLOGY

## Mechanism of Action

- Cardiac glycosides have an inhibitory effect on sodium/potassium ATPase, resulting in an increase in intracellular sodium and decrease in intracellular potassium. This effect is particularly pronounced in cardiac muscle and vascular smooth muscle.
- The cell's resting membrane potential shifts in a positive direction (i.e., the cell becomes relatively less polarized) and eventually a complete loss of normal myocardial electrical function occurs.
- Extracellular potassium rises, leading to a marked hyperkalemia and loss of cardiac excitability.

## Pharmacokinetics

- Absorption is rapid, with signs developing from 30 minutes to a few hours post ingestion.
- Food delays absorption in all species. In cats, the presence of food in the stomach may decrease the total amount absorbed by as much as 50%.
- Widely distributed in body tissues, particularly heart, kidney, liver, stomach, muscle.
- 20–30% protein bound.
- Elimination is primarily renal.
- Some hepatic metabolism and enterohepatic recirculation occur, but the extent to which this is clinically relevant remains somewhat controversial.
- Renal dysfunction may greatly slow the rate of elimination.

## Toxicity

- Digitalis is a steroidal glycoside. The various plant toxins are structurally similar and present the same toxic profile.
- Several hundred different plant toxins have been identified, most specific to a particular plant species.
- The degree of toxicity varies depending on the specific plant, plant part, and amount consumed.
- Most cardiac glycoside plants can cause toxicosis if fresh or dried plant matter is consumed.
- All plant parts are considered toxic.

## Systems Affected

- Gastrointestinal – signs occur most frequently and include hypersalivation, vomiting, and diarrhea with or without blood.
- Cardiovascular – abnormalities include bradycardia, hypotension, all degrees of AV block, and a variety of arrhythmias. Rarely, tachycardia may occur. Death occurs from asystole.
- Neuromuscular – signs are vague and may be secondary to decreased cardiac output and hypotension.
- Ophthalmic – mydriasis can occur.

# SIGNALMENT/HISTORY

- No breed or species predilection for exposure.
- Cats may be more sensitive than dogs; male cats seem to be more sensitive than females.
- Dogs with ABCB1 (formerly referred to as MDR-1) gene mutation (e.g., collies, Australian shepherds, etc.) are reported to be more sensitive to the CNS effects of glycoside toxicity.

## Risk Factors

- Animals with a prior history cardiac disease, especially those currently receiving digoxin or other cardiac drugs.
- Obese animals may experience toxicosis at lower doses than lean animals.

## Historical Findings

- Owner often reports that the animal chewed or dug up relevant plants.

## Location and Circumstances of Poisoning

- Can occur anywhere. Some species of the plants are widely distributed throughout the United States.
- Oleander toxicosis tends to occur with greater frequency in the warmer portions of the country, in particular the South and Southwest.
- Most of the plants are unpalatable but may be ingested by bored or confined animals.

 # CLINICAL FEATURES

- Vomiting with or without blood, diarrhea with or without blood, and hypersalivation are the most reported signs, often occurring within 30–45 minutes of ingestion. Weakness and depression often precede the onset of cardiac abnormalities. Varying degrees of bradycardia or tachycardia, weak and irregular pulses, hypotension, AV block, and arrhythmias can occur. Other signs include mydriasis, tremors, and coma.
- Animals may be found dead.

 # DIFFERENTIAL DIAGNOSIS

- Primary cardiac disease of any origin.
- Calcium channel blocker or beta receptor antagonists.
- Ingestion of other pharmaceuticals with known cardiac effects.
- Ingestion of *Taxus* spp. (yew) or plants in Ericaceae family (azaleas, rhododendrons, others).
- Severe GI disease associated with viral, bacterial, or parasitic infection.

 # DIAGNOSTICS

## Clinical Pathological Changes

- Serum chemistry with early and marked hyperkalemia. May change to hypokalemia as time passes. Elevations in BUN and creatinine secondary to dehydration from vomiting.
- Metabolic acidosis.

## Other Diagnostics

- Torn up plants or plants/plant pieces in emesis.
- Serum digoxin levels may be available from human hospitals. If a plant ingestion is suspected, ensure the laboratory is running an assay that includes the toxin associated with the specific plant in question.
- Detection of cardiac glycosides in tissue or urine is rarely performed but can be done by chromatography if the specific glycoside is known.

## Pathological Findings

- Gross findings depend on the time of death, but plant pieces may be found in the stomach and small intestine. The epicardium may have a mottled appearance with clotted blood in the ventricles.

- Histopathological findings include venous and capillary congestion throughout the body with severe, diffuse hepatic congestion and marked caudal vena cava distension.

 **THERAPEUTICS**

## Detoxification

- Induction of emesis if recent exposure and the animal is not already vomiting.
- In massive ingestions, consider sedation, endotracheal intubation (with a cuffed, inflated tube), and gastric lavage.
- Activated charcoal with a cathartic × 1 dose followed by activated charcoal q 6–8 hours × 2 doses if no risk for aspiration and sodium level can be monitored.

## Appropriate Health Care

- Hospitalize animals with known ingestions for at least 12 hours. Clinical signs are often evident 30–45 minutes post ingestion but may be delayed for several hours, depending on the plant ingested.
- Severely affected patients may require 3–6 days of hospitalization.
- ECG monitoring for a minimum of 24 hours in animals with clinical signs. Treat arrhythmias as they develop.
- Baseline serum chemistry with special attention to potassium concentration and renal indices. Venous blood gases to monitor for metabolic acidosis. Correct electrolyte and acid–base abnormalities as needed.
- Judicious use of IV fluids with close monitoring of patient response. The goal is to support, but not overload, the cardiovascular system.

## Antidote

- Digoxin-specific Fab fragments (digoxin-FAB; Digibind® or DigiFAB®) have been used in dogs to reverse the cardiac effects of digoxin and oleander and may be effective for other cardiac glycoside toxins as well. The high cost may preclude their use. A wide variety of doses have been suggested. If used, the best option is to monitor serum digoxin levels and adjust dose accordingly.

## Drug(s) of Choice

- Early yet cautious use of IV fluids to maintain blood pressure and perfusion.
- Bradycardia.
  - Atropine 0.02–0.04 mg/kg IV, IM, or SQ.
  - Glycopyrrolate 0.01–0.02 mg/kg SQ, IM, or IV.
  - In severe cases of bradycardia unresponsive to medical management, the use of a temporary pacemaker may be indicated.
- The use of antiarrhythmics may be necessary if the patient is persistently tachycardic and non-responsive to sedation, IV fluids, has severe ventricular dysrhythmias, or has evidence of poor perfusion (hypotension, pulse deficits, tachycardia, pale mucous membranes, prolonged CRT).
  - Lidocaine.
    - Dogs: 2–4 mg/kg IV over 1–2 minutes to effect. If effective, follow with CRI at 25–100 mcg/kg/min. ECG must be monitored carefully during use.
    - Cats: 0.25–0.5 mg/kg slow IV while monitoring ECG. If effective, use CRI of 10–20 mcg/kg/min. Use very cautiously in cats.
  - Procainamide.
    - Dogs: 2–4 mg/kg IV over 3–5 minutes (up to 20 mg/kg IV bolus over 15–20 minutes), followed by 20–50 mcg/kg/min CRI or 10–20 mg/kg q 8hours IM or SQ. Rarely used but may be effective if no other drugs are available.

- Other antiarrhythmic agents may be useful, depending on the availability and comfort level of practitioner.
- Antiemetics if vomiting is severe or persistent.
  - Maropitant 1 mg/kg SQ, IV (dogs over 4 months) q 24 hours.
  - Ondansetron 0.5–1 mg/kg IV q 12 hours for dogs; 0.1–1 mg/kg IV, SQ, IM q 6–12 hours for cats.
  - Dolasetron 0.6 mg/kg IV, SQ q 24 hours.
- GI protectants as needed.
  - Famotidine 0.5–1 mg/kg PO, SQ, IM, IV q 12 hours.
  - Omeprazole 0.5–1 mg/kg PO q 24 hours.
  - Sucralfate 0.25–1 g PO q 8 hours for 5–7 days if evidence of active ulcer disease.
- Sedation as needed.
  - Acepromazine 0.01–0.2 mg/kg IV (slowly), IM, SQ; lower doses recommended (0.02–0.03 mg/kg) due to risk of hypotension.
  - Butorphanol 0.1–0.5 mg/kg IV, IM, SQ; lower dose of 0.2 mg/kg recommended.
  - Buprenorphine 0.005–0.03 mg/kg IM, IV or SQ q 6–12 hours.

## Precautions/Interactions

- Calcium channel blockers and beta-blockers can have additive effects on AV conduction and should be avoided as they may result in complete heart block.
- Hawthorn, an herbal supplement, should not be used as it exacerbates the toxicity of cardiac glycosides.

## Alternative Drugs

- Fructose-1,6-diphosphate has been used experimentally to decrease the severity of cardiac effects in dogs. The mechanism of action is not understood, and it is not used in clinical practice.

## Patient Monitoring

- Continuous ECG for first 24 hours and then as needed to monitor effect of cardiac drugs.
- Serial blood pressure monitoring, especially early in toxicity. Hypotension may become severe.
- Baseline and repeat serum electrolytes. Hyperkalemia may be early and marked; hypokalemia has been reported but generally occurs later.
- Good nursing care. Palpation of extremities for coldness; may indicate decreased perfusion secondary to hypotension.

 **COMMENTS**

### Prevention/Avoidance

- Owners should know the common plants in their home, yard, and geographical location.
- Oleander commonly grows wild in the Southwest, especially in California, Arizona, New Mexico, and Texas. Off-leash dogs in these areas should be watched carefully for any signs of exposure.

### Expected Course and Prognosis

- Prognosis is guarded to good with appropriate care and timely intervention.
- Cardiac arrhythmias may complicate recovery but are not insurmountable if treated early.

## See Also

Chapter 22 Beta Receptor Antagonists (Beta-blockers)
Chapter 24 Calcium Channel Blockers
Chapter 108 Azaleas and Rhododendrons
Chapter 121 Yew

## Abbreviations

See Appendix 1 for a complete list.

## Suggested Reading

Atkinson KJ, Fine DM, Evans TJ et al. Suspected lily-of-the-valley (*Convallaria majalis*) toxicosis in a dog. *J Vet Emerg Crit Care* 2008;18(4):399–403.

Bandara V, Weinstein SA, White J et al. A review of the natural history, toxinology, diagnosis and clinical management of *Nerium oleander* (common oleander) and *Thevetia peruviana* (yellow oleander) poisoning. *Toxicon* 2010;56(3):273–281.

Galton AF, Granfone MC, Caldwell DJ. Digoxin-specific antibody fragments for the treatment of suspected *Nerium oleander* toxicosis in a cat. *J Feline Med Surg* 2020;6(2):2055116920969599.

Magnani B, Woolf AD. Cardiotoxic plants. In: Brent J, Burkhart K, Dargan P et al. (eds) *Critical Care Toxicology*. Cham: Springer, 2017; pp. 2187–2203.

Milweski LM, Safda AK. An overview of potentially life-threatening poisonous plants in dogs and cats. *J Vet Emerg Crit Care* 2006;16(1):25–33.

Morsy N. Cardiac glycosides in medicinal plants. In: El-Shemy H (ed.) *Aromatic and Medicinal Plants – Back to Nature*. London: Intechopen, 2017; pp 29–45.

Smith G. Kalanchoe species poisoning in pets. *Vet Med* 2004;99(11):913–936.

## Acknowledgments

The author and editor acknowledge the contributions of James Eucher who edited this chapter in the previous edition.

**Author**: Tyne K. Hovda
**Consulting Editor**: Ahna G. Brutlag, DVM, MS, DABT, DABVT

# Chapter 113

# Cyanogenic Glycosides

## DEFINITION/OVERVIEW

- More than 2500 plant species contain hydrogen cyanide in the form of nontoxic glycosides; amygdalin and prunasin are two of approximately 50 known cyanogenic glycosides.
- Common plants associated with cyanogenic glycosides and human or animal poisoning include the following.
  - *Sorghum* spp: sorghum, Johnson grass, Sudan grass.
  - *Triglochin* spp: arrowgrass.
  - *Trifolium repens*: white clover.
  - *Prunus* spp.
    - Choke cherry (Figures 113.1 and 113.2), black cherry, and cherry laurel pits.
    - Peaches, apricots: kernels (seeds) within pits (Figures 113.3 and 113.4).
    - Almonds (bitter variety).
  - *Sambucus* spp: elderberry (seeds, bark, leaves, and raw berries).
  - *Malus* spp: apple (seeds).
  - *Hydrangea* spp: hydrangeas (Figure 113.5).
  - *Eucalyptus* spp: gum trees.
  - *Manihot esculenta*: cassava (bitter variety), tapioca, yucca.
  - *Pteridium aquilinum*: bracken fern.
  - *Bambusa* spp: bamboo (shoots).
- Cyanide poisoning occurs following exposure to free hydrogen cyanide (i.e., prussic acid) and can be acute or chronic.
- In veterinary medicine, cyanide poisoning following ingestion of cyanogenic glycoside-containing plants is seen almost exclusively in ruminant species and, to a lesser degree, equines.
- Cyanide toxicosis following ingestion of cyanogenic glycoside-containing plants by dogs and cats is **rare** because of the reduced ability of monogastric species to liberate hydrogen cyanide from the glycoside molecule.

## ETIOLOGY/PATHOPHYSIOLOGY

### Mechanism of Action

- Glucosidases and lyases, plant enzymes that cleave cyanide from the glycoside, are structurally separated from cyanogenic glycoside within the plant. Damage to plants by chewing, crushing, drought, wilting, or frost allows glucosidases and lyases contact with cyanogenic glycosides which frees hydrogen cyanide from the glycoside.

*Blackwell's Five-Minute Veterinary Consult Clinical Companion: Small Animal Toxicology*, Third Edition. Edited by Lynn R. Hovda, Ahna G. Brutlag, Robert H. Poppenga, and Steven E. Epstein.
© 2024 John Wiley & Sons, Inc. Published 2024 by John Wiley & Sons, Inc.

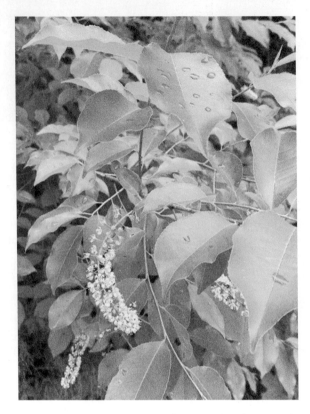

■ **Figure 113.1** Choke cherry (*Prunus virginiana*) produces fragrant, white flowers in the spring. Source: Courtesy of Lynn R. Hovda.

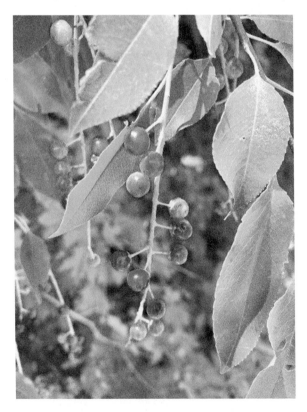

■ **Figure 113.2** Choke cherry berries (*Prunus virginiana*) turn from green to yellowish to dark red as they ripen. The fruit is used for wines, syrups, jams, and jellies. The pits are toxic. Source: Courtesy of Lynn R. Hovda.

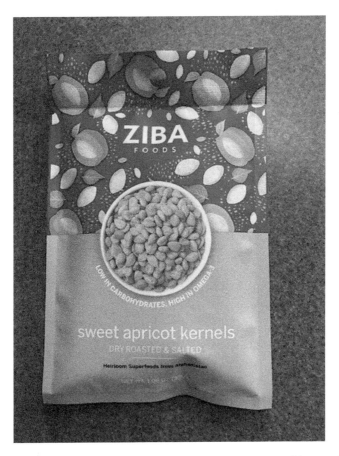

■ **Figure 113.3** Apricot kernels (seeds) for human consumption. Source: Courtesy of Susan Holland.

■ Glucosidase and lyase activity are increased at a neutral rumen pH and decreased at the acidic stomach pH in monogastric species; this encourages the release of hydrogen cyanide in ruminants, greatly increasing their risk for cyanide toxicosis.

■ Hydrogen cyanide reversibly binds to the trivalent iron component of the cytochrome *c* oxidase in mitochondria. This action halts the mitochondrial transport chain and stops cellular respiration, the reduction of oxygen to generate energy in the form of adenosine triphosphate (ATP).

■ Oxygen, blocked from oxidative phosphorylation, supersaturates hemoglobin resulting in cherry-red mucous membranes.

■ Reduction of aerobic metabolism by hydrogen cyanide primarily affects the brain and heart; CNS and cardiovascular clinical signs precede death in acute cyanide poisoning.

■ Chronic cyanide poisoning includes (1) hypothyroidism via disruption of iodide uptake by thiocyanate in lambs; (2) neuropathy due to demyelination in ruminants and horses; (3) skeletal deformities in piglets, calves, and foals of dams ingesting cyanogenic glycoside-containing plants during gestation; and (4) chronic neuropathy (distal limbs, ocular, auditory) in humans associated with a diet high in improperly prepared cassava. Chronic cyanide poisoning has not been reported in small animals.

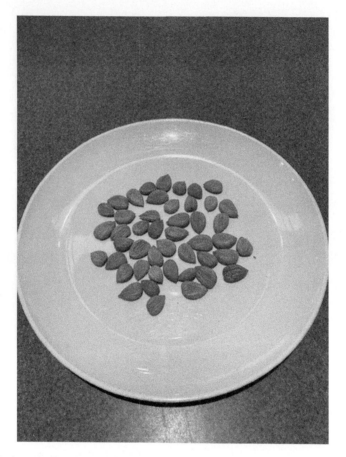

■ **Figure 113.4** Apricot pits. Source: Courtesy of Susan Holland.

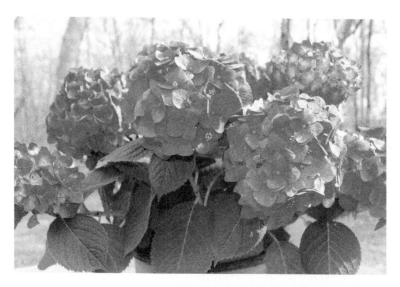

■ **Figure 113.5** *Hydrangea* spp. All parts of the plant, including the showy pink or blue flowers, are poisonous. Source: Courtesy of Lynn R. Hovda.

## Toxicokinetics

- Cyanide, as hydrogen cyanide (HCN) or free cyanide (CN⁻), is rapidly absorbed and distributed following oral, dermal, or respiratory exposure.
- Metabolism of cyanide occurs in the liver. Sulfonation of cyanide with thiosulfate via the enzyme rhodanese (i.e., thiosulfate-rhodanese pathway) creates the nontoxic, major metabolite thiocyanate. 2-Amino-2-thiazoline-4-carboxylic acid (ATCA), a lesser metabolite, and thiocyanate have clinical use as indirect biomarkers of cyanide exposure (human).
- Thiocyanate is water soluble and excreted in the urine.
- The half-life of cyanide is 14–76 minutes (human, pig, goat, rat).

## Toxicity

- Acute lethal dose of hydrogen cyanide is 2–2.5 mg/kg for most species. Severe clinical signs (human data) are noted when blood cyanide levels are ≥40 μmol/L.

## Systems Affected

- Nervous – ataxia, seizure, death (peracute and acute).
- Cardiovascular – tachycardia, arrhythmia, "cherry-red" mucous membranes.
- Respiratory – dyspnea, breath odor: almond.
- Gastrointestinal – hypersalivation, vomiting, fecal incontinence.
- Musculoskeletal – fasciculation progressing to spasm.
- Ocular – excess lacrimation.
- Urinary – incontinence.

 **SIGNALMENT/HISTORY**

## Risk Factors

- Dogs and cats are at **low risk** for developing cyanide poisoning following most oral exposures.
- Small animal risk for acute cyanide poisoning increases with ingestion of massive amounts of damaged cyanogenic glycoside-containing plant foliage (e.g., wet/wilted, frost-damaged, crushed leaves, young regrowth following stunting) or large number of apricot kernels (product for human consumption).

## Historical Findings

- Owners frequently report pets as asymptomatic following ingestion of fruit seeds (apple) or stone fruit pits (cherry, peach).

 **CLINICAL FEATURES**

- Most small animals are asymptomatic following oral exposures to a few small pits, seeds, or leaves.
- Transient emesis following ingestion of plant material or large numbers of pits. Abdominal pain and persistent emesis may occur from foreign body obstruction in small pets ingesting large (peach) intact pits.
- Acute cyanide poisoning causes rapid onset of ataxia, hypersalivation, lacrimation, tachycardia, dyspnea, emesis, bright red mucous membranes, and muscle fasciculations progressing to convulsions, arrhythmias, and death.
  - Reported "bitter almond" odor to breath.
  - Infrequently, clinical signs delayed up to two hours post ingestion.
  - Acute cyanide poisoning in dogs and cats is unanticipated.
- Peracute death possible.

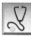

# DIFFERENTIAL DIAGNOSIS

- Carbon monoxide, salicylates, acetaminophen, tricyclic antidepressants, organophosphates, isoniazid.

# DIAGNOSTICS

### Clinical Pathological Findings

- No significant abnormal findings expected for most small animal exposures. Testing not indicated for asymptomatic patient.
- Acute cyanide poisoning (**rare**) – testing indicated for symptomatic patient.
  - Blood gas – elevated plasma lactate, normal arterial $O_2$, elevated venous $O_2$, A-V $O_2$ difference <10%, high anion gap metabolic acidosis.
  - CBC, chemistry, electrolytes: no pathognomonic changes.

### Other Diagnostics

- Toxicology testing – plant material, gastric contents, blood: freeze rapidly and submit to toxicology diagnostic lab for cyanide level. Plant level (gastric contents) >200 ppm or blood level >1 ppm suggestive of cyanide poisoning.

### Pathological Findings

- Associated with acute cyanide poisoning.
- Gross findings.
  - Muscle tissue, internal organs: congested.
  - Heart, lungs, internal organs: hemorrhage.
  - Stomach, small intestine: "bitter almond" odor – inconsistent finding.
- Other: liver or blood cyanide level >1 ppm suggestive of cyanide poisoning; brain or ventricular myocardium cyanide level >100 µg/g is diagnostic of cyanide toxicity.

# THERAPEUTICS

### Detoxification

- Not indicated for most small animals that ingest several leaves, pits, or seeds.
- For very small patient ingesting a large pit – emesis induction advised to reduce risk of foreign body obstruction.
- For exposure to (1) large volume of wet, damaged foliage or (2) large number of apricot kernels (human product).
  - Induce emesis in alert, asymptomatic patient following recent exposure.
  - Administer activated charcoal with sorbitol (1 g/kg PO) to alert, asymptomatic patient following recent exposure.

### Appropriate Health Care

- Veterinary exam is unnecessary for most dogs or cats who ingest small volumes of leaves, pits, or seeds. Home monitor for clinical signs of acute cyanide poisoning.
- Oral exposure to massive volume of leaves or apricot kernels – physical exam and hospitalization for monitoring for clinical signs of acute cyanide poisoning. Monitor vital signs, blood pressure, respiratory effort and lung sounds, mucous membrane color for eight hours.

## Antidotes

- Indicated only for **rare** patient with clinical signs of acute cyanide poisoning.
- Hydroxocobalamin – antidote of choice.
  - MOA: cyanide preferentially binds to hydroxocobalamin forming cyanocobalamin (vitamin $B_{12}$) which is excreted in urine.
  - Adverse reaction: dermal erythema, hypertension.
  - Dose: 75–150 mg/kg IV slowly once.
- Cyanide two-step kit – sodium nitrite and sodium thiosulfate.
  - MOA: nitrite oxidizes iron in hemoglobin to methemoglobin which preferentially attracts cyanide from cytochrome $c$ oxidase returning cells to aerobic metabolism. Sodium thiosulfate provides a sulfur donor for remaining cyanide forming thiocyanate, a water-soluble molecule that is excreted in urine.
  - Adverse effect: nitrite-induced vasodilation and hypotension; methemoglobinemia.
  - Dose: sodium nitrite (3% solution) 10–20 mg/kg IV slowly followed by sodium thiosulfate (25% solution) 150–500 mg/kg IV bolus or CRI.
- Sodium thiosulfate only.
  - Advantage: no induction of methemoglobinemia.
  - Dose: sodium thiosulfate (25% solution) 150–500 mg/kg IV as bolus or CRI.

## Drug(s) of Choice – Acute Cyanide Poisoning (Clinical Patient)

- Oxygen therapy: 100% oxygen encourages the dissociation of cyanide from cytochrome $c$ oxidase.
- IV fluids: rate dependent upon hemodynamic and metabolic status.
- Antiarrhythmic medication: for ventricular tachycardia.
  - Lidocaine (extra-label).
    - ○ Dog: 2–8 mg/kg IV (slowly) initial bolus followed by 25–80 mcg/kg/min IV CRI.
    - ○ Cat (*CAUTION: increased risk for CNS adverse reaction*): 0.2–0.7 mg/kg IV (slowly) initial bolus followed by 10–20 mcg/kg/min IV CRI.
  - Procainamide.
    - ○ Dog: 2–4 mg/kg IV (slowly) to maximum 20 mg/kg followed by 20–50 mcg/kg IV CRI.
- Vasopressors: for life-threatening hypotension nonresponsive to fluid therapy.
  - Norepinephrine: 0.1–2.0 mcg/kg/min IV CRI.
  - Dopamine: 10–20 mcg/kg/min IV CRI to effect.
- Antiemetic.
  - Maropitant: dog, cat: 1 mg/kg SQ or IV slowly q 24 hours.
  - Ondansetron (extra-label).
    - ○ Dog: 0.5–1.0 mg/kg IV (slowly) q 8–12 hours.
    - ○ Cat: 0.1–1.0 mg/kg IV (slowly), IM, SQ q 6–12 hours.
- Anticonvulsant.
  - Diazepam (extra-label).
    - ○ Dog: 0.5–1 mg/kg IV bolus; repeat q 10 min up to three times.
    - ○ Cat: 0.5–2 mg/kg IV.
  - Midazolam (extra-label).
    - ○ Dog: 0.1–0.5 mg/kg IV bolus; may repeat up to 0.5 mg/kg twice; 0.2–0.4 mg/kg/h IV CRI.
    - ○ Cat: 0.5–1.0 mg/kg IV.

- Levetiracetam (extra-label).
  - Dog: 30–60 mg/kg IV.
  - Cat: 20–40 mg/kg IV.
- Phenobarbital (extra-label).
  - Dog: 4–8 mg/kg IV (slowly) after benzodiazepine dosing. Repeat 4 mg/kg q 20 minutes up to 24 mg/kg.
  - Cat: 3 mg/kg IV after benzodiazepine dosing q 20 minutes up to 24 mg/kg in 24 hours.
- Methylene blue.
  - For severe methemoglobinemia (adverse effect of sodium nitrite antidote).
  - Use is controversial; may cause release of free cyanide.
  - *New methylene blue cannot be substituted for methylene blue.*
  - Dog: 1 mg/kg of 1% methylene blue IV slowly over 20 minutes; repeat in 30 minutes.

## Patient Monitoring

- Acute cyanide poisoning – clinical patient.
  - Frequent to continuous monitoring for critical patient.
    - Electrocardiogram.
    - Blood pressure.
    - Respiratory status – be prepared for mechanical or manual ventilation; blood gas monitoring required.
    - Body temperature.
    - Seizure activity.

 **COMMENTS**

### Prevention/Avoidance

- Restrict pet access to stone fruit pits, apple cores (seeds), apricot kernels (human supplement). Remove wet, damaged foliage of cyanogenic glycoside-containing plants from environment.

### Expected Course and Prognosis

- Excellent for most small animal exposures; poor for rare small animal patient that develops clinical signs of acute cyanide toxicity if antidote is not readily available.

### Abbreviations

See Appendix 1 for a complete list.

### Suggested Reading

Barr AC. Household and garden plants. In: Peterson ME, Talcott PA (eds) *Small Animal Toxicology*, 3rd edn. St Louis: Elsevier Saunders, 2013: pp. 357–400.

Burrow GE, Tyri RJ. *Toxic Plants of North America*, 2nd edn. Hoboken: Wiley-Blackwell, 2013.

Fitzgerald KT. Cyanide. In: Peterson ME, Talcott PA (eds) *Small Animal Toxicology*, 3rd edn. St Louis: Elsevier Saunders, 2013: pp. 523–531.

Gupta PK. *Concepts and Applications in Veterinary Toxicology: An Interactive Guide*. New York: Springer, 2019: pp. 259–263.

Panter KE. Cyanogenic glycoside-containing plants. In: Gupta R (ed.) *Veterinary Toxicology Basic and Clinical Principles*, 3rd edn. St Louis: Elsevier, 2018; pp. 935–940.

**Author:** Susan Holland DVM, DABT
**Consulting Editor:** Lynn R. Hovda, RPh, DVM, MS, DACVIM

# Chapter 114

# Lilies

## DEFINITION/OVERVIEW

- Toxicosis is associated with ingestion of many plants in the genera *Lilium* and *Hemerocallis*.
- Accurate identification is crucial to a good outcome. Photos of the lily, especially a direct shot of the flower, as well as the stem, if possible, are best.
- The rose lily (*Lilium orientalis* cultivar) may be difficult to identify as it looks much like a rose attached to a lily stem (Figure 114.1).
- There are many plants with the word "lily" in the name. Most are not in these two genera and are not toxic to the kidneys, but rather primarily cause GI signs.
- Cats are the target species.

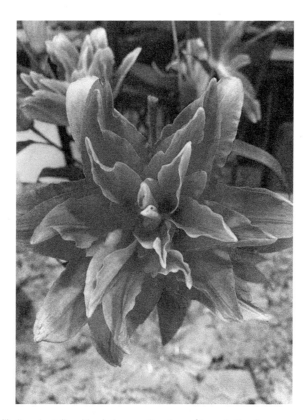

■ **Figure 114.1** Rose lily (*L. orientalis* cultivar). Source: Courtesy of Lynn R. Hovda.

*Blackwell's Five-Minute Veterinary Consult Clinical Companion: Small Animal Toxicology*, Third Edition.
Edited by Lynn R. Hovda, Ahna G. Brutlag, Robert H. Poppenga, and Steven E. Epstein.
© 2024 John Wiley & Sons, Inc. Published 2024 by John Wiley & Sons, Inc.

- Kidneys are the target organs.
- Ingestion of plant parts can result in vomiting, anorexia, lethargy, oliguria or anuria, acute kidney injury, and, rarely, pancreatitis.
- Lilies are frequently cultivated as garden and house plants, found growing in nature, and used in many floral bouquets and baskets.

 ## ETIOLOGY/PATHOPHYSIOLOGY

- Ingestion of plant material (leaves, stems, and flowers).
- Ingestion of pollen and water contaminated with pollen or plant material.
- Aqueous floral extract contains the highest amounts of toxic compound.
- Includes lilies such as the stargazer (*Lilium* spp.), Asiatic lily (*L. asiatic*; Figures 114.2, 114.3), Easter lily (*L. longiflorum*; Figure 114.4), Japanese show lily (*L. speciosum*; Figure 114.5), Madonna lily (*L. candidum*; Figure 114.6), Oriental lily (*L. orientalis*; Figure 114.7), red lily (*L. umbellatum*; Figure 114.8), rose lily (*L. orientalis* cultivar; Figure 114.1), tiger lily (*L. tigrinum* or *L. lancifolium*; Figure 114.9), Western lily (*L. occidentale*), wood lily (*L. philadelphicum*), and daylily (*Hemerocallis* spp.; Figures 114.10, 114.11).

### Mechanism of Action

- Renal tubular necrosis with intact basement membrane.

### Toxicokinetics

- Little is known.

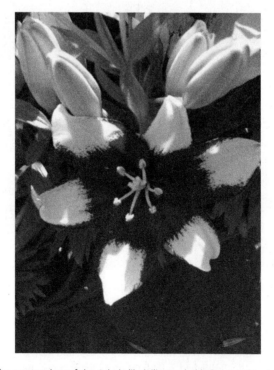

■ **Figure 114.2** One of the many colors of the Asiatic lily (*Lilium asiatic*). Source: Courtesy of Lynn R. Hovda.

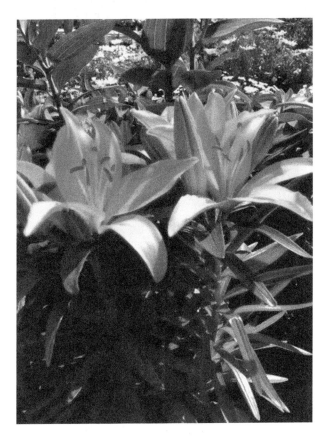

■ **Figure 114.3** Commonly colored Asiatic lily (*Lilium asiatic*). Source: Courtesy of Lynn R. Hovda.

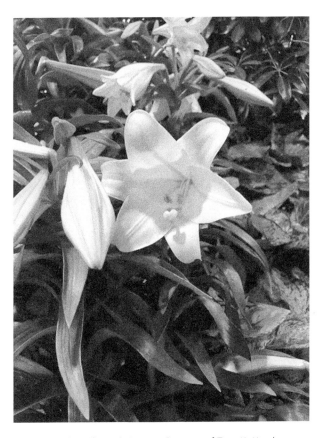

■ **Figure 114.4** Easter lily (*Lilium longiflorum*). Source: Courtesy of Tyne K. Hovda.

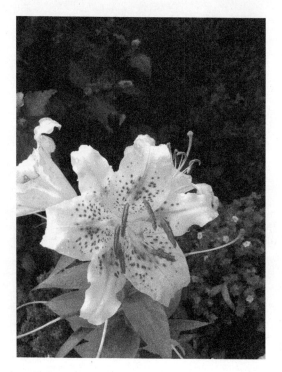

■ **Figure 114.5** Japanese show lily (*Lilium speciosum*). Source: Courtesy of Lynn R. Hovda.

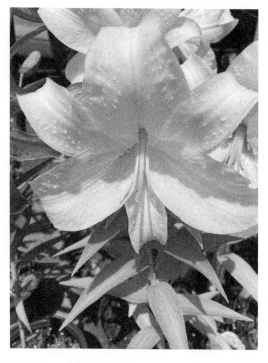

■ **Figure 114.6** Madonna lily (*Lilium candidum*). Source: Courtesy of Lynn R. Hovda.

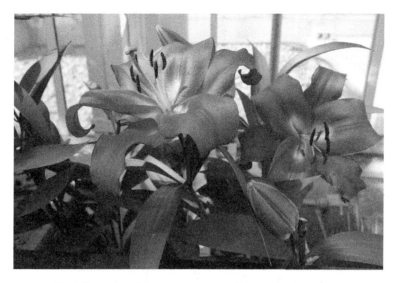

■ **Figure 114.7** Oriental lily (*Lilium orientalis*). Source: Courtesy of Lynn R. Hovda.

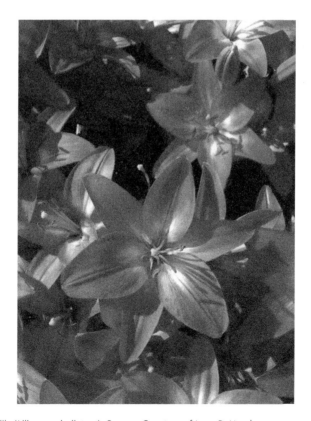

■ **Figure 114.8** Red lily (*Lilium umbellatum*). Source: Courtesy of Lynn R. Hovda.

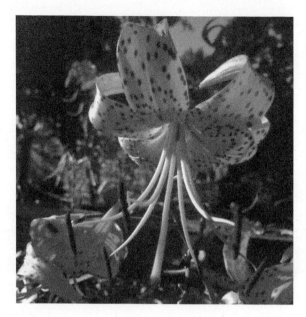

■ **Figure 114.9** Tiger lily (*Lilium tigrinum or L. lancifolium*). The mature tiger lily flower points downward. Source: Courtesy of Lynn R. Hovda.

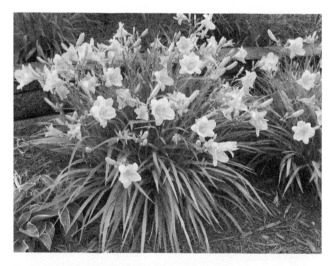

■ **Figure 114.10** Daylily (*Hemerocallis* spp.). Note the many leaves arranged in a grass-like cluster. Source: Courtesy of Tyne K. Hovda.

## Toxicity

- The toxin is known to be water soluble and has tentatively been identified as solasodine-type steroidal glycoalkaloids.
- Doses of 568 mg/kg of aqueous leaf extract and 291 mg/kg of aqueous flower extract of Easter lily have elicited toxicosis in cats.
- Deaths have occurred after ingestion of only one or two plant pieces.

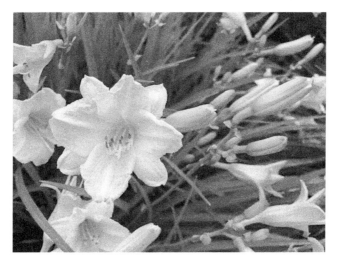

■ Figure 114.11 Close-up of daylily flower (*Hemerocallis* spp.) Source: Courtesy of Tyne K. Hovda.

### Systems Affected
- Renal – acute kidney injury.
- Gastrointestinal – vomiting, diarrhea, anorexia, hypersalivation.
- Neurological – depression, ataxia, tremors, seizures.

## SIGNALMENT/HISTORY
- Most cases are reported in cats.
- Dogs are thought to be affected but attempts to reproduce the reaction in dogs (and rabbits) have been unsuccessful.
- Most exposures occur around holidays or other festive occasions where lilies are used as house plants or found in floral arrangements.

## CLINICAL FEATURES
- All parts of the lily are considered toxic but the leaves are most commonly ingested.
- Signs usually develop within 6–12 hours of exposure.
- Early signs include vomiting, anorexia, and lethargy followed by acute kidney injury.
- Clinical signs of acute kidney injury include polyuria, oliguria, or anuria, dehydration, vomiting, diarrhea, and depression.
- Some cats also present with CNS signs such as ataxia, head pressing, disorientation, tremors, and seizures.
- Severe pancreatitis has also been reported but is considered rare.

## DIFFERENTIAL DIAGNOSIS
- Toxins.
  - Ethylene glycol.
  - Grapes or raisins.
  - Nonsteroidal antiinflammatory drugs and nephrotoxic drugs.

- • Cholecalciferol (rodenticide or vitamin D$_3$ supplements).
- • Soluble oxalate plants.
- ▪ Infectious diseases.
- ▪ Physical abnormalities (ureteral obstruction, nephrolith).

 ## DIAGNOSTICS

### Clinical Pathological Findings

- ▪ Serum chemistry findings include increases in blood urea nitrogen (BUN), creatinine, phosphorus, and potassium. BUN and creatinine generally increase within 18–24 hours of exposure. Creatinine may be disproportionately elevated.
- ▪ Urinalysis typically shows glucosuria, proteinuria, and isosthenuria. Epithelial casts usually can be seen in urine 12 hours after exposure.

### Other Diagnostics

- ▪ Renal ultrasound reveals changes consistent with acute tubular necrosis.

### Pathological Findings

- ▪ Gross examination shows swollen, edematous kidneys and systemic congestion. Pancreatic necrosis may be present.
- ▪ Histopathological examination of the kidneys shows acute proximal convoluted renal tubular necrosis with or without mineralization. The collecting ducts may contain granular or hyaline casts, and the basement membrane, while intact, may contain mitotic figures.

 ## THERAPEUTICS

- ▪ Early and aggressive supportive care including early decontamination, prevention of renal damage, and maintenance of fluid, electrolyte, and acid–base balance.
- ▪ Baseline BUN, creatinine, and electrolytes should be obtained on admission and repeated daily until they have returned to normal.

### Detoxification

- ▪ Bathe cats contaminated with pollen.
- ▪ Emesis within 1–2 hours of ingestion. Hydrogen peroxide is not recommended in cats. Dexmedetomidine (7 mcg/kg IM or 3.5 mcg/kg IV) is an effective emetic in cats. Xylazine (0.44–1.1 mg/kg IM or SQ) is less effective.
- ▪ Activated charcoal with a cathartic × 1 dose.

### Appropriate Health Care

- ▪ Early and aggressive use of IV fluids to prevent renal damage.
- ▪ Baseline serum chemistries to include BUN and creatinine. Monitor daily.
- ▪ Monitor urine output and add diuretics as needed.

### Antidote

- ▪ No antidote available.

### Drug(s) of Choice

- ▪ IV fluid therapy at 2–3 times maintenance for 48 hours, then decrease depending on BUN and creatinine levels.
    - • Choice of fluid therapy depends on electrolyte and glucose levels.
    - • IV fluids should be started within 18 hours of exposure; SQ fluids are not effective.

- Diuresis in oliguric cats once they are well hydrated.
  - Furosemide CRI at 1–2 mg/kg/h IV.
  - Mannitol bolus at 1–2 g/kg IV, followed by CRI if needed.
- Antiemetics.
  - Maropitant 1 mg/kg SQ, IV q 24 hours.
  - Ondansetron 0.5–1 mg/kg IV q 12 hours for dogs; 0.1–1 mg/kg IV, SQ, IM q 6–12 hours for cats.
- GI protectants as needed.
  - H$_2$-blockers: famotidine 0.5–1 mg/kg PO, SQ, IM, IV q 12 hours.
  - Omeprazole 0.5–1 mg/kg PO daily.
  - Sucralfate 0.25–1 g PO q 8 hours × 5–7 days if evidence of active ulcer disease.
- Peritoneal or renal dialysis may be useful in anuric cats.

 **COMMENTS**

### Prevention/Avoidance

- Any exposure to lilies in cats, regardless of the amount, should be considered harmful, and immediate veterinary intervention sought.
- Keep Easter lilies and floral arrangements with lilies out of households with cats.
- Do not plant or maintain lilies in a garden if an outside cat can gain access to them.

### Expected Course and Prognosis

- Delaying treatment 18 hours or longer after exposure usually results in acute kidney injury.
- The prognosis for cats aggressively treated prior to 18 hours post exposure is good. Once oliguria or anuria develops, the prognosis becomes fair to grave. Chronic renal impairment may occur in these cats even after treatment.
- Mortality rate from Easter lily toxicosis is reported to be as high as 100% if treatment is delayed and renal failure occurs.

### See Also

Chapter 9 Ethylene Glycol and Diethylene Glycol
Chapter 72 Grapes and Raisins
Chapter 124 Cholecalciferol

### Abbreviations

See Appendix 1 for a complete list.

### Suggested Reading

Bennett AJ, Reineke EL. Outcome following gastrointestinal tract decontamination and intravenous fluid diuresis in cats with known lily ingestion: 25 cases (2001–2010). *J Am Vet Med Assoc* 2013;242: 1110–1116.
Berg RI, Francey T, Segev G. Resolution of acute kidney injury in a cat after lily (*Lilium lancifolium*) intoxication. *J Vet Intern Med* 2007;21(4):857–859.
Fitzgerald KT. Lily toxicity in the cat. *Top Comp Anim Med* 2010;25(4):213–217.
Hadley RM, Richardson JA, Gwaltney-Brant SM. A retrospective study of daylily toxicosis in cats. *Vet Hum Toxicol* 2003;45(1):38–39.
Uhlig S, Hussain F, Wisloff H. Bioassay-guided fractionation of extracts from Easter lily (*Lilium longiflorum*) flowers reveals unprecedented structural variability of steroidal glycoalkaloids. *Toxicon* 2014; 92:42–49.

**Author**: Amanda L. Poldoski, DVM
**Consulting Editor**: Lynn R. Hovda, RPh, DVM, MS, DACVIM

# Chapter 115

# Mushrooms

## DEFINITION/OVERVIEW

- Several thousand species of mushrooms are found in North America, but only a few hundred are toxic.
- There is no simple test that distinguishes poisonous from nonpoisonous mushrooms.
- The most toxic mushrooms contain amatoxins.
- The number of reported mushroom poisonings in animals is low, likely as a result of the lack of diagnostic work-up and methods to confirm exposure in a majority of cases.
- Amatoxins.
  - The majority of confirmed mushroom poisonings in animals are caused by hepato-toxic mushrooms that contain amatoxins, specifically the hepatotoxic cyclopeptides, alpha-, beta-, gamma- and epsilon-aminitin.
  - Poisoned animals develop gastrointestinal signs between six and 24 hours after inges-tion. After a period of "false recovery," fulminant liver failure develops generally 36–48 hours after exposure. During the final stage, renal failure can also develop.
  - While several mushroom genera (*Amanita*, *Galerina*, *Lepiota*) contain the hepatotoxic cyclopeptides, *Amanita phalloides* (Figure 115.1), also known as death cap or death angel, and *A. ocreata* (Figure 115.2), also known as the destroying angel, are the species most frequently reported in poisonings.
  - Comprehensive therapeutic measures are required to improve prognosis and include decontamination, supportive care, and administration of drugs that may reduce the toxin uptake into hepatocytes.
- Other toxic mushrooms (not further discussed in detail in this chapter).
  - Mushrooms that contain muscarine (e.g., *Inocybe* spp., *Clitocybe* spp.) are relatively common but do not appear to be a major risk for poisoning in animals. Poisoned ani-mals show signs of salivation, lacrimation, vomiting, diarrhea, bradycardia, and miosis generally within 2 hours. Atropine and decontamination procedures are important treatment strategies.
  - Mushrooms that contain muscimol and ibotenic acid (e.g., *Amanita muscaria*, *A. pan-therina*) are common in the Pacific Northwest. Ingestion can result in ataxia, sedation, muscle spasms, and seizures within 30 to 120 minutes, but with aggressive supportive care, full recovery is expected within 1–2 days.
  - False morel (*Gyromitra* spp.) ingestion can lead to vomiting, abdominal pain, and diarrhea followed by convulsions 6 to 12 hours after ingestion. With supportive care, poisoned animals are likely to recover within several days of exposure.

*Blackwell's Five-Minute Veterinary Consult Clinical Companion: Small Animal Toxicology*, Third Edition.
Edited by Lynn R. Hovda, Ahna G. Brutlag, Robert H. Poppenga, and Steven E. Epstein.
© 2024 John Wiley & Sons, Inc. Published 2024 by John Wiley & Sons, Inc.

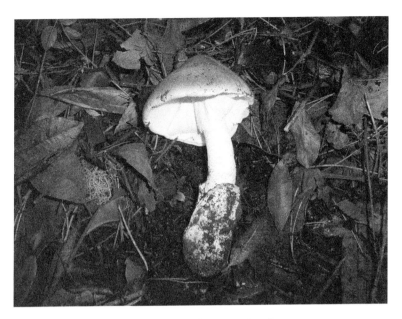

■ **Figure 115.1** *Amanita phalloides*. Source: Courtesy of R. Michael Davis.

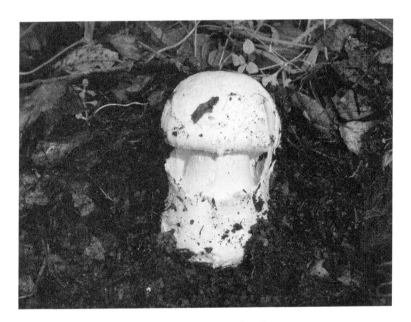

■ **Figure 115.2** *Amanita ocreata*. Source: Courtesy of R. Michael Davis.

- Hallucinogenic mushrooms (*Psilocybe, Panaeolus, Conocybe,* and *Gymnopilus* spp.) contain psilocybin. Poisoned animals can develop ataxia, vocalization, overt aggression, nystagmus, and increased body temperature within 30 to 60 minutes. The management is essentially supportive and in most cases, treatment is not necessary.
- Many mushrooms are capable of causing gastrointestinal irritation (*Agaricus, Boletus, Chlorophyllum, Entoloma, Lactarius, Omphalotus, Rhodophyllus, Scleroderma,* and *Tricholoma* spp.). In most exposures, vomiting and diarrhea develop between one and six hours after ingestion, with complete recovery within 24–48 hours.

**ETIOLOGY/PATHOPHYSIOLOGY**

- *A. phalloides* (commonly known as death cap; Figure 115.1) is found throughout North America and grows most commonly under oak, birch, pine, and other hardwoods. It can also be found in open pastures.
- *A. ocreata* (commonly known as western North American destroying angel; Figure 115.2) grows from Baja California, Mexico, along the Pacific Coast to Washington. *A. ocreata* is most often found in sandy soils under oak or pine.
- Amanitins (alpha-, beta-, gamma-, and epsilon-amanitins) are bicyclic octapeptides that are found in approximately 35 mushroom species from three different genera: *Amanita*, *Galerina*, and *Lepiota*. The toxins are not degraded by cooking, freezing, or the acidic environment of the stomach.

### Mechanism of Action

- Amanitins inhibit nuclear RNA polymerase II, resulting in decreased protein synthesis and cell death. Hepatocytes, crypt cells, and proximal convoluted tubules are especially susceptible to the effect because of their high metabolic rate.
- Other toxic mechanisms are likely to play an important role in the toxicity of amanitins.

### Toxicokinetics

- After exposure, amanitins are rapidly absorbed from the gastrointestinal tract and quickly exert their toxic effects on intestinal cells. Following absorption, amanitins are distributed (not plasma protein bound) to liver and kidney. The plasma half-life of amanitins in dogs is short, ranging from 25 to 50 minutes. Amanitins are largely excreted unchanged in urine and can be detected in urine well before clinical signs occur. Only a small amount of amanitins is excreted in the bile.
- Species-specific data on the bioavailability of amanitins are largely unavailable, but it appears that the absorption rate in dogs is much greater than in mice and rabbits and much less than in people. Rodents appear resistant to the effects of amanitins.

### Toxicity

- Amanitins are extremely toxic. The IV $LD_{50}$ of alpha-amanitin in dogs is 0.1 mg/kg BW. An oral $LD_{50}$ for methyl-gamma-amanitin was estimated to be 0.5 mg/kg BW. In humans, the estimated oral $LD_{50}$ of alpha-amanitin is 0.1 mg/kg BW.
- Toxin concentrations in *Amanita* spp. vary depending on growing conditions, moisture, and time of year. Hence, it is very difficult to estimate the minimum amount of mushroom material needed to cause poisoning. Considering the average concentration of amanitins per mushroom of 4 mg/g, the ingestion of two *A. phalloides* has the potential to be lethal to an adult dog, while a smaller amount may kill a puppy.

### Systems Affected

- Gastrointestinal – vomiting, diarrhea, and severe abdominal pain begin approximately 8–12 hours after exposure.
- Hepatobiliary – fulminant liver failure develops approximately 36–48 hours after exposure.
- Renal/urological – if the animal survives liver failure, renal and multiorgan failure can develop.
- Hemic – coagulopathy can develop as a result of liver failure.
- Nervous – encephalopathy can develop as a result of liver failure.

# SIGNALMENT/HISTORY

- All breeds and genders are equally susceptible.
- There are no known genetic predispositions.
- Severe gastrointestinal signs such as vomiting, diarrhea, and abdominal pain occurring hours after an observed mushroom ingestion or after unobserved roaming in the woods, especially during mushroom season.
- Liver failure occurring after a period of recovery, although gastrointestinal signs were present prior to the recovery phase.

## Location and Circumstances of Poisoning

- Amanitin-containing mushrooms are very common in the San Francisco Bay area, the Santa Cruz Mountains, the Pacific Northwest, and the Northeast.
- Toxic mushrooms are most abundant in warm, wet years and are often found under certain trees (oak, cork, spruce, birch, pine).
- In California, toxic mushrooms are typically found from mid-autumn through late winter.
- In the Northeast, toxic mushrooms are most commonly found from late September through late October.

# CLINICAL FEATURES

- The chief complaints of amanitin poisoning are vomiting and diarrhea within 24 hours of mushroom exposure and icterus, lethargy, ataxia, seizures, and coma approximately 36–48 hours after exposure.
- The clinical course of amanitin toxicosis can be separated into four phases, with characteristic clinical features for each phase. However, not every case presents with the classic four stages and identification of distinct phases of toxicosis should not be attempted to screen dogs for toxicosis.
    - The first phase is a latency period of approximately 6–12 hours after ingestion of amanitin-containing mushrooms without any clinical signs.
    - The second phase begins approximately 6–24 hours after mushroom exposure and is characterized by vomiting, diarrhea, and abdominal pain.
    - The third phase is a period of false recovery during which the animal appears to have recovered. This phase can last from several hours to a few days. During this third phase, close monitoring of liver and kidney function is essential to prevent misdiagnosis. In this phase, the breakdown of liver glycogen can lead to severe hypoglycemia.
    - The last phase is characterized by fulminant liver failure and begins between 36 and 84 hours after exposure to amanitins. In this stage, renal and multiorgan failure can also occur and affected animals are icteric, lethargic, and ataxic and have polyuria, polydypsia, anorexia, clotting abnormalities, seizures, or coma. If large amounts of amanitin-containing mushrooms are ingested, or if a puppy ingested a toxic mushroom, it is possible that the animal may die acutely within 24 hours or just be found dead.

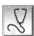

# DIFFERENTIAL DIAGNOSIS

- Caustics.
- Viral, bacterial, rickettsial, and parasitic diseases.
- Mushrooms that cause gastrointestinal signs (without liver involvement) – collect mushrooms in area of exposure and have them identified.
- Dietary indiscretion such as ingestion of garbage or spoiled food.

- Other causes of acute liver failure.
- Severe acute pancreatitis.
- Toxicants.
  - Acetaminophen overdose.
  - Aflatoxins.
  - Cocklebur (*Xanthium* spp.).
  - Cycad palms (*Cycas* spp.).
  - Heavy metals (e.g., lead, zinc).
  - Microcystins (hepatotoxic blue-green algae toxins).
  - Organophosphate and carbamate insecticides.
  - Ricin and abrin.
  - Xylitol.

# DIAGNOSTICS

## Clinical Pathological Findings

- Serum chemistry: beginning with the second or third phase, see increases in AST, ALT, ALP, and bilirubin; hypoglycemia develops.
- Coagulation panel: beginning with the third phase, see prolonged PT and PTT.

## Other Diagnostics

- Identification of mushrooms found in the environment or gastric contents. Accurate mushroom identification will require consultation with an experienced mycologist. DNA sequencing of mushroom material is also possible.
- Detection of amanitin in serum, urine, gastric contents, liver, or kidney. This testing is provided by select veterinary toxicology laboratories but a point-of-care (POC) lateral flow immunoassay for aminitins in urine (http://amatoxtest.com) is available.
  - In live animals, urine is considered of superior diagnostic use compared to serum. Amanitins can be detected in urine well before any clinical sign has developed, whereas routine laboratory tests such as serum chemistry profiles are unremarkable until liver or kidney damage has occurred. Amanitins are excreted in urine for several days (up to 72 hours) post exposure. Because of the short half-life of amanitins in plasma, amanitins are usually only detected for approximately 36 hours post exposure. Plasma and urine amanitin concentrations do not seem to correlate with clinical severity or outcome.
  - If the POC is negative but clinical signs strongly suggest amatoxicosis, confirmation with veterinary diagnostic laboratory testing should be pursued.
  - Postmortem, kidney contains higher amanitin concentrations than liver and is considered the sample of choice, especially if the animal survived for a longer period of time.

## Pathological Findings

- The liver may be swollen and distended. No other significant gross abnormalities may be noticed. Histopathologically, the liver has massive hepatocellular necrosis with collapse of hepatic cords. Acute tubular necrosis is seen in dogs that develop renal failure.

# THERAPEUTICS

- No specific therapy has proven to be effective. Even with supportive measures, the mortality rate from amanitin poisoning in dogs is high. Amanitin poisoning requires immediate and aggressive treatment to improve prognosis. The key components of therapy are close monitoring, fluid replacement, and supportive care.

## Detoxification

- Emesis in animals where exposure occurred less than two hours prior to presentation.
- Activated charcoal: multidose activated charcoal at 1–4 g/kg PO q 2–6 hours until 2–3 days post ingestion.

## Appropriate Health Care

- Monitoring in the clinical setting for the first 2–3 days in suspected amanitin exposure.

## Antidote

- No specific antidote is available.

## Drug(s) of Choice

- Intravenous fluids – maintain hydration, induce diuresis, correct hypoglycemia.
- 50% dextrose 1 mL/kg IV slow bolus (1–3 min).
- Furosemide 2–4 mg/kg IV q 8–12 hours.
- Vitamin K$_1$ 0.5–1.5 mg/kg SQ or IM q 12 hours; 1–5 mg/kg PO q 24 hours.
- Blood products – dependent on hemostatic test results.
- Silibinin – may be beneficial, but controlled studies are lacking. Experimentally, silibinin was shown to be effective when given twice to dogs at a dose of 50 mg/kg IV, five and 24 hours after exposure to *A. phalloides*. An oral form is available that can be given at 2–5 mg/kg PO q 24 hours (silibinin complexed with phosphatidylcholine).
- Penicillin G – reduces the uptake of amanitins into hepatocytes; 1000 mg/kg IV as soon as possible after exposure.

## Precautions/Interactions

- A variety of decontamination procedures are used in humans, including hemodialysis, hemoperfusion, plasmapheresis, forced diuresis, and nasoduodenal suctioning. Controversy remains about the efficacy of these procedures, as specific data do not exist.
- The use of steroids, thioctic acid, and cimetidine is no longer recommended in the treatment of amanitin poisoning.

## Alternative Drugs

- N-acetylcysteine (NAC) – antioxidant; no data on efficacy in amanitin toxicosis available. This glutathione precursor can be included in the treatment regimen for acute fulminant hepatic failure at 140 mg/kg IV load, followed by 70 mg/kg IV q 6 hours for seven treatments.
- S-adenosylmethionine (SAMe) – antioxidant and hepatoprotectant; no data on efficacy in amanitin toxicosis available. 20 mg/kg PO q 24 hours.
- Ascorbic acid – hepatocyte protector; no data on efficacy in amanitin toxicosis available. Can be given for supportive therapy.

## Surgical Considerations

- Biliary drainage through serial cholecystocentesis or cannula placement has been proposed as a means of removing amatoxins from enterohepatic circulation. Risk for the development of bile peritonitis or other bleeding complications must be considered. A study in pigs found that amatoxins were no longer present in the enterohepatic circulation 24 hours after exposure, suggesting that biliary drainage after such time may be poorly effective as a treatment.

## Patient Monitoring

- Monitor blood glucose, electrolytes, CBC, serum biochemistry, and coagulation parameters at least daily.
- Prevent hypothermia.
- Monitor urine output.

## Diet

- Oral intake should be discontinued in severe cases in which patient is at risk of aspiration. Trickle feeding via NG or NE is advised at 25% RER to prevent mucosal atrophy.
- Low-protein diet if hepatic encephalopathy is present.

 **COMMENTS**

### Prevention/Avoidance

- Advise owner to closely scrutinize the environment for mushrooms. Suggest that owner have mushrooms identified by mycology expert and get additional information on the seasonality of amanita mushrooms in their geographic region.

### Possible Complications

- DIC.
- Hepatic encephalopathy.
- Progressive hepatic failure.
- Renal failure.

### Expected Course and Prognosis

- Progressive worsening of liver and kidney function and unresponsiveness to supportive treatments are negative indicators.
- Prompt decontamination and aggressive supportive treatment improve chances of survival.

### Synonyms

*Amanita* toxicosis, death cap intoxication, amatoxin poisoning, hepatotoxic mushroom poisoning, amanitin poisoning.

### See Also

Chapter 45 Acetaminophen
Chapter 101 Organophosphorus and Carbamate Anticholinesterase Pesticides
Chapter 118 Sago Palm (Cycads)

### Abbreviations

See Appendix 1 for a complete list.

### Suggested Reading

Bever CS, Swanson KD, Hamelin EI et al. Rapid, sensitive, and accurate point-of-care detection of lethal amatoxins in urine. *Toxins* 2020;12(2):123.

Kaae JA, Poppenga RH, Hill AE. Physical examination, serum biochemical, and coagulation abnormalities, treatments, and outcomes for dogs with toxicosis from α-amanitin-containing mushrooms: 59 cases (2006–2019). *J Am Vet Med Assoc* 2021;258(5):502–509.

Puschner B. Mushroom toxins. In: Gupta RC (ed.) *Veterinary Toxicology: Basic and Clinical Principles*, 3rd edn. San Diego: Elsevier, 2018: pp. 955–966.

Puschner B, Rose HH, Filigenzi MS. Diagnosis of amanita toxicosis in a dog with acute hepatic necrosis. *J Vet Diagn Invest* 2007;19:312–317.

Puschner B, Wegenast C. Mushroom poisoning cases in dogs and cats: diagnosis and treatment of hepatotoxic, neurotoxic, gastroenterotoxic, nephrotoxic, and muscarinic mushrooms. *Vet Clin North Am Small Anim Pract* 2018;48(6):1053–1067.

## Acknowledgment

The author and editors acknowledge the prior contributions of Birgit Puschner, DVM, PhD, DABVT, who co-authored this topic in the previous edition.

**Author**: Adrienne Bautista, DVM, PhD, DABVT
**Consulting Editor**: Lynn R. Hovda, RPh, DVM, MS, DACVIM

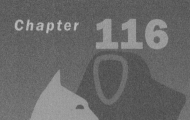

# Chapter 116

# Oxalates (Insoluble)

## DEFINITION/OVERVIEW

- Insoluble oxalate crystals are found naturally in plants of the Araceae family.
- Roughly 200 species worldwide contain insoluble oxalate crystals.
- *Dieffenbachia* spp. is most associated with problems in animals.
  - Oxalate crystals occur in several layers in leaves and stems.
  - Plants are present in many homes and offices.
- Common names vary tremendously from plant to plant and accurate plant identification must include the scientific name.
- Common plants associated with toxicity include the following.
  - Anthurium, flamingo flower (*Anthurium* spp.; Figure 116.1).
  - Arrowhead vine (*Syngonium* spp.; Figure 116.2).
  - Calla lily (*Zantedeschia* spp.; Figure 116.3).
  - Chinese evergreen (*Aglaonema commutatum*; Figure 116.4).
  - Dumbcane (*Dieffenbachia* spp.; Figure 116.5).
  - Fruit salad plant (*Monstera deliciosa*; Figure 116.6).
  - Peace lily (*Spathiphyllum* spp.; Figure 116.7).
  - Philodendron, sweetheart vine (*Philodendron* spp.; Figure 116.8).
  - Pothos, hunter's robe, devil's ivy (*Epipremnum* spp.; Figure 116.9).
  - Umbrella plant (*Schefflera actinophylla*; Figure 116.10).
  - Upright elephant's ear (*Xanthosoma* spp.; Figure 116.11).

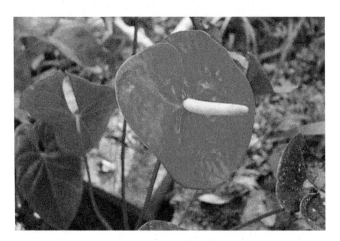

■ **Figure 116.1** Anthurium (*Anthurium* spp.). Source: Courtesy of Tyne K. Hovda.

*Blackwell's Five-Minute Veterinary Consult Clinical Companion: Small Animal Toxicology*, Third Edition.
Edited by Lynn R. Hovda, Ahna G. Brutlag, Robert H. Poppenga, and Steven E. Epstein.
© 2024 John Wiley & Sons, Inc. Published 2024 by John Wiley & Sons, Inc.

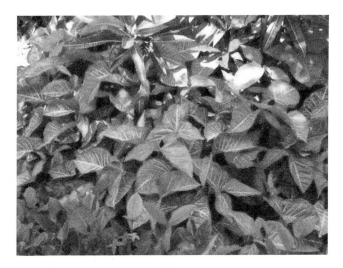

■ **Figure 116.2** Arrowhead (*Syngonium* spp.). Source: Courtesy of Tyne K. Hovda.

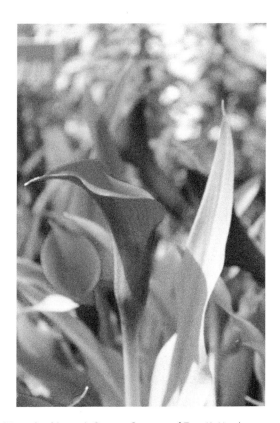

■ **Figure 116.3** Calla lily (*Zantedeschia* spp.). Source: Courtesy of Tyne K. Hovda.

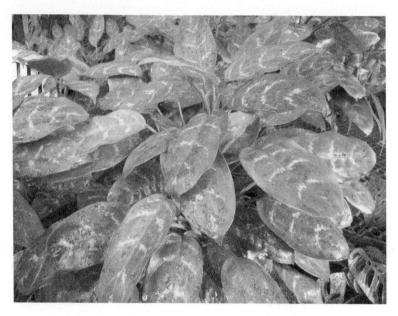

■ **Figure 116.4** Chinese evergreen (*Aglaonema commutatum*). Source: Courtesy of Tyne K. Hovda.

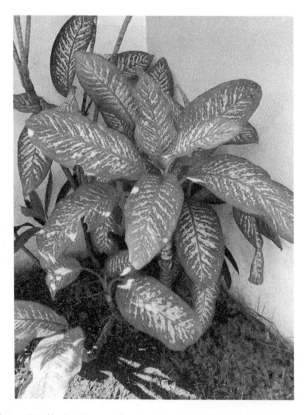

■ **Figure 116.5** Dumbcane (*Dieffenbachia* spp.). Source: Courtesy of Tyne K. Hovda.

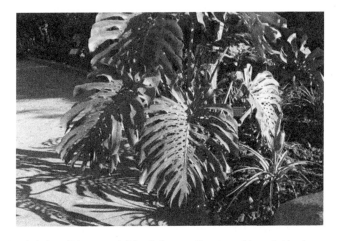

■ **Figure 116.6** Fruit salad plant (*Monstera deliciosa*). Source: Courtesy of Lynn R. Hovda

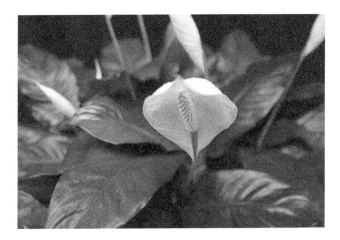

■ **Figure 116.7** Peace lily (*Spathiphyllum* spp.). Source: Courtesy of Tyne K. Hovda.

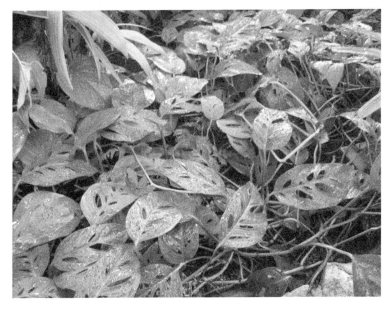

■ **Figure 116.8** Philodendron vine (*Philodendron* spp.). Source: Courtesy of Tyne K. Hovda.

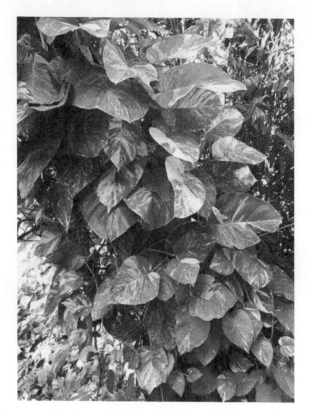

■ **Figure 116.9** Golden pothos (*Epipremnum aureum*). Source: Courtesy of Lynn Rolland Hovda.

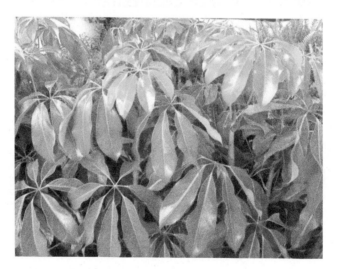

■ **Figure 116.10** Umbrella plant (*Schefflera actinophylla*). Source: Courtesy of Tyne K. Hovda.

- Pets chewing on plants or ingesting plant pieces show immediate evidence of oral pain.
- Human beings, especially young children and vulnerable adults, are equally at risk if they chew or ingest plant pieces.

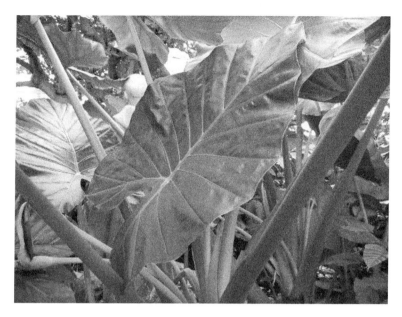

■ Figure 116.11 Upright elephant ear (*Xanthosoma* spp.). Source: Courtesy of Tyne K. Hovda.

 **ETIOLOGY/PATHOPHYSIOLOGY**

### Mechanism of Action

■ Insoluble crystals are needle sharp and arranged in bundles called raphides. In many plants, bundles of raphides are organized into specialized cells called idioblasts.
■ Chewing or biting into plant material rapidly releases the crystals until the idioblast is emptied.
  • The double-edged crystals act much like miniature spears or needles and function primarily as mechanical irritants to the mucous membranes.
  • They also act as chemical irritants, penetrating cells and allowing the entrance of other substances such as prostaglandins, histamine, proteolytic enzymes, or oxalic acid.

### Toxicokinetics

■ Onset of action is very rapid, occurring within minutes of chewing on the plant.

### Toxicity

■ Generally are all regarded as mild-to-moderate toxicants.
■ Severe cases have occurred and, rarely, death has been reported.
■ *Dieffenbachia* spp. has been associated with more serious outcomes, including death, in dogs and cats.
■ Cats ingesting philodendrons may exhibit a wider array of clinical signs.

### Systems Affected

■ Gastrointestinal – immediate onset of oral pain with vocalization, pawing at the muzzle, and hypersalivation; anorexia and vomiting; and edema of lips, tongue, and/or pharynx.
■ Respiratory – rarely dyspnea from inflammation and laryngeal swelling.
■ Ophthalmic – plant juices in the eye are associated with severe pain, photophobia, and conjunctival swelling; crystals may be present on the corneal epithelium.

# SIGNALMENT/HISTORY

- Indoor dogs and cats are at a higher risk, as most poisonings are associated with houseplants.
  - Dogs tend to chew and destroy the entire plant, often ingesting leaves and stems.
  - Cats are generally fastidious and tend to nibble on the leaves.
- All ages can be affected, although ingestions by younger pets, curious or bored by confinement, tend to occur more often.
- The most common immediate signs are related to the severe pain in the oropharynx and include hypersalivation, head shaking, and pawing at the muzzle area. Signs occurring shortly after exposure include edema of the lips and tongue, vomiting, and anorexia. Airway obstruction and dyspnea are more rare occurrences. Ophthalmic exposure results in severe pain, photophobia, lacrimation, blepharospasm, and swelling of the lids.

## Risk Factors

- Presence of plants in animal's environment.
- Boredom, confinement.

# CLINICAL FEATURES

- Gastrointestinal – evidence of immediate oral pain (hypersalivation, head shaking, pawing at muzzle) within minutes of exposure; redness or irritation to mucous membranes in oropharynx occurring a short time later; vomiting minutes to hours after exposure.
- Respiratory – dyspnea and airway obstruction if inflammation is severe (rare).
- Ophthalmic – issues only if plant juices have been squirted or rubbed into the eye.

# DIFFERENTIAL DIAGNOSIS

- Systemic diseases associated with oral lesions and GI signs.
- Toxicants.
  - Other agents causing oral irritation (capsaicin, topically applied permethrins, detergents).
  - Caustic agents (alkalis, acids in household, and drain cleaners).
  - Plants containing bitter volatile oils.
  - Stinging nettle ingestion.

# DIAGNOSTICS

- Rarely performed as crystals are insoluble and not absorbed; signs are primarily local in nature and self-limiting. Consider serum electrolytes and chemistry if vomiting persists.

## Pathological Findings

- Death rarely occurs, and in the few reported cases, severe and extensive erosive and ulcerative glossitis was present.

# THERAPEUTICS

- Therapy is generally limited and includes appropriate detoxification and supportive care. Many animals respond in 2–4 hours, while some may take 12–24 hours for a complete response.

## Detoxification

- Wash the mouth and oral cavity with copious amounts of cool fluids.
- Provide small amounts of milk, yogurt, or other calcium-containing products to bind the oxalate crystals. Give enough to coat the oropharynx but not to cause GI upset and diarrhea.
- If ophthalmic exposure is evident, lavage the eye for 15 minutes and treat as needed.

## Appropriate Health Care

- Observe closely for evidence of dyspnea, especially in those animals that chewed or ingested large amounts of plants.
- Thorough ophthalmic examination after lavage; fluorescein dye or slit lamp examination.

## Antidote

- No specific antidote is available.

## Drug(s) of Choice

- IV fluids if dehydration occurs secondary to hypersalivation and vomiting.
- Antiemetic agents as needed.
    - Maropitant 1 mg/kg SQ, IV q 24 hours.
    - Ondansetron 0.5–1 mg/kg IV q 12 hours for dogs; 0.1–1 mg/kg IV, SQ, IM q 6–12 hours for cats.
    - Dolasetron 0.6 mg/kg SQ, IV q 24 hours.
- GI protectants as needed.
    - Famotidine 0.5 mg/kg PO, SQ, IM, IV q 12–24 hours (cautious IV use in cats).
    - Omeprazole 0.5–1 mg/kg daily.
    - Sucralfate 0.25–1 g PO q 8 hours × 5–7 days if evidence of active ulcer disease.
- Nonsteroidal antiinflammatory agents if needed for pain and inflammation.
    - Carprofen 2.2 mg/kg PO q 12–24 hours (dogs).
    - Deracoxib 1–2 mg/kg PO q 24 hours (dogs).
    - Robenacoxib 1 mg/kg PO q 24 hours (cats only) × maximum of three doses.
- Corticosteroid use is controversial, but dexamethasone phosphate 0.125–0.5 mg/kg IV, IM, or SQ may be useful in cases with severe inflammation.

## Diet

- NPO or soft diet until signs have resolved.

 **COMMENTS**

## Prevention/Avoidance

- Identify plants presently in the household and place them far out of the animal's reach.

## Expected Course and Prognosis

- Prognosis is excellent as most signs are mild to moderate, have a short duration of action, and require no therapy.

## Abbreviations

See Appendix 1 for a complete list.

## Suggested Reading

Botha CJ, Penrith M. Potential plant poisonings in dogs and cats in southern Africa: review article. J S Afr Vet Assoc 2009;80(2):63–74.

Burrows GE, Tyrl RJ. *Toxic Plants of North America*, 2nd edn. Ames,: Wiley-Blackwell, 2012.

Ellis W, Barfort T, Mastman GJ. Keratoconjunctivitis with corneal crystals caused by Dieffenbachia plant. *Am J Ophthalmol* 1973;76:143–146.

Knight AP. *A Guide to Poisonous House and Garden Plants*. Jackson Hole: Teton NewMedia, 2006.

Peterson K, Beymer J, Rudloff E et al. Airway obstruction in a dog after Dieffenbachia ingestion. *J Vet Emerg Crit Care* 2009;19(6):635–639.

Savage GP, Vanhanen L, Mason SM, Ross AB. Effect of cooking on the soluble and insoluble oxalate content of some New Zealand foods. *J Food Comp Anal* 2000;13(3):201–206.

Severino L. Toxic plants and companion animals. *CAB Reviews* 2009;4:1–6. www.cabdirect.org/cabdirect/abstract/20093068261

**Author**: Lynn R. Hovda, RPh, DVM, MS, ACVIM
**Consulting Editor**: Lynn R. Hovda, RPh, DVM, MS, AVCIM

# Chapter 117

# Oxalates (Soluble)

 ## DEFINITION/OVERVIEW

- Oxalate toxicity includes both oxalic acid and oxalate salts.
  - Oxalic acid is a dicarboxylic acid found naturally in plants of the Araceae, Oxalidaceae, Liliaceae, Polygonaceae, Chenopodiaceae, and Amaranthus families.
  - Soluble salts (ammonium, calcium, potassium, sodium) of oxalic acid are also found in several plants in these families.
- Most of these plants are weeds growing in pastures and are only associated with problems in livestock grazing on them. A few have been cultivated as houseplants and if ingested in large enough quantities, are a potential source of poisoning to dogs and cats.
- Common household plants or fruits with soluble oxalates include the following.
  - Common or garden rhubarb (*Rheum rhabarbarum*; Figure 117.1).
  - Hybrid plants, *Oxalis* spp.
  - Purple shamrock plant (*Oxalis* spp.; Figure 117.2).
  - Shamrock plant (*Oxalis* spp.; Figure 117.3).
  - Star fruit (*Averrhoa carambola*; Figures 117.4–117.6).

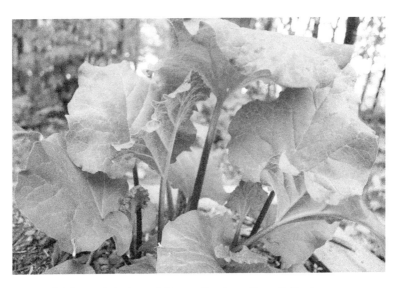

■ **Figure 117.1** Rhubarb (*Rheum rhabarbarum*). Source: Courtesy of Lynn R. Hovda.

*Blackwell's Five-Minute Veterinary Consult Clinical Companion: Small Animal Toxicology*, Third Edition.
Edited by Lynn R. Hovda, Ahna G. Brutlag, Robert H. Poppenga, and Steven E. Epstein.
© 2024 John Wiley & Sons, Inc. Published 2024 by John Wiley & Sons, Inc.

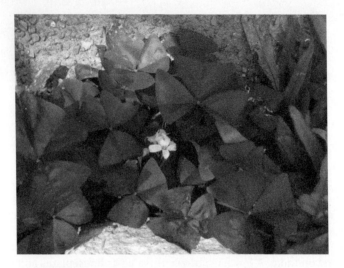

■ **Figure 117.2** Purple shamrock (*Oxalis* spp.). Source: Courtesy of Lynn R. Hovda.

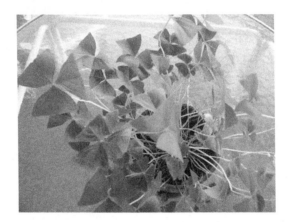

■ **Figure 117.3** Shamrock (*Oxalis* spp.). Source: Courtesy of Tyne K. Hovda.

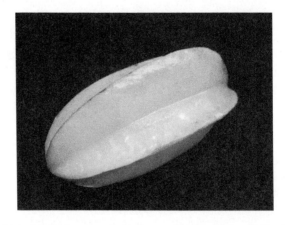

■ **Figure 117.4** Star fruit intact (*Averrhoa carambola*). Source: Courtesy of Tyne K. Hovda.

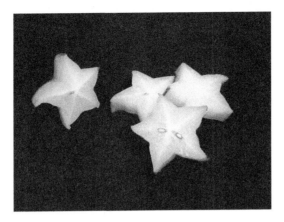

■ **Figure 117.5** Edible star fruit cut sections (*Averrhoa carambola*). Source: Courtesy of Tyne K. Hovda.

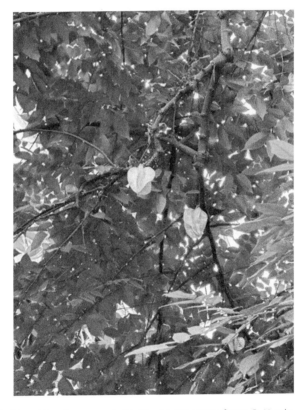

■ **Figure 117.6** Star fruit tree (*Averrhoa carambola*). Source: Courtesy of Lynn R. Hovda.

 ## ETIOLOGY/PATHOPHYSIOLOGY

### Mechanism of Action

- Soluble oxalates and free oxalic acid are present to varying degrees in all parts of the plant. Total oxalate material in many of the pasture plants is about 16%, with 7–10% of this in the form of an oxalate salt.

- Rhubarb stems (also known as the stalk) are edible, the leaves are not.
- Star fruit presents an interesting dilemma, with soluble oxalates found in much greater concentrations in the sour fruit versus sweet fruit.
  - The sour fruit is generally recognized as *inedible*, the sweet fruit and juices as edible.
  - Acute kidney injury may be due to oxalate crystals, although some believe another unknown toxin or mechanism is responsible.
  - A neurotoxin present in star fruits may be responsible for the neurological signs.
- Ingestion of plants results in both free oxalic acid and soluble salts.
- Soluble oxalate salts are absorbed through the GI tract and bind with systemic calcium, resulting in a sudden drop in serum calcium. The accumulation of calcium oxalate crystals causes nephrosis and renal failure.
- Free oxalic acid may be responsible for GI irritation.

## Toxicokinetics

- Little is known about the toxicokinetics in animals.

## Toxicity

- Unlikely to be an issue with most plants unless substantial amounts are ingested. The sap is very bitter tasting, and this may limit absorption in most animals.
- Stems (often referred to as stalks) of rhubarb are edible and often used for jams or baking; the leaves contain soluble oxalate crystals and are not edible.
- Limited access to star fruit and sweet star fruit juices purchased at a grocery store is usually not a problem when ingested. An animal with access to lesser amounts of inedible, *sour* star fruits or juice, eating many edible star fruits, drinking a large amount of edible star fruit juice, or with underlying kidney disease is at higher risk for toxicosis.

## Systems Affected

- Gastrointestinal – GI irritation with vomiting (with or without blood) and diarrhea (with or without blood).
- Renal/urological – kidney failure from formation of calcium oxalate crystals.
- Neuromuscular – signs associated with hypocalcemia.
- Musculoskeletal – tetany secondary to hypocalcemia.

 **SIGNALMENT/HISTORY**

- All small animals, indoors and out, are susceptible.

## Risk Factors

- Preexisting GI or chronic renal disease.
- Boredom in confined animal.

## Historical Findings

- Confirmation of chewed-up plant in animal's environment.
- Leaves from rhubarb plants that have not been adequately disposed of and are ingested.

# CLINICAL FEATURES

- Hypersalivation and anorexia are the earliest signs, followed by vomiting with or without blood and diarrhea with or without blood.
- Depression, weakness, tremors, tetany, and coma follow if the ingestion is large enough to result in systemic hypocalcemia.
- Acute kidney failure secondary to calcium oxalate crystal formation results in polydipsia and polyuria, or oliguria with oxaluria, hematuria, and albuminuria. Signs develop at 24–36 hours post ingestion.

 # DIFFERENTIAL DIAGNOSIS

- Diabetes mellitus (ketoacidosis or hypoglycemic shock).
- Toxicants.
  - Calcipotriene (Dovonex®, others).
  - Cholecalciferol rodenticides.
  - Ethylene glycol.
  - Other plant ingestions, including lilies in cats.
- Underlying diseases such as chronic kidney failure, pancreatitis, or diabetes mellitus.
- Viral or bacterial gastroenteritis.

 # DIAGNOSTICS

### Clinical Pathological Findings

- Hypocalcemia, increases in BUN/creatinine in severe cases.
- Urinalysis initially may be normal but later will show crystalluria (oxaluria), hematuria, and albuminuria.

### Pathological Findings

- Gross pathology yields only renal lesions (swollen and edematous kidneys) and systemic congestion. Histopathological lesions include moderate-to-severe, diffuse acute renal tubular necrosis.

 # THERAPEUTICS

### Detoxification

- Emesis early after ingestion.
- Activated charcoal with cathartic × 1 dose.

### Appropriate Health Care

- In severe cases with systemic hypocalcemia and oxaluria, aggressive IV fluid therapy for a minimum of 48 hours to preserve renal function.
- Monitor serum calcium and electrolytes, BUN, and creatinine daily until they have returned to normal limits.

## Antidotes

- No true specific antidote, although some may consider the administration of IV calcium an antidote.

## Drug(s) of Choice

- Hypocalcemia.
    - 10% calcium gluconate IV at 0.5–1.5 mL/kg over 20–30 minutes.
    - Stop if bradycardia or arrhythmias develop; once CV system is stable, reinstitute at a slower rate.
- IV fluid therapy at 1.5–2X maintenance and adjust as needed for dehydration, electrolyte changes, and urine output. SQ fluids will not be effective in preventing renal damage if oxaluria is present.
- Monitor urine output for development of oliguria (0.5 mL/kg/h of urine) or anuria (<0.5 mL/kg/h of urine). If decreased urinary output, consider individually or in combination.
    - Furosemide 2–4 mg/kg IV intermittent boluses in both dogs and cats.
    - Dopamine 2–5 mcg/kg/min IV.
    - Mannitol 0.25–1 g/kg IV over 10–40 minutes.
- Antiemetics if vomiting is severe or persists.
    - Dolasetron 0.6 mg/kg SQ, IV q 24 hours.
    - Maropitant 1 mg/kg SQ, IV q 24 hours.
    - Ondansetron 0.5–1 mg/kg IV q 12 hours for dogs; 0.1–1 mg/kg IV, SQ, IM q 6–12 hours for cats.
- GI protectants as needed.
    - Famotidine 0.5–1 mg/kg PO, SQ, IM, IV q 12 hours (cautious IV use in cats).
    - Omeprazole 0.5–1 mg/kg daily PO.
    - Sucralfate 0.25–1 g PO q 8 hours × 5–7 days if evidence of active ulcer disease.
- Nonsteroidal antiinflammatory agents or other analgesics for pain.
    - Carprofen 2.2 mg/kg PO q 12–24 hours (dogs).
    - Deracoxib 1–2 mg/kg PO q 24 hours (dogs).
    - Robenacoxib 1 mg/kg PO q 24 hours (cats). Limit dosing to three days.

 # COMMENTS

### Prevention/Avoidance

- Keep these and other toxic plants out of the reach of animals.
- Properly dispose of rhubarb leaves after removing and saving the stems.

### Possible Complications

- Chronic kidney disease.

### Expected Course and Prognosis

- In general, few problems other than GI irritation occur with ingestion of these plants by healthy animals, and the prognosis for recovery is excellent.
- Rarely, systemic hypocalcemia with secondary renal disease develops. If treated early, the prognosis is very good for a full recovery. The prognosis decreases considerably for those animals treated after acute renal disease has occurred.

## See Also

Chapter 9 Ethylene Glycol and Diethylene Glycol
Chapter 23 Calcipotriene/Calcipotriol
Chapter 124 Cholecalciferol

## Abbreviations

See Appendix 1 for a complete list.

## Suggested Reading

Abeysekera RA, Wijetunge S, Nanayakkara N et al. Star fruit toxicity: a cause of both acute kidney injury and chronic kidney disease: a report of two cases. *BMC Res Notes* 2015;8:796.
Burrows GE, Tyrl RJ. *Toxic Plants of North America*, 2nd edn. Ames: Wiley-Blackwell, 2012.
Chen CL, Fang HC, Chou KJ. Acute oxalate nephropathy after ingestion of a star fruit. *Am J Kidney Dis* 2001;37:418–422.
Knight AP. *A Guide to Poisonous House and Garden Plants*. Jackson Hole: Teton NewMedia, 2006.
Nakata PA. Plant calcium oxalate crystal formation, function, and its impact on human health. *Front Biol* 2012;7(3):254–266.
Pamodh Y, Umesh J, Ishan D et al. Mechanisms of star fruit (*Averrhoa carambola*) toxicity: a mini-review. *Toxicon* 2020;187:198–202.

**Author**: Lynn R. Hovda, RPh, DVM, MS, DACVIM
**Consulting Editor**: Lynn R. Hovda, RPh, DVM, MS, DACVIM

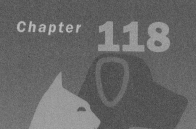

# Sago Palm (Cycads)

## DEFINITION/OVERVIEW

- Cycads (order Cycadales) refers to a plant in one of three families – Cycadaceae, Stangeriaceae, and Zamiaceae. There are about 300 species in this order.
- The term "cycads" is generally used describe sago palms, although all species of cycads cause toxicosis if ingested.
- Sago palms grow in tropical and subtropical environments and can also be found in garden stores as landscape and household plants. Some zoological and personal gardeners grow them in a more compact bonsai form.
  - *Cycas revoluta* (king sago) is a common sago palm popular throughout the United States.
  - *Zamia furfuracea* (cardboard palm) and others are beginning to appear in garden stores, and they are just as toxic as sago palms.
- Sago palms are not really palms, nor are they ferns. They are a woody, seed-producing plant with large stiff leaves that reproduce by production of male (elongated) and female (round and "fuzzy") cones (Figures 118.1, 118.2). Once fertilized, the female plant produces seeds (nuts) containing substantial amounts of toxin. *Zamia* spp. reproduces in a like manner, although both the female and male plant have elongated cones (Figures 118.3, 118.4).
- Toxicosis occurs when *any* part of a cycad plant is ingested, although the seeds (nuts) contain a higher level of toxin.
- The target species is the dog with reported mortality ranging from 12.5% to 67%.
- Clinical signs occur about 15 minutes to four hours after ingestion but may be delayed for up to 24 hours. The GIT, liver, and CNS are most often affected.
- Dogs presenting with an ALT >125 U/l and <200 000 platelets/microliter have an increased risk of mortality.

## ETIOLOGY/PATHOPHYSIOLOGY

- Historically, most cases occurred in the southern United States and Hawaii due to the natural geographic location of sago palms.
- Popularity as household plants has led to toxicity being widespread around the country, including the colder regions.

---

*Blackwell's Five-Minute Veterinary Consult Clinical Companion: Small Animal Toxicology*, Third Edition. Edited by Lynn R. Hovda, Ahna G. Brutlag, Robert H. Poppenga, and Steven E. Epstein.
© 2024 John Wiley & Sons, Inc. Published 2024 by John Wiley & Sons, Inc.

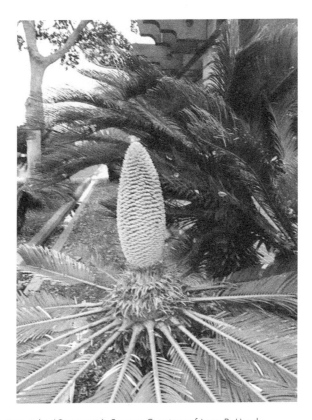

■ **Figure 118.1** Male sago palm (*Cycas* spp.). Source: Courtesy of Lynn R. Hovda.

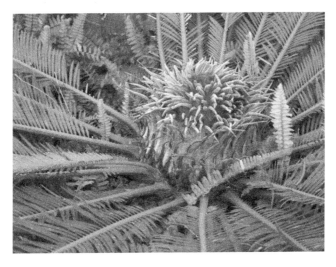

■ **Figure 118.2** Female sago palm (*Cycas* spp.). If fertilized by the male palm, the round cone present in the middle produces seeds containing large amounts of toxins.

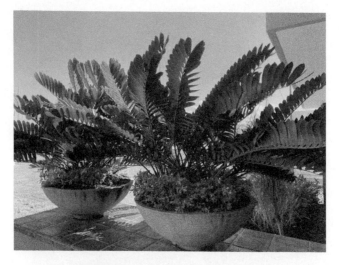

■ **Figure 118.3** Cardboard palm (*Zamia* spp.). Source: Courtesy of Lynn R. Hovda.

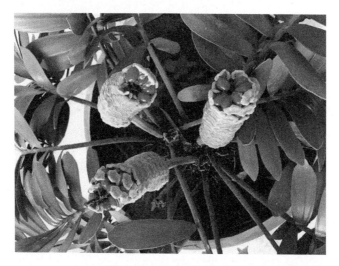

■ **Figure 118.4** Seeds of female cardboard palm (*Zamia* spp.) Source: Courtesy of Lynn R. Hovda.

## Mechanism of Action

- Three toxins.
  - Azoglycosides (cycasin, macrozamin, and neocyasin), with cycasin the main glycoside. After ingestion, they are metabolized and converted into toxic metabolite methylazo-oxymethanol (MAM). MAM is responsible for the GI signs and hepatotoxicity.
  - Beta-methylamino-L-alanine (BMAA) is a neurotoxic amino acid associated with weakness, tremors, and seizures.
  - Unidentified high molecular weight compound may also be responsible for neurological signs.

## Toxicokinetics

- Absorption is rapid, with clinical signs occurring in 15 minutes to four hours. Signs may be delayed up to 24 hours in some dogs. Signs of hepatotoxicity may be delayed for up to 72 hours.
- Azoglycosides are converted into the toxic metabolite MAM by intestinal bacteria. MAM is water soluble, low molecular weight and undergoes enterohepatic recirculation.

## Toxicity

- All parts of the plant are toxic, with the seeds containing the highest concentration of toxins.
- As few as 1–2 seeds can result in toxicosis and death in dogs.

## Systems Affected

- Gastrointestinal – acute vomiting, hematemesis, diarrhea within 15 minutes to hours of ingestion.
- Hepatobiliary – acute, severe hepatic necrosis within 24–72 hours.
- Nervous – acute CNS signs occur less commonly and in only 30–53% of dogs. Ataxia, abnormal mentation, tremors, seizures. CNS signs may develop secondary to hepatic failure as well.

 **SIGNALMENT/HISTORY**

### Risk Factors

- Dogs are the primary species affected. All dogs are affected, regardless of age, medical history, or current medications.
- No breed or sex predilections.

### Historical Findings

- Owners report history of ingesting sago palm or seeing evidence of plant material in vomitus/feces.

### Location and Circumstances of Poisoning

- Naturally occurring sago palms are present in the sandy soils and tropical-subtropical climates of the southern United States and Hawaii.
- Sago palms are also prevalent in colder climates as ornamental bonsai or houseplants.

 **CLINICAL FEATURES**

- Roughly 90% of dogs spontaneously vomit within 15 minutes to four hours of ingestion.
- Other gastrointestinal signs include hypersalivation, regurgitation, anorexia, hematemesis, diarrhea, and melena.
- Hepatic changes (abdominal pain, icterus, coagulopathies) can be seen in 24–72 hours.
- Roughly 30–53% of dogs develop nervous system signs, including ataxia, abnormal mentation, lethargy, tremors, and seizures in the acute stage. CNS signs may also develop following liver failure.

 **DIFFERENTIAL DIAGNOSIS**

- Any toxin or disease process resulting in vomiting and acute hepatic failure.
- Common toxicants.

- Acetaminophen.
- *Amanita* (cyclopeptide) mushrooms.
- Blue-green algae.
- Nonsteroidal antiinflammatory drugs.
- Xylitol.
- Disease processes.
    - Hepatopathy.
    - Leptospirosis.
    - Necrotizing pancreatitis.
    - Septicemia.

 **DIAGNOSTICS**

### Clinical Pathological Findings

- Significant elevation in ALT.
- Elevations in ALP, AST.
- Prolonged PT, PTT.
- Thrombocytopenia.
- With liver failure: hypoalbuminemia, hypoglycemia, increased bile acids, elevated ammonia, low cholesterol, elevated bilirubin.
- Secondary to vomiting/dehydration: elevated lactate, electrolyte disturbances, leukocytosis, pre-renal azotemia.

### Other Diagnostics

- Abdominal imaging may help determine if further plant material is in stomach.
- Liver injury may be evaluated by ultrasound.

### Pathological Findings

- Gross findings include icterus, petechial and ecchymotic hemorrhages, dark, tarry ingesta in the stomach, evidence of liver damage.
- Histopathological findings include cirrhosis with focal centrilobular and midzonal necrosis and evidence of generalized hemorrhagic disease.

 **THERAPEUTICS**

- Prompt early decontamination, liver protectants, supportive therapy.
- Treat aggressively and promptly.

### Detoxification

- Induce emesis ASAP.
- Plant material may cause delayed gastric emptying, so emesis/gastric lavage can be performed hours after ingestion if vomiting has not occurred spontaneously.
- If emesis is ineffective or patient cannot protect airway, consider gastric lavage.
- Activated charcoal with a cathartic (ACC) at 1–2 g/kg PO × 1 dose.
- Follow ACC with multidose cholestyramine 0.3–1 g/kg PO q 8 hours for three days for enterohepatic recirculation. Avoid cholestyramine products that contain xylitol.
- Consider feeding tube if patient will not take medications orally.
- Warm water enemas can be used to expel plant material from intestines if warranted.

## Appropriate Health Care

- Hospitalization for aggressive treatment and close liver monitoring is recommended, even if patient is asymptomatic.
- Some patients may need long-term liver support.

## Antidote

- There is no antidote.

## Drug(s) of Choice

- Fluid therapy.
  - Balanced crystalloid.
  - Colloid or FFP if needed for oncotic support.
- Liver protectants.
  - N-acetylcysteine (NAC) loading dose 140 mg/kg, followed by 70 mg/kg PO/IV q 6 hours for 7–17 doses. Dilute and give through 0.22 micron filter if giving IV.
  - S-adenosylmethionine (SAM-E) 40 mg/kg loading dose, followed by 20 mg/kg PO daily × 4–6 weeks.
  - Silymarin (milk thistle) 50–250 mg/kg PO q 12 hours.
  - Vitamin E 400 IU PO q 24 hours.
- GI support.
  - Antiemetics.
    - Maropitant 1 mg/kg SQ, IV q 24 hours.
    - Ondansetron 0.5–1 mg/kg IV q 12 hours for dogs; 0.1–1 mg/kg IV, SQ, IM q 6–12 hours for cats.
    - Dolasetron 0.6 mg/kg IV, SQ q 24 hours.
  - GI protectants.
    - Famotidine 0.5–1 mg/kg PO, SQ, IM, IV q 12 hours.
    - Omeprazole 0.5–1 mg/kg PO q 24 hours.
    - Sucralfate 0.25–1 g PO q 8 hours for 5–7 days if evidence of active ulcer disease.
- Liver failure support.
  - Fresh frozen plasma (FFP) 10–20 mL/kg as needed for thrombocytopenia and coagulation deficits.
  - Dextrose supplementation in IVF at 2.5–5% CRI.
  - Vitamin $K_1$ 2–5 mg/kg PO or SQ q 24 hours or divided every 12 hours as needed for clotting disorders.
  - Broad-spectrum antibiotics (ampicillin 15–25 mg/kg IV/PO q 8–12 hours).
  - Lactulose enema if concern for hepatic encephalopathy.
- Neurological support.
  - Lowest effective dose anticonvulsants .
    - Diazepam 0.25–0.5 mg/kg IV PRN. Other benzodiazepines may be used depending on availability and comfort level of treating DVM.
    - Levetiracetam 30–60 mg/kg IV q 8 hours.
  - Methocarbamol 55–220 mg/kg IV bolus to effect for tremors. Do not exceed 330 mg/kg/day.

## Precautions/Interactions

- Avoid cimetidine as it inhibits cytochrome P450 oxidation in liver.

## Alternative Drugs

- Over-the-counter N-acetylcysteine may be available if injectable formulation unavailable.

### Extracorporeal Therapy

■ Extracorporeal therapies have not been evaluated for this toxicity.

### Surgical Considerations

■ Patients may develop coagulopathy.

### Patient Monitoring

■ Liver enzymes, platelet count, +/- PT/PTT should be monitored at baseline, 24, and 48 hours. If no abnormalities seen within 48 hours, toxicity is unlikely to occur.
■ Patients who develop liver enzyme elevations should be monitored daily until clinical signs have resolved, then every 1–2 weeks until they normalize or plateau. Some patients may develop chronic hepatopathies.

### Diet

■ Resume feedings once vomiting is controlled. Consider feeding tube in anorexic animals if no clotting abnormalities. Consider liver diet if chronic hepatopathy develops.

 **COMMENTS**

### Prevention/Avoidance

■ Remove sago palms access or ensure that access is prevented.
■ Do not place around swimming pools or other areas where dogs routinely have access.

### Possible Complications

■ Acute: DIC, sepsis, AKI, coagulopathy.
■ Chronic: chronic active hepatitis, hepatic fibrosis, permanent hepatic dysfunction, acquired liver shunts.

### Expected Course and Prognosis

■ Fair to good prognosis if decontaminated immediately following ingestion and initiation of aggressive therapy prior to clinical signs. Patients that present asymptomatic and are decontaminated quickly have the best chance of survival.
■ Guarded prognosis once clinical signs develop (mortality rate up to 50–67%). Patients with baseline elevated ALT, prolonged clotting times, or thrombocytopenia have high risk of a poor outcome.
■ Many animals survive with supportive care but may require prolonged hepatic support.
■ Frequent death and euthanasia reported.

### Synonyms

■ Coontie plant, queen sago, fern palm, Japanese cycad.

### See Also

Chapter 45 Acetaminophen
Chapter 110 Blue-green Algae (Cyanobacteria): Microcystins
Chapter 115 Mushrooms
Chapter 79 Xylitol

### Abbreviations

See Appendix 1 for a complete list.

## Suggested Reading

Albretsen JC, Khan SA, Richardson JA. Cycad palm toxicosis in dogs: 60 cases (1987–1997). *J Am Vet Med Assoc* 1998;213(1):99–101.

Burrows GE, Tyrl RJ. Cycadaceae. In: *Toxic Plants of North America*, 2nd edn. Ames: John Wiley & Sons, 2013; pp. 402–409.

Clarke C, Burney D. Cycad palm toxicosis in 14 dogs from Texas. *J Am Anim Hosp Assoc* 2017;53:159–166.

Fatourechi L, DelGiudice LA, Sookhoo N. Sago palm toxicosis in dogs. *Compendium* 2013;35(4):E1–E8.

Ferguson D, Crowe M, McLaughlin L et al. Survival and prognostic indicators for cycad intoxication in dogs. *J Vet Intern Med* 2011;25(4):831–837.

Lake BB, Edwards T, Atiee G et al. The characterization of cycad palm toxicosis and treatment effects in 130 dogs. *Aust Vet J* 2020;98:555–562.

**Author:** Jessie Barber, DVM
**Consulting Editor:** Lynn R. Hovda, RPh, DVM, MS, DACVIM

# Chapter 119

# Spring Bulbs

## DEFINITION/OVERVIEW

- Poisoning is associated with exposure to many plants belonging to several genera including *Crocus, Hippeastrum, Hyacinthus, Narcissus,* and *Tulipa.*
- Gastrointestinal signs predominate but CV, respiratory, and neurological signs may also occur, depending on the amount and genus ingested.
- In much of the US, bulbs are generally planted in the fall with blooms occurring in the spring, although many varieties are shipped and planted in spring with equal success. In growing zones in the southern US, bulbs may be shipped and planted at virtually any time of the year.
- May be found in gardens, as potted houseplants, or in cut flower arrangements.

## ETIOLOGY/PATHOPHYSIOLOGY

- Ingestion of plant material (leaves, stems, flowers, and bulbs).
- Includes *Crocus* spp. (spring-blooming crocus; Figure 119.1), *Hippeastrum* spp. (amaryllis; Figure 119.2), *Hyacinthus* spp. (hyacinth; Figure 119.3), *Narcissus* spp. (daffodil, jonquil, narcissus, paperwhite; Figures 119.4, 119.5), and *Tulipa* spp. (tulip; Figure 119.6).

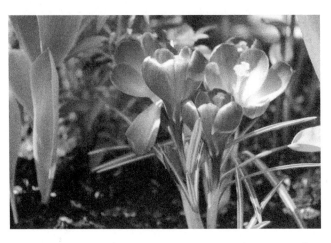

■ **Figure 119.1** Spring-flowering crocus (*Crocus* spp.). Source: Courtesy of Lynn R. Hovda.

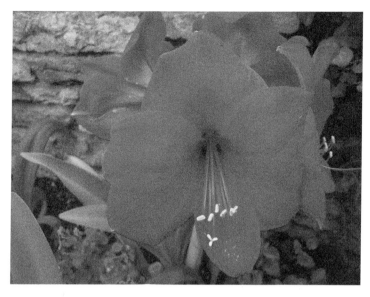

■ **Figure 119.2** Amaryllis (*Hippeastrum* spp.). Source: Courtesy of Lynn R. Hovda.

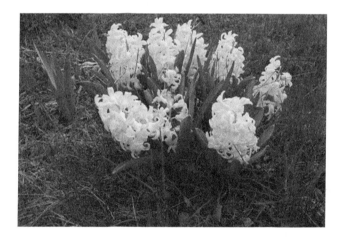

■ **Figure 119.3** Hyacinth (*Hyacinthus* spp.). Source: Courtesy of Tyne K. Hovda.

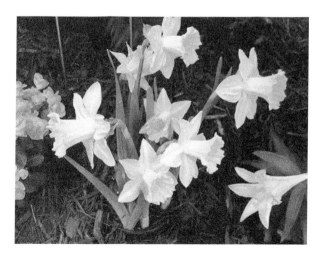

■ **Figure 119.4** Daffodils (*Narcissus* spp.). Source: Courtesy of Lynn R. Hovda.

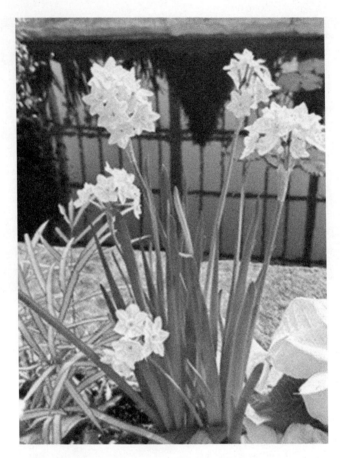

■ **Figure 119.5** Paperwhite (*Narcissus* spp.). Source: Courtesy of Lynn R. Hovda.

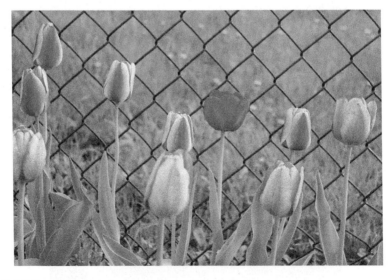

■ **Figure 119.6** Tulips (*Tulipa* spp.). Source: Courtesy of Lynn R. Hovda.

## Mechanism of Action

- *Crocus* spp. – GI irritation (not to be confused with autumn-blooming crocus or *Colchicum* spp. which contains colchicine).
- *Hippeastrum* spp. and *Narcissus* spp. – phenanthridine alkaloids (mainly lycorine) lead to GI signs, hypotension, arrhythmias, and rarely CNS signs; calcium oxalate raphides (needle-like crystals) lead to oral and GI irritation, possible contact dermatitis, and dyspnea.
- *Hyacinthus* spp. – GI irritation and possible contact dermatitis due to calcium oxalate raphides and unknown compounds.
- *Tulipa* spp. – irritant and allergenic lactones tuliposides A and B along with calcium oxalate raphides cause GI signs and possible contact dermatitis, dyspnea, and tachycardia.

## Toxicokinetics

- Onset of signs is typically rapid, occurring within minutes of ingestion; rarely delayed up to 24 hours.

## Toxicity

- Ingestion of small amounts of plant material tends to cause mild signs; ingestion of large amounts of foliage and/or bulbs may cause moderate-to-severe signs.
- Toxins tend to occur in higher concentrations in the bulbs.
- Exposure to plants in the *Narcissus* spp. has been associated with more serious outcomes. Deaths have been reported but are considered rare.

## Systems Affected

- Gastrointestinal – hypersalivation, vomiting, diarrhea, abdominal pain, oral irritation, anorexia.
- Cardiovascular – hypotension, arrhythmias.
- Nervous – ataxia, depression, tremors, seizures (rare).
- Respiratory – dyspnea rarely occurs secondary to oropharyngeal swelling.
- Skin – contact dermatitis and erythema may occur but this is more common in humans.

# SIGNALMENT/HISTORY

- Dogs and cats are at risk for toxicosis if plant material is ingested.
- Dogs tend to ingest larger amounts of foliage and/or bulbs than cats and are at higher risk for moderate-to-severe clinical signs.

## Risk Factors

- Presence of plants in the animal's environment (either indoor or outdoor).
- Boredom, curiosity.

## Historical Findings

- Observations and signs often reported by the owner.
  - Ingestion may or may not be witnessed by the owner but damage to plants, missing, or dug-up bulbs may be noted.
  - Initial reported signs tend to be GI in nature with possible progression to weakness, dyspnea, and CNS signs in severe cases.

### Location and Circumstances of Poisoning

- Indoors – ingestion of leaves and flowers from potted plants, bouquets, or floral arrangements.
- Outdoors – ingestion of plants in gardens or bulbs freshly planted or left unattended.

 ## CLINICAL FEATURES

- Signs may be noted within minutes of exposure but rarely may be delayed up to 24 hours.
- Gastrointestinal – evidence of oral irritation or pain (hypersalivation, pawing at the mouth, head shaking) within minutes; redness or irritation to the mucous membranes and oropharynx; vomiting, diarrhea, and abdominal pain within minutes to hours. GI bleeding may occur in *Narcissus* spp. exposures.
- Cardiovascular – lethargy and weakness may be noted in patients experiencing hypotension or arrhythmias following large exposure, especially to *Narcissus* spp.
- Nervous – ataxia, tremors, and seizures are possible following large ingestion of *Narcissus* spp. but rarely occur.
- Respiratory – dyspnea and airway obstruction if severe inflammation of the oropharynx occurs (rare).
- Skin – erythema, pruritus, edema, and pustular rash are rarely reported in animals.

 ## DIFFERENTIAL DIAGNOSIS

- Other toxins.
  - Plants containing irritants including insoluble calcium oxalate crystals.
  - Household products causing oral irritation (dilute cleaning agents, topical insecticides, many fertilizers).
  - Caustic agents (strong acids or alkalis, drain cleaners, batteries, some detergents).
- Foreign body obstruction.
- Systemic diseases associated with GI signs.

 ## DIAGNOSTICS

- Diagnosis is most often made by identification of the plant ingested.

### Clinical Pathological Findings

- Clinical laboratory tests (serum chemistry and CBC) are not specifically diagnostic. Changes related to dehydration and persistent GI signs may be noted.

### Pathological Findings

- Deaths are rare but reddened GI mucosa may be noted, possible cardiac ventricular dilation with exposure to *Narcissus* spp.

 ## THERAPEUTICS

- Treatment of spring-blooming plant or bulb poisoning consists primarily of symptomatic and supportive care, including management of GI signs, correction of dehydration, and treatment of cardiovascular and CNS signs in severe cases. Small exposures typically only require at-home monitoring and nursing care.

## Detoxification

- Extensive decontamination is generally not required in cases involving minimal exposure.
- Rinse the oral cavity with cool water to dilute irritants from the mouth.
- Early emesis should be employed in cases where substantial amounts of plant material and/or bulbs were ingested, provided the patient is not already vomiting.
- Activated charcoal with a cathartic × 1 dose (following large ingestion only).

## Appropriate Health Care

- Minor exposures can often be managed at home with dilution and monitoring.
- SQ or IV fluid therapy as needed depending upon hydration status and severity of GI signs.
- Frequent monitoring of blood pressure and ECG for 12–24 hours in severe cases.
- Close monitoring of CNS status following large ingestion.
- Monitor for dyspnea and airway obstruction in cases involving significant oropharyngeal swelling.

## Antidote

- No specific antidote.

## Drug(s) of Choice

- Fluid therapy.
  - SQ fluids in cases with minor signs.
  - IV fluids as needed to correct dehydration, support perfusion, and maintain adequate blood pressure.
- Antiemetic agents as needed.
  - Maropitant 1 mg/kg SQ, IV q 24 hours.
  - Ondansetron 0.5–1 mg/kg IV q 12 hours for dogs; 0.1–1 mg/kg IV, SQ, IM q 6–12 hours for cats.
- GI protectants.
  - $H_2$-blocker: famotidine 0.5 mg/kg PO, SQ, IM, IV q 12–24 hours.
  - Proton pump inhibitors.
    - Omeprazole 0.5–1 mg/kg PO q 24 hours.
    - Pantoprazole 0.7–1 mg/kg IV over 15 minutes q 24 hours.
  - Sucralfate 0.25–1 g PO q 8 hours × 5–7 days if evidence of active ulcer disease.
- Antiarrhythmics may be necessary if the patient is persistently tachycardic and nonresponsive to IV fluids, has severe ventricular dysrhythmias, or evidence of poor perfusion (hypotension, pulse deficits, tachycardia, pale membranes, prolonged CRT).
  - Lidocaine.
    - Dogs: 2–4 mg/kg IV over 1–2 minutes while monitoring ECG. If effective, switch to CRI at 25–100 mcg/kg/min.
    - Cats: 0.25–0.5 mg/kg slow IV while monitoring ECG. If effective, switch to CRI of 10–20 mcg/kg/min. Use judiciously in cats.
  - Procainamide.
    - Dogs: 2–4 mg/kg IV over 2–5 minutes (may repeat up to 20 mg/kg IV total), followed by 20–50 mcg/kg/min CRI.

## Diet

- Depending on the severity of GI signs, consider keeping the patient NPO initially then feeding a bland or highly digestible diet.

## COMMENTS

### Prevention/Avoidance

- Identify plants presently in the household or on the property and limit exposure by placing them out of the animal's reach or restricting access to gardens and flowerbeds.
- Do not leave unplanted bulbs unattended while gardening or in areas that are generally accessible to pets, especially dogs.

### Expected Course and Prognosis

- Prognosis is generally excellent to good as most cases develop only mild-to-moderate signs of short duration and require minimal therapy.

### See Also

Chapter 116 Oxalates (Insoluble)

### Abbreviations

See Appendix 1 for a complete list.

### Suggested Reading

Burrows GE, Tyrl RJ. *Toxic Plants of North America*, 2nd edn. Ames: John Wiley & Sons, 2013.
Knight AP. *A Guide to Poisonous House and Garden Plants*. Jackson Hole: Teton NewMedia, 2006.
Kretzing S, Abraham G, Seiwart B et al. Dose-dependent emetic effects of the Amaryllidaceous alkaloid lycorine in beagle dogs. *Toxicon* 2011;57(1):117–124.
Lieske CL. Spring-blooming bulbs: a year-round problem. *Vet Med* 2002;97:580–588.

**Author**: Amanda L. Poldoski, DVM
**Consulting Editor**: Lynn R. Hovda, RPh, DVM, MS, DACVIM

# Chapter 120

# Yesterday, Today, and Tomorrow Plant

 ## DEFINITION/OVERVIEW

- The *Brunfelsia* genus consists of 30–50 species within the nightshade family (Solanaceae) and the subfamily Petunioideae.
- The plants are shrubs or small trees with distinctive tri-colored flowers. Over the course of approximately three days, the blooms progress from a deep blue/purple (Figure 120.1) to a lighter hue of blue/purple and then to white (Figure 120.2). The common name "yesterday, today, and tomorrow" references these tri-colored blooms.
- Native species are present in the West Indies, South America, and Central America.
- Various species have become popular as ornamental plants and may be encountered worldwide. *Brunfelsia* may be grown outside in warmer climates, and in transportable planters or indoors in cooler areas.

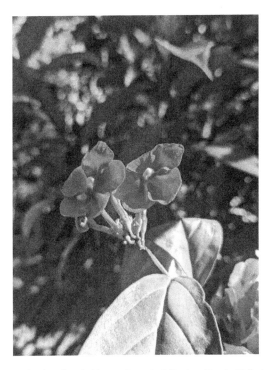

■ Figure 120.1 *Brunfelsia* spp. bud and early bloom. Botanical Garden, Puerto Vallarta, Mexico. Source: Courtesy of Stephanie Jenson.

---

*Blackwell's Five-Minute Veterinary Consult Clinical Companion: Small Animal Toxicology*, Third Edition. Edited by Lynn R. Hovda, Ahna G. Brutlag, Robert H. Poppenga, and Steven E. Epstein. © 2024 John Wiley & Sons, Inc. Published 2024 by John Wiley & Sons, Inc.

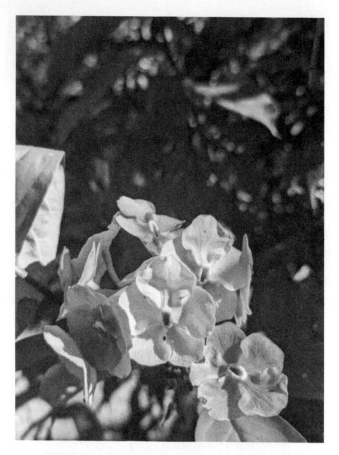

■ **Figure 120.2** Three colors of *Brunfelsia* spp. Botanical Gardens, Puerto Vallarta, Mexico. Source: Courtesy of Stephanie Jenson.

■ *Brunfelsia* spp. associated with toxicity include *Brunfelsia americana*, *B. australis*, *B. calycina* var. *floribunda*, *B. grandiflora*, *B. pauciflora*, and *B. uniflora*. Further research is required to assess toxicity in additional species.

■ Toxicity often includes initial gastrointestinal signs (vomiting, diarrhea), followed by severe life-threatening neurological and neuromuscular signs including ataxia, tremors, and seizures.

■ *Brunfelsia* spp. have been used by indigenous peoples for medicinal purposes. Further study is being conducted to evaluate components from *Brunfelsia* spp. and potential effects.

## Mechanism of Action

■ Brunfelsamidine – a pyrrolidine alkaloid and most likely to be a significant toxicant.
  • Neurological/neuromuscular (excitation, seizures, death).
■ Hopeanine – an alkaloid of possible clinical significance.
  • Neurological/neuromuscular (lethargy, depression, paralysis, seizures, hyperesthesia).
■ Scopoletin – a tropane alkaloid, the first component identified, but does not appear to be primary toxic component.
  • Cardiovascular (hypotensive agent, bradycardia, decreased cardiovascular strength).
  • Neuromuscular (smooth muscle relaxant, neuromuscular block).
  • Antiinflammatory properties.

- Other components include cuscohygrine, scopolamine, scopoletin, and esculetin; the significance of these and additional components requires further examination.
- All parts of the plant are potentially toxic.
- Not all *Brunfelsia* spp. are toxic.
- Incidence has a high degree of regional variability.

## Toxicokinetics

- No known specific toxicokinetics exists in dogs or cats.

## Toxicity

- Specific toxicity values have not been established.

## Systems Affected

- Gastrointestinal – hypersalivation, vomiting, diarrhea, anorexia, abdominal discomfort.
- Nervous – lethargy, depression, agitation, hyperesthesia, vocalization, nystagmus.
- Neuromuscular – ataxia, weakness, fasciculations, tremors, seizures, opisthotonos.
- Cardiovascular – arrhythmias, bradycardia, hypotension, decreased cardiovascular output, cardiac arrest.
- Respiratory – coughing, hypoventilation.

# SIGNALMENT/HISTORY

## Risk Factors

- Dogs are the most commonly affected small animal due to their propensity for dietary indiscretion.
- Variably seasonal toxicity has not been established in small animals. Increased toxicity in sheep and donkeys ingesting *Brunfelsia uniflora* when the plant was flowering has been demonstrated.

## Historical Findings

- Ingestion of plant material prior to onset of clinical signs may be reported by the owner.
- Rapid onset of initial gastrointestinal signs followed by neurological involvement may be noted by the owner.
- Plant material may be identified in vomitus or diarrhea.

## Location and Circumstances of Poisoning

- *Brunfelsia* spp. are typically encountered outside in warmer climates.
  - In the US, regions such as Florida, the Gulf Coast, and California are suitable climates for growing *Brunfelsia* spp. outside year round.
- *Brunfelsia* spp. may be grown indoors or transported indoors/outdoors with season changes in any climate.

# CLINICAL FEATURES

- Onset of signs is typically rapid, within minutes to hours of an ingestion.
- Early signs include agitation, vomiting, diarrhea, coughing, opisthotonos, and nystagmus.

- Several hours following exposure, clinical signs may progress to ataxia, tremors, and seizures (typically repeated extensor rigidity).
  - Seizure activity is often in response to external stimulation. As it is much like seizure activity following strychnine exposure, clinical signs have been described as strychnine-like.
  - Dysrhythmias, hypotension, cardiac failure, and other clinical signs as listed previously under Systems Affected have been reported.
- Clinical signs may persist for days.

 **DIFFERENTIAL DIAGNOSIS**

- Toxicants.
  - Pesticides including strychnine, metaldehyde, bromethalin, phosphide, and organophosphates/carbamates.
  - Tremorgenic mycotoxins.
  - Cane toad (*Rhinella marina*) intoxication.
  - Cyanobacteria.
  - Medications (amphetamines, baclofen, ivermectin, 5-fluorouracil, pseudoephedrine, and phenylephrine).
  - Stimulants including methylxanthines and illicit drugs including amphetamines and methamphetamine.
  - Ethanol.
  - Tetrahydrocannabinol (THC).
- Nontoxicant-related causes may include other dietary indiscretion; neurological disorders including epilepsy; fulminant hepatic necrosis or other hepatic failure; infectious and parasitic disease; neoplasia; and trauma.

 **DIAGNOSTICS**

- History of known or suspected plant ingestion.
- Presence of plant material in emesis, diarrhea, or upon necropsy.

### Clinical Pathological Findings

- Clinical laboratory tests are not specifically diagnostic, though changes secondary to clinical signs (such as dehydration, hyperthermia, or prolonged seizure activity) may occur.

### Other Diagnostics

- Endoscopy is not typically indicated but evidence of plant material may be identified if performed.

### Pathological Findings

- Presence of plant material may occur throughout the gastrointestinal tract.
- There are no pathognomonic changes identified but the following changes may be present in some cases.
  - Reddening and other inflammatory signs in the gastrointestinal tract.
  - Lung congestion.
  - Lymph node congestion.

# THERAPEUTICS

- Treatment is focused on initial decontamination, monitoring, and largely supportive and symptomatic care in symptomatic patients.

## Detoxification

- Home induction of emesis is not recommended due to the rapid potential onset of neurological signs.
- Emesis or gastric lavage may be considered as deemed safe by the treating clinician if a significant amount of plant material remains in the stomach.
- Single dose of activated charcoal with a cathartic as deemed safe by the treating clinician.
- Radiographs may allow for evaluation of ingesta location and amount.
- Warm water enema if plant material has progressed to the lower gastrointestinal tract.

## Appropriate Health Care

- Hospitalization for decontamination and monitoring is recommended following *Brunfelsia* spp. exposure.
- Continued hospitalization if neurological, neuromuscular, or cardiovascular signs are present.
- Cool as needed if hyperthermic.
- If the patient is asymptomatic or displays only mild gastrointestinal signs, home monitoring for development of neurological signs may be appropriate.

## Antidote

- No specific antidote is available.

## Drug(s) of Choice

- Fluid therapy.
  - Intravenous balanced crystalloid fluids as needed to maintain hydration and perfusion in cases with more than mild gastrointestinal signs or large ingestion of plant material. Adjust rate as needed.
  - Subcutaneous fluids in asymptomatic patients or those with mild gastrointestinal signs.
- Antiemetic agents.
  - Maropitant 1 mg/kg SQ, IV q 24 hours.
  - Ondansetron 0.5–1 mg/kg IV q 12 hours for dogs; 0.1–1 mg/kg IV, SQ, IM q 6–12 hours for cats.
- Anticonvulsant agents.
  - Benzodiazepines (diazepam 0.5–1 mg/kg IV or per rectum; midazolam 0.25–0.5 mg/kg IV). Can administer either as bolus IV or CRI depending on clinician preference and response to treatment. Adjust doses as needed.
  - Barbiturates (phenobarbital 2–8 mg/kg IV PRN).
  - Levetiracetam (30–60 mg/kg IV slow bolus over 5–15 minutes).
- Antitremorgenic agent: methocarbamol 55–220 mg/kg IV. Recommend not to exceed a maximum total dose of 330 mg/kg/day.
- Note: dosages above are for dogs, unless otherwise specified. Appropriate drugs and dosages should be confirmed for other species.

## Precautions/Interactions

- Atropine use is controversial and should be used with caution, if at all.

## Surgical Considerations

- Cardiovascular and respiratory status should be evaluated and treated accordingly if anesthesia is considered.

## Patient Monitoring

- Monitor vitals, electrocardiogram, blood pressure, and neurological status.
- Frequency of monitoring depends on clinical status.

## Diet

- If the patient is unable to swallow or otherwise protect their airway, temporarily discontinue oral feeding and water oral intake. Otherwise, no dietary changes are required.

 **COMMENTS**

### Prevention/Avoidance

- *Brunfelsia* spp. are popular as ornamental plants and education regarding potential toxicity is required to minimize potential exposure.
- Animal owners should prevent further access to the *Brunfelsia* spp. plants directly or to clippings from the plants.

### Possible Complications

- Aspiration may occur with subsequent development of aspiration pneumonia.
- If neurological, neuromuscular, and cardiovascular signs cannot be controlled, death may occur or humane euthanasia may be indicated.

### Expected Course and Prognosis

- Excellent prognosis in patients who are asymptomatic or develop mild signs.
- Worsening prognosis with development of significant neurological or cardiovascular signs.

### Synonyms

Kiss me quick, morning-noon-and-night, Brazil rain-tree, chiricaspi, uva silvestre.

### See Also

Chapter 68 Toads
Chapter 127 Strychnine

### Abbreviations

See Appendix 1 for a complete list.

### Suggested Reading

Burrows GE, Tyrl RJ. Brunfelsia L. In: *Toxic Plants of North America*. Ames: John Wiley & Sons, 2013; pp. 1134–1136.
Clipsham R. *Brunfelsia australis* (yesterday, today, and tomorrow tree) and Solanum poisoning in a dog. *J Am Anim Hosp Assoc* 2012;48(2):139–144.

Crowley JD, Thomas KA, Donahoe SL et al. Hypoventilation, cardiac dysrhythmia, and cardiac arrest following acute *Brunfelsia* species (yesterday, today, tomorrow) intoxication in a dog. *Aust Vet J* 2019;97(6):202–207.

Luzuriaga-Quichimbo CX, Hernandez del Barco M, Blanco-Salas J et al. Chiricaspi (*Brunfelsia grandiflora*, Solanaceae), a pharmacologically promising plant. *Plants* 2018;7(3):67.

Mello GW, Riet-Correa F, Batista MC et al. Poisoning by *Brunfelsia uniflora* in sheep and donkeys. *J Vet Diag Invest* 2018;30(3):476–478.

**Author**: Sarah R. Alpert, DVM, DABT
**Consulting Editor**: Lynn R. Hovda, RPh, DVM, MS, DACVIM

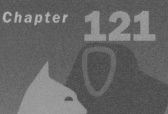

# Chapter 121

# Yew

## DEFINITION/OVERVIEW

- The term "yew" refers to plants in the genus *Taxus*. There are three species native to North America and numerous introduced species, hybrids, and cultivars. Native species grow in forested areas of the Northwest. Cultivars are common landscape plants throughout the continent, often found along fencerows and building foundations.
- Yews are easily identified by their 2–3 cm long needle-like leaves that are simple, alternate, and spirally arranged. Leaves are dark green on top with yellow longitudinal stripes underneath (Figure 121.1).

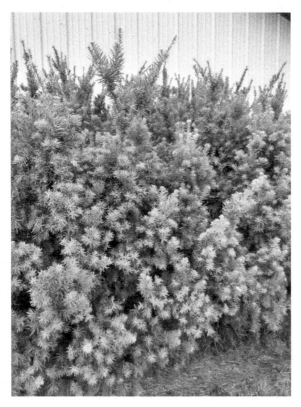

■ **Figure 121.1** Yew (*Taxus* spp.) Yew shrub planted alongside the foundation of a building. Source: Courtesy of Rebecca Anderson.

*Blackwell's Five-Minute Veterinary Consult Clinical Companion: Small Animal Toxicology*, Third Edition. Edited by Lynn R. Hovda, Ahna G. Brutlag, Robert H. Poppenga, and Steven E. Epstein.
© 2024 John Wiley & Sons, Inc. Published 2024 by John Wiley & Sons, Inc.

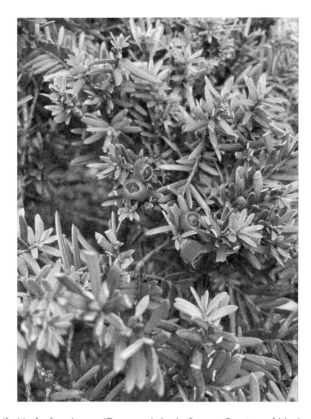

■ **Figure 121.2** Arils (fruit) of a female yew (*Taxus* spp.) shrub. Source: Courtesy of Meghan Jerden.

- Yews are dioecious, with individual specimens being either male or female. Female plants will have green, red-orange, or scarlet red fruit called arils (Figure 121.2). Male trees/shrubs may be more toxic than females.
- Ingestion of the leaves, bark, and seeds can result in toxicosis. The flesh of the aril is not toxic. Fresh and dried plant material are both toxic. Toxicosis has been reported in pets that have chewed on branches.
- Clinical signs of toxicosis include nausea, vomiting, diarrhea, gastritis, trembling, ataxia, aggressive behavior, seizures, bradycardia, collapse, hypothermia, and sudden death.
- Case management consists of decontamination, cardiovascular monitoring, antiarrhythmic therapies, GI support, and general nursing care.
- Unexpected death within minutes to days of ingestion is often the only sign of toxicosis.

# ETIOLOGY/PATHOPHYSIOLOGY

## Mechanism of Action

- Taxines A and B are the primary toxic components.
- Taxine B is more toxic than taxine A.
- Taxines are potent direct calcium and sodium channel antagonists primarily affecting the cardiovascular system, causing coronary arterial vasodilation, decreased cardiac contractility, and decreased rate of cardiac depolarization leading to significant arterial vasodilation-mediated hypotension.
- Acute death is due to diastolic cardiac standstill.
- Yews also contain volatile oil irritants that cause acute gastritis.
- Mechanism of CNS excitation is unknown.

## Toxicokinetics

- Absorption is rapid. Taxines are extensively distributed throughout body tissues apart from the CNS and testes.
- Metabolism is by hepatic P450 enzymes. Excretion is via bile as numerous metabolites including benzoic acid.
- Coadministration of compounds that affect P450 enzymes may affect metabolism of taxines.

## Toxicity

- $LD_{(min)}$ in dogs is 2.3 g leaves/kg BW or 11.5 mg/kg BW taxine alkaloids. Leaves contain approximately 5 mg/g taxine alkaloids.

## Systems Affected

- Cardiovascular – bradycardia, depressed or absent P wave, wide QRS complexes, cardiovascular collapse.
- Gastrointestinal – nausea, vomiting, diarrhea secondary to gastritis.
- Nervous – trembling, ataxia, aggressive behaviors, seizures.

 # SIGNALMENT/HISTORY

### Risk Factors

- Dogs and cats of any age, breed, or sex can be affected by this toxicosis.
- Plant has an unpleasant taste due to volatile oils which may limit ingestion, especially of fresh leaves.
- Taxines are more concentrated in plant material in the winter, increasing the risk of toxicosis during colder months.
- Toxicosis occurs more frequently in grazing animals than companion animal species.

### Historical Findings

- Presence of plant or plant clippings in animal's environment.
- Witnessed ingestion of leaves or playing with sticks.
- Presence of plant material in vomitus.

### Location and Circumstances of Poisoning

- Yew plants are widely distributed in North America. Toxicity varies with yew species. The Pacific yew (*Taxus brevifolia*) has lower levels of taxines than other species and therefore less potential for toxicity. However, most species of yew visually appear very similar, so exercise caution when making risk assessments based on species identification.

 # CLINICAL FEATURES

- Nausea, vomiting, diarrhea, gastritis, bradycardia, trembling, ataxia, aggressive behavior, seizures, collapse, hypothermia, and sudden death.

 # DIFFERENTIAL DIAGNOSIS

- Antiarrhythmic drug ingestion, especially digoxin.
- Other cardiovascular drugs (beta-blockers, calcium channel blockers).
- Other pharmaceuticals with known cardiovascular effects (baclofen, imidazoline decongestants, benzodiazepines, others).
- Cardiac glycoside-containing plants (oleander, foxglove, kalanchoe, lily of the valley, others).

- Other toxic plants known to cause cardiovascular effects (azaleas, rhododendrons, *Brunfelsia* spp., others).
- Organophosphorus and carbamate insecticides.
- Cardiac disease.

# DIAGNOSTICS

## Clinical Pathological Findings

- Baseline CBC, chemistry, electrolytes, and venous blood gases recommended. Specific abnormalities not expected. Hepatic insufficiency may increase susceptibility to toxin.

## Other Diagnostics

- Examination of vomitus/GI contents to identify plant material. Microscopic exam may be warranted since toxicity can occur at low doses.
- Taxines identified in GI contents or blood using gas or liquid chromatography and mass spectroscopy.
- ECG findings.
  - Depression or absence of P wave.
  - Widening of QRS complex due to AV conduction delay.

## Pathological Findings

- Minimal pathological changes expected.
- Reddening and edema of stomach and small intestine mucosa from volatile irritant oils.
- Mild-to-moderate pulmonary congestion and edema with ecchymoses.

# THERAPEUTICS

Sudden death is often reported with no opportunity for treatment. Cardiovascular support is central. Arrhythmias refractory to standard therapies have been reported. Supportive care may be required for several weeks.

## Detoxification

- Induce emesis within 30–60 minutes of ingestion if no ECG abnormalities are present.
- Gastric lavage.
- Activated charcoal with cathartic, one dose.

## Appropriate Health Care

- Continuous ECG monitoring for several days post exposure.
- Supplemental oxygen or positive pressure ventilation may be needed with severe respiratory depression.
- Avoid cardiovascular stressors including exercise, transportation, and excitement for several weeks after exposure.

## Antidote

- There is no antidote.

## Drug(s) of Choice

- IV fluids for maintenance of hydration and perfusion. Fluid diuresis will not aid excretion. Adjust rate based on cardiovascular status to avoid fluid overload.

- Anticholinergic drugs for bradycardia in early exposures. Use with caution to avoid increased myocardial oxygen demand.
  - Atropine 0.02–0.04 mg/kg IV, IM, or SQ.
  - Glycopyrrolate 0.011 mg/kg IV, IM, or SQ.
- Antiarrhythmics for persistent tachycardia not responsive to IV fluids, ventricular arrhythmias, or evidence of poor perfusion.
  - Lidocaine.
    - Dogs: 2–4 mg/kg IV bolus over 30 seconds while monitoring ECG. If effective, follow by CRI of 25–80 mcg/kg/min, not to exceed 8 mg/kg/h.
    - Cats: 0.25–0.5 mg/kg IV as slow bolus while monitoring ECG. Follow with 10–20 mcg/kg/min CRI if effective. Use with caution due to high sensitivity to CNS effects.
  - Procainamide can be considered if lidocaine is ineffective.
    - Dogs: 2–4 mg/kg IV bolus over 2–5 minutes while monitoring ECG. If effective, follow with 20–50 mcg/kg/min IV CRI or 7–10 mg/kg IM q 6–8 hours.
    - Cats: 1–2 mg/kg IV bolus slowly over 20 minutes. For maintenance, 3–8 mg/kg PO q 6–8 hours. Rarely used but can be considered with refractory arrhythmias.
- Antiemetics prior to activated charcoal to decrease aspiration risk and control severe or persistent vomiting.
  - Maropitant 1 mg/kg SQ or IV over 1–2 minutes q 24 hours.
  - Ondansetron 0.1–1 mg/kg IV q 12 hours for dogs; 0.1–1 mg/kg IV, SQ, IM q 6–12 hours for cats.
- GI protectants as needed for gastritis.
  - $H_2$-blockers: famotidine 0.5–1 mg/kg PO, SQ, IM, IV q 12–24 hours.
  - Proton pump inhibitors.
    - Omeprazole 0.5–1 mg/kg PO q 24 hours.
    - Pantoprazole 0.7–1 mg/kg IV q 24 hours.
  - Sucralfate 0.25–1 g PO q 8 hours if evidence of GI ulcers.
- Seizure and aggression control as needed.
  - Diazepam 0.25–0.5 mg/kg IV PRN up to three doses.
  - Midazolam 0.1–0.5 mg/kg IV, IM PRN up to two doses or 0.25–0.4 mg/kg/h CRI.
  - Phenobarbital 4–8 mg/kg IV PRN or levetiracetam 30–60 mg/kg IV over 5–15 minutes if not responsive to benzodiazepines.

## Alternative Drugs

- Intravenous lipid emulsion has been used successfully in human patients with arrhythmias refractory to antiarrhythmic therapies.

## Extracorporeal Therapy

- Extracorporeal membrane oxygenation and external cardiac pacing have been used successfully in human patients.

## Patient Monitoring

- Continuous ECG monitoring for several days post exposure for widening of QRS complexes, third-degree AV block, sinus or supraventricular bradycardia, ventricular tachycardia or fibrillation, and cardiac arrest. Control of arrhythmias indicates effectiveness of treatment.

## Diet

- A bland diet may be necessary until gastritis resolves.

**COMMENTS**

### Prevention/Avoidance

- Prevention is paramount.
- Avoid planting *Taxus* spp. in areas accessible to pets.
- Do not use yew branches as chew sticks or playthings.
- Discard clippings from yew shrubs and trees away from pets. Do not use leaves or clippings for bedding.

### Expected Course and Prognosis

- Acute death is possible.
- Prognosis is fair to guarded in symptomatic patients.
- Prognosis improves with early decontamination and intervention.

### See Also

Chapter 22 Beta Receptor Antagonists (Beta-blockers)
Chapter 24 Calcium Channel Blockers
Chapter 101 Organophosphorus and Carbamate Anticholinesterase Pesticides
Chapter 108 Azaleas and Rhododendrons
Chapter 112 Cardiac Glycosides
Chapter 120 Yesterday, Today, and Tomorrow Plant

### Abbreviations

See Appendix 1 for a complete list.

### Suggested Reading

Burrows GE, Tyrl, RJ. *Toxic Plants of North America*, 2nd edn. Ames: John Wiley & Sons, 2013.
Cope RB. The dangers of yew ingestion. *Vet Med* 2005;100(9):646–650.
Rutkiewicz A, Schab P, Kibicius A. Yew poisoning – pathophysiology, clinical picture, management and perspective of fat emulsion utilization. *Anaesthesiol Intens Ther* 2019;51:404–408.
Wilson CR, Hooser SB. Toxicity of yew (*Taxus* spp.) alkaloids. In: Gupta RC (ed.) *Veterinary Toxicology: Basic and Clinical Principles*, 3rd edn. St Louis: Elsevier, 2018; pp. 947–954.

### Acknowledgment

The authors and editors acknowledge the prior contribution of Catherine M. Adams, DVM, who authored this topic in the previous edition.

**Author**: Rebecca Anderson, DVM
**Consulting Editor**: Lynn R. Hovda, RPh, DVM, MS, DACVIM

# Rodenticides

# Chapter 122

# Anticoagulant Rodenticides

## DEFINITION/OVERVIEW

- Anticoagulant rodenticide (AR) toxicosis is a coagulopathy caused by reduced circulation of vitamin $K_1$-dependent clotting factors.
- Newer second-generation anticoagulant rodenticides (SGARs) are generally more toxic and some persist longer than older first-generation anticoagulant rodenticides (FGARs), often requiring a longer duration of treatment.
- ARs are commonly marketed as pellets or paraffin blocks under a variety of trade names (Figure 122.1).
- EPA restrictions, issued in 2008 and fully implemented in 2011, regarding availability of SGARs in consumer outlets were designed to decrease exposure of nontarget species such as dogs and cats to products containing them. Some states have further restricted the use of SGARs.

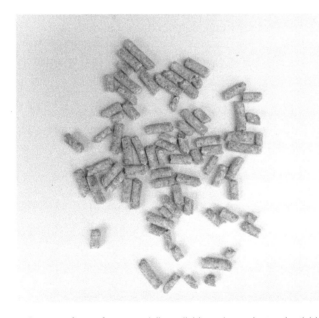

■ Figure 122.1 Common form of commercially available anticoagulant rodenticide bait pellets.

---

*Blackwell's Five-Minute Veterinary Consult Clinical Companion: Small Animal Toxicology*, Third Edition.
Edited by Lynn R. Hovda, Ahna G. Brutlag, Robert H. Poppenga, and Steven E. Epstein.
© 2024 John Wiley & Sons, Inc. Published 2024 by John Wiley & Sons, Inc.

# ETIOLOGY/PATHOPHYSIOLOGY

## Mechanism of Action

- Reduced vitamin $K_1$ is required for carboxylation of vitamin K-dependent clotting factors II, VI, IX, and X; uncarboxylated clotting factors do not bind calcium sufficiently to participate in clot formation.
- Carboxylation of these clotting factors oxidizes vitamin $K_1$ to the inactive epoxide form.
- ARs inhibit vitamin $K_1$ epoxide reductase, DT-diaphorase, and possibly other enzymes involved in the reduction of vitamin $K_1$-epoxide to vitamin $K_1$.
- After exposure to a toxic dose of AR, circulating carboxylated clotting factors decline sufficiently for hemorrhage and potentially death to occur in untreated animals.

## Pharmacokinetics – Absorption, Distribution, Metabolism, Excretion

- Readily absorbed (90%) from the gastrointestinal tract.
- Peak plasma concentrations occur 1–12 hours post ingestion.
- Bind to plasma proteins, providing an inactive reservoir until released and transported to the liver.
- Concentrated in the liver; this may involve enterohepatic recycling.
- Some are metabolized in the liver to hydroxyl metabolites that are excreted in urine.
- Plasma half-life ranges from hours for some FGAR products like warfarin to days for SGARs like brodifacoum, bromadiolone, or difethialone.
- Warfarin passes into human milk. Limited evidence of AR in the milk of animals has also been reported. Clinically, it is best to assume that nursing puppies or kittens may be exposed if the dam has been exposed.
- Limited cases of transplacental transfer of some AR have also been reported.

## Toxicity

- General.
  - FGARs (i.e., warfarin, pindone, diphacinone, and chlorophacinone) had historically been replaced by more potent SGARs; however, following EPA and select state governments (e.g., California) reducing access to or banning use of SGARs, FGARs made a commercial resurgence. The most common currently used is diphacinone.
  - SGARs (i.e., brodifacoum, bromadiolone, difethialone, and difenacoum) are generally more toxic and some are more persistent in the body than FGARs.
  - Consumption of bait often precedes clinical hemorrhage by 2–5 days.
- Dogs and cats.
  - Brodifacoum: oral $LD_{50}$ for dogs = 0.25 mg/kg; oral $LD_{50}$ for cats = 25 mg/kg.
  - Bromadiolone: oral $LD_{50}$ for dogs = 10–15 mg/kg; oral $LD_{50}$ for cats = >25 mg/kg.
  - Chlorophacinone: oral $LD_{50}$ for dogs = 0.9–9 mg/kg; oral $LD_{50}$ for cats = 15 mg/kg.
  - Difenacoum: oral $LD_{50}$ for dogs = 50 mg/kg; oral $LD_{50}$ for cats = 100 mg/kg.
  - Difethialone: oral $LD_{50}$ for dogs = 4 mg/kg; oral $LD_{50}$ for cats = >16 mg/kg.
  - Diphacinone: oral $LD_{50}$ for dogs = 0.9–9 mg/kg; oral $LD_{50}$ for cats = 15 mg/kg.
  - Warfarin: oral $LD_{50}$ for dogs = 20–50 mg/kg; oral $LD_{50}$ for cats = 5 mg/kg.

## Systems Affected

- Hemic/lymphatic/immune – depletion of activated clotting factors resulting in hemorrhage.
- Gastrointestinal – oral, gastric, intestinal, or colonic bleeding.
- Respiratory – massive pulmonary hemorrhage and hemothorax can cause sudden death.

- Neuromuscular – hemorrhage within the CNS compresses neural tissue in the cranium or spinal canal, causing ataxia, tetraparesis, and seizures in rare cases.
- Musculoskeletal – large intramuscular hematomas following injection, lameness secondary to hemarthrosis; muscle hemorrhage occurs in response to trauma.
- Renal hemorrhage – leads to hematuria.
- Reproductive – placental hemorrhage can lead to abortion; vaginal bleeding may also occur.

 # SIGNALMENT/HISTORY

## Risk Factors

- Rodenticide products are more commonly used in the spring and fall, so exposure increases during these times.
- Dogs and cats are primarily affected, with a much higher prevalence in dogs.
- No breed or gender predilections.
- Younger animals may ingest bait more readily than older animals due to their curious nature.
- SGARs persist in the body for months to years so subsequent exposures lead to added risk.
- Per Pet Poison Helpline, a national 24/7 animal poison control center, exposures to SGARs have been steadily declining since 2011 due to the EPA restriction of consumer rodenticide products to those containing FGARs or non-ARs. Instead, exposures to bromethalin have increased. See Suggested Reading for details of the decision.

## Historical Findings

- Baits are often sold as pellets or blocks of various sizes.
- Most baits are colored to distinguish them as a pesticide. However, specific identification of one type of product is difficult based on color alone. Common bait colors: green, blue-green, red, or brown/tan.
- Coughing, dyspnea, tachypnea, or exercise intolerance are often the first clinical signs.
- Less commonly, SQ swellings, joint swelling, or bleeding from body orifices are observed.
- Rarely, death is the first evidence of poisoning.

## Location and Circumstances of Poisoning

- Often in or around buildings where rodent baits are placed.
- Prevalence increased by careless placement without protective bait stations (which are required).
- Exposure may be acute with a single large dose or multiple small doses.

 # CLINICAL FEATURES

## Physical Examination

- Evidence of hemorrhagic shock (i.e., tachycardia, hypovolemia, hypotensive, poor pulse quality, pallor).
- Coughing, dyspnea, tachypnea, pale mucous membranes.
- Hemarthrosis, lameness, presence of SQ hematomas.

- Exercise intolerance, lethargy, depression.
- Hematomas – often ventral and at venipuncture sites.
- Bleeding from body orifices, periorbital bleeding.
- Epistaxis, vaginal or rectal bleeding.
- Muffled heart or lung sounds.

## Systemic Signs

- Clotting factor depletion results in generalized ecchymotic hemorrhages and often frank bleeding from many body sites.
- Oral, gastric, intestinal, or colonic bleeding characterized by epistaxis, hemoptysis, hematemesis, melena, or hemorrhagic diarrhea; severe hemorrhage can result in anemia.
- Coughing, dyspnea, abnormal auscultation (i.e., moist rales, increased bronchovesicular sounds, dull ventral lung sounds, etc.), muffled heart sounds, massive pulmonary hemorrhage, hemothorax, exercise intolerance.
- Acute anemia, hypoxemia, respiratory arrest, and sudden death may follow acute pulmonary bleeding.
- Evidence of hemorrhagic shock secondary to blood loss, hypovolemia, or poor cardiac filling may be seen.
- Pericardial effusion (evidenced by muffled heart sounds, presence of VPCs, pulse deficits, vomiting, collapse, etc.) may be seen with toxicosis, resulting in poor cardiac filling and signs of hypovolemic shock.
- Hemarthrosis results in general or asymmetrical lameness.
- Rarely, hemorrhage compresses neural tissue in the cranium or spinal canal, resulting in CNS signs including ataxia, lethargy, blindness, and occasionally seizures. Spinal bleeding can cause paraplegia or quadriplegia.
- Muscle hemorrhage occurs in response to trauma or IM injection.
- Hematuria.
- Placental hemorrhage can lead to abortion; vaginal bleeding possible.

# DIFFERENTIAL DIAGNOSIS

- IMT – platelet count <10 000–15 000 × 10³/microliter.
- Coagulation factor deficiency from acute or chronic liver disease. Assay for related factor deficiencies, for example, factor VII, liver function, bile acids.
- DIC – association with neoplasia, sepsis, pancreatitis, other concurrent disease; laboratory evidence of elevated PT, PTT, FDP, d-dimers with thrombocytopenia.
- Hemophilia – congenital clotting factor deficiencies. Assay for related factor deficiencies, for example factor VIII.
- Fat malabsorption.
- Hemorrhagic shock from trauma, neoplasia, bone marrow suppression, IMHA.

# DIAGNOSTICS

## Clinical Pathological Findings

- Anemia – with marked hemorrhage, often acute and nonregenerative.
- Thrombocytopenia from consumptive bleeding (typically 50 000–150 000 × 10³/microliter).

- Prolonged PT and PTT support exposure to AR; PT/PTT prolongation seen at 36–48 hours after ingestion but will normalize within 12–18 hours of vitamin $K_1$ therapy. Typically, PT is prolonged more extensively and earlier (6–18 hours earlier) than PTT.
- Activated clotting time (ACT) >120 seconds supports coagulopathy.
- AR analysis of blood/serum or liver confirms exposure to a specific product.
  - Blood/serum concentrations do not necessarily correlate with likelihood of poisoning; positive results need to be correlated with clinical information.
- Anticoagulant assay of stomach or intestinal contents is rarely reliable because of the 2–3-day delay between consumption of bait and appearance of clinical signs.

## Other Diagnostics

- Thoracic radiography may detect pleural effusion (i.e., hemothorax), multilobular, alveolar infiltration (i.e., pulmonary hemorrhage), or an enlarged cardiac silhouette (i.e., pericardial effusion).
- Thoracocentesis in dyspneic patients can confirm hemothorax.
- Preliminary ultrasound of both the pleural and peritoneal cavities can reveal effusion consistent with hemorrhage.

## Pathological Findings

- Free blood in the thoracic cavity, lungs, and abdominal cavity is a common finding.
- Hemorrhage into the cranial vault, gastrointestinal tract, and urinary tract is less common; can also see hemorrhage in the subcutaneous space or within muscle bellies.

 # THERAPEUTICS

## Detoxification

- If recent ingestion has occurred, immediate emesis induction, potentially followed by administration of one dose of activated charcoal with a cathartic (if needed based on AR dose).
- If clinical signs have already developed or if the patient is already coagulopathic (based on diagnostic testing), oral detoxification is often ineffective.

## Appropriate Health Care

- Inpatient care necessary for acute crisis – provide active clotting factors.
- Correct acute signs of hemorrhagic shock with IV crystalloids, colloids, and blood products as needed. Initial shock boluses of 20 mL/kg of crystalloids can be given over 15–20 minutes during initial stabilization. Repeat 2–3 times as needed to increase blood pressure.
- The use of pRBC, WB, FFP, or FP might be necessary to increase oxygen-carrying capacity (increasing RBC count) and/or replace coagulation factors. Patients should be blood-typed prior to transfusion.
- Correct life-threatening cardiac tamponade or hemothorax. If volume resuscitation (listed above) does not improve clinical signs of hemorrhagic shock, or if dyspnea is severe, pericardiocentesis or thoracocentesis may be indicated. If the patient is stable and responding to therapy, these procedures should be avoided due to the coagulopathic state of the patient. With time, the blood will be reabsorbed and clinical signs should improve. However, if there is no response to therapy, an autotransfusion of the patient's blood from the pericardial sac or thoracic cavity can be performed via aseptic technique.
- Outpatient care can be considered once the coagulopathy is stabilized.

## Antidote

- Administration of vitamin $K_1$: oral administration is preferred if there are no contraindications such as vomiting, recent charcoal administration, or GI bleeding that may affect absorption. Bioavailability is enhanced by the concurrent feeding of a small amount of a fatty meal, such as canned dog food. Alternatively, it may be administered SQ with a small needle, in multiple locations if needed. Do not administer IM.
- Vitamin $K_1$ – 2.5–5.0 mg/kg PO divided q 12 hours (preferred) or PO q 24 hours for two weeks (warfarin) or four weeks (all others, even if they are an FGAR).

## Precautions/Interactions

- Sulfonamides, many NSAIDs, and other highly protein-bound compounds may displace AR from plasma-binding sites, leading to more free rodenticide.
- Concurrent use of NSAIDs or other drugs that inhibit platelet function is discouraged due to exacerbation of coagulopathy.
- Vitamin $K_3$ – not efficacious in the treatment of toxicosis; contraindicated.
- Intravenous vitamin $K_1$ – reported anaphylactic reactions; avoid this route of administration.
- Avoid unnecessary surgical procedures and unnecessary parenteral injections until coagulation parameters are within normal limits (e.g., ACT, PT, PTT).
- Minimize stress, trauma, and jugular venipuncture or cystocentesis. Catastrophic bleeding can occur as a result.
- Use the smallest possible needle when giving an injection or collecting samples. Phlebotomy sites should be held off adequately to ensure appropriate clot formation.

## Diet

- Feed a nutritious high-quality protein diet to support coagulation factor synthesis.

## Surgical Considerations

- Thoracocentesis may be important for removing free thoracic blood, which causes dyspnea and respiratory failure, but should only be performed when life-threatening, severe dyspnea or hypoxemia is evident.
- Coagulopathies must be corrected prior to surgery.

## Patient Monitoring

- Confine patient during the early stages; activity enhances blood loss.
- PT – assess efficacy of therapy; monitor for 48–72 hours after discontinuation of vitamin $K_1$ therapy; if PT is still prolonged, an additional two weeks of vitamin $K_1$ therapy should be given. Recheck PT again following final dose as before.
- There is no need to check PT, ACT, or PTT while patients are on vitamin $K_1$ therapy as these coagulation panels should be normal while on therapy. Follow-up blood work should be monitored upon discontinuing vitamin $K_1$ therapy.
- Do not discontinue vitamin $K_1$ medication, even if the patient appears completely healthy, without checking coagulation parameters to ensure treating for the adequate duration of time.

**COMMENTS**

## Prevention/Avoidance

- Do not allow animals to have access to AR; place out of reach of pets and children.
- Bait stations are now required although their effectiveness at preventing toxicosis in nontarget species is unknown and some may be readily torn apart by pets.
- Baits transported and hoarded by rodents could be consumed by nontarget species.

## Possible Complications

- Warn client that reexposure could be a serious problem; remove all bait from the environment before sending the patient home.
- Stress importance of continuing vitamin $K_1$ for the full prescribed period otherwise recurrence of serious hemorrhage can occur.
- Pregnant animals can abort after acute crisis due to placental hemorrhage and detachment.
- A nursing mother that ingested a toxic amount should be treated; the puppies or kittens will also need to be treated for the full duration of time with vitamin $K_1$ therapy.

## Expected Course and Prognosis

- If the patient survives the first 48 hours of acute coagulopathy, the prognosis improves.
- Ensure vitamin $K_1$ therapy is administered for the advised duration based on the specific AR.
- Early decontamination after exposure most often precludes the need for vitamin $K_1$ therapy, but coagulation parameters need to be checked 48–72 hours after decontamination if no vitamin $K_1$ is administered.

## Abbreviations

See Appendix 1 for a complete list.
- AR = anticoagulant rodenticide
- FGAR = first-generation anticoagulant rodenticide
- SGAR = second-generation anticoagulant rodenticide
- FFP = fresh frozen plasma

## Suggested Reading

EPA Risk Mitigation Decision for Ten Rodenticides. May 28, 2008.

Haines B. Anticoagulant rodenticide ingestion and toxicity: a retrospective study of 252 canine cases. *Aust Vet Pract* 2008;38:38–50.

Lawson C, O'Brien M, McMichael M. Upper airway obstruction secondary to anticoagulant rodenticide toxicosis in five dogs. *J Am Anim Hosp Assoc* 2017;52:236–241.

Murphy MJ, Talcott PA. Anticoagulant rodenticides. In: Peterson ME, Talcott PA (eds) *Small Animal Toxicology*, 3rd edn. St Louis: Elsevier, 2013; pp. 435–446.

Pachtinger GE, Otto CM, Syring RS et al. Incidence of prolonged prothrombin time in dogs following gastrointestinal decontamination for acute anticoagulant rodenticide ingestion. *J Vet Emerg Crit Care* 2008;18:285–291.

## Acknowledgment

The author and editors acknowledge the prior contributions of Michael Murphy, DVM, JD, PhD, DABVT, DABT, who authored this chapter in previous editions and provided expertise for the current version.

Author: Ahna G. Brutlag, DVM, MS, DABT, DABVT
Consulting Editor: Robert H. Poppenga, DVM, PhD, DABVT

# Chapter 123

# Bromethalin

## DEFINITION/OVERVIEW

- Bromethalin is a rodenticide that produces marked CNS effects. Rodenticide baits often contain 0.01% or 0.025% bromethalin.
- Minimal lethal doses are approximately 0.25 and 1 mg/kg in cats and dogs, respectively.
- Chemical name: N-methyl-2,4-dinitro-N-[2,4,6-tribromophenyl]-6-[trifluoromethyl] benzeneamine.

## ETIOLOGY/PATHOPHYSIOLOGY

- Poisonings arising from exposure to bromethalin-based rodenticides are increasingly observed in veterinary medicine. Most veterinary cases will involve accidental ingestion but deliberate exposures have also been reported.
- Trade names for rodenticdes that contain bromethalin include Tomcat®, Talpirid Mole Bait®, Top Gun®, Fastrac®, and others.

### Mechanism of Action

- Bromethalin is not an anticoagulant rodenticide and vitamin $K_1$ is not an antidote.
- Bromethalin uncouples oxidative phosphorylation, resulting in reduced ATP production, impaired sodium and potassium pump function, cerebral edema, and elevated CSF pressure.
- Lipid peroxidation also occurs.

### Pharmacokinetics – Absorption, Distribution, Metabolism, Excretion

- Bromethalin is rapidly absorbed from the gastrointestinal tract.
- Peak plasma concentrations occur within 4–6 hours of ingestion.
- Bromethalin is highly lipophilic and is widely distributed to the brain, fat, liver, and kidney.
- Hepatic metabolism to an N-demethylated intermediate (desmethylbromethalin) is required for toxicosis to occur. Species with limited N-demethylase activity (e.g., guinea pigs) are generally resistant to bromethalin poisoning.
- Bromethalin is excreted in the bile and undergoes enterohepatic recirculation that can delay clearance from the body (half times of elimination >3–6 days).

*Blackwell's Five-Minute Veterinary Consult Clinical Companion: Small Animal Toxicology*, Third Edition.
Edited by Lynn R. Hovda, Ahna G. Brutlag, Robert H. Poppenga, and Steven E. Epstein.
© 2024 John Wiley & Sons, Inc. Published 2024 by John Wiley & Sons, Inc.

## Toxicity

### Dogs

- $LD_{50}$ in dogs is 2.4–3.7 mg bromethalin/kg BW.
- Minimum lethal dose is approximately 1 mg bromethalin/kg BW.

### Cats

- $LD_{50}$ in cats is 0.54 mg bromethalin/kg BW.
- Minimum lethal dose is approximately 0.25 mg bromethalin/kg BW.

## Systems Affected

- Nervous – CNS depression, ataxia, muscle tremors, seizures, paresis/paralysis, hyperthermia, coma.
- Ophthalmic – abnormal PLR, anisocoria, nystagmus.
- Gastrointestinal – anorexia, nausea, vomiting (uncommon).
- Respiratory – respiratory depression (may contribute to morbidity).

 # SIGNALMENT/HISTORY

- Canines are more commonly reported to ingest rodenticides, including bromethalin-based products, than felines.
- Younger animals tend to be more likely to consume rodenticides.
- No breed or age specificity is seen.
- Also a concern in birds and wildlife.

## Risk Factors

- Cats are more sensitive to toxicosis than dogs.
- Cats may be at risk of relay toxicity from the ingestion of poisoned rodents.
- Repeated ingestions may produce clinical signs of toxicosis.

## Historical Findings

- Owners may report tan, green, or greenish blue material in the feces.
- Owners may observe the exposure or see evidence of exposure (e.g., damaged bait boxes, rodenticide packages).
- The pet owner often notes clinical signs including ataxia, CNS depression, and lethargy.

## Location and Circumstances of Poisoning

- Often occurs in the garage and other locations where rodenticides are used or stored.

 # CLINICAL FEATURES

- Ingestion of supralethal doses of bromethalin ($\geq LD_{50}$) may result in an acute onset of CNS excitation, muscle tremors, and seizures.
- Ingestion of lower doses of bromethalin ($<LD_{50}$) may result in a delayed syndrome that develops within 2–7 days following ingestion; however, delays of up to two weeks may occur.

- Common clinical signs include anorexia, progressive ataxia, paresis and hindlimb paralysis, moderate-to-severe CNS depression, fine muscle tremors, and focal motor or generalized seizures. Abnormal PLR, anisocoria, and nystagmus are often seen.
- Forelimb extensor rigidity and decerebrate postures are often seen when an animal is placed in dorsal recumbency.
- With mild poisoning, clinical signs may resolve within 1–2 weeks of onset of clinical signs, although signs can persist for up to 4–6 weeks in some animals.
- Prognosis is very guarded in severely affected animals.

# DIFFERENTIAL DIAGNOSIS

- Other toxicants with sedative and/or CNS depressant effects.
- Primary neurological disease (e.g., inflammatory, infectious, infiltrative).
- Primary metabolic disease (e.g., hypoglycemia, hepatic encephalopathy).

# DIAGNOSTICS

## Clinical Laboratory Findings

- Diagnosis is dependent upon a history of exposure to a potentially toxic dose of a bromethalin-based rodenticide and the development of consistent clinical signs, the presence of diffuse white matter vacuolization on postmortem examination, and analytical confirmation of bromethalin or its desmethyl metabolite in tissues.
- Alterations in routine serum electrolytes and chemistries are not anticipated unless dehydration is present.
- CSF from bromethalin-poisoned dogs generally reveals normal cytology, protein concentration, specific gravity, and cell count.
- EEG abnormalities may include spike and spike-and-wave activity, marked voltage depression, and abnormal high-voltage, slow-wave activities.
- Neuroimaging (MRI) may reveal T2 hyperintensity of brain and spinal cord white matter.
- Detection of desmethyl metabolite in serum/plasma and tissues.

## Pathological Findings

- Lesions are generally confined to the CNS.
  - Gross evidence of cerebral edema may occur but is often mild.
  - Histopathological changes include spongy degeneration (white matter vacuolization) in the cerebrum, cerebellum, brainstem, spinal cord, and optic nerve white matter due to myelin edema.
  - Some lethal exposures result in an absence of spongy degeneration of the white matter.
- Analytical chemical confirmation of bromethalin or its desmethyl metabolite in fresh frozen fat, liver, kidney, and brain tissue.
- Bromethalin has been detected in formalin-fixed human liver and brain samples by gas chromatography with mass spectrometry detection.

# THERAPEUTICS

## Detoxification

- Gastrointestinal tract decontamination including early induction of emesis in asymptomatic animals.
- Repeated administration of activated charcoal (0.5–1 mg/kg PO q 4–8 hours for at least 2–3 days). An osmotic cathartic (sodium sulfate 125 mg/kg PO) is given once with the first dose of activated charcoal. Discontinue activated charcoal if hypernatremia occurs.
- The ASPCA Animal Poison Control Center (APCC) has recommended the judicious use of intravenous lipid emulsions (ILE) in cases of severe intoxication with bromethalin. Use 20% intravenous lipid emulsions: bolus dose of 1.5 mL/kg over 2–3 minutes or a continuous rate infusion of 0.25 mL/kg/min for 30–60 minutes. Check serum q 2 hours until it becomes clear; repeat as needed; if no clinical improvement after three doses, discontinue. Adverse effects of ILE may relate to contamination of the lipid product or direct reaction to the emulsion. Efficacy of ILE is not proven.

## Drugs and Antidotes of Choice

- There are no known effective antidotes for bromethalin.
- Control of cerebral edema with mannitol (250 mg/kg, q 6 hours IV), dexamethasone (2 mg/kg, q 6 hours IV), and furosemide (1–2 mg/kg, q 6 hours IV) has been recommended but shown to have limited clinical efficacy.
- Diazepam (1–2 mg/kg, as needed, IV) and/or phenobarbital (5–15 mg/kg, as needed, IV) may be given to control severe muscle tremors and seizures.
- Methocarbamol (55–220 mg/kg IV, to effect PRN) for control of muscle tremors in the absence of seizures. Do not exceed 330 mg/kg in 24 hours. Monitor for excessive sedation and respiratory depression with high-dose therapy.

## Appropriate Health Care

- Hospitalization is often required to manage severe CNS and respiratory depression.
- If respiratory function is compromised, a cuffed endotracheal tube should be placed and ventilation supported mechanically as required.
- Maintaining normal body temperature is important.
- Monitor blood pressure and blood glucose frequently and treat appropriately.
- Bromethalin toxicosis can result in severe CNS depression/coma, and appropriate nursing care is imperative. Patients should be kept in a padded cage and should be turned q 6 hours to prevent atelectasis.
- Ophthalmic lubrication may be necessary q 6 hours.
- Keep the patient clean and dry.

## Precautions/Interactions

- Contraindications for the use of mannitol include renal disease, pulmonary edema, dehydration, and intracranial hemorrhage.
- Animals receiving mannitol therapy may become dehydrated during treatment.
- Rehydration of some animals is associated with a worsening of clinical signs, possibly due to rebound cerebral and pulmonary edema. Maintenance of hydration is important and can be more safely accomplished through the administration of oral fluids.

## Patient Monitoring

- Acid–base monitoring is recommended in symptomatic animals.
- Blood glucose concentrations should be monitored frequently.

## Diet

- Moderately to severely affected animals should have food and water withheld to prevent aspiration pneumonia.
- Enteral or parenteral feeding if prolonged neurological complications preclude oral nutrition.

## Activity

- Patients should be restricted from activity until clinical signs resolve, as ataxia and CNS depression will be apparent. Once clinical signs resolve, no exercise restriction is necessary.

# COMMENTS

### Prevention/Avoidance

- Prevent access of pets to all pesticides, including bromethalin-based rodenticides.
- Early treatment is also important. Clients should be encouraged to contact their veterinarian if a pesticide exposure has occurred or an animal is displaying unusual clinical signs.

### Expected Course and Prognosis

- Cases involving only mild signs may resolve with close monitoring and supportive care within a 3–7-day period.
- Follow-up is generally unnecessary, as patients are clinically normal once signs resolve.
- The prognosis is guarded to poor in cases involving severe CNS or respiratory system depression, coma, or paralysis.

### Abbreviations

See Appendix 1 for a complete list.

### Suggested Reading

Feldman R, Stanton M, Borys D, Kostic M, Gummin D. Medical outcomes of bromethalin rodenticide exposures reported to US poison centers after federal restriction of anticoagulants. *Clin Toxicol* 2019;57(11):1109–1114.

Gwaltney-Brant S, Meadows I. Use of intravenous lipid emulsions for treating certain poisoning cases in small animals. *Vet Clin North Am Small Anim Pract* 2012;42:251–262.

Kent M, Glass EN, Boozer L et al. Correlation of MRI with the neuropathologic changes in two cats with bromethalin intoxication. *J Am Anim Hosp Assoc* 2019;55(3):e55302.

Murthy VD, McLarty E, Woolard KD et al. Case report: MRI, clinical, and pathological correlates of bromethalin toxicosis in three dogs. *Front Vet Sci* 2022;9:879007.

Pasquale-Styles MA, Sochaski MA, Dorman DC. Fatal bromethalin poisoning. *J Forensic Sci* 2006;51(5):1154–1157.

Peterson ME. Bromethalin. *Top Compan Anim Med* 2013;28(1):21–23.

Romano MC, Loynachan AT, Bolin DC et al. Fatal bromethalin intoxication in 3 cats and 2 dogs with minimal or no histologic central nervous system spongiform change. *J Vet Diagn Invest* 2018;30:642–645.

Seguel M, McManamon R, Reavill D et al. Neuropathology of feral conures with bromethalin toxicosis. *Vet Pathol* 2022;59:489–492.

**Author**: David C. Dorman, DVM, PhD, DABVT, DABT
**Consulting Editor**: Robert H. Poppenga, DVM, PhD, DABVT

# Chapter 124

# Cholecalciferol

## DEFINITION/OVERVIEW

- Vitamin D is part of dietary requirements. Its sources include foods, vitamin supplements, and biosynthesis with dermal sun exposure.
- It maintains physiological serum calcium and phosphate concentrations within reference ranges.
- The important vitamin D compounds include ergocalciferol (vitamin $D_2$), produced by plants, fungi and yeasts, and cholecalciferol (vitamin $D_3$), produced by animals. Ergocalciferol has a much wider safety margin than cholecalciferol.
- The primary cholecalciferol intoxication sources for dogs and cats are rodenticides and human dietary supplements and medications (e.g., antipsoriasis creams), and less commonly, improperly formulated commercial or homemade pet foods and certain calcitriol glycoside-containing plants (e.g., *Cestrum* [jasmine] spp.).
- Vitamin $D_3$ is expressed as mg/kg or international units (IU); 1 IU is equivalent to 0.025 mcg while 1 mcg is equivalent to 40 IU.
- Cholecalciferol-containing rodenticides are available under a variety of proprietary names, as granules, flakes, tablets, cakes, or briquettes, most often containing cholecalciferol at 0.075% w/v.

## ETIOLOGY/PATHOPHYSIOLOGY

### Mechanism of Action

- Cholecalciferol intoxication leads to hypercalcemia, and associated clinical signs.
- 1,25-Dihydroxycholecalciferol (calcitriol) is the most active cholecalciferol metabolite.
- Following ingestion, cholecalciferol is rapidly absorbed in the intestines, transported to the liver, bound to vitamin D-binding protein (gc-globulin), and undergoes hepatic 25-hydroxylation to 25-hydroxycholecalciferol (calcifediol), followed by renal 1-alpha-hydroxylation to 1,25-dihydroxycholecalciferol (calcitriol), the active form.
- In toxic exposures, calcitriol exerts negative feedback, suppressing renal 1-alpha-hydroxylase, but minimal negative feedback on hepatic 25-hydroxylase by calcium and calcitriol, resulting in persistent calcifediol production.
- Calcitriol increases intestinal absorption, renal tubular reabsorption, and bone resorption, of calcium, decreasing parathyroid hormone (PTH) synthesis.

*Blackwell's Five-Minute Veterinary Consult Clinical Companion: Small Animal Toxicology*, Third Edition. Edited by Lynn R. Hovda, Ahna G. Brutlag, Robert H. Poppenga, and Steven E. Epstein.
© 2024 John Wiley & Sons, Inc. Published 2024 by John Wiley & Sons, Inc.

- Intoxication therefore induces unregulated hypercalcemia and hyperphosphatemia. When serum calcium X phosphorus product exceeds 60 mg/dL, soft tissue mineralization occurs, particularly in the heart, kidney, and gastrointestinal tract, in dogs, and pulmonary and soft tissues in cats, manifested clinically by acute kidney injury (AKI) and cardiac arrhythmias.

## Pharmacokinetics – Absorption, Distribution, Metabolism, Excretion

- Cholecalciferol and calcifediol half-lives are 19–25 hours and ≥10 days, respectively. Cholecalciferol and its metabolites are highly lipid soluble, resulting in extremely long, week to months, terminal half-lives.
- Cholecalciferol undergoes enterohepatic recirculation.
- Following a single exposure, serum calcifediol reaches up to 20-fold its reference concentration within 24 hours. This metabolic step is unregulated, and dependent upon substrate concentration.
- Calcitriol concentration peaks within 48–96 hours post ingestion and normalizes within one week of a single exposure, primarily due to its tight regulation. The calcitriol plasma half-life is 3–7 days.
- The minimum chronic toxic dose and toxicokinetics in dogs and cats are unknown.

## Toxicity

- Individual variation; not necessarily dose dependent.
- The cholecalciferol $LD_{50}$ in dogs is 88 mg/kg (calculated based on its 0.075% concentration in rodenticides).
- Clinical signs can occur with an oral cholecalciferol dosage of 0.1 mg/kg (4000 IU/kg).
  - Dosages >0.5 mg/kg can induce hypercalcemia, hyperphosphatemia, and AKI.
- Some vitamin D analogs are potently calcemic and phosphatemic, and are potentially lethal when ingested at much lower dosages compared to cholecalciferol.

## Systems Affected

- Renal lesions – acute renal tubular necrosis, impaired calcium and phosphorus homeostasis, and metastatic calcification.
- Cardiovascular – bradycardia, ventricular arrhythmias, ECG abnormalities (e.g., shortened QT interval and ST segment, prolonged PR interval, widened QRS complex and T wave), and metastatic calcification.
- Gastrointestinal – increased gastric acid secretion and smooth muscle intestinal atony, predisposing to ulcers and hemorrhage; metastatic gastric muscularis calcification.
- Respiratory – pulmonary metastatic calcification, decreased lung compliance, edema, and hemorrhage.
- Central nervous system – variable, ranging from lethargy, ataxia, obtundation, listlessness, muscle twitching, up to seizures and coma.
- Musculoskeletal – excessive calcium bone mobilization, metastatic and periarticular calcification.

 **SIGNALMENT/HISTORY**

- All cat and dog breeds and ages are susceptible.
- Animals aged <6 months are more sensitive than adults.
- Cats are more resistant than dogs.

## Risk Factors

- Preexisting diseases (e.g., neoplasia, hyperparathyroidism, granulomatous diseases, hypoadrenocorticism, and primary kidney disease).
- Animals fed high-calcium and -phosphorus diets.

# CLINICAL FEATURES

- The latent period between exposure to appearance of clinical signs partly depends on the involved vitamin D form, the time required for its metabolic activation and overcoming physiological calcium homeostasis.
- Clinical signs become apparent usually within 12–36 hours post ingestion.
- Initial clinical signs include depression, weakness, and anorexia, followed by vomiting, melena, hemorrhagic diarrhea, polyuria, polydipsia, constipation, dehydration, and death.
- Laboratory abnormalities include hypercalcemia, hyperphosphatemia, hyposthenuria, azotemia (i.e., AKI), and metabolic acidosis.
- AKI develops within 12–36 hours post ingestion. Cardiac arrhythmias are common.
- Clinical signs may persist for weeks due to slow vitamin D product release from fat stores.
- Surviving animals might sustain ongoing chronic renal impairment and dystrophic mineralization-induced cardiac and gastrointestinal complications.

# DIFFERENTIAL DIAGNOSIS

- Hypercalcemia of malignancy.
- Chronic or acute kidney disease.
- Primary hyperparathyroidism.
- Hypoadrenocorticism.
- Osteolytic bone disease.
- Ethylene glycol toxicosis.
- Grape/raisin toxicosis.
- Feline idiopathic hypercalcemia.
- Calcium overdose (oral or injectable).
- Ingestion of calcipotriene- or tacalcitol-containing skin products.
- Granulomatous disease.
- Pheochromocytoma.
- Juvenile hypercalcemia.
- Hypervitaminosis A.

# DIAGNOSTICS

## Laboratory Findings

- Serum chemistry abnormalities: severe hyperphosphatemia and hypercalcemia (total and ionized), followed by hyperproteinemia, azotemia, hyperkalemia, and metabolic acidosis.
- Hyperphosphatemia often precedes hypercalcemia by up to 12 hours.
- Urinalysis: isosthenuria or hyposthenuria and calciuria.

- Toxicosis becomes life-threatening with serum total and ionized calcium concentrations >13 mg/dL and >6.6 mg/dL, respectively, and serum phosphorus concentration >8 mg/dL.
- Calcium X phosphorus product may exceed 130 mg/dL (values >60 pose high risk of soft tissue mineralization).

## Other Diagnostics

- Radiography or ultrasonography might show renal, gastrointestinal, and other tissue mineralization.
- Confirmatory tests, to differentiate between various etiologies of hypercalcemia, include serum PTH with total and ionized calcium concentrations, and calcifediol and calcitriol concentrations.
  - Serum PTH is low (suppressed), with high total and ionized calcium and calcifediol concentrations and normal to low calcitriol concentration.
- Specific assays for vitamin $D_3$ analogs such as calcipotriene and tacalcitol are unavailable. Such intoxications should be considered in the event of hyperphosphatemia and total and ionized hypercalcemia calcium, while PTH concentration is low, and when the history suggests possible exposure to these products.

## Pathological Findings

- Characteristic but nonpathognomonic histopathological lesions include kidney, lung, stomach, atria and major blood vessel mineralization, renal tubular degeneration and necrosis, and gastric mucosal ulceration and hemorrhage.
- Bile and kidney tissue can be tested postmortem or antemortem for 25-hydroxycholecalciferol levels.

 # THERAPEUTICS

## Detoxification

- Early gastrointestinal decontamination (within six hours post ingestion): induced emesis and/or gastric lavage.
- Activated charcoal with a cathartic initially, followed by activated charcoal *without* a cathartic, q 8 hours, for 1–2 days, to decrease enterohepatic circulation.

## Appropriate Health Care

- Baseline laboratory work: CBC, routine serum chemistry, venous blood gas analysis, and urinalysis.
- Daily serum calcium and phosphorus concentration monitoring for 5–7 days, followed by three times weekly for two additional weeks.
- The treatment goal is maintaining serum total calcium concentration <12.5 mg/dL and serum phosphorus concentration <7 mg/dL.

## Antidote

- No specific antidote is available for vitamin D intoxication.

## Drug(s) of Choice

- Administer IV 0.9% NaCl (4–6 mL/kg/h) to correct dehydration, provide moderate volume expansion and induce calciuresis.

- If urine output decreases despite adequate hydration, diuretics are indicated.
  - Furosemide 1–2 mg/kg IV, followed by IV CRI 0.5–1 mg/kg/h.
  - Mannitol bolus 0.25–1 g/kg IV.
- Enhancing renal calciuresis.
  - Furosemide 0.5–1 mg/kg/h IV, *or* 2–4 mg/kg for dogs, and 1–2 mg/kg for cats, IV/SQ/PO q 8–12 hours, as necessary.
  - Glucocorticoids: dexamethasone 0.1–0.2 mg/kg IV/SQ q 12 hours *or* prednisolone 1.0–2.2 mg/kg SQ/PO q 12 hours.
- Bisphosphonates decrease osteoclastic activity, thereby decreasing bone resorption and hypercalcemia.
  - Pamidronate is the most commonly used bisphosphonate in veterinary medicine for managing hypercalcemia, at 1.3–2.0 mg/kg, administered IV in 150–250 mL 0.9% saline, over 2–4 hours per single dose.
  - Expect serum calcium and phosphorus concentrations to decrease within 24–48 hours.
  - If their concentrations decrease, and later rebound, a second pamidronate dose might be needed, after 5–7 days. Anecdotally, extremely large vitamin D ingestions required earlier pamidronate redosing, at 3–4 days.
- Sodium bicarbonate might be considered for crisis therapy, with risk of death, to decrease serum ionized and total calcium concentrations, at 1 mEq/kg IV, as a slow bolus (up to 4 mEq/kg total dose).
- Phosphate binders are given to maintain the calcium X phosphorus product <60 mg/dL.
  - Aluminum hydroxide 10–30 mg/kg PO q 6 hours, when hyperphosphatemia persists.
- Antiemetics might be needed for persistent vomiting.
  - Maropitant 1 mg/kg SQ/IV q 24 hours.
  - Ondansetron 0.1–0.2 mg/kg IV q 8–12 hours.
  - Metoclopramide 0.2–0.5 mg/kg IV/IM/SQ/PO q 6–8 hours.
- Gastric protectants.
  - Famotidine 1 mg/kg IV slowly followed by 8 mg/kg/day IV CRI.
  - Pantoprazole *or* omeprazole 0.7–1 mg/kg IV/PO q 12 hours.
  - Sucralfate 0.25–1 g PO q 8 hours for 5–7 days, when active gastric ulceration is evident.

## Alternative Drugs

- Salmon calcitonin (Calcimar®, Micalcin®), at 4–7 IU/kg SQ q 6–12 hours.
  - Currently, calcitonin treatment is not routinely recommended due to inconsistent results, high cost and dosing frequency, limited efficacy, and tachyphylaxis.
  - Pamidronate is the first-line treatment. In nonresponders, salmon calcitonin can be considered instead of pamidronate, while all other treatment recommendations remain unchanged.

## Precautions/Interactions

- Thiazide diuretics, which induce calcium retention, are contraindicated.
- Excessive pamidronate dosing might cause hypocalcemia, hypophosphatemia, hypokalemia, and hypomagnesemia.
- Combined bisphosphonates and calcitonin should rarely be used, only in the most refractory cases. Some evidence shows that such combination might increase soft tissue mineralization.

## Diet

- Dietary calcium restriction is recommended to reduce gastrointestinal calcium uptake.

## Extracorporeal Therapy

- Hemodialysis and peritoneal dialysis (although its effect is slower than hemodialysis), with little or no calcium in the dialysis fluid, are both effective for hypercalcemia, and considered as last-resort therapies.
- Dialysis might be indicated with severe hypercalcemia and renal insufficiency or heart failure, when aggressive IV fluid therapy cannot be safely administered.

## Patient Monitoring

- Serum calcium and phosphorus concentration should be monitored daily for 5–7 days, followed by three times weekly for two additional weeks.
- The treatment goal is maintaining calcium concentration <12.5 mg/dL and phosphorus concentration <7 mg/dL.

 **COMMENTS**

### Expected course and prognosis

- The outcome depends on the duration and severity of hypercalcemia. The prognosis is good if treatment is initiated early, before hypercalcemia, hyperphosphatemia, and dystrophic mineralization ensue.
- If cardiac, renal, pulmonary or gastrointestinal tract calcification has already occurred, the prognosis is guarded to poor.
- Hematemesis is associated with a poor prognosis.
- The full treatment course might require one to several weeks.

### Abbreviations

See Appendix 1 for a complete list.
- Calcifediol = 25-hydroxy-vitamin D3 = 25-monohydroxycholecalciferol
- Calcitriol= 1,25 dihydroxy-vitamin D3 = 1,25-dihydroxycholecalciferol

### Suggested Reading

Bates N. Vitamin D toxicosis. *Compan Anim* 2017;22:700–706.
Groman RP. Acute management of calcium disorders. *Top Compan Anim Med* 2016;27:167–171.
Hostutler RA, Chew D, Jaeger J et al. Uses and effectiveness of pamidronate disodium for treatment of dogs and cats with hypercalcemia. *J Vet Intern Med* 2005;19:29–33.
Peterson ME, Fluegeman K. Cholecalciferol. *Top Compan Anim Med* 2013;28:24–27.
Rumbeiha WK, Fitzgerald S, Kruger J et al. Use of pamidronate disodium to reduce cholicalciferol-induced toxicosis in dogs. *Am J Vet Res* 2000;61:9–13.

**Authors:** Sigal Klainbart, DVM, DACVECC and Itamar Aroch, DVM, DECVIM-CA
**Consulting Editor:** Robert H. Poppenga, DVM, PhD, DABVT

# Chapter 125

# Sodium Monofluoroacetate (Compound 1080®)

## DEFINITION/OVERVIEW

- Sodium monofluoroacetate (Compound 1080®) is an odorless, water-soluble compound used as a pesticide to control rodents and other pests.
- Used in New Zealand for aerial control of opossums.
- It is currently used in livestock protection collars for sheep and goats in the United States; its use is highly regulated.
- Sodium monofluoroacetate has been found as the toxic agent of plants found in Brazil, South Africa, West Africa, and Australia.
- Compound 1080 is also a potent metabolite of 5-fluorouracil.
  - Adverse effects of 5-fluorouracil are similar to sodium monofluoroacetate intoxication.
- Intoxication in dogs results in frenzied, vocalized excitation with rapid GI evacuation.

## ETIOLOGY/PATHOPHYSIOLOGY

### Mechanism of Action

- Sodium monofluoroacetate is converted to fluorocitrate, an inhibitor of the Krebs cycle.
  - Inhibition of this cycle results in depletion of cellular energy stores, leading to cell death and dysfunction.
- Elevated plasma citrate levels occur, resulting in metabolic acidosis and chelation of serum calcium.
  - Hypocalcemia from chelation may be the cause of rapid onset of seizures.

### Pharmacokinetics – Absorption, Distribution, Metabolism, Excretion

- Hydrophilic.
- Readily absorbed by the gastrointestinal tract, lungs, and through abrasions in the skin.
- Distributed into soft tissue and organs.
- Metabolized into fluorocitrate in the liver.
- Urinary excretion.

### Toxicity

- $LD_{50}$ values.
  - Canine $LD_{50}$: 0.05–1 mg/kg BW.
  - Feline $LD_{50}$: 0.20 mg/kg BW.
  - Rodent $LD_{50}$: 2–8 mg/kg BW.
- Most products contain 0.2% sodium fluoroacetate.

---

*Blackwell's Five-Minute Veterinary Consult Clinical Companion: Small Animal Toxicology*, Third Edition.
Edited by Lynn R. Hovda, Ahna G. Brutlag, Robert H. Poppenga, and Steven E. Epstein.
© 2024 John Wiley & Sons, Inc. Published 2024 by John Wiley & Sons, Inc.

## Systems Affected

- Gastrointestinal – emesis, salivation, defecation, tenesmus.
- Cardiovascular – ventricular tachycardia or fibrillation, bradycardia (cats).
- Neuromuscular – tremors, seizures, convulsions.
- Nervous – hyperexcitability, agitation, vocalization.
- Renal/urological – inappropriate urination.
- Respiratory – respiratory failure secondary to pulmonary edema or bronchopneumonia.
- Multiple organ failure is possible secondary to hyperthermia and convulsions.

# SIGNALMENT/HISTORY

### Risk Factors

- Dogs are more likely to be poisoned than cats.
- Breed, age, or sex predilections are not known.

### Historical Findings

- Recent ingestion of carcass of animal poisoned by sodium fluoroacetate.
- Baits not protected from access by pets.
- Malicious administration to pets.

### Location and Circumstances of Poisoning

- Current registered use for sodium fluoroacetate is in livestock protection collars for sheep and goats in the United States.
- Aerial pesticide in New Zealand.

# CLINICAL FEATURES

- Clinical signs may occur as early as 30 minutes or be delayed 2–4 hours after ingestion.
- Progression of clinical signs is rapid as cellular energy levels decline.
- Dogs display CNS excitation and GI hypermotility.
- Convulsions begin after hyperexcitability.
    - Patients are usually nonresponsive to external stimuli.
- Death from ventricular tachycardia or fibrillation and/or respiratory failure secondary to pulmonary edema.
    - Anoxia that occurs during convulsions causes respiratory failure.
- Eventually patient becomes comatose, with death occurring within 2–12 hours of ingestion.

# DIFFERENTIAL DIAGNOSIS

- Strychnine – patients extremely sensitive to noise and external stimuli.
- Chlorinated hydrocarbons – hyperthermia and convulsions.
- Lead – CNS signs, GI pain and vomiting.
- Hypomagnesemia – hypocalcemia and CNS signs.
- Hypoglycemia – seizures.
- Garbage intoxication – tremorgenic mycotoxins causing CNS signs, hyperthermia, and GI upset.
- Japanese yew – CNS stimulation and GI upset.

- Methylxanthines – GI upset and CNS stimulation.
- Seizures – result of nontoxic conditions (trauma, neoplasia, infection, metabolic disorders, and congenital disorders).

# DIAGNOSTICS

## Clinical Pathological Findings

- Monitor serum calcium, potassium, BUN, creatinine, and liver enzymes.
- Hyperglycemia; two-fold serum increase.
- Metabolic acidosis.
- Citrate levels elevated at least two or more times in the heart and serum.
- Hypocalcemia is common.
  - Research in cats has shown iCa is elevated instead of total calcium.

## Other Diagnostics

- Testing can be performed on vomitus or stomach contents with a minimum of 50 g required for analysis.
- Detectable levels in urine and kidneys have been found in dead animals.
- Few laboratories offer testing; testing is available at the California Animal Health and Food Safety Laboratory (https://cahfs.vetmed.ucdavis.edu/lab-tests-fees).

## Pathological Findings

- No pathognomonic lesions.
- Rigor mortis has rapid onset.
- Cyanosis.
- Congestion of visceral organs.
- Agonal petechial hemorrhage on myocardium.
- Pulmonary congestion.
- Empty stomach.
- Enteritis.
- Flaccid pale heart in diastole.

# THERAPEUTICS

## Detoxification

- Emesis if patient is asymptomatic.
- At home, use hydrogen peroxide at 1–3 mL/kg BW; if unsuccessful, refer to veterinary hospital.
- In hospital, recommend apomorphine 0.03 mg/kg IV (preferred) or 0.04 mg/kg IM or ropinirole topically 3.75 mg/m$^2$ in dogs.
  - Do not administer to patients with seizures or that are comatose or hyperesthetic.
- In cats, xylazine 0.44 mg/kg IM can be used as emetic.
- In symptomatic patients, recommend gastric lavage with water 3–5 mL repeated until lavage fluid is clear.
- Follow gastric lavage with activated charcoal (1 g/kg BW PO) with sorbitol (4g/kg BW PO).
- Symptomatic patients should have their clinical signs controlled and once stable, gastric lavage can be performed under sedation or general anesthesia. Airway should be protected with inflated ETT, and stomach lavaged to remove product.

## Appropriate Health Care

- Emergency inpatient intensive care until clinical signs are controlled.
- Antiemetic to prevent aspiration of vomitus.
- Aggressive IV fluid therapy with NaCl 0.9%.
    - Supplement calcium and potassium based on laboratory evaluation.
    - Aid in cooling measures and perfusion.
- Control hyperthermia with ice packs, IV fluids until temperature reaches 103.5 °F.
- If acetamide is available, dissolve 15 g acetamide in 1 litre of warm 5% glucose solution and administer 10 mL/kg BW over 15 minutes. Reduce to 8 mL/kg/h CRI until the first liter is infused.
- Continue acetamide at 5 mL/kg/h until CS resolved.
- If acetamide not available, infuse 300 mg/kg sodium bicarbonate (8.4% w/v) IV CRI over 15–30 minutes or give 50% of dose as IV bolus and infuse the remaining IV slowly.
- Charcoal hemoperfusion has been successful in experimentally induced sodium fluoroacetate toxicosis in dogs.

## Antidote

- No antidote available.

## Drug(s) of Choice

- Convulsions are controlled with benzodiazepines, barbiturates, muscle relaxers, injectable or general anesthesia.
    - Phenobarbital 2–8 mg/kg IV to effect.
    - Diazepam 0.13–1 mg/kg IV or 0.5 mg/kg rectally.
    - Midazolam 0.05–0.3 mg/kg/h IV as CRI.
    - Methocarbamol 50–220 mg/kg IV to effect; do not exceed 330 mg/kg/day.
    - Propofol 3-6 mg/kg IV or 0.1 mg/kg/min CRI.
    - Inhalation anesthesia.

## Precautions/Interactions

- Never induce emesis in a convulsing patient.

## Patient Monitoring

- Monitor calcium, BUN, potassium, creatinine, and liver enzymes.
- Allow anticonvulsants to wear off to reevaluate seizure condition.

 **COMMENTS**

### Prevention/Avoidance

- Do not allow dogs to scavenge carcasses in areas where product is known to be or has been used.
- Use of dog muzzles to prevent ingestion of carcasses, especially in New Zealand and Australia.

### Possible Complications

- Liver or renal dysfunction secondary to convulsion and hyperthermia.
- Aspiration pneumonia in a convulsing patient.

## Expected Course and Prognosis

- Most cases have a poor or grave prognosis.
- Prognosis ultimately depends on amount ingested and severity of signs at presentation.
- Dogs that survive the initial 12–18 hours are not expected to have residual effects.
- Improved prognosis with early acetamide or sodium bicarbonate administration and supportive care.
- Delayed or nonaggressive treatment may result in death within hours of ingestion.

## Synonyms

Compound 1080.

## Abbreviations

See Appendix 1 for a complete list.

## Suggested Reading

Collicchio-Zuanaze RC, Sakate M, Langrafe L, Takahira RK, Burini C. Hematological and biochemical profiles and histopathological evaluation of experimental intoxication by sodium fluoroacetate in cats. *Hum Exp Toxicol* 2010;29(11):903–913.

Eason CT, Ross J, Miller A. Secondary poisoning risks from 1080-poisoned carcasses and risk of trophic transfer – a review. *N Z J Zool* 2013;40:217–225.

Goh CSS, Hodgson DR, Fearnside SM et al. Sodium monofluoroacetate (Compound 1080) poisoning in dogs. *Aust Vet J* 2005;83(8):474–479.

Parton K. Sodium monofluoroacetate. In: Peterson ME, Talcott PA (eds) *Small Animal Toxicology*, 3rd edn. St Louis: Elsevier, 2013; pp. 811–816.

**Author**: Erica J. Howard, DVM
**Consulting Editor**: Robert H. Poppenga, DVM, PhD, DABVT

# Chapter 126

# Phosphides

## DEFINITION/OVERVIEW

- Zinc phosphide has been used as a rodenticide since the 1930s and is used to control rats, mice, voles, ground squirrels, prairie dogs, nutria, muskrats, feral rabbits, and gophers.
- Aluminum phosphide is also used as a fumigant in grain storage silos and grain transport vehicles.
- OTC products containing 2% zinc phosphide are available in many states; often they are labeled only for below-ground use to control gophers and moles.
- Zinc phosphide is a gray crystalline powder commonly available in 2–10% concentrations as grain- or sugar-based baits in powder, pellet, paste, or tablet formulations.
- Formulations of phosphides commonly have a distinctive odor described as similar to acetylene, rotten fish, or garlic.
- Toxicity is secondary to the production of phosphine gas following ingestion which leads to GI, respiratory, and CNS effects.

## ETIOLOGY/PATHOPHYSIOLOGY

- Zinc (or aluminum and magnesium) phosphide exerts toxic effects due to ingestion, inhalation, or by absorption through broken skin. The most common type of exposure is ingestion with subsequent phosphine gas production.
- Phosphine gas is produced by hydrolysis in a moist or acid environment. The phosphine gas is considered a corrosive and is a direct irritant to the gastrointestinal tract (GIT), leading to anorexia, vomiting, and possible hematemesis or melena. The production of phosphine gas within the stomach may lead to gastric or abdominal distension ("bloat") and often pain.
- Profound cardiovascular and respiratory effects can lead to circulatory collapse, cardiac arrhythmias, pulmonary edema, or pleural effusion.
- The smell of rotten fish or acetylene might be noted on the patient's breath or from the vomitus.

### Mechanism of Action

- Phosphine gas is produced by hydrolysis in a moist or acid environment.
- Significant hydrolysis of zinc phosphide occurs at a pH of less than 4, whereas aluminum or magnesium phosphide will undergo hydrolysis at a neutral pH.
- Phosphine gas is considered to have direct corrosive effects on the GIT (esophagus, stomach, and duodenum).

*Blackwell's Five-Minute Veterinary Consult Clinical Companion: Small Animal Toxicology*, Third Edition.
Edited by Lynn R. Hovda, Ahna G. Brutlag, Robert H. Poppenga, and Steven E. Epstein.
© 2024 John Wiley & Sons, Inc. Published 2024 by John Wiley & Sons, Inc.

- Phosphine is rapidly absorbed from the GIT mucosa and systemically distributed.
- Phosphine can lead to the production of free radicals and oxidative stress, which cause cellular damage and inhibit aerobic respiration.

### Pharmacokinetics – Absorption, Distribution, Metabolism, Excretion

- Kinetics of phosphides are not well described.
- Given the rapid onset of clinical signs and the broad range of effects typically seen, there is presumed rapid GIT absorption and broad tissue distribution of phosphine gas.
- Significant elimination occurs in expired air after oral exposure; available information suggests this might occur within 12 hours after ingestion.

### Toxicity

- The approximate toxic dosage of zinc phosphide is believed to be 20–40 mg/kg.
- Several factors affect toxicity, including the amount of food in the stomach, the gastric acid level, and the formulation of zinc phosphide; therefore, the toxic dose varies depending on when the animal last ate.
- Anecdotally, animals that have ingested up to 300 mg/kg on an empty stomach have survived. Consumption of much lower dosages is toxic when consumed with food as a result of increased gastric acid production that promotes hydrolysis.
- Zinc phosphide ingestion can lead to emesis; therefore, the toxicity may be self-limiting in some cases.
- A dose that may produce clinical signs is estimated to be 1/10 of a lethal dose.
- Clinical signs often occur within 15 minutes to four hours; death has been reported to occur within 3–48 hours.

### Systems Affected

- Gastrointestinal – anorexia, vomiting, hematemesis, melena.
- Cardiovascular – direct myocardial damage, arrhythmias, decreased contractility, hypotension.
- Respiratory – pulmonary edema, pleural effusion.
- Hemic/lymphatic/immune – methemoglobinemia, Heinz body production.
- Nervous – ataxia, weakness, tremors, hyperesthesia, seizures.
- Renal/urological – azotemia, acute renal failure.
- Hepatobiliary – increased ALT, AST, and total bilirubin.
- Endocrine/metabolic – metabolic acidosis; electrolyte imbalances (e.g., potassium and magnesium).
- Musculoskeletal – weakness, ataxia.

 # SIGNALMENT/HISTORY

- No known breed or sex predilection.
- Common presenting complaints may include the following.
  - Acute GIT signs of vomiting, hematemesis, anorexia, bloating, abdominal pain, and melena.
  - Respiratory distress.
  - Neurological signs of ataxia, tremors, seizures, coma, or sudden death.

### Risk Factors

- Ingestion of food will decrease the gastric pH and lead to rapid phosphine gas release.
- Pet owners should be told not to feed their affected pet after exposure (e.g., piece of bread).

## Historical Findings

- Determine if there has been potential exposure to rodenticide, and if so, determine the active ingredient of the product used.
- Owners may report acute abdominal distension, pain, emesis, and a malodor noted on the animal's breath.
- In severe cases, respiratory distress, ataxia, seizures, and sudden death have occurred.

## Location and Circumstances of Poisoning

- These may be used as household, environmental, or commercially placed baits.

## Interactions with Drugs, Nutrients, or Environment

- The toxicity of this product varies depending on the exposure parameters.
- Zinc phosphide will remain stable when placed in a dry environment for two weeks, but excessive heat will lead to decreased efficacy of the baits (>122 °F).
- Exposure to moisture will cause deterioration of the product.
- Exposure to acid will lead to rapid hydrolysis and phosphine production.
- Some products are formulated to preserve stability in outdoor environments, so occasionally toxicity can persist for extended periods.

 **CLINICAL FEATURES**

- The most common initial clinical signs are vomiting, nausea, and hematemesis.
- The animal may have considerable abdominal distension or pain on palpation.
- A rotten fish odor from the animal's breath or the vomitus is characteristic.
- As phosphine gas is absorbed, there is progression to respiratory distress with labored or raspy breathing and tachypnea.
- Signs may progress to include neurological signs such as ataxia, agitation, aimless wandering or pacing, wild running and barking, tremors, and seizures.
- On PE, the gums may appear cyanotic (hypoxemia) or brown (methemoglobinemia).
- On thoracic auscultation, crackles may be noted.
- Heart rate may be rapid or slow, and arrhythmias may be evident.
- Shock can occur, as demonstrated by rapid heart rate, decreased pulse quality, and cool extremities.
- Neurological assessment will vary depending on the degree of CNS effects.

 **DIFFERENTIAL DIAGNOSIS**

- Cholinesterase-inhibiting insecticides (e.g., organophosphorus or carbamates).
- Metaldehyde.
- Serotonin syndrome.
- NSAIDs.
- Tremorgenic mycotoxins.
- Primary gastrointestinal disease (e.g., HGE, acute gastroenteritis, parvovirus, etc.).
- Primary cardiac disease (e.g., congestive heart failure).
- Secondary cardiopulmonary disease (e.g., noncardiogenic pulmonary edema from near drowning, seizures, electrocution, ARDS).
- Metabolic disease (renal, hepatic, pancreas).

# DIAGNOSTICS

- There is no in-house confirmatory test for phosphide rodenticide exposure.
- A suspected exposure, along with consistent clinical signs and an acetylene or rotten fish smell, can support the diagnosis.
- Confirmation using gas chromatography or a Dräger detector tube test can be performed through a diagnostic laboratory. The Dräger test has been validated using canine stomach contents and vomitus. Other postmortem samples for detection of phosphine include the liver and kidney.
- Blood work findings may include the following.
  - Methemoglobinemia or Heinz body formation with evidence of secondary hemolysis.
  - Clinical chemistry panel may reveal azotemia, increased liver enzymes (ALT, AST, and total bilirubin).
  - Electrolyte abnormalities, such as hypokalemia and hypomagnesemia.
  - Other changes may include decreased cholinesterase activity, increased myocardial troponin, metabolic acidosis, and hypoxemia.

## Pathological Findings

- Postmortem findings are nonspecific and include venous congestion, capillary breakdown, pulmonary congestion, interlobar lung edema, pleural effusion, hepatic and renal congestion, renal tubular necrosis (in some cases), myocardial necrosis with mononuclear infiltration and fragmentation of fibers, valvular (mitral and aortic) inflammation, and desquamated respiratory epithelium.

# THERAPEUTICS

- Treatment goals are to perform a safe and effective decontamination followed by symptomatic and supportive care.
- Given the risk of phosphine gas exposure to veterinary staff (and owners), clinical judgment and treatment in a well-ventilated area are important considerations. Depending on the patient's clinical presentation, detoxification may include induction of emesis or gastric lavage.
- Administration of an oral liquid antacid might increase gastric pH and thus limit the production of phosphine gas.
- Treatment should include gastroprotectants; monitoring for any respiratory, CNS, electrolyte, liver, or kidney effects; and subsequent supportive care.

## Detoxification

- Increasing the gastric pH via administration of an oral liquid antacid may decrease or stop the production of phosphine gas.
- Activated charcoal may help decrease the toxicity of zinc phosphide.

## Drug(s) and Antidotes of Choice

- There is no antidote available.
- Liquid antacids (such as aluminum hydroxide, magnesium hydroxide, or calcium carbonate) or 5% sodium bicarbonate administered at a dose of 0.5–1 mL/kg orally may help increase the gastric pH, which may slow or stop the production of phosphine gas. These given prior to emesis induction or at the time of gastric lavage can also protect veterinary staff due to decreased phosphine gas production.

- Single dose of charcoal at 1–4 g/kg PO.
- Respiratory – if there is evidence of hypoxemia, then oxygen supplementation or mechanical ventilation might be indicated.
- In the presence of shock and for renal protection, IV fluid therapy with either crystalloids or colloids is warranted.
- Gastroprotectants should be used due to the corrosive effects of phosphine gas on the GI mucosa.
  - Famotidine 0.5–1 mg/kg IV q 12 hours.
  - Omeprazole 0.5–1 mg/kg PO q 24 hours.
  - Misoprostol (synthetic prostaglandin analog) may be helpful, 2–5 mcg/kg PO q 8 hours.
  - Sucralfate 0.25–1 g PO q 8–12 hours.
- Anticonvulsants to control seizures.
  - Diazepam 0.5 mg/kg IV to effect or CRI at 0.5–1 mg/kg/h IV.
  - Phenobarbital 4–16 mg/kg IV to effect.
  - Propofol 1–8 mg/kg IV to effect followed by a CRI at 0.1–0.6 mg/kg/h IV.
- Methocarbamol 50–220 mg/kg IV, to effect; up to 330 mg/kg/day may be effective for tremors.
- Hepatic support.
  - S-adenosyl-methionine 18 mg/kg PO q 24 hours.
  - Silymarin/milk thistle 50–250 mg/day PO q 24 hours.
  - Vitamin $K_1$ 2–3 mg/kg PO q 12–24 hours.
  - Low-protein diet.
- Antioxidants (free radical scavengers and antioxidants can protect tissues from damage).
  - N-acetylcysteine (NAC) can help replace depleted glutathione stores, be directly cyto-protective to the myocardium, and can prevent damage by reactive oxygen species formed due to phosphine gas.
- Methemoglobinemia can be treated with NAC.
  - NAC: loading dose 140 mg/kg IV or PO, followed by intermittent dosing 70 mg/kg IV or PO q 4–6 hours for up to 72 hours.
- Analgesics may be indicated.

## Alternative Drugs

- Magnesium supplementation – there are some reports of hypomagnesemia as a result of zinc phosphine toxicosis and controversy regarding supplementation exists.
  - Magnesium plays a key role in the synthesis and activity of glutathione and other antioxidants, which may help counteract some of the damage caused by phosphine gas.
- Pralidoxime (2-PAM).
  - Rat studies have shown that phosphine causes some acetylcholinesterase inhibition.
  - Improved survival is reported with administration of pralidoxime (and atropine) in rats poisoned with aluminum phosphide.
- Melatonin has been shown to decrease tissue damage caused in several organs (brain, heart, liver, kidney, and lungs) by phosphine gas.
- Lipids.
  - There are a few clinical reports of the use of coconut oil to decrease phosphine gas production.
  - The administration of oil (vegetable or paraffin) has been shown *in vitro* to decrease phosphine gas release.

## Appropriate Health Care

- Symptomatic and supportive care.
- Hospitalization and care should be continued until life-threatening symptoms resolve.

## Precautions/Interactions

- Examination and emesis should be performed in a well-ventilated area to avoid human exposure to the phosphine gas.
- Do not feed these animals prior to induction of emesis as it may lead to increased phosphine gas production due to lowering of gastric pH.

## Patient Monitoring

- Monitoring for the development of signs in the asymptomatic patient for 12 hours is warranted.
- Close monitoring of the patient in hospital will help guide treatment.
  - Evaluation of respiratory status and hypoxemia should be done frequently on initial presentation.
  - Pulse oximetry monitoring and arterial blood gas analysis may help direct therapy.
  - Presence of hypoxemia and brown-appearing blood should alert the clinician to possible methemoglobinemia.
  - Monitoring of the acid–base status and electrolytes (i.e., ionized calcium, ionized magnesium, sodium, potassium, and chloride) may be indicated.
  - Evaluation of liver and kidney function should be repeated to assess for delayed injury.
- At-home monitoring post treatment for any evidence of GI ulceration or possible perforation.
  - Signs such as weakness, lethargy, anorexia, vomiting, retching, malaise, labored breathing, painful abdomen, etc. should prompt an immediate recheck.
  - Delayed hepatic insults have been reported.
  - Owners should watch for PU/PD, anorexia, vomiting, weight loss, icterus, etc.
  - Acute tubular necrosis is also possible.
  - Animals should be monitored for evidence of renal failure, PU/PD, vomiting, anorexia, and decreased urine production.

## Diet

- Due to the GIT effects and irritation, a bland diet is indicated for 5–7 days.

 ## COMMENTS

- This can be a very serious or lethal toxicosis.
- Decontamination should take priority, followed by symptomatic and supportive care.
- Risk of exposure to phosphine gas by owners (or veterinary staff) if emesis is induced at home, occurs in the car or clinic and not in a well-ventilated area. The owner should drive with windows down to prevent exposure to phosphine gas should the dog vomit during transport. Veterinary staff should exercise caution and perform any decontamination procedures in a well-ventilated area.

## Prevention/Avoidance

- Client education to allow safe use or placement of baits in the animal's environment.
- Discontinue use and remove baits or discontinue access to bait.

## Possible Complications

■ Acute renal failure and hepatic damage may follow sublethal exposures.
  • A follow-up clinical chemistry should be evaluated following discharge.

## Expected Course and Prognosis

■ Asymptomatic patients should be monitored for up to 12 hours.
■ Symptomatic patients should be monitored for 48–72 hours or until life-threatening signs resolve and the dog is stable enough for at-home care.

## Abbreviations

See Appendix 1 for a complete list.

## Suggested Reading

Fessesswork GG, Stair EL, Johnson BW et al. Laboratory diagnosis of zinc phosphide poisoning. *Vet Hum Toxicol* 1994;36:517–518.

Gray SL, Lee JA, Hovda LR et al. Potential zinc phosphide rodenticide toxicosis in dogs: 362 cases (2004–2009). *J Am Vet Med Assoc* 2011;239(5):646–651.

Knight MW. Zinc phosphide. In: Peterson ME, Talcott PA (eds) *Small Animal Toxicology*, 3rd edn. St Louis: Elsevier, 2013; p. 853.

Proudfoot AT. Aluminum and zinc phosphide poisoning. *Clin Toxicol* 2009;47:89–100.

Schwartz A, Walker R, Sievert J et al. Occupational phosphine gas poisoning at veterinary hospitals from dogs that ingested zinc phosphide – Michigan, Iowa, and Washington, 2006–2011. *MMWR* 2012;61(16):286–288.

**Author**: Sarah L. Gray, DVM, DACVECC
**Consulting Editor**: Robert H. Poppenga, DVM, PhD, DABVT

# Strychnine

Chapter **127**

## DEFINITION/OVERVIEW

- Strychnine is a very potent alkaloid toxin, derived from the seeds of *Strychnos nux-vomica* and *S. ignatii*. It is used to kill/control ground squirrels, mice, chipmunks, prairie dogs, rats, moles, gophers, birds, and occasionally larger predators (e.g., coyotes, wolves, dogs).
- Strychnine is very rapidly absorbed, with onset of clinical signs within 10 minutes to two hours.
- Strychnine reversibly blocks the binding of the inhibitory neurotransmitter glycine, resulting in an unchecked reflex stimulation.
- Clinical signs progress from hyperextension of all limbs, extensive muscle rigidity (i.e., with the extensor muscles being more severely affected due to more dominant tone), seizures, and finally respiratory arrest from paralysis of muscles or respiration.
- Strychnine is eliminated as hepatic metabolites; the parent compound is eliminated in the urine.
- Cause of death is due to apnea, hypoxemia, and respiratory arrest.
- Baits are available in multiple forms and concentrations, and typically range from <0.5% to >0.5%. Lower concentrations are available to the general public in some states, but concentrations >0.5% are limited to use by certified applicators.

## ETIOLOGY/PATHOPHYSIOLOGY

- Malicious poisoning is a relatively common means of exposure.
- Direct exposure to bait is more common in dogs than other domestic species, due to their indiscriminate feeding behavior.
- Relay toxicosis can occur via the ingestion of poisoned rodents and birds.
- Due to more rigid state control and regulation, strychnine toxicosis is less commonly seen.

### Mechanism of Action

- Strychnine reversibly blocks the binding of glycine, an inhibitory neurotransmitter in the dorsal horn of the spinal cord and in the CNS.
- Loss of the inhibitory effect in the nervous system results in unchecked spinal reflexes and nerve excitability to the skeletal muscles.
- Muscle tremors, extensor rigidity, seizures, and respiratory failure develop secondary to toxicosis.

*Blackwell's Five-Minute Veterinary Consult Clinical Companion: Small Animal Toxicology*, Third Edition.
Edited by Lynn R. Hovda, Ahna G. Brutlag, Robert H. Poppenga, and Steven E. Epstein.
© 2024 John Wiley & Sons, Inc. Published 2024 by John Wiley & Sons, Inc.

## Pharmacokinetics – Absorption, Distribution, Metabolism, Excretion

- Strychnine absorption is very rapid and occurs primarily from the small intestine. A significant amount may also be absorbed from the stomach as well.
- It is widely distributed in the tissues.
- Strychnine is actively metabolized by the liver.
- Parent compound is excreted in the urine.
- Complete elimination should occur by 48–72 hours post ingestion.

## Toxicity

- Oral lethal dosage.
  - Dogs: 0.5 mg/kg.
  - Cats: 0.5–2.0 mg/kg.
  - Rodents: 1–20 mg/kg.

## Systems Affected

- Neuromuscular – uninhibited nerve stimulation leads to continuous muscle stimulation and eventually to tetanic contracture
- Nervous – uninhibited nerve stimulation leads to seizures.
- Metabolic – continual muscle stimulation leads to metabolic acidosis.
- Musculoskeletal – trauma from the seizure activity can lead to musculoskeletal damage.
- Respiratory – terminal rigidity of respiratory musculature results in apnea and death.

 # SIGNALMENT/HISTORY

## Risk Factors

- Dogs and cats are quite susceptible, as well as all other species.
- All ages of animals are equally susceptible.
- Unsupervised, outdoor dogs that roam pastures, fields, etc. are at higher risk.

## Historical Findings

- The most common clinical sign is seizure activity.
- Often, owners do not see the initial signs of muscle tremors.
- Hyperthermia and metabolic acidosis are commonly observed, secondary to the extreme muscle exertion.
- Strychnine contamination of illicit drugs has been reported, primarily with LSD, heroin, and cocaine.
- Occasional history of "rodenticide exposure" or suspicions for malicious poisoning but more commonly owners do not know of the exposure.
- Occasionally, histories of carcass ingestion are reported.

## Location and Circumstances of Poisoning

- Most strychnine poisonings occur in rural areas and agricultural communities. However, it could occur in any area.

 # CLINICAL FEATURES

- Clinical signs can develop within 10–120 minutes of ingestion.
- Violent tetanic seizures may be initiated by physical, visible, or auditory stimuli.

- Extensor rigidity.
- Muscle stiffness.
- Opisthotonus.
- Tachycardia.
- Hyperthermia.
- Metabolic acidosis.
- Apnea.
- Vomiting – very rare.
- Death.
- Recovery should be less than 48–72 hours.

# DIFFERENTIAL DIAGNOSIS

- Other toxicants.
  - 1080 (fluoroacetate).
  - 4-Aminopyridine.
  - Acetylcholineseterase-inhibiting insecticides.
  - Amphetamines.
  - Antidepressants.
  - Bromethalin.
  - Caffeine.
  - Chocolate (theobromine).
  - Cocaine.
  - Lead.
  - LSD.
  - Metaldehyde.
  - Neurotoxic cyanobacteria.
  - Nicotine.
  - Pyrethrins or pyrethroids.
  - Tremorgenic mycotoxins.
  - Zinc phosphide.
- Systemic diseases: uremia, electrolyte abnormalities (e.g., hypocalcemia) and hepatic encephalopathy, CNS neoplasia, hypoglycemia, CNS disorders, heat stroke, trauma, ischemia, tetanus.

# DIAGNOSTICS

- Analysis of stomach contents, liver, kidney, blood, or urine for the presence of strychnine
  - If death is too rapid, kidney and urine might be negative.
- Death from strychnine intoxication is often rapid, with significant bait material still present in the stomach on autopsy.
  - Often, the color-coded grains or pellets (red or green) are obvious in the stomach contents.
  - The sample of choice for testing is generally stomach contents.

## Clinical Pathological Findings

- Serum chemistries will identify high CK and lactate dehydrogenase, as well as a systemic metabolic acidosis on venous blood gas analysis.
- Evidence of myoglobinuria may be present on UA.

## Pathological Findings

- Gross and histological pathology is associated with trauma from the seizure activity.
- Red or green pellets or bait stations are often found in the stomach contents.

 **THERAPEUTICS**

- Inpatient therapy may require treatment for as long as 48–72 hours.
- Primary goals are preventing dehydration, controlling seizures, maintaining cerebral perfusion, reducing ICP, preventing hypoxemia, and treating muscle rigidity. This often requires care in a 24/7 facility, mechanical ventilation with aggressive sedation, the use of mannitol (to decrease ICP), oxygen therapy, IV fluid therapy, thermoregulation, and nursing care.

### Detoxification

- Early decontamination is imperative to minimize duration and severity of clinical signs.
  - Decontamination – activated charcoal (2 g/kg PO); cathartic (sorbitol at 2.1 g/kg PO; magnesium sulfate at 0.5 g/kg PO given only once).
- In asymptomatic patients, immediate emesis induction should be performed, followed by activated charcoal with a cathartic. Because strychnine undergoes enterohepatic recirculation, an additional dose of activated charcoal, this time without a cathartic, should be given orally q 6–8 hours for 24 hours.
- In symptomatic patients, sedation, control of the airway (with an inflated ETT), and gastric lavage are imperative for recent ingestion. Activated charcoal should be administered with a gastric tube once the stomach has been thoroughly lavaged.

### Appropriate Health Care

- Strychnine poisoning is *not* treatable at home.
- Patients should be sedated in a quiet, dimly lit room, with cotton earplugs in place to prevent auditory stimulation.
- Patients should be treated with IV fluid therapy q 8 hours for 24 hours to maintain hydration, perfusion, and aid in strychnine elimination and urinary excretion.
- Control tremors and seizures. The use of anticonvulsants is imperative with strychnine toxicosis.
- Supportive care and nursing care.
  - Minimize animal stimulation to avoid inducing a seizure.
  - Control hyperthermia. Monitor temperature q 2–4 hours; implement cooling measures when temperatures exceed 105.5 °F. Cooling measures should be stopped when temperatures reach 103.5 °F.
  - Change body position and lubricate eyes q 4–6 hours.
  - Avoid nutritional feeding (orally) until clinical signs resolve in order to prevent aspiration pneumonia.

### Antidote

- No specific antidote.

### Drug(s) of Choice

- Seizure control.
  - Phenobarbital 4–16 mg/kg IV q 2–6 hours PRN.
  - Potassium bromide 100 mg/kg PO or rectally q 6 hours × 4 doses.
  - Diazepam 0.5–1 mg/kg IV to effect.

- Tremor control.
  - Methocarbamol 55–100 mg/kg IV q 2–6 hours PRN
  - Glycerol guaiacolate 100 mg/kg IV, repeated as needed.

## Precautions/Interactions

- Do not induce emesis in symptomatic patients due to risks of aspiration pneumonia and seizure stimulation.
- Do not acidify with ammonium chloride if the patient is acidotic, based on venous blood gas analysis.

## Patient Monitoring

- Monitoring for secondary renal damage from myoglobinuria and possible tubular cast development. Aggressive treatment with IV fluids should be used to prevent this.
- With use of sedation/anesthesia to control seizures, the animal can be gradually withdrawn periodically to evaluate the reoccurrence of seizure activity as a means of determining how long the treatment must be continued.
- Early significant decontamination will shorten the duration of required treatment.
- Normal activity should resume upon recovery, unless traumatic injuries limit activity.

 **COMMENTS**

- Although anesthetic intervention does not directly treat the cause of the seizures, it provides the time necessary for the animal to eliminate the strychnine.
- CAUTION: Do not induce a seizure with a stimulus as a means of diagnosing strychnine. This is *not* diagnostic and may be lethal.
- Due to potential exposure to and poisoning of children, the source of the exposure should be investigated and eliminated.
- Strychnine is degraded by soil organisms.
- Strychnine poisoning is *not* treatable at home. If exposure has occurred, have the owner bring the animal to the clinic immediately. If clients wait until clinical signs occur, the animal may be dead before it reaches the clinic.

### Prevention/Avoidance

- Prevention is limited to keeping animals away from baits or poisoned carcasses, and supervising dogs at all times (instead of free roaming).
- Prevent reexposure by removing the source of the toxin.

### Possible Complications

- Dependent on the initiation of therapy, hypoxemia that occurred prior to therapy can have permanent neurological effects.
- Renal damage secondary to myoglobinuria will gradually repair.

### Expected Course and Prognosis

- Prognosis is poor until seizures are controlled.
- Prognosis is good after seizures are controlled, but prior hypoxemia and secondary renal effects should be discussed with the owner.
- Animals that have normal neurological function at 48–72 hours should have no permanent effect.

## See Also

Chapter 1 Decontamination and Detoxification of the Poisoned Patient
Chapter 2 Emergency Management of the Poisoned Patient

## Abbreviations

See Appendix 1 for a complete list.

## Suggested Reading

Cowan VE, Blakely BR. A retrospective study of canine strychnine poisonings from 1998 to 2013 in Western Canada. *Can Vet J* 2015;56(6):587–590.

Gupta RC. Non-anticoagulant rodenticides. In: Gupta RC (ed.) *Veterinary Toxicology: Basic and Clinical Principles*, 3rd edn. San Diego: Elsevier, 2018; pp. 613–626.

Osweiler GD. Strychnine poisoning. In: Kirk RW (ed.) *Current Veterinary Therapy VIII*. Philadelphia: Saunders, 1983; pp. 98–100.

Talcott PA. Strychnine. In: Peterson ME, Talcott PA (eds) *Small Animal Toxicology*, 3rd edn. St Louis: Elsevier, 2013; pp. 827–831.

## Acknowledgment

The author and book editors acknowledge the prior contribution of Jeffery O. Hall.

**Author**: Chelsea Sykes, DVM
**Consulting Editor**: Robert H. Poppenga, DVM, PhD, DABVT

# Toxic Gases

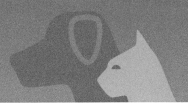

# Chapter 128

# Carbon Monoxide

## DEFINITION/OVERVIEW

- Carbon monoxide (CO) is a tasteless, colorless, and odorless gas produced by incomplete combustion of carbon compounds.
- The main source of CO is fire-related smoke inhalation, but also malfunctioning heating devices, and fuel burning systems (motor vehicle, stoves) in insufficiently ventilated areas.
- Carbon monoxide binding to hemoglobin forms carboxyhemoglobin (COHb) which impairs oxygen transport and release to tissues, resulting in severe hypoxic injury predominantly in the central nervous system and myocardium.
- Typical symptoms include acute and delayed neurological signs (agitation, seizures), arrhythmia, tachycardia, and occasionally bright red mucous membranes and skin.

## ETIOLOGY/PATHOPHYSIOLOGY

### Mechanism of Action

- CO binds to ferrous heme-containing proteins (hemoglobin, myoglobin, and mitochondrial cytochromes), altering their function.
- CO affinity for hemoglobin is 200–270 times that of oxygen. Hemoglobin's preferential binding to CO impairs transport of oxygen to the tissues, resulting in tissue hypoxia.
- COHb shifts the oxyhemoglobin dissociation curve to the left and prevents oxygen offloading to tissues.
- CO binding to mitochondrial cytochromes causes disruption of oxidative phosphorylation, subsequent decreased ATP production, and cellular death.
- CO can also directly cause oxidative damage in the central nervous system, resulting in local inflammation.

### Pharmacokinetics – Absorption, Distribution, Metabolism, Excretion

- Once inhaled, CO diffuses rapidly into the blood where it binds onto hemoglobin preferentially. It can also accumulate in the muscles by binding to myoglobin and cellular cytochromes.
- High alveolar ventilation promotes CO elimination via exhalation.

### Toxicity

- Lethality may be related to duration of exposure and concentration of CO in inhaled gas (for example in humans, inhalation of 40 000 ppm for two minutes is as lethal as 1500 ppm for 60 minutes). Experimentally, dogs can tolerate 200 ppm for 90 days without signs of toxicity. However, the CO concentration in inhaled gas is difficult to estimate clinically.

---

*Blackwell's Five-Minute Veterinary Consult Clinical Companion: Small Animal Toxicology*, Third Edition. Edited by Lynn R. Hovda, Ahna G. Brutlag, Robert H. Poppenga, and Steven E. Epstein.
© 2024 John Wiley & Sons, Inc. Published 2024 by John Wiley & Sons, Inc.

- Fatal poisoning is reported with COHb concentration >40% in humans, 54–90% in dogs, and 41–57% in cats. It is unclear whether COHb concentration directly correlates with severity of clinical signs or mortality in veterinary patients given the paucity of studies available.

## Systems Affected

- Tissues with high oxygen demand (myocardium, central nervous system) are primarily affected.
- Central nervous system – decreased oxygen delivery can cause cerebral hypoxia leading to neuronal ischemia responsible for the acute neurological signs noted. However, CO also causes direct cellular effects leading to alteration of ATP synthesis, inflammation, oxidative damage and neuronal demyelination leading to delayed neurological signs.
- Cardiovascular – myocardial ischemia, systolic dysfunction, and arrhythmias contribute the large number of prehospital deaths in humans.
- Hematological/immunological – platelet activation and neutrophil degranulation participate to cause endothelial damage, inflammation, and thrombosis and may worsen hypoxic and oxidative injuries.

# SIGNALMENT/HISTORY

## Risk Factors

- Humans with low hemoglobin concentration tend to have a higher COHb levels after CO exposure, though the significance of this phenomenon in anemic cats and dogs is unknown.
- Since alveolar ventilation is the route of elimination, patients with impaired lung function could have increased COHb concentration.
- Increasing age, history of illness, and longer duration of unresponsiveness may correlate with development of more severe or delayed clinical signs.

## Historical Findings

- Development of neurological signs ranging from ataxia to loss of consciousness, within a few hours or exposure.

## Location and Circumstances of Poisoning

- History of being in a fire or in poorly ventilated spaces with fuel-burning devices (stoves, motor vehicles, charcoal grills).

# CLINICAL FEATURES

- Acute (within few hours) and delayed (2–240 days post exposure) neurological signs such as altered mentation, ataxia, agitation, deafness, tremors, seizure, coma, and death.
- Cardiovascular abnormalities can be profound with signs such as arrhythmia, systemic vasodilation, and systolic dysfunction leading to hypotension and death.
- COHb has a bright red color, therefore "cherry red" mucous membranes and skin are possible, though its absence does not rule out CO poisoning.
- Can see concurrent smoke inhalation or fire-related injuries (burns, respiratory signs) as well as increased respiratory effort.

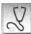

# DIFFERENTIAL DIAGNOSIS

- Primary intracranial (epilepsy, inflammatory brain disease, etc.) and extracranial (hepatic shunts, electrolyte/glycemic derangements) diseases.
- Other neurotoxic compounds causing seizures, agitation, and ataxia (bromethalin, permethrin in cats, tricyclic antidepressants, ivermectin, metaldehyde, baclofen, etc.). Exposure to such compounds can be determined by thorough questioning of the owners.
- Cyanide poisoning secondary to smoke inhalation, can also cause tissue hypoxia, neurological signs and bright red mucous membranes. Measurement of COHb levels can help differentiate CO from cyanide poisoning.

# DIAGNOSTICS

## Clinical Pathological Findings

- COHb can be detected in the blood via cooximetry. Carbon monoxide can be endogenously produced during heme catabolism, but generally does not result in COHb levels >1–4% in dogs and cats. In humans, clinical signs of CO toxicity seem to develop with COHb levels >15–20%, but correlation between COHb levels and severity of signs is controversial.
- Routine laboratory testing (complete blood count, biochemistry profile) is generally unremarkable or may reflect hypoxic tissue damage (mild stress leukogram and hyperglycemia).
- Arterial blood gas analysis might be normal in the absence of significant lung disease, since CO does not affect the amount of oxygen dissolved in the blood ($PaO_2$).
- Conventional two wavelength pulse oximeters are unable to distinguish between oxyhemoglobin and COHb. Therefore, oxygen saturation via pulse oximetry is erroneously normal despite high levels of COHb and this method should not be used to rule out CO poisoning.
- Specialized pulse oximeters are available that can measure COHb (SpCO) but they have not been validated in veterinary species.

## Other Diagnostics

- Cardiac ultrasound, electrocardiogram, and biomarker measurement could be considered in patients suspected to have signs of myocardial injury secondary to CO poisoning.

## Pathological Findings

- Histopathological findings can be suggestive, but not pathognomonic of CO poisoning. Gross pathological findings range from normal to diffusely bright red discoloration of the skin, mucosal surfaces, and muscles.
- Microscopically, cerebral necrosis has been noted in humans, although not reported in veterinary medicine. Diffuse pulmonary congestion, interstitial and alveolar edema and basophilic discoloration of cardiomyocytes was noted in two cats.

# THERAPEUTICS

## Detoxification

- Oxygen supplementation (increasing $FiO_2$) is the treatment of choice and can accelerate CO elimination by exhalation. It should be implemented as soon as possible, regardless of the patient's $PaO_2$ or respiratory status. In humans, the half-life of COHb breathing room air at normal atmospheric pressure is 320 minutes, which can be further reduced to 37 minutes with the use of high-flow nasal oxygen therapy. In dogs, the half-life of COHb was 167 minutes with high-flow nasal oxygen therapy in one case report.

### Appropriate Health Care

■ Oxygen supplementation can also increase the dissolved oxygen content high enough to reverse the patient's hypoxic state and minimize the deleterious effects on the myocardium and central nervous system.
■ Supportive care to correct neurological and cardiovascular signs is also recommended.

### Drug(s) of Choice

■ Increased $FiO_2$.

### Precautions/Interactions

■ While oxygen supplementation is recommended to accelerate CO elimination, care should be taken to avoid oxygen toxicity. A $FiO_2$ >60% for more than 12 hours is not recommended.

### Alternative Drugs

■ By increasing $PaO_2$ as high as 1800 mmHg, hyperbaric oxygen therapy can subsequently reduce the COHb half-life down to 20 minutes in humans. However, there is insufficient evidence of its beneficial effects regarding its routine use in human and veterinary medicine.

### Patient Monitoring

■ Serial COHb measurement via cooximetry could be performed to allow titration of oxygen supplementation. In human medicine, patients typically receive oxygen therapy until COHb <10% and clinical signs have resolved (~6 hours).
■ Cardiovascular monitoring (blood pressure, ECG, etc.) can be implemented in a selected population of patients.

 **COMMENTS**

■ Carbon monoxide is often called the "silent killer" so any pets exposed to a fire should be rapidly evaluated by a veterinarian even in the absence of overt clinical signs. Since respiratory distress is not a main clinical feature of CO poisoning, a common mistake would be to withhold oxygen supplementation in these patients. It is important to note that with CO poisoning, the primary purpose of oxygen therapy is promoting elimination of CO. Education of first responders to provide supplemental oxygen to pets found in house fires may be beneficial.

### Prevention/Avoidance

■ Prevention relies on avoiding exposure to carbon monoxide. Avoid leaving pets in a poorly ventilated area with fuel-burning devices.

### Expected Course and Prognosis

■ The true mortality rate of CO poisoning is unknown due to the high level of preadmission mortality.
■ Some patients may initially show clinical improvement following oxygen therapy and further develop severe delayed neurological signs. Morbidity and mortality appear to correlate with the severity of initial neurological signs.

## See Also

Chapter 129 Smoke Inhalation

## Abbreviations

- CO = carbon monoxide
- COHb = carboxyhemoglobin
- $PaO_2$ = arterial partial pressure of oxygen
- $FiO_2$ = fraction of inspired oxygen
- SPCO = saturation of arterial blood with carbon monoxide as measured by pulse oximetry

## Suggested Reading

Berent AC, Todd J, Sergeeff J, Powell LL. Carbon monoxide toxicity: a case series. *J Vet Emerg Crit Care* 2005;15(2):128–135.

Garg J, Krishnamoorthy P, Palaniswamy C et al. Cardiovascular abnormalities in carbon monoxide poisoning. *Am J Ther* 2018;25(3):e339–348.

Gazsi K, Goic JB, Butler AL. Successful treatment of carbon monoxide toxicity with high flow nasal oxygen compared to mechanical ventilation. *Vet Rec Case Rep* 2022;10(3):e388.

Sobhakumari A, Poppenga RH, Pesavento JB, Uzal FA. Pathology of carbon monoxide poisoning in two cats. *BMC Vet Res* 2018;14(1):67.

**Author**: Laurence M. Saint-Pierre, DVM, DACVECC
**Consulting Editor**: Steven E. Epstein, DVM, DACVECC

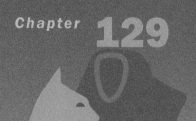

# Smoke Inhalation

## DEFINITION/OVERVIEW

- Smoke inhalation injury can occur in animals entrapped in a confined space in the presence of fire and smoke.
- Clinical signs are primarily respiratory and neurological and can have an acute and/or delayed onset.
- Severity of initial clinical signs is extremely variable and is directly dependent on the length of exposure, amount of heat generated by the fire, and type of materials combusted.
- Oxygen supplementation is considered mandatory in all patients exposed to smoke to minimize the risk of delayed neurological signs.

## ETIOLOGY/PATHOPHYSIOLOGY

### Mechanism of Action

- Smoke is generally composed of a mixture of superheated particles (soot) and fire gases. The composition of the smoke produced during combustion is unique for each fire site and depends on factors such as the type of material combusted, oxygen level, and temperature reached.
- Smoke inhalation injury has a multifactorial pathophysiology. The main processes that lead to the insurgence of clinical signs are:
    - burn injuries.
    - soot inhalation.
    - chemical irritants inhalation.
    - systemic toxicant inhalation.
- Increased environmental temperatures can result in inflammation and edema of the tissues of the oral cavity, nasal cavity, larynx, and trachea. Upper airway edema can lead to various levels of obstruction. Edema severity can be variable and can peak up to 24 hours from the initial exposure.
- Soot and chemical irritants inhalation promote the development of a severe pulmonary inflammatory response that could lead to bronchoconstriction, pulmonary vasodilation, and airway fluid accumulation. Within a few hours from the initial insult, inflammatory and epithelial component accumulation could lead to the formation of obstructive airway casts.
- Pulmonary structure disruption and the associated inflammatory process can promote the insurgence of delayed pulmonary injuries as secondary bacterial infection and/or acute respiratory distress syndrome (ARDS).

*Blackwell's Five-Minute Veterinary Consult Clinical Companion: Small Animal Toxicology*, Third Edition. Edited by Lynn R. Hovda, Ahna G. Brutlag, Robert H. Poppenga, and Steven E. Epstein.
© 2024 John Wiley & Sons, Inc. Published 2024 by John Wiley & Sons, Inc.

■ Systemic toxicity is promoted by exposure to toxic gases. The most commonly reported compounds present in smoke are carbon monoxide (see Chapter 128) and hydrogen cyanide.

■ Neurological signs can be observed in the acute phase as a consequence of decreased brain oxygenation from respiratory disease and toxin exposure. Delayed neurological signs can be observed up to days following the initial smoke exposure.

■ Smoke inhalation can promote myocardial dysfunction and lead to congestive heart failure. Additionally, exposure to CO can promote a hypercoagulable state, predisposing to the risk of thrombosis.

## Pharmacokinetics – Absorption, Distribution, Metabolism, Excretion

■ Carbon monoxide is an odorless and colorless gas, thus cannot be detected in the environment without specialized equipment (see Chapter 128).

■ Cyanide is a colorless gas, whose odor has been compared to bitter almonds although its presence might be difficult to detect at fire sites. Cyanide is a physiological metabolite in the body and is normally converted into thiocyanate by the liver and excreted by the kidneys. Large concentrations of cyanide might overcome liver metabolic function and thus result in tissue accumulation.

■ Chemical irritants present in the smoke can be inhaled at the fire site. Irritants can distribute through the tracheobronchial tree and pulmonary alveoli. Additionally, irritants can be absorbed by ingestion during grooming.

## Toxicity

■ The most toxic compounds present in the smoke are carbon monoxide and hydrogen cyanide.

■ Hydrogen cyanide toxicosis manifests at the mitochondrial level, with inhibition of the electron transport chain and impairment of cellular ATP production. Currently, there are no documented reports of hydrogen cyanide toxicity in small animal species, but it is reasonable to suspect that this toxin influences prehospital mortality.

## Systems Affected

■ Respiratory.
  • Upper airway obstruction.
    ○ Oropharyngeal, nasopharyngeal, and laryngeal burns, inflammation, and/or edema.
    ○ Tracheal necrosis with secondary airflow obstruction.
  • Lower airway damage.
    ○ Bronchitis, bronchoconstriction, and/or bronchospasm.
    ○ Mucociliary apparatus dysfunction.
  • Pulmonary parenchymal disease.
    ○ Hypoxemia.
    ○ Pulmonary edema.
    ○ Chemical pneumonitis.
    ○ ARDS.
    ○ Bacterial pneumonia (secondary).
■ Nervous.
  • Cerebral hypoxia.
  • Seizures/ataxia/aggressive behavior/blindness/deafness/stupor/coma.

- Cardiovascular.
  - Left ventricular dysfunction can occur secondary to direct myocardial damage.
  - Increased myocardial oxygen demand occurs secondary to sympathetic activation by compensatory mechanisms.
  - Carbon monoxide can lead to decreased oxygen delivery to myocardial tissue and consequently predispose to arrhythmias, congestive heart failure, and systemic hypotension.
- Ophthalmic: corneal irritation and corneal ulceration can occur secondary disruption of the natural corneal film from exposure to gaseous irritants, soot, and heat.
- Hemic/lymphatic/immune: hypercoagulability and thromboembolic disease.

 **SIGNALMENT/HISTORY**

### Risk Factors

- There are no specific species, breed, or sex predilections.
- Brachycephalic breeds could be predisposed to develop early signs of upper airway obstruction.

### Historical Findings

- Dyspnea.
- Increased respiratory rate and/or effort.
- Coughing, gagging.
- Loss of consciousness.
- Seizures.
- Ataxia.
- Superficial thermal injuries.
- Smoke odor and soot on the haircoat.
- Foaming from the mouth and/or hypersalivation.

### Location and Circumstances of Poisoning

- Animals trapped in small confined spaces in the presence of fire and/or smoke.

 **CLINICAL FEATURES**

- Respiratory system.
  - Respiratory distress.
  - Upper airway obstruction.
  - Wheezes.
  - Fine crackles.
  - Nasal discharge.
- Nervous system.
  - Altered mentation (obtundation, stupor, coma).
  - Ataxia.
  - Excitement/agitation.
  - Vocalization.
  - Seizures.
- Cardiovascular system.
  - Hyperemic mucous membranes.
  - Cyanotic mucous membranes.

- Tachycardia.
- Decreased pulse quality.
- Arrhythmias.
- Gallop rhythm (cats).
■ Ophthalmic.
  - Corneal abrasion/ulceration.
  - Conjunctival hyperemia.
  - Blepharospasm.
  - Epiphora.
■ Skin/exocrine.
  - Thermal injuries.
  - Smoke odor, soot on the haircoat, and burnt fur.

# DIFFERENTIAL DIAGNOSIS

■ Exposure to respiratory irritants could lead to pulmonary signs similar to what is observed during smoke exposure.
■ Upper airway obstruction.
■ Hypoxemia: other primary pulmonary parenchymal diseases.
■ Altered mentation.
  - Primary neurological diseases.
  - Systemic inflammatory or metabolic conditions (e.g., sepsis).
■ Excitement/agitation.
  - Stress.
  - Pain.
■ Seizures: primary structural brain diseases or metabolic causes.

# DIAGNOSTICS

## Clinical Pathological Findings

■ A rapid diagnostic test to measure cyanide plasmatic concentration is currently unavailable.
■ Pulse oximetry for oxygen saturation level should be interpreted cautiously as it can be altered by carbon monoxide.
■ Blood gas analysis.
  - Elevated $PCO_2$ (hypoventilation) may be present.
  - Low $PaO_2$ (hypoxemia) may be present. In the presence of carbon monoxide, $PaO_2$ is not expected to be decreased.
  - Hyperlactatemia, when present in the face of adequate perfusion parameters, should raise the suspicion of carbon monoxide intoxication.

## Other Diagnostics

■ Thoracic radiographs.
  - Diffuse broncho to interstitial to alveolar patterns, or a combination of those.
  - Airways (bronchial and/or tracheal) narrowing.
■ Tracheal wash cytology and aerobic culture could be considered to confirm the presence of particulate matter and of pneumonia.
■ ECG should be performed to rule out cardiac arrhythmias.
■ Echocardiography, cardiac troponin, and/or NT-proBNP could be considered in those patients in which myocardial dysfunction is suspected.

- Viscoelastic coagulation testing could be used to confirm the presence of hypercoagulability.
- Complete ophthalmological examination including tear production test (Schirmer's test) and fluorescein test should be performed.
- Serial neurological examinations are warranted to monitor the progression of clinical signs and/or the insurgence of delayed neurological signs.

## Pathological Findings

- The gross and histopathological findings are determined by the degree and nature of injury (e.g., thermal injury, inhaled toxins, soot inhalation).
- Nasopharyngeal, oropharyngeal, and laryngeal burns, erosions, ulcerations, inflammation, and edema may be present.
- Tracheal inflammation, edema, and particulate matter deposition may be present.
- Mucosal edema, mucosal sloughing, and pseudomembranous casts may also be seen.
- Histological evaluation of the pulmonary parenchyma may show particulate matter, edema, hyaline casts, intraalveolar hemorrhage, purulent material consistent with pneumonia, and atelectasis.

 # THERAPEUTICS

- During the first hours after the smoke exposure, supplemental oxygen therapy is considered mandatory, even if hypoxemia is not suspected.
- Oropharyngeal, nasopharyngeal, and laryngeal burns, inflammation, and/or edema with consequent airway obstruction might require endotracheal intubation and/or tracheostomy to bypass the obstructive area.
- In patients with hypoventilation and/or hypoxemia refractory to conventional therapies, mechanical ventilation might be necessary.

## Detoxification

- Oxygen therapy effectively decreases carbon monoxide half-life and should be used to minimize the risks of acute and delayed neurological signs.
- Fur should be accurately washed to remove any residual soot.
- Eyes should be cleaned with an appropriate rinsing solution.

## Appropriate Health Care

- Hospitalization and close monitoring are recommended in all cases. Patients should be closely observed for worsening respiratory or neurological signs.
- Supportive care that might be necessary in smoke inhalation cases includes:
  - saline nebulization for 15–20 minutes, every 4–6 hours as needed.
  - ophthalmic ointment application q 4–6 hours.

## Antidote

- Hydroxocobalamin (vitamin $B_{12a}$) is currently considered the antidote of choice for the treatment of suspected or confirmed cyanide toxicity. Recommended dosage in humans is 70–100 mg/kg IV.

## Drug(s) of Choice

- The prophylactic use of antimicrobial therapy is not recommended.
- The routine use of systemic steroids is not recommended.

- Fluid therapy should be titrated to optimize perfusion and hydration parameters, while closely monitoring for signs of fluid overload.
- Terbutaline (0.01 mg/kg IV) could be considered in cases with suspected bronchoconstriction.
- Antiemetic drugs should be considered in vomiting patients or those with a decreased level of mentation.
  - Maropitant 1 mg/kg SQ, IV q 24 hours.
  - Ondansetron 0.1–0.5 mg/kg IV q 8–12 hours.

### Precautions/Interactions

- In the past, amyl nitrate and sodium thiosulfate have been recommended to treat cyanide toxicities. The use of these drugs leads to a reduction of the overall oxygen-carrying capacity as methemoglobin formation is promoted.

### Surgical Considerations

- Patients with severe upper airway obstruction may require a tracheostomy to ensure adequate ventilation.

### Patient Monitoring

- Pulmonary function should be closely monitored via serial pulse oximetry (results might be falsely elevated in the presence of CO) or arterial blood gases. Repeated radiographs might be necessary to assess disease progression.
- Serial neurological examinations are warranted to monitor the progression of clinical signs and/or the insurgence of delayed neurological signs.

### Diet

- In patients with decreased mentation or swallowing difficulties, oral food intake should be temporarily limited. Feeding devices (e.g., nasogastric tube) should be considered in patients with or expected prolonged reduction of food intake.

 **COMMENTS**

- First responders should provide oxygen supplementation prior to arrival at the hospital.

### Possible Complications

- There is limited information about long-term complications in veterinary medicine.
- Neurological dysfunction might be permanent.
- Long-term pulmonary complications might include pulmonary fibrosis, asthma, and chronic obstructive pulmonary disease.

### Expected Course and Prognosis

- The overall mortality rate in small animal patients is difficult to estimate, as reports are scarce and highly affected by the elevated prehospital mortality and financial considerations.
- The incidence of neurological signs is variable, and delayed signs can occur within 10 hours to six days after the initial smoke exposure. In the veterinary literature, successful outcome has been reported despite significant neurological complications.
- Acute and delayed respiratory signs may vary in severity and type.

## See Also

Chapter 128 Carbon Monoxide

## Abbreviations

- ARDS = acute respiratory distress syndrome
- CO = carbon monoxide

## Suggested Reading

Ashbaugh EA, Mazzaferro EM, McKiernan BC, Drobatz KJ. The association of physical examination abnormalities and carboxyhemoglobin concentrations in 21 dogs trapped in a kennel fire. *J Vet Emerg Crit Care* 2012;22(3):361–367.

Drobatz KJ, Walker LM, Hendricks JC. Smoke exposure in cats: 22 cases (1986–1997). *J Am Vet Med Assoc* 1999;215(9):1312–1316.

Drobatz KJ, Walker LM, Hendricks JC. Smoke exposure in dogs: 27 cases (1988–1997). *J Am Vet Med Assoc* 1999;215(9):1306–1311.

Guillaumin J, Hopper K. Successful outcome in a dog with neurological and respiratory signs following smoke inhalation. *J Vet Emerg Crit Care* 2012;23(3):328–334.

Rosati T, Hopper K. Smoke inhalation. In: Silverstein DC, Hopper K (eds) *Small Animal Critical Care Medicine*, 3rd edn. St Louis: Saunders, 2022; pp. 804–809.

**Author:** Tommaso Rosati, DVM, DACVECC, DECVECC
**Consulting Editor:** Steven E. Epstein, DVM, DACVECC

# Abbreviations

| | |
|---|---|
| 2-PAM | Pralidoxime |
| 2,4-D | 2,4-Dichlorophenoxyacetic acid |
| 5-FU | 5-Flurouracil |
| 5-HT$_2$ | 5-Hydroxytryptamine |
| 5-HTP | 5-Hydroxytryptophan |
| A-V | Arterial to venous difference |
| AAFCO | Association of American Feed Control Officials |
| AAPCC | American Association of Poison Control Centers |
| AAVLD | American Association of Veterinary Laboratory Diagnosticians |
| ABCB-1 | ATP binding cassette subfamily B member 1 |
| AC | Activated charcoal |
| ACC | Activated charcoal with cathartic |
| ACEI | Angiotensin-converting enzyme inhibitors |
| ACT | Activated clotting time |
| ACTH | Adrenocorticotrophic hormone |
| ADD | Attention deficit disorder |
| ADH | Antidiuretic hormone |
| ADHD | Attention deficit hyperactivity disorder |
| ADWD | Automatic dishwashing detergents |
| AFAST | Abdominal focused assessment with sonography for trauma, triage, and tracking |
| AIVR | Accelerated idioventricular rhythm |
| AKI | Acute kidney injury |
| ALI | Acute lung injury |
| ALP | Alkaline phosphatase |
| ALT | Alanine aminotransferase |
| AngII | Angiotensin II |
| ANP | Atrial natriuretic peptide |
| APCC | Animal Poison Control Center |
| aPTT | Activated partial thromboplastin time |
| AR | Anticoagulant rodenticide |
| ARB | Angiotensin receptor blocker |
| ARDS | Acute respiratory distress syndrome |
| ARF | Acute renal failure |
| ASA | Acetylsalicylic acid, aspirin |

---

*Blackwell's Five-Minute Veterinary Consult Clinical Companion: Small Animal Toxicology*, Third Edition.
Edited by Lynn R. Hovda, Ahna G. Brutlag, Robert H. Poppenga, and Steven E. Epstein.
© 2024 John Wiley & Sons, Inc. Published 2024 by John Wiley & Sons, Inc.

| | |
|---|---|
| ASPCA | American Society for the Prevention of Cruelty to Animals |
| AST | Aspartate aminotransferase |
| ASX | Asymptomatic |
| ATCA | 2-amino-2-thiazoline-4-carboxylic acid |
| ATP | Adenosine triphosphate |
| ATSDR | Agency for Toxic Substances and Disease Registry |
| AV | Atrioventricular |
| BAL | British anti-Lewisite (dimercaprol) |
| BBB | Blood–brain barrier |
| BE | Base excess |
| BG | Blood glucose |
| BID | Twice daily |
| BMAA | Beta-N-methylamino-L-alanine |
| BMBT | Buccal mucosal bleeding time |
| BP | Blood pressure |
| BPM | Beats per minute, breaths per minute |
| BUN | Blood urea nitrogen |
| BW | Body weight |
| BZD | Benzodiazepine |
| Ca | Calcium |
| cAMP | Cyclic adenosine monophosphate |
| CaNa2 EDTA | Calcium disodium ethylene diamine tetraacetate |
| CB receptor | Cannibinoid receptor |
| CBC | Complete blood count |
| CBD | Cannabidiol |
| CBDA | Cannabidiolic acid |
| CCA | Chromated copper arsenate |
| CCB | Calcium channel blocker |
| CHF | Congestive heart failure |
| CK | Creatine kinase |
| CNS | Central nervous system |
| CO | Carbon monoxide |
| COA | Certificate of analysis |
| COHb | Carboxyhemoglobin |
| COPD | Chronic obstructive pulmonary disease |
| COX | Cyclooxygenase |
| CRI | Constant rate infusion |
| CRRT | Continuous renal replacement therapy |
| CRT | Capillary refill time |
| CSF | Cerebrospinal fluid |
| CTZ | Chemoreactive trigger zone |
| CV | Cardiovascular |
| CVM | Center for Veterinary Medicine |
| CYP | Cytochrome P |
| d | Day |
| D2 | Dopamine |
| D5W | Dextrose 5% in water |
| DCM | Dilated cardiomyopathy |

| | |
|---|---|
| DEA | Dog erythrocyte antigen |
| DEET | diethyltoluamide |
| DEG | Diethylene glycol |
| DGA | Diglycolic acid |
| DIC | Disseminated intravascular coagulation |
| dL | Deciliter |
| DMSA | Dimercaptosuccinic acid |
| DMSO | Dimethylsulfoxide |
| DMT | N,N-dimethyltryptamine |
| DNA | Deoxyribonucleic acid |
| DOR | Delta opioid receptor |
| DPH | Diphenhydramine |
| DVM | Veterinarian (Doctor of Veterinary Medicine) |
| ECG | Electrocardiogram |
| ECS | Endocannabinoid system |
| ECT | Extracorporeal therapy |
| EDTA | Ethylenediaminetetraacetic acid |
| EEG | Electroencephalogram |
| EG | Ethylene glycol |
| ELISA | Enzyme-linked immunosorbent assay |
| EPA | Environmental Protection Agency |
| ER | Extended release |
| ERG | Electroretinogram |
| $ETCO_2$ | End-tidal carbon dioxide |
| ETT | Endotracheal tube |
| Fab | Fragment antigen-binding region |
| FBAL | Alpha-fluoro-beta-alanine |
| FBO | Foreign body obstruction |
| FCE | Fibrocartilaginous embolism |
| FDA | Food and Drug Administration |
| FDPs | Fibrin degradation products |
| FFP | Fresh frozen plasma |
| FFPA | Free from prussic acid |
| FGAR | First-generation anticoagulant rodenticide |
| Fib | Fibrinogen |
| FIP | Feline infectious peritonitis |
| FP | Frozen plasma |
| g | Gram |
| GABA | Gamma-aminobutyric acid |
| GC/MS | Gas chromatography/mass spectrometry |
| GDV | Gastric dilation and volvulus |
| GFAAS | Graphite furnace atomic absorption spectrometry |
| GFR | Glomerular filtration rate |
| GGT | Gamma-glutamyl transferase |
| GHB | Gamma-hydroxybutyric acid |
| GI | Gastrointestinal |
| GIT | Gastrointestinal tract |
| GPCR | G protein-coupled receptor |

| | |
|---|---|
| GRAS | Generally regarded as safe |
| $H_2$ | Histamine 2 |
| Hb | Hemoglobin |
| HCM | Hypertrophic cardiomyopathy |
| HD | Hemodialysis |
| HDI | High-dose insulin |
| HE | Hepatic encephalopathy |
| HF | Hydrofluoric acid |
| HGE | Hemorrhagic gastroenteritis |
| HP | Hemoperfusion |
| HPLC | High-pressure liquid chromatography |
| HR | Heart rate |
| HSDB | Hazardous Substances Data Bank |
| IBD | Inflammatory bowel disease |
| ICP | Intracranial pressure |
| ICP-MS | Inductively coupled plasma-mass spectrometry |
| IgG | Immunoglobulin G |
| ILE | Intralipid emulsion |
| IM | Intramuscular |
| IMHA | Immune-mediated hemolytic anemia |
| IMTP | Immune-mediated thrombocytopenia |
| INR | International normalized ratio |
| IOP | Intraocular pressure |
| IP | Intraperitoneal |
| IR | Immediate release |
| IU | International unit |
| IV | Intravenous |
| IVDD | Intervertebral disc disease |
| IVIS | International Veterinary Information Service |
| KBr | Potassium bromide |
| KCS | Keratoconjunctivitis sicca |
| Kg | Kilogram |
| KOR | Kappa opioid receptor |
| L | Liter |
| LC/MS | Liquid chromatography/mass spectrometry |
| $LC_{50}$ | Median lethal concentration |
| LD min | Minimum lethal dose |
| $LD_{50}$ | Median lethal dose |
| LDH | Lactate dehydrogenase |
| $LD_{LO}$ | Lethal dose low |
| LDP | Laundry detergent pod |
| LSA | Lysergic acid amide substances |
| LSD | Lysergic acid diethylamide |
| M | Mole |
| MAM | Methylazooxymethanol |
| MAO | Monoamine oxidase |
| MAOI | Monoamine oxidase inhibitor |
| MAP | Mean arterial blood pressure |

| | |
|---|---|
| MC | Microcystin |
| mcg | Microgram |
| MCPA | 2-methyl-4-chlorophenoxyacetic acid |
| MCPP | 2-(4-chloro-methylphenoxy) propionic acid |
| MDI | Diphenylmethane diisocyanate |
| MDMA | 3,4-methylenedioxymethamphetamine |
| MDPV | Methylenedioxypyrovalerone |
| MDR | Multi-drug resistant |
| MDR1 | Multi-drug resistance 1 |
| mEq | Milliequivalent |
| MetHb | Methemoglobinemia |
| mg | Milligram |
| mL | Milliliter |
| MLD | Minimum lethal dose |
| mM | Millimole |
| MOA | Mechanism of action |
| MODS | Multiple organ dysfunction syndrome |
| MOR | Mu opioid receptor |
| mOSM | Milliosmole |
| MRI | Magnetic resonance imaging |
| MRSA | Methicillin-resistant *Staphylococcus aureus* |
| MSDS | Material safety data sheets |
| MTD | Minimum toxic dose |
| NAC | N-acetylcysteine |
| NADPH | Nicotinamide adenine dinucleotide phosphate |
| NAPQI | N-acetyl-p-benzoquinone imine |
| NAT | N-acetyltransferase |
| NBZD | Nonbenzodiazepine |
| NE | Norepinephrine |
| NET | Norepinephrine transporter |
| NIEHS | National Institute for Environmental Health Sciences |
| ng | Nanogram |
| NLM | National Library of Medicine |
| NMDA | N-methyl-D-aspartate |
| NOAEL | No observed adverse lethal effect level |
| NOEL | No observed effect level |
| NPDS | National Poison Data System |
| NPIC | National Pesticide Information Center |
| NPO | Nil *per os* (nothing by mouth) |
| NSAID | Nonsteroidal antiinflammatory drug |
| OAT | Organic anion transporter |
| OP | Organophosphate |
| OSHA | Occupational health and safety administration |
| OTC | Over the counter |
| OTM | Oral transmucosal |
| Oz | Ounce |
| P-GP | P-glycoprotein |
| PaCO$_2$ | Partial pressure of arterial carbon dioxide |

| | |
|---|---|
| $PaO_2$ | Partial pressure of arterial oxygen |
| $PCO_2$ | Partial pressure of carbon dioxide |
| PCP | Phencyclidine |
| PCV | Packed cell volume |
| PCR | Polymerase chain reaction |
| PD | Polydipsia |
| PDB | Paradichlorobenzene |
| PDE | Phosphodiesterase |
| PE | Phenylephrine, physical examination |
| PEG | Polyethylene glycol |
| PIVKA | Protein induced by vitamin K absence or antagonism |
| PGE2 | Prostaglandin E2 |
| PK | Pharmacokinetics |
| PLR | Pupillary light response |
| Plt | Platelet |
| PO | *Per os* (by mouth) |
| POC | Point of care |
| PPA | Phenylpropanolamine |
| ppb | Parts per billion |
| PPE | Personal protective equipment |
| PPH | Pet Poison Hotline |
| ppm | Parts per million |
| PPV | Positive pressure ventilation |
| PRN | *Pro re nata* (as needed) |
| PSE | Pseudoephedrine |
| PT | Prothrombin time |
| PTH | Parathyroid hormone |
| PTT | Partial thromboplastin time |
| PU | Polyuria |
| PVA | Polyvinyl acetate |
| $PvCO_2$ | Partial pressure of venous carbon dioxide |
| q | Every |
| QID | Four times a day |
| RAAS | Renin-angiotensin-aldosterone system |
| RBC | Red blood cell |
| RNA | Ribonucleic acid |
| ROMK | Renal outer medullary potassium |
| RR | Respiratory rate |
| SAMe | S-adenosyl-methionine |
| $SaO_2$ | Arterial oxygen saturation |
| SCB | Synthetic cannabinoids |
| SGAR | Second-generation anticoagulant rodenticide |
| SID | Once daily |
| SNRI | Serotonin and norepinephrine reuptake inhibitor |
| sp. | Species |
| SPCO | Saturation of arterial blood with carbon monoxide as measured by pulse oximetry |
| $SpO_2$ | Saturation of arterial blood with oxygen as measured by pulse oximetry |

| | |
|---|---|
| spp. | Multiple species |
| SQ | Subcutaneous |
| SSRI | Selective serotonin reuptake inhibitor |
| STT | Schirmer tear test |
| SVT | Supraventricular tachycardia |
| SX | Symptomatic |
| T3 | Liothyronine |
| T4 | Thyroxine |
| TCA | Tricyclic antidepressant |
| TENS | Toxic epidermal necrolysis |
| TEPP | Tetraethyl pyrophosphate |
| TETA | Trientine |
| TFAST | Thoracic focused assessment with sonography for trauma, triage, and tracking |
| THC | Tetrahydrocannabinol |
| THCA | Tetrahydrocannabinolic acid |
| THCP | Tetrahydrocannabiphorol |
| THCV | Tetrahydrocannabivarin |
| TIBC | Total iron binding capacity |
| TID | Three times a day |
| TLC | Thin-layer chromatography |
| TP | Total protein |
| TPE | Therapeutic plasma exchange |
| TPP | Total plasma protein |
| TPR | Temperature, pulse, and respiration |
| TRPV | Transient receptor potential cation channel |
| TS | Total solids |
| U | Unit |
| UA | Urinalysis |
| UOP | Urine output |
| USDA | United States Department of Agriculture |
| UV | ultraviolet |
| Vd | Volume of distribution |
| VIN | Veterinary Information Network |
| VPC | Ventricular premature contraction |
| WB | Whole blood |
| WBC | White blood cell count |
| XR | Extended release |
| ZOR | Zeta opioid receptor |

# Anthelmintics

Anthelmintics are used to treat infections from several common small animal helminths including varieties of flukes, hookworms, roundworms, tapeworms, and whipworms. This appendix covers common veterinary OTC and prescription anthelmintics used in cats and dogs in the United States which are not covered in individual chapters.

*Blackwell's Five-Minute Veterinary Consult Clinical Companion: Small Animal Toxicology*, Third Edition.
Edited by Lynn R. Hovda, Ahna G. Brutlag, Robert H. Poppenga, and Steven E. Epstein.
© 2024 John Wiley & Sons, Inc. Published 2024 by John Wiley & Sons, Inc.

| Class and active ingredients | Toxicity | Clinical signs | Treatment/ prognosis |
|---|---|---|---|
| **Benzimidazoles**<br><br>Fenbendazole and febantel (prodrug that is metabolized to fenbendazole). Febantel is most commonly found in combination parasiticides.<br><br>Albendazole is not commonly used in dogs and cats due to concern for anorexia and bone marrow toxicosis.<br><br>Mebendazole and oxibendazole have caused acute hepatic injury in dogs and are no longer used. | **Fenbendazole**<br><br>**Therapeutic dosages:**<br><br>Dogs: 50–100 mg/kg PO. Safe for use in pregnant dogs.<br><br>Cats (extra-label): 25–100 mg/kg PO.<br><br>**Toxicity studies:**<br><br>Dog oral LD$_{50}$ ≥500 mg/kg.<br><br>Dog: No adverse effects at 250 mg/kg × 6 days.<br><br>Dog: 80–250 mg/kg/day × 30 days leads to gastric mucosa changes and fatty degeneration of the liver. 125 mg/kg/day for 6 months lead to cerebellar changes.<br><br>**Febantel**<br><br>**Therapeutic dosage:**<br><br>Dogs and cats: 10 mg/kg PO.<br><br>**Toxicity studies:**<br><br>Dog: Oral LD$_{50}$ ≥10 000 mg/kg.<br><br>Dog: Oral NOEL = 50–66 mg/kg/day. 110 mg/kg/day × 9 d = anorexia, vomiting, depression, death in 2 of 4 dogs.<br><br>Cats: 66 mg/kg × 9 d = vomiting, minor weight loss. 110 mg/kg × 9 d = no signs in some cats while death occurred in 2 of 4 cats that had preexisting liver or renal disease. | Adverse effects are rare at therapeutic doses and may include vomiting, diarrhea, and anorexia.<br><br>**Other:**<br><br>Hypersensitivity reactions due to antigen released from dying parasites (rare).<br><br>Pancytopenia in 1 dog following fenbendazole 50 mg/kg PO q 12 h for 11 days. Suspected to be idiosyncratic. | Wide margin of safety in acute doses. Greater risk with chronic overdose.<br><br>In case of overdose, do not feed as food increases systemic absorption. Most acute overdoses, especially if within 2–3 × therapeutic dose, will not require treatment.<br><br>Induce emesis if appropriate and, depending on extent of decontamination, consider 1 dose of activated charcoal with a cathartic.<br><br>Supportive care as needed for other signs.<br><br>**Prognosis:**<br><br>Excellent for acute overdoses. |

(Continued)

| Class and active ingredients | Toxicity | Clinical signs | Treatment/ prognosis |
|---|---|---|---|
| **Tetrahydropyrimidines:**<br><br>Pyrantel pamoate<br><br>Pyrantel tartrate<br><br>Often included in combination antiparasitic drugs. | Labeled dosages should specify whether dose is based on the salt (e.g., pyrantel pamoate) or pyrantel base. Check the product label to confirm the dose is listed. Each gram of pyrantel pamoate is ≈347 mg (34.7%) of the base.<br><br>**Therapeutic dosages:**<br><br>Pyrantel base:<br><br>Dogs: 5–10 mg/kg, depending on body weight.<br><br>Pyrantel pamoate:<br><br>Dogs: 5–20 mg/kg,<br><br>cats: 20 mg/kg.<br><br>Because of its low absorption from the gut, pyrantel pamoate has a higher safety margin. Pyrantel tartrate is better absorbed than pamoate and signs occur at lower dosages.<br><br>**Toxicity dosages:**<br><br>Dogs: <70 mg/kg pyrantel pamoate is generally considered nontoxic.<br><br><200 mg/kg pyrantel pamoate, possible GI effects but can usually monitor at home without intervention.<br><br>Acute $LD_{50}$ >690 mg/kg (pyrantel pamoate).<br><br>50 mg/kg/day pyrantel tartrate × 3 months = increased respiratory rates, ataxia and other cholinergic effects.<br><br>Cats: <70–100 mg/kg pyrantel pamoate is generally considered nontoxic.<br><br>Single dose of 230.6 mg/kg pyrantel pamoate produced vomiting and diarrhea in 2/92 cats. | Adverse effects are rare at therapeutic doses. Vomiting, diarrhea, lethargy, and anorexia can occur but may also be due to expulsion of parasites.<br><br>Signs are usually mild and transient. | Wide margin of safety in acute doses. Greater risk with chronic overdose.<br><br>Most acute overdoses, if <2–3 × labeled dose will not require treatment.<br><br>If needed, induce emesis if appropriate and, depending on extent of decontamination, consider 1 dose of activated charcoal with a cathartic.<br><br>Provide supportive care as needed for other signs for vomiting, dehydration, and persistent GI signs.<br><br>Anticholinergic signs are very rare and not expected unless overdoses are massive but can be treated with atropine.<br><br>**Prognosis:**<br><br>Excellent for acute overdoses. |

## Piperazine

Includes the following salts and their corresponding percentage of piperazine base:

Piperazine adipate 37%

Piperazine chloride 48%

Piperazine citrate 35%

Piperazine dihydrochloride 50–53%

Piperazine hexahydrate 44%

Piperazine phosphate 42%

Piperazine sulfate 46%.

### Toxicity studies:

121.8 mg/kg/day PO (61.3 mg/kg/day piperazine base) × 6 weeks = no clinical signs or histopathological lesions

In cats, piperazine hexahydrate at 50–300 mg/kg IV led to a reduction in heart rate and blood pressure, followed by an increase in both values.

### Therapeutic dosages:

Labeled dosages should specify whether dose is based on the salt (e.g., piperazine citrate) or piperazine base. Check the product label to confirm the dose is listed.

Dogs/cats: 50–110 mg/kg (base) PO.

### Toxic dosages and study data:

Dogs: <500 mg/kg piperazine base is generally considered low risk.

≥500 mg/kg and <1 gram/kg, decontamination warranted.

Cats: <150 mg/kg piperazine base is generally considered low risk.

≥150 mg/kg, decontamination warranted.

Clinical signs begin 2–24 hours from ingestion and may take a few days to resolve.

In dogs, the following signs were reported with both overdose and therapeutic dosing: vomiting, diarrhea, ataxia, muscle weakness, head pressing, hyperesthesia, and myoclonus.

In cats, the following signs were reported with both overdose and therapeutic dosing: vomiting, diarrhea, ataxia, muscle weakness, intention tremors of the head and neck, head pressing, severe epileptiform seizures, hyperesthesia, tetanic spasms, slow pupillary light reflexes, and lethargy.

The rapid paralysis of roundworms in young animals with a heavy parasite burden, particularly kittens, may result in GI obstruction.

If necessary, induce emesis if appropriate and consider 1 dose of activated charcoal with a cathartic.

Provide supportive care such as antiemetics and fluid therapy as needed for vomiting, dehydration, and persistent GI signs.

Neurological signs are more likely compared to other anthelmintics described in this appendix and may respond to fluid therapy, anticonvulsants (e.g., benzodiazepines, phenobarbital, levetiracetam), and methocarbamol (tremors). Monitor HR and blood pressure, especially for hypotension, and correct.

### Prognosis:

Good for acute overdoses if treated early.

*(Continued)*

| Class and active ingredients | Toxicity | Clinical signs | Treatment/ prognosis |
|---|---|---|---|
| **Prazinoisoquinolines:**<br><br>Praziquantel<br><br>Often included in combination antiparasitic drugs. | **Therapeutic dosages:**<br><br>FDA-approved dosage varies by weight with smaller animals requiring larger dosages. Refer to a veterinary drug label or formulary for specifics.<br><br>Dogs: 5–12.5 mg/kg PO (FDA approved) based on body weight; up to 40 mg/kg PO (extra-label).<br><br>5.0–11.4 mg/kg IM or SQ (FDA approved).<br><br>Cats: 4.6–10 mg/kg (FDA approved) based on body weight; up to 35 mg/kg PO (extra-label).<br><br>5–10 mg/kg IM or SQ (FDA approved); up to 25 mg/kg SQ (extra-label).<br><br>12–30 mg/kg topically q 30 d<br><br>**Toxicity dosages:**<br><br>Dogs: 150–200 mg/kg caused vomiting, salivation, and depression.<br><br>33.8–40 × the labeled dosage in adult dogs resulted in vomiting, excessive salivation, and depression, but no deaths.<br><br>5× FDA-approved dosages for both dogs and cats resulted in no signs IM or SQ.<br><br>Cats: Doses 10–20 times the labeled rate in adult cats induced vomiting, depression, muscle tremors, and incoordination. Deaths occurred in 5 of 8 cats treated subcutaneously and in all 8 injected intramuscularly at doses greater than 20 times the label rate. | Dogs: Oral administration of praziquantel can cause anorexia, vomiting, lethargy, or diarrhea. Parenteral administration can lead to pain at injection site, vomiting, diarrhea, staggering gate. Large overdoses may cause GI signs with muscle tremors and ataxia.<br><br>Cats: Oral administration may cause salivation and diarrhea; transient ataxia has also been reported at therapeutic dosages. Following parenteral administration, diarrhea, weakness, vomiting, salivation, sleepiness, transient anorexia, and/or pain at the injection site have been demonstrated. | Wide margin of safety in acute oral doses.<br><br>Most acute overdoses, regardless of route, will require no or minimal treatment.<br><br>If needed for oral exposure, induce emesis if appropriate and, depending on extent of decontamination, consider 1 dose of activated charcoal with a cathartic.<br><br>Provide supportive care such as antiemetics and fluid therapy as needed for vomiting, dehydration, and persistent GI signs.<br><br>Ataxia in cats tends to self-resolve but keep cats safe/confined until asymptomatic.<br><br>Methocarbamol can be used for muscle tremors in either species, if required.<br><br>**Prognosis:**<br><br>Excellent for acute overdoses. |

Abbreviations: see Appendix 1 for a complete list.

**Author:** Ahna G. Brutlag, DVM, MS, DABT, DABVT

# Information Resources for Toxicology

## DEFINITION/OVERVIEW

- The tens of thousands of metals, minerals, natural products, and synthetic chemicals used in modern civilization provide numerous opportunities for exposure of small companion animals to potentially toxic materials.
- Of the hundreds of drugs and products used in a veterinary practice, many can interact with one another to either increase or mitigate the desired effects.
- Veterinarians receive questions and calls daily about the safety of a variety of products to which pets are exposed.
- Beyond the personal experience and knowledge gained from frequent encounters with the most familiar products, veterinarians need resources to bolster their personal knowledge when less frequently known chemical exposures or questions occur.
- This appendix presents several sources of information that can help veterinarians extend their service to clients by effectively using information resources in toxicology.
- Principal categories of assistance include the following.
  - Persons with in-depth experience relevant to specific toxicants or circumstances. Examples include agronomists, botanists, chemists, limnologists, mycologists, pest control specialists, pharmacists, pharmacologists, pathologists, veterinary extension faculty, wildlife specialists, state and federal regulatory professionals, among others.
  - Textbooks and reference books prepared by knowledgeable experts and provided by reliable publishers.
  - Selected peer-reviewed, scientific veterinary journals that routinely accept original reports of toxicology clinical cases or toxicology research.
  - Animal poison control centers that maintain a staff of skilled and knowledgeable veterinary specialists 24/7 for consultation when veterinary toxicology questions arise.
  - Government agencies with emphasis on toxicology scientific, regulatory, or educational services
  - Reliable internet resources for quick and easy access to useful toxicology information on a 24/7 basis.

## VETERINARY AND TOXICOLOGY INFORMATION RESOURCES

- As with all professional services, critical evaluation of resources available is essential to gathering reliable information for toxicology support.
- Sources that are well documented and subject to some form of peer review are usually most reliable.

*Blackwell's Five-Minute Veterinary Consult Clinical Companion: Small Animal Toxicology*, Third Edition. Edited by Lynn R. Hovda, Ahna G. Brutlag, Robert H. Poppenga, and Steven E. Epstein.
© 2024 John Wiley & Sons, Inc. Published 2024 by John Wiley & Sons, Inc.

- If regulatory or legal aspects of toxicology are important, official government sources often provide helpful and reliable information.
- Of course, the veterinarian must carefully and critically determine how the information applies to the needs of any given case.

## Specialists with In-Depth Expertise Relevant to Veterinary Toxicology

- Examples include agronomists, botanists, chemists, limnologists, mycologists, pest control specialists, pharmacists, pharmacologists, pathologists, veterinary extension faculty, wildlife specialists, state and federal regulatory professionals and many others.
- Knowing about these highly skilled and focused individuals can be invaluable when an infrequently encountered question or exposure demands special knowledge on short notice.
- Prior contact or arrangements with experts that one already knows are often invaluable when a quick and thorough response is required to support a toxicology incident in small animals.
- Keep in mind that many situations are complex and might require expert advice from several disciplines.

## Principal Reference Books and Textbooks

The most recent editions are provided. Often, earlier editions have useful toxicology information as well.

- Bonagura J, Twedt D. *Kirk's Current Veterinary Therapy XV*, Saunders, 2014.
- Peterson ME, Talcott PA (eds). *Small Animal Toxicology*, 3rd edn. Elsevier Saunders, 2013.
- Burrows GE, Tyrl RJ. *Handbook of Toxic Plants of North America*, 2nd edn. Wiley- Blackwell, 2006.
- Hovda L, Brutlag A, Poppenga R, Peterson K. *Blackwell's Five-Minute Veterinary Consult Clinical Companion: Small Animal Toxicology*, 2nd edn. Wiley-Blackwell, 2016.
- Hooser S, Khan S. *Veterinary Clinics of North America Small Animal Practice: Common Toxicologic Issues in Small Animals: An Update*. Elsevier, 2018.
- Gupta RC (ed.). *Veterinary Toxicology: Basic and Clinical Principles*, 3rd edn. Academic Press, 2018.
- Knight AP. *A Guide to Poisonous House and Garden Plants*. Teton NewMedia, 2006.
- Plumlee KH (ed.). *Clinical Veterinary Toxicology*. Mosby-Elsevier, 2004.
- Tilley LP, Smith FWK, Sleeper, MM, Braindard, BM (eds). *Blackwell's Five-Minute Veterinary Consult: Canine and Feline*, 7th edn. Wiley-Blackwell, 2021.

## Supportive Reference Books and Textbooks

- Papich MG. *Saunders Handbook of Veterinary Drugs*, 5th edn. Saunders Elsevier, 2020.
- Plumb DC. *Plumb's Veterinary Drug Handbook*, 9th edn. Wiley-Blackwell, 2018.
- Riviere JE, Papich MG (eds). *Veterinary Pharmacology and Therapeutics*, 10th edn. Wiley-Blackwell, 2018.

There are numerous veterinary emergency and critical care textbooks that contain relevant small animal toxicology information.

## Selected Veterinary Journals Containing Small Animal Toxicology Information

- *American Journal of Veterinary Research*
- *Australian Veterinary Journal*
- *Canadian Journal of Veterinary Research*
- *Journal of the American Animal Hospital Association*
- *Journal of the American Veterinary Medical Association*

- *Journal of Small Animal Practice*
- *Journal of Veterinary Diagnostic Investigation*
- *Journal of Veterinary Emergency and Critical Care*
- *Journal of Veterinary Internal Medicine*
- *Journal of Veterinary Pharmacology and Therapeutics*
- *Research in Veterinary Science*
- *Veterinary Journal*
- *Veterinary Quarterly*
- *Veterinary Record*

## Animal Poison Control Centers (US)

24/7 consultations with trained veterinary toxicologists/staff.
- ASPCA Animal Poison Control Center
  - www.aspca.org/pet-care/poison-control/
  - (888) 426-4435
  - Consultation fee
- Pet Poison Helpline
  - www.petpoisonhelpline.com/
  - (855) 764-7661
  - Consultation fee

## Internet-Based Toxicology Resources

The internet has a wealth of relevant information applicable to veterinary toxicology. An internet search is perhaps the easiest way to determine what active ingredients are in a given product, the category of an active ingredient (e.g., insecticide, rodenticide, drug agent), and some idea of relative toxicity based upon $LD_{50}$ information. Of course, it is important to understand that there is much information on the internet that is not based upon the best available evidence and should not be used to guide case management decisions.

Some of the more relevant internet resources pertaining to general toxicology, human toxicology (information that can often be extrapolated to veterinary patients, but not always), or veterinary toxicology include the following.
- Agency for Toxic Substances and Disease Registry (ATSDR)
  - www.atsdr.cdc.gov/
  - ATSDR, based in Atlanta, Georgia, is a federal public health agency of the US Department of Health and Human Services. ATSDR protects communities from harmful health effects related to exposure to natural and man-made hazardous substances.
  - The site contains toxicologic profiles for many toxic chemicals.
- American Board of Veterinary Toxicology
  - www.abvt.org
  - Established in 1967, the ABVT is one of 22 veterinary specialty organizations recognized by the American Veterinary Medical Association. It was the first professional organization to provide certification in the field of toxicology. As a nonprofit educational organization, the board administers a specialty certification examination to qualified veterinarians. The credentialing process ensures that animal and human lives will be protected by veterinarians with expertise in veterinary toxicology.
- American Association of Poison Control Centers (AAPCC)
  - www.aapcc.org/
  - American Association of Poison Control Centers assists 60 poison centers in the United States on a 24/7 basis.

- Poison Help hotline at 1-800-222-1222 can be dialed from anywhere in the United States and will be automatically routed to an appropriate center.
- Certifies poison control center personnel and owns and maintains the National Poison Data System (NPDS).
- Consultant
  - https://consultant.vet.cornell.edu/
  - Consultant is a diagnostic support system to assist in possible differential diagnoses based on clinical signs entered. When clinical signs are entered, it enables a wide selection of potential toxic differential diagnoses.
  - Consultant is free of charge, but monetary support is welcome to help defray expenses. It is species specific, provides a brief synopsis of a selected diagnosis/cause, and is supported by 3–6 recent references pertinent to the diagnosis selected.
  - Supported by a database of approximately 500 signs/symptoms, 7000 diagnoses/causes, and 18 000 literature references, of which 3000 are web sources.
- Cornell University Poisonous Plants
  - www.ansci.cornell.edu/plants/index.html
  - Maintained by the Animal Science Department at Cornell University as a reference only.
  - Includes plant images, pictures of affected animals, and presentations concerning botany, chemistry, toxicology, diagnosis, and prevention of poisoning of animals by plants and other natural flora.
  - The images are copyrighted but may be printed, downloaded, or copied, provided it is in an educational setting and proper attribution is provided.
- FDA Center for Veterinary Medicine (FDA-CVM)
  - www.fda.gov/about-fda/fda-organization/center-veterinary-medicine
  - Official website for the Center for Veterinary Medicine.
  - Provides current information on pet food regulations, labeling, product recalls, and food safety for pets.
  - Monitors and investigates outbreaks of suspected toxicoses related to pet foods.
  - Recent examples have included aflatoxins in dogs, melamine/cyanuric acid nephrosis in dogs and cats, and safety of imported pet treats.
  - Maintains a safety reporting portal for animal drugs and foods: www.safetyreporting.hhs.gov/SRP2/en/Home.aspx?sid=c8b65b6e-4ba6-48e1-8004-946f570b3ec1
- InChem
  - www.inchem.org
  - Rapid access to internationally peer-reviewed information on chemicals, including contaminants in the environment and food.
  - Primarily human and environment oriented.
  - Consolidates information from a number of intergovernmental organizations to assist in sound management of chemicals.
  - Includes environmental health criteria as well as health and safety guidelines.
  - Provides poison information monographs.
- International Veterinary Information Service (IVIS)
  - www.ivis.org
  - Free service to veterinarians, veterinary students, and animal health professionals.
  - Provides online peer-reviewed references.
  - Access to a variety of toxicology and pharmacology information.
- Merck Veterinary Manual
  - www.merckvetmanual.com/mvm/index.jsp

- Medline
  - http://medlineplus.gov/
  - Service provided by the National Library of Medicine and National Institutes of Health.
  - Updated daily.
  - Human focused, but can be a good source of information about human drugs encountered by animals.
  - Also a source of information about human antidotes useful in veterinary medicine.
  - Public access is allowed.
- MSDS Search
  - http://sdsmanager.com/us/search
  - A database service specializing in providing a digital source of MSDS (material safety data sheets) required by many commercial businesses and manufacturing companies.
  - MSDS sheets contain information about the characteristics and nature of thousands of chemicals to which animals could be exposed.
  - The information is often not assembled consistently in standard references.
  - The MSDS provides a relatively consistent and detailed documentation of composition, use, and potential adverse effects.
- National Institute for Environmental Health Sciences (NIEHS)
  - www.niehs.nih.gov/
  - The NIEHS's mission is to reduce the burden of human illness and disability by understanding how the environment influences the development and progression of human disease. Some of the NIEHS activities include:
    - rigorous research in environmental health sciences, and to communicating the results of this research to the public.
    - alphabetical listing of major health topics that are related to or affected by environmental exposures.
    - access to materials and guidance for use by health professionals in educating, diagnosing, and treating patients with conditions and diseases influenced by environmental agents.
- National Pesticide Information Center
  - http://npic.orst.edu/
  - NPIC provides objective, science-based information about pesticides and pesticide-related topics to enable people to make informed decisions. NPIC is a cooperative agreement between Oregon State University and the US Environmental Protection Agency.
  - NPIC provides fact sheets for many pesticides that discuss their toxicology in terms pet owners are likely to understand.
- PubMed
  - www.ncbi.nlm.nih.gov/pubmed/medline.html
  - PubMed is a search service of the US National Library of Medicine.
  - It comprises more than 19 million citations for biomedical articles from Medline and life science journals.
  - Citations include links to full-text articles from PubMed Central or publisher websites.
  - Numerous major scientific and applied veterinary journals can be reliably accessed through PubMed.
- TOXNET (National Library of Medicine Toxicology Information)
  - https://infocus.nlm.nih.gov/2015/11/04/toxnet-the-nlm-toxicology-databases/
  - TOXNET is a collection of toxicology and environmental health databases.

- o Hazardous Substances Data Bank (HSDB) is a database of potentially hazardous chemicals.
- o Household Products Database identifies the chemicals used in over 15 000 consumer products.
- o TOXLINE offers 4 million citations to articles from scientific journals and other authoritative sources about the biochemical, pharmacological, physiological, and toxicological effects of drugs and other chemicals.
- o ChemIDplus offers an online dictionary of chemical substances cited in NLM databases and other internet resources. It lists over 400 000 chemicals with their common names, synonyms, and structures.
- USP Veterinary Drug Information
  - www.usp.org/audiences/veterinary/
  - USP is an independent, scientific nonprofit organization focused on ensuring the supply of safe, quality medicines.
- Veterinary Information Network
  - www.vin.com
  - A veterinary organization and system of education and databases to help veterinary professionals keep up to date through:
    - o bringing veterinarians together worldwide as colleagues.
    - o providing instant access to vast amounts of up-to-date veterinary information.
    - o bringing instant access to "breaking news" that affects veterinarians, their patients, and their practice.
    - o bringing easy access to colleagues who have specialized knowledge and skills including veterinary toxicologists.
    - o providing ongoing, easily available continuing education.

**Author**: Robert H. Poppenga, DVM, PhD, DABVT

# Other Metallic Toxicants

For information on more frequent and serious metallic toxicants for small animals, see individual chapters on iron, lead, and zinc.

*Blackwell's Five-Minute Veterinary Consult Clinical Companion: Small Animal Toxicology*, Third Edition.
Edited by Lynn R. Hovda, Ahna G. Brutlag, Robert H. Poppenga, and Steven E. Epstein.
© 2024 John Wiley & Sons, Inc. Published 2024 by John Wiley & Sons, Inc.

| Metal and sources | Toxicity | Clinical effects | Diagnostics | Therapy/prevention |
|---|---|---|---|---|
| **Arsenic (As)** | | | | |
| Trivalent (+3) and pentavalent (+5) sources are of concern. | Absorbed via GIT, intact skin, inhalation. | Immediately post absorption – oral irritation, dysphagia. | Liver, kidney: >10 ppm As is toxic. | No emetics or gastric lavage unless very early and asymptomatic. |
| Natural +5 sources are found in soil, coal, mine tailings, and seafoods (2–22 ppm). | +3 is 3–10 times more toxic than +5 valence. | Acute toxicosis 1–3 hours – abdominal pain, salivation, vomiting, hematochezia, melena, rice-water stools, hypovolemia from capillary dilation and vascular transudation. | Urine: current exposure = 2–100 ppm. | Charcoal is not an effective adsorbent. |
| | Storage in liver, kidney, GIT, spleen, skin, hair. | | Hair: chronic levels ≥25 ppm. | Intensive care with IV fluids, demulcents, treat for shock, maintain body temp, hemodialysis for renal failure. |
| Both +3 and +5 valence in pesticides. | Excreted 50% in urine within 48 hours. | | Blood: unreliable for arsenic concentration. | Sucralfate, proton pump inhibitors, $H_2$-blockers, antiemetics, antidiarrheals. |
| Other: | | | CBC: hemoconcentration secondary to dehydration, hemolysis, anemia, ± basophilic stippling, possible pancytopenia, leukopenia, or thrombocytopenia. | |
| Pre-2004 treated wood (CCA). | Lethal dosage range 1–25 mg/kg. | Oral erosions and ulceration. | | Monitor renal function. |
| Well water ≤21 ppm. | More toxic to cats than dogs. | Subacute – renal tubular necrosis, renal failure, azotemia. | | Prognosis guarded in acute intoxications. |
| Weed and insect killers. | Toxicity order is As+3 (arsenite) > As+5 (arsenate) > trivalent organics. | | Urinalysis: monitor for whole cells, casts, protein, evidence of hemolysis, hematuria. | Best chelator is succimer (DMSA); less toxic, more expensive, more effective than dimercaprol (BAL). |
| Medical: immiticide (melarsomine) adult heartworm treatment (thiacetarsamide). | Melarsomine = severe toxicosis at 7.5 mg/kg. | | | See dosages at end of table. |
| **Barium (Ba)** | | | | |
| Rodenticide (obsolete), welding fluxes, depilatories, dyes, glass manufacture, explosive detonators. | Acid- or water-soluble barium salts act as strong cardiac suppressants and cause severe hypokalemia by blocking exit channels for K+ in muscle cells. Barium also stimulates skeletal, smooth, and cardiac muscle. | Acute – vomiting, colic, salivation, diarrhea, ventricular tachycardia/fibrillation, dyspnea, weakness. | Hypokalemia, from blocking cellular K+ exit. | Emesis and activated charcoal not recommended. |
| | | Violent peristalsis, arterial hypertension, and arrhythmias. | ECG changes from hypokalemia (QRS or QTc interval changes). | Consider gastric lavage if patient is stabilized and airway protected. |
| | | Additional signs may include seizures, tremors, mydriasis. | Tissue levels – primarily in bones (replacing Ca++); soft tissue normal values generally less than 1 ppm. | Magnesium sulfate (250 mL/kg PO) to form insoluble $BaSO_4$ and reduce absorption. |
| | Toxic dose, canine: 50 mg/kg BW. | | Blood values from acute poisoning are 2–10 ppm. | Saline diuresis, intravenous K+ to control hypokalemia and tachycardia is critical. |
| | | | | Lidocaine recommended in humans if refractory to potassium. |

## Cadmium (Cd)

| | | |
|---|---|---|
| Ores, mine tailings, smelters. Also in foods (shellfish), cigarettes, fertilizers, solders, batteries, art pigments, automotive paints, semiconductors, solar cells. | Multisystem effects. Accumulates in kidneys and very slowly excreted – oxidative damage and lysosomal release → renal damage. Competes with Ca and Zn. Dogs tolerate 10 ppm in diet; chronic toxicity occurs at 50 mg/kg. | Acute – dyspnea, vomiting, colic, diarrhea (mucosal damage), weakness, renal failure. Chronic – rhinitis, anorexia, renal tubular dysfunction, sodium retention, osteomalacia/osteoporosis enlarges joints, testicular damage, potential copper deficiency. | Blood levels ≥100 mcg/dL reflect acute exposure; urine levels represent chronic exposure, but blood or urine values for small animals are poorly defined. Liver accumulates 1–2 ppm and kidney from 3–10 ppm. Diagnosis depends on history of exposure, typical clinical signs, and elevated cadmium in blood, urine, or tissue. | Treat symptomatically; supportive therapy for gastroenteritis and renal insufficiency. Zinc supplementation may reduce accumulation or persistence of Cd residues. CaNa$_2$EDTA or d-penicillamine. *See dosages at end of table.* |

## Copper (Cu)

| | | |
|---|---|---|
| Liver accumulation in dogs is enhanced by autosomal recessive trait in Bedlington terriers; also high risk in West Highland, Skye, Dalmatian, Doberman, and Labrador. Sources include coins, wiring, garden sprays, feeds, copper oxide capsules. | Absorbed readily from GIT, stored mainly in liver cell lysosomes, excreted in bile complexed with molybdenum. Excess accumulation causes hepatic cell necrosis. Hereditary copper accumulation is a liver disease. Acute release from liver may cause hemolytic crisis. | Acute exposure to concentrated copper salts – moderate to severe gastroenteritis. Chronic accumulations – hepatic insufficiency, possible encephalopathy, and occasional acute hemolytic crisis with icterus and hemoglobinuria. | Chemistry panel –elevated LDH, ALT, AST, bilirubin, bile acids. CBC – anemia, hemoglobinemia, hypoproteinemia. Urine – hemoglobinuria. Liver biopsy for histopathology and copper analysis may be diagnostic. Liver normal <400 ppm dry weight. Secondary Cu accumulation 400–800 ppm. Toxicosis >800 ppm. | Treat acute signs of liver disease and anemia symptomatically. If chronic toxicity – chelation of copper with d-penicillamine. Continue therapy with monitoring up to 1 year; biopsy for liver Cu concentrations again after 1 year. *See dosages at end of table.* |

## Chromium (Cr)

| | | |
|---|---|---|
| Occurs in nature in 4 oxidation states. Cr+6 is made and used in various industrial processes. Cr+3 is used in leather tanning, pigments, and wood preservation. Few sources are generally available to small animals. | Cats tolerate 100 mcg/day or 16 mcg/kg/day. Dogs tolerate 50 mcg/kg/day. Cr supports glucose tolerance and modulates serum triglycerides and cholesterol. | Reports of poisoning in small animals are rare. Signs in other species include vomiting, profuse diarrhea with mucosal sloughing, and dermatitis. | Cr is widely distributed in mammalian species at very low (ng/g) concentrations. Normal values in rats are 6 ppm (liver) and 8 ppm (kidney). Dosage of 100 mg/kg raises Cr values to 90 and 700 ppm in liver and kidney, respectively. Excreted mainly in urine. | Minimal toxicity is expected after ingestion. Some sources suggest activated charcoal adsorbs Cr, others do not. Overdose, if it occurs, is treated with general detoxification, fluids, and GIT therapy to manage potential or real gastroenteritis and dermatitis. |

*(Continued)*

| Metal and sources | Toxicity | Clinical effects | Diagnostics | Therapy/prevention |
|---|---|---|---|---|
| **Gold (Au)** | | | | |
| Gold-containing drugs are used primarily to manage rheumatoid arthritis. Forms include gold sodium thioglucose, gold sodium thiomalate, gold thiosulfate. | Rat IM $LD_{50}$ = 35–440 mg/kg.<br><br>Gold drugs are generally not available in a way that would expose small animals unless by malicious intent or extreme carelessness. | Most data are for parenteral exposure. Signs include ventricular tachycardia, vasodilation, hypotension, stomatitis, glossitis, ocular inflammation, pneumonitis, encephalopathy, and polyneuropathy. | Urine assay for gold would establish exposure, but diagnostic values are not established.<br><br>Human therapeutic use produces approximately 1 mcg/mL blood levels. | Gold toxicosis has been treated in humans with steroids, BAL, and N-acetylcysteine (NAC).<br><br>Animal treatment regimens are not established.<br><br>*See dosages at end of table.* |
| **Lithium (Li)** | | | | |
| Used in human medicine to treat manic depressive illness. Standard and sustained-release products available. Adult therapy range is 300–1800 mg/day. Tablet strength typically is 300 mg.<br><br>Lithium batteries low risk: pass through GIT and contain limited lithium. | Rat oral $LD_{50}$ = 525 mg/kg.<br><br>Feline: Toxic dose >85 mg/kg.<br><br>Animals with renal disease, dehydration, sodium depletion, cardiovascular disease, severe debilitation, or receiving diuretics are at higher risk.<br><br>Crosses the placenta, concentrates in fetus, may be teratogenic. | CNS – drowsiness, tremors, weakness, confusion, ataxia, seizures, or coma.<br><br>GIT – vomiting, diarrhea, nausea, anorexia.<br><br>Other – blurred vision, PU/PD, T-wave ECG changes.<br><br>Signs prolonged if sustained-release product ingested. | History: excessive and/or sustained high dosages.<br><br>Human serum values:<br><br>Moderate toxicity = 1.5–2.5 mEq/L.<br><br>Severe toxicity = 2.5–3 mEq/L.<br><br>Fatal = >3 mEq/L.<br><br>Recheck serum Li as needed.<br><br>Follow clinical course with baseline electrolytes, BUN, and creatinine. | Activated charcoal not effective.<br><br>Consider gastric lavage if <1 h post ingestion.<br><br>Whole-bowel irrigation if >1 h post ingestion, using PEG at 25–50 mg/kg followed by 0.5 mg/kg/h oral infusion until effluent is clear.<br><br>IV fluids at 1.5–2 × maintenance with 0.9% NaCl to aid renal excretion.<br><br>Acetazolamide (10 mg/kg q 8 h) and aminophylline to enhance renal excretion.<br><br>Hemodialysis may be option in some cases. |
| **Mercury (Hg)** | | | | |
| Current sources are limited. Ointments, leather preservatives, thermometers, fungicides, barometers, anti-mildew paints, fluorescent bulbs, mercury vapor lamps.<br><br>Fish-based diets potentially contain methyl mercury which has a long half-life and can potentially bioaccumulate. | Vapors and organic mercurials absorbed by inhalation and from GIT. Metallic mercury concentrates in GIT and kidney.<br><br>Organic mercury concentrates in brain. All forms pass the placenta.<br><br>Cats considered to be highly sensitive. | Organic mercurials cause erythema, conjunctivitis, stomatitis, depression, ataxia, incoordination, proprioceptive deficits, abnormal postures, paresis, and blindness.<br><br>Hypoproteinemia, proteinuria, and azotemia typical in inorganic Hg poisoning. | Blood (>6.0 ppm) and urine (>1.5 ppm) are good samples for acute to subacute exposure. Hair (>45 ppm) for chronic exposure.<br><br>Liver (>30 ppm) and kidney (>20 ppm) associated with toxicosis in cats. | Acute inorganic mercury – egg white to inactivate mercury; activated charcoal results variable but evidence in humans suggests administration is warranted. Whole-bowel irrigation with PEG recommended.<br><br>Antidotes: oral d-penicillamine or succimer are chelators of choice.<br><br>*See dosages at end of table.* |

## Selenium (Se)

| | | | | |
|---|---|---|---|---|
| Selenium dietary supplements, gun bluing compounds, pigments, photocells, photography developing products. | Canine lethal dosage is 1.5–3 mg/kg both oral and parenteral. Dietary levels of 10–20 ppm are toxic. Selenium causes glutathione depletion, lipid peroxidation, and replaces sulfur in amino acids. May also depress ATP formation. | Acute – vomiting, diarrhea, dyspnea, ataxia, hypovolemia and collapse result from acute exposure. Signs are similar to acute arsenic or iron toxicosis. Chronic – exposure may cause rough, dull haircoat, alopecia, weight loss, and infertility. | A normal blood Se value in dogs is approximately 0.22 ppm. Blood Se >1–2 ppm is suggestive of toxicosis. Kidney and liver values >12 ppm are considered toxic. Chronic exposure can be detected with hair analysis. | Symptomatic therapy for gastroenteritis and shock in acute intoxications. Activated charcoal is recommended by some, not by others. N-acetylcysteine. *See dosages at end of table.* |

## Tin (Sn)

| | | | | |
|---|---|---|---|---|
| Food preparation, toothpaste, pigments for ceramics and textiles. Organotins (alkyl tins) used as fungicides, insecticides, and in wood, leather, textile, preservatives. | Two valence forms (+2 and +4). Organic tins are toxic and well absorbed from GIT, but inorganic forms are highly tolerated. | Organotin target organs are brain, liver, immune system, and skin. Causes skin and eye irritation, colic, diarrhea, hepatotoxicity, and neurotoxicity (seizures, ataxia). | Myelin edema (status spongiosis) and demyelization in CNS. Blood levels >0.3 ppm and liver levels ≥0.6 ppm have been associated with organotin toxicosis. | Acute exposures not likely. If occurs, activated charcoal is recommended. BAL for 4 days effective in experimental animals. Control fever and hypotension. *See dosages at end of table.* |

# ANTIDOTES AND DOSAGES

For more details, consult Plumb DC. *Plumb's Veterinary Drug Handbook*, 10th edn. Wiley-Blackwell, 2023.

- CaNa$_2$EDTA: as an alternative to succimer for lead and zinc intoxications, extra-label: 25 mg/kg q 6 hours SQ diluted in D5W to a concentration of 10 mg/mL. Some sources indicate not to exceed 2 grams per animal per day. Treat for 5 days and reevaluate metal concentration in 5–14 days to determine if additional course of therapy is necessary.
- BAL (dimercaprol): dogs/cats, extra-label use, scant evidence to support any dosage regimen: 2.5–5 mg/kg IM q 4 hours for first 2 days of treatment then q 12 hours until recovery. 5 mg/kg doses are typically only given on the first day of treatment and only to acutely affected patients then q12 until recovery. Succimer, extra-label: 10 mg/kg PO q 8 hours for 5 to 10 days and reevaluate metal concentration several days after course of therapy to determine if additional course of therapy is necessary.
- d-Penicillamine, extra-label: for copper-associated hepatopathy, 7–15 mg/kg PO q 12 hours. Drug may cause vomiting. Give 1 hour before feeding. Lower dosage of 7 mg/kg PO might be efficacious while reducing drug cost and incidence of vomiting. For lead intoxication in dogs, extra-label: as an alternative or adjunct to Ca$_2$EDTA give penicillamine 110 mg/kg/day divided every 6 to 8 hours PO 30 minutes before feeding for 1 to 2 weeks. If vomiting is a problem, may premedicate with dimenhydrinate 2 – 4 mg/kg PO. Alternatively, may give penicillamine 33 – 55 mg/kg/day divided as above. For lead intoxication in cats, extra-label: 125 mg/cat (NOT mg/kg) PO every 12 hours for 5 days. Do not administer if any lead remains in the GI tract since it will increase systemic lead absorption.
- NAC, extra-label: initial dose of 140 to 180 mg/kg IV (5% solution and give via slow IV over 15 to 20 minutes) or 280 mg/kg PO initially, then 70 mg/kg q 6 hours PO or IV for a minimum of 7 treatments (IV preferred in serious intoxications).

## Abbreviations

- ATP = adenosine triphosphate
- BAL = British anti-Lewisite (dimercaprol)
- CaNa$_2$EDTA = calcium disodium ethylene diamine tetraacetate
- CCA = chromated copper arsenate
- LD$_{50}$ = median lethal dose
- NAC = N-acetylcysteine
- PEG = polyethylene glycol

**Author**: Robert H. Poppenga, DVM, PhD, DABVT
**Consulting Editor**: Steven E. Epstein, DVM, DACVECC

# Calculations for the Evaluation of Toxicity

The dose, dosage, route, and duration of exposure for a given toxicant determines the potential clinical outcome or toxidrome(s) that may present to a veterinary clinician and will guide the course of action for treatment and prognosis.

An accurate calculation of potential exposure to a toxicant(s) is the foundational reasoning behind the judgment necessary to limit the damage to an individual or group of animals, and the public's health.

The basic information needed to determine the potential toxicity of an exposure is as follows.

- Body weight (BW) of the patient in kilograms (kg).
- Weight or volume of the substance potentially ingested, inhaled, or applied topically.
- Concentration of a potential toxicant in the substance ingested, inhaled, or applied topically (weight of toxicant/weight or volume of the potentially toxic substance or product).
  - This will typically be provided by either laboratory analysis performed on the product or be identified on the product label in parts per million (ppm), parts per billion (ppb), amount per serving, or percent (%).
  - Concentrations of toxicants in liquids are typically shown as the mass of toxicant (milligram (mg) or microgram (mcg) per volume of liquid (e.g., liter [L]).
  - Concentrations of toxicants in foods, powders, or solid medications such as pills are shown as the mass of the toxicant (mg, mcg) per mass of the food or other delivery system (e.g., kg).
- Minimum toxic *dose* (mg) of a given toxicant known to elicit a harmful effect.
- Minimum toxic *dosage*, or rate of exposure, of a toxicant known to elicit a harmful effect = mg toxicant/kg BW.
- The actual or potential maximum dosage, or rate of exposure to a toxicant, for a specific patient = mg, g, or kg of a toxicant/kg BW of the affected animal.

## ESTIMATE OF TOXICOLOGIC EXPOSURE

- Toxic dose/lethal dose.
  - Determine the actual or potential maximum exposure dose to a toxicant. For a given animal species and average weight, one can compare this to any precedent for a minimum toxic dose (MTD), or minimum lethal dose (MLD), that has been shown to cause harm.
  - Typically expressed in mg.
  - Calculated by multiplying the concentration of a toxicant in a given substance by the weight or volume of the toxic substance ingested, inhaled, or applied topically to an animal.
  - Example: acetaminophen toxicity.

---

*Blackwell's Five-Minute Veterinary Consult Clinical Companion: Small Animal Toxicology*, Third Edition.
Edited by Lynn R. Hovda, Ahna G. Brutlag, Robert H. Poppenga, and Steven E. Epstein.
© 2024 John Wiley & Sons, Inc. Published 2024 by John Wiley & Sons, Inc.

- ○ Feline: minimum toxic dosage is 10 mg acetaminophen/kg BW.
- ○ The average weight of an adult cat is approximately 10 pounds or 4.5 kg BW.
- ○ Thus, 50 mg is the minimum toxic dose for an average cat.
- ○ Conclusion: any size tablet consumed by a cat is potentially toxic.
- Toxic dosage.
  - The toxic dosage is a reflection of the potential toxicity of a substance.
  - The toxic dosage is obtained by dividing the toxic dose by the patient's BW in kg.
  - Typically expressed in mg toxicant/kg BW of the patient.
  - It is used to assess whether the dosage that the animal was exposed to, based on mg toxicant/kg BW of the patient, meets the level of known toxicity that has previously caused harm.
- Example for how to use both the toxic dose and dosage: methylxanthine case study.
  - Three-year-old, 9 kg BW dog consumed the contents of a new box of dark chocolate candy.
  - The minimum lethal dosage (MLD) of dark chocolate in dogs is 0.7 oz dark chocolate/kg BW. The potential minimum lethal dose that could be potentially life-threatening for a 9 kg BW dog is:
    - ○ 0.7 oz dark chocolate/kg BW multiplied by 9 kg BW = 6.3 oz dark chocolate.
  - There are 7 of 25 pieces left in the box, uneaten.
  - A total of 18 pieces of candy were consumed.
  - The total weight of the dark chocolate candy in the box is 10 ounces (oz).
    - ○ 10 oz dark chocolate/25 pieces candy = 0.4 oz dark chocolate/piece.
    - ○ 18 pieces eaten multiplied by 0.4 oz/piece = 7.2 oz dark chocolate ingested.
  - Conclusion: 7.2 oz dark chocolate is greater than the potential minimum lethal dose of 6.3 oz for this patient.
  - Prognosis: Critical.
    - ○ Start decontamination and treatment immediately.

## STEPS FOR CALCULATING THE POTENTIAL FOR TOXICOSIS

- Convert % to mass per unit volume or mass per unit mass ratio (ppm, ppb, ppt), i.e., mg toxicant/kg or mg toxicant/L of a potential toxic substance.
  - 1% = 10 000 ppm.
- Determine the total weight (kg) or volume (L) of the potentially toxic substance that a patient ate, drank, inhaled, or was topically exposed to, and multiply this by the concentration of the toxicant in the toxic substance to find the weight (mg) of the toxicant (i.e., potential toxic dose).
- Divide the weight of the toxicant (dose [mg]) that the animal was exposed to by the weight of the patient (kg BW) (i.e., potential toxic dosage).
- Compare the minimum known toxic dosage of a given toxicant that will elicit a clinical response (mg toxicant/kg BW) to the calculated weight of the toxicant/kg BW of your patient.
- If the potential toxic dosage of the patient (mg toxicant/kg BW of patient) is less than the known, minimum, toxic dosage (mg toxicant/kg BW of an animal) needed to elicit harm, then an exposure, in all probability, did not rise to the level of concern. Therefore, there would not be an expectation of a significant adverse, toxic effect(s) at the level consumed, inhaled, or applied topically, in an otherwise healthy patient at the time of the event.

### Example #1

- A 10 kg BW dog has a cough.
- The dog was exposed to a bait that contains 0.005% brodifacoum (B).

- The known lethal dose of brodifacoum (B) for dogs is 0.25 mg B/kg BW.
- How many grams of bait would the dog have to eat for it to be lethal?

(Note: To avoid confusion, always label units of measurement.)

*Step 1*: concentration equivalent of toxicant in bait in metric units: 0.005% B multiplied by 10 000 ppm/per1% = 50 ppm B = 50 mg B/kg bait.

*Step 2*: potentially lethal dose for this dog: 0.25 mg B/kg BW multiplied by 10 kg BW of the dog = 2.5 mg B is a potentially lethal dose.

*Step 3*: amount of bait needed to provide a lethal dose of 2.5 mg B. The concentration of B in the bait is 1 kg bait/50 mg B, multiplied by the lethal dose of 2.5 mg B = 0.05 kg or 50 grams of bait would be potentially lethal to this dog.

## Example #2

- A 36 kg Labrador consumed a 1-ounce chunk of bait containing 0.01% bromethalin.
- The minimum toxic dosage of bromethalin (B) is 1.67 mg B/kg BW in dogs.
- What is the dosage ingested by the dog in mg B/kg BW?
- What is the prognosis?

*Step 1*: conversion of imperial to metric units: 1 ounce = 28.4 grams = 0.0284 kg of a 0.01% B-containing product was eaten.

*Step 2*: concentration equivalent in metric units: 0.01% B in the product = 0.01% multiplied by 10 000 ppm/1% = 100 ppm B = 100 mg B/kg product.

*Step 3*: total amount of the toxicant, bromethalin, consumed by the Labrador: 100 mg B/kg product multiplied by 0.0284 kg product = 2.84 mg B consumed.

*Step 4*: actual dosage consumed by patient: 2.84 mg B/36 kg BW Labrador = 0.08 mg B/kg BW Labrador.

*Step 5*: compare dosage consumed by patient to minimum toxic dosage: 0.08 mg B/kg BW Labrador is less than 1.67 mg B/kg BW.

*Step 6*: prognosis is good.

## CONVERSION EQUIVALENTS FOR WEIGHT (MASS), LIQUID (VOLUME), CONCENTRATION, AND TEMPERATURE

### Equivalents for Unit of Mass to Unit Volume

1 gram = 1 cubic centimeter = 1 milliliter (mL)
1 kilogram (kg) = 1 liter (L)

### Weight (Plumb 2015; Peterson and Talcott 2013)

1 ounce = 28.4 grams
1 pound (lb) = 0.454 kg = 454 grams = 16 ounces
1 microgram (mcg or μg) = 1000 nanograms (ng)
1 milligram (mg) = 1000 micrograms (mcg or μg)
1 gram = 1000 mg
1 kilogram (kg) = 2.2 pounds = 1000 grams
1 grain (gr.) = 64.8 milligram (mg) (often rounded to 60 or 65 mg)
1 gram = 15.43 grains = 1000 mg

### Liquid

1 teaspoon (tsp.) = 5 mL
1 tablespoon (tbsp.) = 15 mL = 3 teaspoons (tsp.)

1 fluid ounce (fl. oz.) = 30 mL
1 cup (c.) = 8 fl. oz. = 237 mL = 16 tablespoons (tbsp.)
1 quart (qt.) = 2 pints (pts.) = 32 fluid ounces (fl. oz.) = 473 mL
1 gallon (gal.) = 4 quarts (qts.) = 8 pints (pts.) = 128 fluid ounce (fl. oz.) = 3.785 liters (L) = 3785 milliliters (mL)
1 milliliter (mL) = 1 cubic centimeter (cc) = 1000 microliters (μL or mcL)
1 deciliter (dL) = 100 mL
1 liter (L) = 1000 mL = 10 deciliters (dL) = 1.06 qts.
4 liters = 1.07 gals.

## Concentration

1% = 10 000 ppm
1 part per million (ppm) = 1 mg/kg = 1 mg/L
1 ppb = 1 mcg/kg
1 ppm = 1000 parts per billion (ppb)
1 ppb = 1000 parts per trillion (ppt)

# ADDITIONAL RESOURCES

Food Animal Residue Avoidance & Depletion Species Pages (FARAD). 2016. Calculations and Conversions for Drugs, Forage, Feed and Water Consumptions. www.farad.org/publications/vfd/farad_vfd_calculator.pdf

### Suggested Reading

Blodgett DJ. How to evaluate toxicant exposures. *Vet Clin North Am Small Anim Pract* 2002;32:341–355.
Osweiler GD. General toxicologic principles for clinicians. In: Peterson ME, Talcott PA (eds) *Small Animal Toxicology*, 3rd edn. St Louis: Elsevier, 2013; pp. 1–12.
Plumb DC. *Plumb's Veterinary Drug Handbook*, 10th edn. Ames: Wiley-Blackwell, 2023.

**Author**: Sandra James-Yi, DVM, PhD, DABT, DABVT
**Consulting Editor**: Robert H. Poppenga, DVM, PhD, DABVT

# Topical Toxins: Common Human OTC Dermatological Preparations

This appendix covers common commercial human OTC dermatological products to which cats and dogs may be exposed through either accidental ingestion or therapeutic use, which are not covered elsewhere in this book. Other common prescription and OTC topical preparations in both human and veterinary markets that also pose a risk for toxicosis in small animals detailed in the following chapters: 5-fluoruracil (5-FU), amitraz, calcipotriene/calcipotriol (vitamin D analogs), cyclosporine, essential oils, estrogen/hormone replacement therapy products, imidazoline decongestants, ivermectin (see Macrocyclic Lactones), minoxidil, nicotine and fentanyl transdermal patches (see Opiates and Opioids), NSAIDs (e.g., diclofenac), pyrethroid insecticides, retinoids (vitamin A analogs; see Vitamins and Minerals), tacrolimus, salicylates (see Aspirin), and tea tree oil (melaleuca oil), xylitol, and zinc.

## XYLITOL IN TOPICAL PRODUCTS

Xylitol, a natural sugar alcohol toxic to dogs, is increasingly being used in topical personal care products. While used for its humectant (moisture retention) and antifermentation/molding properties, it is reputed to also have beneficial moisturizing effects on skin and hair. Examples of products that contain xylitol include baby wipes; body lotion; deodorant; face cleansers, creams, masks, and antiaging products; hair and scalp tonics, serums or treatments; hair detanglers and other leave-in products; personal lubricants; shaving cream; and skin gels. The use of xylitol in personal care products is expected to grow.

*Blackwell's Five-Minute Veterinary Consult Clinical Companion: Small Animal Toxicology*, Third Edition. Edited by Lynn R. Hovda, Ahna G. Brutlag, Robert H. Poppenga, and Steven E. Epstein.
© 2024 John Wiley & Sons, Inc. Published 2024 by John Wiley & Sons, Inc.

| Product category and trade name (all ®) | Active ingredients | Toxicity | Clinical signs | Treatment | Prognosis |
|---|---|---|---|---|---|
| **Analgesics (camphor):** Absorbent Rub AleveX Campho-Phenique Carmex Rub A535 Antiphlogistine Salonpas Tiger Balm Arthritis Rub; White; Red Vicks VapoRub Vicks VapoSteam | Camphor, up to 11% May have other actives such as menthol, salicylates, etc. added. | Toxicity is not well established in cats/dogs. <1 g of camphor has caused death in children. Mouse LD$_{50}$ (oral) = 1310 mg/kg. Camphor is readily absorbed across the skin. | Onset of signs is 5–20 minutes. Dermal application can cause local irritation. Any ingestion can cause GI distress: vomiting, diarrhea, abdominal discomfort, gastrointestinal ulceration, oral/pharyngeal irritation or ulceration have been reported. Large ingestion can cause CNS depression and seizures (humans). Death from respiratory depression/ seizures. | No antidote. GI protectants if needed. Benzodiazepines, levetiracetam, or barbiturates for seizures. Respiratory support. Monitor blood pressure and vitals. | Good with treatment/mild signs. Severe signs without treatment have a poorer prognosis. If no signs by 60 min, toxicosis unlikely. |
| **Antibiotics:** Lanabiotic Lumi-Sporyn Medi-Quik Neosporin Polysporin Triple Antibiotic | Bacitracin Neomycin Polymyxin B Some versions may have added glucocorticoids or local anesthetics. | Toxicity is not well established in cats/dogs. Severe toxicosis is not expected from acute ingestion/application although anaphylactoid reactions have been reported. | Self-limiting vomiting and diarrhea (partly from the petroleum-based carrier) is most common. Neomycin or polymyxin may result in dermal sensitization. Anaphylaxis/ anaphylactoid reactions have been reported, particularly in cats following ocular administration. | Supportive GI care. Treat for anaphylaxis with O$_2$, epinephrine, fluids, diphenhydramine, possible steroids. | Excellent with acute ingestions and appropriate treatment for anaphylaxis if needed. |

| | | | | |
|---|---|---|---|---|
| **Antifungals:**<br>Femstat<br>Lamisil AT<br>Lotrimin AF<br>Lotrimin Ultra<br>Mentax<br>Monistat<br>Neosporin AF<br>Nizoral A-D<br>Spectazole<br>Tinactin<br>Vagistat | Butenafine, 1%<br>Butoconazole, 2%<br>Clotrimazole, 1–2%<br>Econazole, 1%<br>Ketoconazole, 1–2%<br>Miconazole, 2–4%<br>Terbinafine, 1%<br>Tioconazole, 1–6.5%<br>Tolnaftate, 1%<br>Undecylenic acid | Generally, most OTC antifungal preparations have a wide margin of safety, especially in acute ingestions. | Self-limiting vomiting and diarrhea (partly from the carriers) is the most likely reaction.<br><br>Anaphylactoid reactions in cats or dogs have been associated with butenafine although the route of exposure was not listed. | Supportive GI care. | Excellent with acute ingestions. |
| **Antihistamines:**<br>Benadryl Itch Cooling Spray<br><br>Benadryl Itch Relief Stick<br><br>Benadryl Itch Stopping Gel<br><br>Dermamycin | Diphenhydramine (DPH), 1–2%<br>Diphenhydramine, 2% and zinc acetate, 1% | Diphenhydramine (DPH): toxicosis unlikely following significant topical application (poor transdermal absorption).<br><br>DPH, oral: 2–4 mg/kg (therapeutic dose), mild CNS depression and anticholinergic effects.<br><br>Large DPH oral overdoses may cause severe CNS stimulation.<br><br>Zinc (Zn): an LD$_{50}$ of 100 mg/kg acute Zn salt ingestion in dogs has been reported; source of study supporting this LD$_{50}$ is unknown.<br><br>Zn is an essential nutrient. Oral zinc acetate is used therapeutically in dogs to reduce hepatic copper toxicosis. The therapeutic dose of elemental Zn is 2–15 mg/kg/day (dogs) and 2–10 mg/kg/day (cats).<br><br>Zn acetate contains 30% elemental zinc (100 mg Zn acetate = 30 mg elemental zinc). | Following ingestion:<br><br>Common – vomiting and diarrhea, especially from carriers and/or Zn.<br><br>Lethargy, dry mouth, urinary retention from DPH.<br><br>Uncommon – CNS stimulation, agitation, and tachycardia from large oral overdoses of DPH.<br><br>Zn toxicosis (e.g., Heinz body formation, hemolytic anemia, etc.) is not expected with acute ingestions because most animals self-decontaminate by spontaneously vomiting. Smaller chronic ingestions, such as daily reapplication directly to the pet with subsequent oral grooming, could result in toxicosis. See Zn chapter for details. | Emesis and activated charcoal (large ingestions of DPH only).<br><br>Sedation and GI support as needed.<br><br>Additional treatment for Zn exposure is not expected to be needed in acute ingestions. See Zn chapter for details. | Excellent following acute ingestion of topical preparations.<br><br>Chronic ingestion of the zinc-containing product could lead to toxicosis and require treatment although this is extremely rare. See Zn chapter for details. |

(Continued)

| Product category and trade name (all ®) | Active ingredients | Toxicity | Clinical signs | Treatment | Prognosis |
|---|---|---|---|---|---|
| **Antiseptics (benzoyl peroxide):**<br>Acne-Clear<br>Benzac<br>Clearasil<br>Clearplex<br>Loroxide<br>NeoBenz<br>Oxy 10<br>PanOxyl<br>Persa-Gel<br>Seba-Gel<br>Zeroxin | Benzoyl peroxide, 2.5–10% | Minimal systemic absorption occur from topical administration. Severe toxicosis is not expected from small, acute ingestions/ applications. Risk for toxicosis is greater in preparations with higher concentrations.<br><br>Large ingestions may cause tissue irritation.<br><br>Mouse oral $LD_{50}$ = 5700 mg/kg<br><br>Rat oral $LD_{50}$ = 7710 mg/kg (cyanosis, other changes in urine composition and liver) | Dermal and ocular irritation, including erythema/ hyperemia, pruritus, pain, and blistering or ulceration (rare) following topical exposure.<br><br>GI irritation (vomiting, pain, gas, diarrhea) likely with small ingestions. Erosion/ulceration possible with massive ingestions. | Dermal or ocular decontamination. Dilution or gas decompression if ingested. Supportive GI care and GI protectants. | Good with acute ingestions or topical reactions. |
| **Corticosteroids:**<br>Anusol HC<br>Cortaid<br>Cortisone<br>Cortizone 10<br>Dermacort<br>Nutracort<br>Penecort<br>Procort<br>Proctozone-HC<br>Salacort | Hydrocortisone, 0.5–1% | Ingestion, even in massive doses, is unlikely to cause serious effects.<br><br>Therapeutic dose = 5 mg/kg PO. | Self-limiting vomiting, diarrhea (partly from carriers) with possible PU/PD. | Supportive GI care. Access to water. | Excellent with acute ingestions. |

| Local anesthetics (amides): | Benzocaine, 5–20%<br>Dibucaine, 1%<br>Lidocaine, 0.5–2.5%<br>Prilocaine, 2.5% | Oral toxic dose is not established. 1–2 licks are unlikely to cause toxicosis. Larger ingestions pose greater risk.<br><br>Dibucaine is more toxic than lidocaine.<br><br>Topical lidocaine is systemically absorbed; toxicity unlikely unless used chronically. High first-pass effect makes oral toxicity less likely. | Anesthetization of the pharynx can lead to aspiration.<br><br>Methemoglobinemia and Heinz bodies can occur with ingestion.<br><br>Cats are more sensitive and can develop methemoglobinemia or seizures more readily than dogs.<br><br>Dibucaine can cause seizures, arrhythmias, hypotension, death. | Emesis of questionable efficacy. Charcoal if no risk of aspiration (give via stomach tube). Treat for methemoglobinemia if present.<br><br>More aggressive treatment needed for some exposures and species. | Good with appropriate care. |
|---|---|---|---|---|---|
| Anacaine | | | | | |
| Cetacaine | | | | | |
| Chigger X Plus | | | | | |
| Goodwinol | | | | | |
| Lidoderm | | | | | |
| Nupercainal | | | | | |
| Solarcaine | | | | | |
| Xylocaine | | | | | |
| **Local anesthetics (other):** | Pramoxine, 1% | Pramoxine is not structurally related to procaine-type anesthetics.<br><br>The oral toxic dose in cats/dogs is not known but small ingestions are not expected to result in significant harm.<br><br>Of 177 ingestions in people, transient mouth irritation developed in 5 patients and oral numbness in 3. Ingestions in children up to 11 mg/kg resulted in minor signs only. | Anesthetization of the pharynx can lead to aspiration.<br><br>Localized dermatitis has been reported in animals and people following therapeutic use.<br><br>The drug has been used in veterinary preparations for more than 15 years.<br><br>Oral exposures reported to Pet Poison Helpline typically involve minor GI upset only. | Cessation if dermatitis occurs.<br><br>Supportive GI care. | Good with acute ingestions or topical reactions. |
| Curasore | | | | | |
| Prax | | | | | |
| Proctofoam-NS | | | | | |
| Tronolane | | | | | |
| Sarna Sensitive | | | | | |
| Proctofoam | | | | | |
| PramoxGel | | | | | |
| Vagisil | | | | | |

## Acknowledgments

We acknowledge Catherine Adams, DVM, for her contribution to this chapter in the previous edition.

## Suggested Reading

Tater KC, Gwaltney-Brant S, Wismer T. Dermatological topical products used in the US population and their toxicity to dogs and cats. *Vet Dermatol* 2019;30:474–e140.

Welch S. Local anesthetic toxicosis. *Vet Med* 2000;95(9):670–673.

Welch S. Oral toxicity of topical preparations. *Vet Clin North Am Small Anim Pract* 2002;32:443–453.

**Author**: Ahna G. Brutlag, DVM, MS, DABT, DABVT

# Toxic Plants: Clinical Signs, Antidotes, and Treatment

*Blackwell's Five-Minute Veterinary Consult Clinical Companion: Small Animal Toxicology*, Third Edition.
Edited by Lynn R. Hovda, Ahna G. Brutlag, Robert H. Poppenga, and Steven E. Epstein.
© 2024 John Wiley & Sons, Inc. Published 2024 by John Wiley & Sons, Inc.

| Plant and characteristics | Clinical signs | Antidotes and/or treatment |
|---|---|---|
| **Air plant, Cathedral bells (*Kalanchoe* spp.)** | Cardiac glycoside causes acute signs 1–3 hours after ingestion. Signs include depression, salivation, diarrhea, bradycardia, tachypnea, ataxia, tremors, and paralysis. | Emesis and/or activated charcoal early after ingestion. Treat as a cardiac glycoside. (see Chapter 102). |
| Bright red-orange to pink blooms; umbel flower pattern. | | |
| Plant contains cardiotoxins similar to azalea and rhododendrons, concentrated mainly in flowers. | | |
| **Aloe, Octopus plant, Candelabra plant (*Aloe* spp.)** | Anorexia, depression, vomiting, colic, diarrhea, tremors (uncommon), and change in urine color. | Drugs for abdominal pain/diarrhea. |
| Succulent plant, used in folk and herbal medicine. | Generally mild in nature. | Protect airway, treat locally for pharyngitis associated with oxalate crystals (rare). |
| Toxic fraction is anthraquinone glycoside; disrupts water and electrolyte balance in large intestine. | | |
| **American bittersweet (*Celastrus scandens*)** | Gastric irritation, vomiting, diarrhea. | Fluids, supportive care as needed. |
| Weed, vine with red berries. | | |
| Immature fruits are toxic. | | |
| Toxins are sesquiterpene alkaloids (celapanine, celastrine, paniculatine). | | |
| **Angel's trumpet (*Brugmansia* spp.)** | Typical anticholinergic effects: restlessness, dilated pupils, tachycardia, dyspnea, dry mouth, GI atony, rarely seizures. | GI decontamination if early after ingestion. |
| Potted ornamental or garden plant in tropical climates. Large pendulous flowers, similar to jimsonweed (*Datura* spp.). | Rarely lethal. | Parasympathomimetic drug (e.g., physostigmine). |
| Tropane alkaloid scopolamine causes anticholinergic effects. | | |
| **Autumn crocus (*Colchicum autumnale*)** | Acute onset 2–12 hours post ingestion. Initial signs are nausea, salivation, vomiting, colic, diarrhea, incoordination, and weakness. Multiple organ systems (heart, lungs, and kidneys) also may be involved. Potential for coagulopathy and elevated serum enzymes. | Induce emesis if not vomiting. Activated charcoal if early. Evaluate CBC and serum chemistries, including prothrombin, LDH, CK. |
| Houseplant, garden plant. | | IV fluids, analgesics, anticonvulsants as needed. |
| Typically blooms in fall, different from most other bulbs. Dosages above 6 g/kg BW considered lethal. | | |
| Although the whole plant is toxic, the toxin (colchicine) is highest in bulbs. | | |

| Plant | Clinical signs | Treatment |
|---|---|---|
| **Baneberry, Doll's eye, Cohosh (*Actaea* spp.)** Native shrub found in woodlands of eastern North America. Toxic principle is protoanemonin glycoside, as well as irritant essential oils. | Clinical response ranges from dermatitis and blistering of skin to oral irritation, drooling, pawing at face or mouth, emesis, diarrhea, and hematuria. Neurological and cardiovascular signs are occasionally reported. | Cleanse mouth thoroughly with water; apply appropriate local demulcents; control emesis and diarrhea as necessary; monitor for organ dysfunction, especially renal damage. |
| **Belladonna lily (*Amaryllis* spp.)** Other common names: surprise lily, naked lady lily, March lily, August lily, resurrection lily. Potted plant, garden plant. Bulbs are most toxic. Contains both lycorine alkaloid (systemic effects) and insoluble oxalates (local pharyngitis). | Nausea, vomiting, diarrhea, hypotension, depression. Oxalate crystals can cause direct pharyngeal irritation. | Gastric lavage, activated charcoal, fluids, and supportive treatment. |
| **Bleeding heart, Dutchman's breeches (*Dicentra* spp.)** Garden, woods, potted plant. Roots more toxic than leaves. Toxins are isoquinoline alkaloids (apomorphine, cularine, protoberberine). | Vomiting, diarrhea, muscle tremors, convulsions, or paralysis. May have repeated episodes of neurological signs interspersed with periods of apparent normalcy. | Fluids and seizure control. |
| **Calla lily (*Zantedeschia aethiopica*)** Landscape ornamental or potted plant. Tubular flowers with one prominent central pistil. Toxic principle is insoluble oxalate. | Chewing on the plant releases oxalate spicules causing immediate irritation, pain, salivation, and inflammation. Rarely, upper airway involvement occurs. | Cleanse mouth thoroughly with water. Apply local and/or systemic antinflammatory agents and offer soft diet if needed. |
| **Castor bean (*Ricinus communis*)** Garden shrub or ornamental grows to 2 meters. Seeds are 1 cm, dark and light mottled, and highly toxic. Chewing the seed greatly increases toxicity. Toxin is ricin. | Severe, dangerous if seeds chewed before swallowing. Latent period 6–48 hours. Emesis, severe and hemorrhagic diarrhea, colic, muscle tremors, sudden collapse. Dehydration, hypotension, hemolysis and/or hemoglobinuria. | Emesis for recent exposure; sorbitol if diarrhea not present; charcoal, fluids, and electrolytes. Monitor electrolytes, liver, kidney, adrenal function up to 6 days; H$_2$-blockers for GI signs; diazepam for seizures. Antibiotics, lactulose, SAMe for liver damage. |

(Continued)

| Plant and characteristics | Clinical signs | Antidotes and/or treatment |
|---|---|---|
| **Cherry, Chokecherry, Peach, Plum, Apricot, Bitter almond (*Prunus* spp.) and/or Apples, Crabapples (*Malus* spp.)**<br><br>Deciduous trees and shrubs distributed across North America in orchards, woodlands, and landscapes.<br><br>Cyanogenic glycosides in leaves, twigs, seeds released by chewing or crushing. Toxicity varies among species and cultivars and is not common in small animals. | Rapid onset and progression of weakness, ataxia, labored breathing, collapse, cardiac arrhythmias, seizures, and death with toxicity. Bitter almond odor on breath, bright cherry red blood, and reddened mucus membranes may also be noted. | GI decontamination and activated charcoal if early after ingestion. Symptomatic and supportive care including IV fluids, oxygen supplementation, anticonvulsants, antiarrhythmics.<br><br>Antidote available, rarely used in small animals: sodium nitrite followed by sodium thiosulfate IV. |
| **Chinaberry tree (*Melia azedarach*)**<br><br>Other common names are Persian lilac, white cedar, Texas umbrella tree.<br><br>Ornamental tree in temperate to subtropical areas: southern coastal states, Mexican border.<br><br>Berry is most toxic.<br><br>Toxins are meliatoxins. | Salivation, anorexia, vomiting, diarrhea. May be followed by weakness, ataxia, excitement, or seizures. Fatalities have occurred, generally within 2 days post ingestion. | Early emesis, GI lavage and charcoal are considered beneficial. Fluid and electrolyte replacement, anticonvulsants, and supportive care. |
| **Christmas rose (*Helleborus niger*)**<br><br>House and garden plant. Entire plant is toxic, but fruits are most dangerous.<br><br>Small amounts considered dangerous.<br><br>Contains several toxins, including ranunculin that is converted to protoanemonin when chewed, cardenolides, and bufadienolides. | Hypersalivation, vomiting, anorexia, diarrhea followed by cardiac arrhythmias, heart block with premature beats, slow irregular pulse.<br><br>Potent cardenolide action is greatest risk. | Gastric lavage or emesis; activated charcoal or saline cathartics to decontaminate the GI tract.<br><br>Atropine may be helpful as for other cardenolide plants such as *Digitalis* spp. |
| **Daphne, Spurge olive (*Daphne mezereum*)**<br><br>Landscape shrub; evergreen or deciduous.<br><br>Entire plant is toxic. Bitter or acid taste discourages consumption, may reduce toxic effects.<br><br>Toxins are tricyclic daphnane and diterpenes. | Vesication and edema of the lips and oral cavity. Signs progress to salivation, thirst, abdominal pain, emesis, hemorrhagic diarrhea. | Analgesics to control pain. General GI detoxification, medical treatment for vomiting and diarrhea. Fluid and electrolyte replacement as needed. Monitor hydration status and electrolytes. |

| Plant | Clinical signs | Treatment |
|---|---|---|
| **Delphinium, Larkspur (_Delphinium_ spp.) and/or Pheasant's eye, Yellow oxeye (_Adonis_ spp.)** | Small animal poisoning unlikely unless seeds are ingested. | GI detoxification; GI protectants and antidiarrheal therapies; physostigmine to treat muscarinic signs. |
| Outdoor perennial: gardens, mountains; tall with blue, purple, or pinkish flowers. | Early signs are vomiting, colic, and diarrhea. May progress to trembling, ataxia, weakness, lateral recumbency. | |
| Seeds more toxic than leaves. | | |
| Toxins are diterpenoid alkaloids. | | |
| **English holly (_Ilex_ spp.)** | Nausea, vomiting, diarrhea most common from consumption of berries. Some animals may be depressed. | Relief of digestive distress; activated charcoal may be helpful. Fluid and electrolyte replacement as needed. |
| Landscape plant; glossy green leaves with marginal spicules. Fruit (drupe) white, yellow, black, red, orange. Occurs in forested areas of eastern North America, elsewhere as an ornamental. | Clinical response most often mild/moderate and transient. | |
| Fruit is most likely portion consumed. | | |
| Fruit and leaves contain potentially toxic saponins. Leaves contain caffeine and theobromine | | |
| **English ivy, Atlantic ivy, Irish ivy, Common ivy (_Hedera helix_)** | Salivation, thirst, emesis, gastroenteritis, diarrhea, dermatitis. Mild to moderate GI irritation most common. | Symptomatic relief of GI distress; supportive care for vomiting and diarrhea. |
| Houseplant or ground cover in mild climates. Commonly grown throughout North America. | | |
| Occurs as a woody, climbing or creeping vine. | | |
| Toxins are triterpenoid saponins. | | |
| **Horse chestnut, Buckeye (_Aesculus_ spp.)** | Gastroenteritis, diarrhea, dehydration, electrolyte imbalance. | Fluid and electrolyte replacement, GI protectants. |
| Landscape, ornamental, or forest tree; palmate leaves. Numerous species native across most of North America. | Neurological signs possible, including ataxia, hypermetria, staggering. Usually transient, rarely fatal. Recovery usual within 24–48 hours. | Confine animals during neurological phase. |
| Nuts, early green foliage, and buds most toxic. | | |
| Horse chestnut more toxic; various Buckeye varieties less toxic. | | |
| Contain several toxins including saponins, anthraquinones, and a coumarin glycoside. | | |

(Continued)

| Plant and characteristics | Clinical signs | Antidotes and/or treatment |
| --- | --- | --- |
| **Iris, Flag, Fleur-de-lis, Sword lily (*Iris* spp.)** | Hypersalivation, vomiting, colic, diarrhea which may be hemorrhagic. Occasionally irritation of the lips and muzzle. | GI decontamination early. |
| Perennial garden flower – very commonly available. | | Fluid and electrolyte therapy as needed. |
| Rootstock (rhizome) most toxic; most risk at transplantation. Close to soil surface, may be dug up by dogs. | | |
| Advise clients of potential risk. | | |
| Rootstock contains purgative toxin irisin and terpenoids. | | |
| **Irish potato (*Solanum tuberosum*) and/or Tomato (*Solanum lycopersicum*)** | Vomiting, diarrhea, depression, rapid heart rate, mydriasis, muscle tremors. Signs may vary from atropine-like to cholinesterase inhibition. Use antidotes accordingly and with caution. | GI decontamination. |
| Vegetable garden plants. | | If atropine-like signs predominate, use physostigmine. If salivation and diarrhea are present, use atropine cautiously. |
| Vines, sprouts, green skin, and fruit are toxic. | | |
| Toxins vary but are solanine and other glycoalkaloids. | | |
| **Jerusalem cherry, Winter cherry (*Solanum pseudocapsicum*)** | Severe GI irritation characterized by drooling, vomiting, diarrhea, ulceration, depression, and sometimes seizures. | GI decontamination if exposure is recent. |
| Common ornamental houseplant. | | If salivation and diarrhea are present and severe, use atropine cautiously. |
| Toxin is the glycoalkaloid solanine similar to other plants of the nightshade (Solanaceae) family. | | Provide fluid therapy based on condition of patient and results of laboratory tests. |
| **Lantana, Shrub verbena (*Lantana camara* and *L. montevidensis*)** | Weakness, lethargy, vomiting, diarrhea, mydriasis, dyspnea. | GI decontamination, activated charcoal for acute exposures. Provide fluids and respiratory support. |
| Occurs wild and in gardens in mild temperate to tropical areas. Potted plant in colder climates. Bright orange, yellow, red, purple, or pink flowers. Foliage and immature berries are most toxic. | Continued ingestion can lead to chronic disease. | Protect from sunlight and treat for hepatic insufficiency. |
| Toxins are pentacyclic triterpenoid lantadenes A, B, and C. | Advanced signs: cholestasis, hyperbilirubinemia. Liver changes predispose to photosensitization. | |
| **Lily of the valley (*Convallaria majalis*)** | Multiorgan failure. Tremors, thirst, vomiting, diarrhea, cardiac arrhythmia/bradycardia, weakness, shock. | Emesis or gastric lavage. Control dehydration, maintain electrolytes; control diarrhea; monitor ECG and serum potassium. Cardiac signs generally responsive to atropine. |
| Ornamental garden plant. Prefers moist, shaded areas. Blossoms nodding/drooping on stem. | Monitor for cardiac arrhythmias, shock, and hyperkalemia. | |
| Toxic principle (cardenolides) persists in dried plants; highest concentration in roots. | | |

| Plant | Signs | Treatment |
|---|---|---|
| **Lupine, Bluebonnet (*Lupinus* spp.)**<br><br>Common garden ornamental throughout USA; wild plants abundant in some regions, primarily western USA.<br><br>Seeds more toxic than leaves, but plant, seeds, and pods are toxic.<br><br>Toxic principle: quinolizidine alkaloids; varies among species and location. | Signs begin 1–24 hours post exposure. Salivation, ataxia, mydriasis, depression or seizures, disorientation, dyspnea.<br><br>Liver and kidney damage may develop from continued ingestion.<br><br>Lupins are teratogenic in ruminants. Risk in small animals is not well known. | GI decontamination with activated charcoal for acute exposure.<br><br>Anticonvulsants may be needed if neurological signs are severe. |
| **Mexican breadfruit, Swiss cheese plant, Hurricane plant (*Monstera deliciosa*)**<br><br>Stems and leaves contain insoluble calcium oxalate spicules (raphides). | Chewing on the plant releases oxalate spicules into mouth, tongue, and lips.<br><br>Response is immediate irritation, pain, salivation, and inflammation. Signs include pawing at face, drooling, and vomiting; potential interference with upper airway. | Cleanse mouth thoroughly with water.<br><br>Apply local and/or systemic antiinflammatory agents based on clinical condition of patient. Soft diet if needed. |
| **Mistletoe (*Phoradendron* spp.)**<br><br>Hemiparasitic shrub found growing on other trees. Oval evergreen leaves with white berries. Accessed by pets when used in homes as holiday decorations.<br><br>Leaves, stems, and berries are moderately toxic – contain toxic amines and proteins. | Vomiting, GI pain, diarrhea; ataxia, hypotension, occasional seizures, cardiovascular failure.<br><br>Principal risk may be from use during holiday season. | Fluid and electrolyte replacement; GI protectants. |
| **Monkshood, Wolf's-bane, Blue rocket (*Aconitum* spp.)**<br><br>Several species native to North America found in wooded areas. Perennial garden ornamental.<br><br>Entire plant is toxic; contains diterpene alkaloids that are primarily neurotoxic. | Interferes with inactivation of Na+ channels in nerves.<br><br>Salivation, vomiting, diarrhea. Muscle tremors, weakness, cardiac arrhythmia and/or heart failure; respiratory depression. | GI decontamination, fluid and electrolyte replacement. Manage similar to digitalis glycoside overdose, with caution for potassium administration. |

*(Continued)*

| Plant and characteristics | Clinical signs | Antidotes and/or treatment |
|---|---|---|
| **Morning glory (*Ipomoea* spp.)** | Nausea, mydriasis, ataxia, muscle tremors, hallucinations, decreased reflexes, diarrhea, hypotension. | Dark, quiet surroundings; tranquilization as needed. |
| Garden annual, potted plant. | | |
| Seeds most toxic. Increased risk when seeds are presoaked, consumed by dogs. Toxicity varies among plant species and varieties. Toxicity can occur after a single large ingestion or multiple smaller one. | | GI decontamination is not routinely recommended. |
| Indole alkaloid toxin similar to ergot alkaloids; abused as hallucinogen. | | |
| **Mountain laurel (*Kalmia* spp.)** | Oral irritation, salivation, projectile vomiting, diarrhea, weakness, impaired vision, bradycardia, hypotension, AV block. | Activated charcoal, fluid replacement, atropine, antiarrhythmics, and respiratory support as needed. |
| Native of eastern and southeastern woods, mountains of North America. Both leaves and flowers are toxic. Honey from nectar also toxic. | | See Azaleas and Rhododendrons (Chapter 108) for additional treatment information. |
| Toxins are diterpenoids, in particular grayanotoxins I and II. | | |
| **Narcissus, Daffodil, Jonquil, Paper-white (*Narcissus* spp.)** | Nausea, vomiting, salivation, hypotension, diarrhea. | Gastric lavage, activated charcoal, fluid replacement, supportive treatment for gastroenteritis. |
| Garden ornamental bulb, potted plant. Bulb is most toxic. | Prolonged signs may cause dehydration. | |
| Contains lycorine alkaloid. | | |
| **Nettle (*Urtica* spp.)** | Oral irritation and pain, hypersalivation, swelling and edema of nose and periocular areas or other areas of skin contact. | Antihistamines and analgesics. Local or systemic antiinflammatory supportive therapy to treat affected contact areas. |
| Garden or waste area weed. | | |
| Hairs on leaves contain toxin that enters skin on contact. | | |
| Most common in hunting or outdoor free-roaming dogs. | | |
| Toxins are biogenic amines (acetylcholine, histamine, etc.). | | |
| **Persian violet, Sowbread (*Cyclamen persicum*)** | Chewing plant parts causes oral irritation with drooling, vomiting, and diarrhea. Occasional hemoglobinuria may color urine red-brown. | Control vomiting and diarrhea if severe; administer fluids as needed. |
| Popular florist's plant; widely available. | | Monitor for hemoglobinuria. |
| Irritant saponins in all parts of the plant, especially tubers or roots. | Large amounts may cause cardiac arrhythmias, seizures, and rarely mortality. | Control seizures and cardiac arrhythmias as needed. |

| | | |
|---|---|---|
| **Philodendron, Sweatheart vine, Hope plant (*Philodendron* spp.) and/or Pothos, Devil's ivy (*Epipremnum* spp.)** | Chewing on the plant releases oxalate spicules into mouth, tongue, and lips. Response is immediate irritation, pain, salivation, and inflammation. | Cleanse mouth thoroughly with water. |
| Very common indoor ornamental vine or upright potted plant. | Signs include pawing at face, drooling, and vomiting; potential interference with upper airway. | Apply local and/or systemic antinflammatory agents based on clinical condition of patient. Soft diet if needed. |
| Toxic principle is insoluble oxalate. | | |
| **Poinsettia (*Euphorbia pulcherrima*)** | Irritation of mouth: may cause vomiting, diarrhea, and dermatitis. | Demulcents for local lesions; fluids to prevent dehydration. |
| Garden or potted plant, especially during the holiday season. | Usually transient and not life-threatening. | |
| Sap of stem and leaves mild irritant. | | |
| Contains a variety of diterpenoid euphorbol esters. | | |
| **Rosary pea, Precatory bean (*Abrus precatorius*)** | Signs may be delayed up to two days after ingestion. Early signs are nausea, vomiting, watery diarrhea (often hemorrhagic) followed by weakness, tachycardia, fever, seizures, coma, death. | Emesis or lavage followed by activated charcoal, GI protectants, fluids, and electrolytes. |
| Native of India. Seeds used in ornamental jewelry. Illegal to import into USA. Previously cultivated as an ornamental; has escaped and naturalized in southeast USA. Seeds are highly toxic when broken or chewed. Reportedly one of the most toxic plants in the world. | | Early and thorough detoxication is important for survival. |
| Toxin is abrin, nearly identical to ricin from castor bean. | | |
| **Thorn apple, jimsonweed (*Datura* spp.)** | Thirst, disturbances of vision, delirium, mydriasis, thirst, tachycardia, hyperthermia, GI atony/constipation. | GI decontamination if early after ingestion. |
| Annual weed, some species are ornamental. | | Parasympathomimetic drug (e.g., physostigmine). |
| Entire plant is toxic, but seeds are most toxic and available. | Commonly described as "Hot as a pistol, blind as a bat, red as a beet, mad as a hatter." | |
| Toxins are tropane alkaloids (hyoscyamine and scopolamine) with effects similar to atropine. | | |
| **Tulips (*Tulipa* spp.). Hyacinths (*Hyacinthus* spp.)** | Signs reflect direct irritation and include drooling, nausea, vomiting, diarrhea, dyspnea, tachycardia, and hyperpnea. | GI decontamination if early after ingestion. |
| Poisoning usually occurs when dogs consume bulbs. | | Apply local and/or systemic antinflammatory agents based on clinical condition of patient. Monitor and control gastrointestinal effects; medicate as needed for tachycardia and dyspnea. |
| Toxic principle includes allergenic lactones and similar alkaloids. | | |

(*Continued*)

| Plant and characteristics | Clinical signs | Antidotes and/or treatment |
| --- | --- | --- |
| **Tobacco (*Nicotiana tabacum*)**<br><br>Garden plant, weed, cigarettes.<br><br>Entire plant toxic.<br><br>Nicotine alkaloid is toxic principle. | Rapid onset of salivation, nausea, emesis, tremors, incoordination, ataxia, collapse, and respiratory failure. | Assist ventilation, provide vascular support. Gastric lavage with activated charcoal. |
| **Wisteria (*Wisteria* spp.)**<br><br>Woody vine or shrub with bluish purple to white legume flowers.<br><br>Seeds are greatest toxicity risk.<br><br>Toxin is a glycoprotein lectin. | Nausea, abdominal pain, prolonged vomiting; diarrhea.<br><br>Signs may persist for 2–3 days. | GI decontamination and activated charcoal if early after ingestion.<br><br>Antiemetics and fluid replacement therapy. |
| **Yellow jessamine, Woodbine (*Gelsemium sempervirens*)**<br><br>Mild temperate to subtropical climates; mainly SE United States. Yellow trumpet-shaped flowers grow on evergreen vines.<br><br>Neurotoxic alkaloids and semipervirine, and indole, are toxins. | Abrupt onset of weakness, ataxia, clonic/tonic seizures, paralysis, respiratory failure. | GI decontamination early in course of toxicosis. Symptomatic and supportive therapy for respiration.<br><br>Fluid replacement therapy as needed. |

## Suggested Reading

Barr AC. Household and garden plants. In: Peterson ME, Talcott PA (eds) *Small Animal Toxicology*, 3rd edn. St Louis: Elsevier, 2013; pp. 357–400.

Burrows GE, Tyrl RJ. *Toxic Plants of North America*, 2nd edn. Ames: Wiley-Blackwell, 2013.

Frohne D, Pfander HJ. *Poisonous Plants*, 2nd edn. Portland: Timber Press, 2005.

Williams MC, Olsen JD. Horse chestnut: a multidisciplinary clinical review. *Am J Vet Res* 1984;45(3):539–542.

**Authors**: Rebecca Anderson, DVM and Lynn R. Hovda, RPh, DVM, MS, DACVIM

# Index by Toxins and Toxicants

Note: Chapter titles and page numbers are in **bold**. Page numbers followed by 't' refer to tables; page numbers followed by 'f' refer to figures.

Specific clinical signs/symptoms are NOT included in this index. Please refer to the **Clinical Signs and Syndromes Index**.

*Blackwell's Five-Minute Veterinary Consult Clinical Companion: Small Animal Toxicology*, Third Edition.
Edited by Lynn R. Hovda, Ahna G. Brutlag, Robert H. Poppenga, and Steven E. Epstein.
© 2024 John Wiley & Sons, Inc. Published 2024 by John Wiley & Sons, Inc.

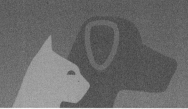

# Index by Clinical Signs and Syndromes

**Abdominal discomfort**
acetaminophen, 289
bone and blood meal, 512
   chocolate and caffeine, 456
   fertilizers, 524
   tacrolimus, 207
   *see also* **Abdominal pain**
**Abdominal distension**
   bread dough, 450
   mycotoxins (aflatoxin), 473
   phosphides, 814
   *see also* **Bloating**; **Gastric distension**
**Abdominal pain**
   acids, 560
   alcohols, 63
   alkalis, 567
   aspirin, 295
   batteries, 573
   cyanogenic glycosides, 719
   diquat and paraquat, 517
   fluoride, 674, 675
   foreign objects, 505
   grapes and raisins, 461
   iron, 651
   lead, 658
   methionine, 534
   mothballs, 585
   mushrooms, 734, 735
   NSAIDs (human), 320, 321
   NSAIDs (veterinary), 387
   onions and garlic, 484, 485
   phosphides, 814
   sago palm (cycads), 759
   spring bulbs, 767, 768
   toxic plants causing, 878t
   vitamins and minerals, 347
   *see also* **Abdominal discomfort**
**Abdominal rigidity/tensing**
   acetaminophen, 289
   black widow spider, 395

**Abnormal behavior**, glow jewelry and toys (dibutyl phthalate), 671
**Acidemia**, acids causing, 559
**Acidosis**
   metabolic *see* **Metabolic acidosis**
   renal tubular, topiramate ingestion, 121
**Acute hepatic failure** *see* **Liver failure**
**Acute hepatic necrosis** *see* **Liver damage/necrosis**
**Acute kidney injury (AKI)/acute renal failure (ARF)**
   ACEIs, 111, 113
   aspirin, 294
   calcipotriene, 154
   calcium channel blockers, 160
   cholecalciferol, 802, 803
   crotalids (pit vipers) venom, 408
   diquat and paraquat, 519
   ethylene glycol causing, 66, 70
   grapes and raisins, 460, 461, 462
   hydrocarbons, 88
   lilies, 729
   mycotoxins (aflatoxin), 473
   NSAIDs (human), 320, 321
   oxalates (soluble), 752, 753
   phencyclidine (PCP), 274
   phosphides, 813
   vitamins and minerals, 346, 347
**Acute pulmonary edema** *see* **Pulmonary edema**
**Acute respiratory distress syndrome** (ARDS)
   smoke inhalation, 832
   *see also* **Respiratory distress**
**Aggression**
   benzodiazepines, 136
   glow jewelry and toys (dibutyl phthalate), 671
   opiates and opioids (illicit), 266, 268
   yew, 780
**Agitation**, 18
   amphetamines, 108
   atypical antipsychotics, 125, 127
   baclofen, 130, 132

*Blackwell's Five-Minute Veterinary Consult Clinical Companion: Small Animal Toxicology*, Third Edition.
Edited by Lynn R. Hovda, Ahna G. Brutlag, Robert H. Poppenga, and Steven E. Epstein.
© 2024 John Wiley & Sons, Inc. Published 2024 by John Wiley & Sons, Inc.